Essentials of
Human Nutrition

Essentials of
Human Nutrition

Third Edition

Edited by

Jim Mann
Professor of Human Nutrition, University of Otago,
New Zealand

A. Stewart Truswell
Emeritus Professor of Human Nutrition, University of
Sydney, Australia

OXFORD
UNIVERSITY PRESS

OXFORD
UNIVERSITY PRESS

Great Clarendon Street, Oxford OX2 6DP

Oxford University Press is a department of the University of Oxford.
It furthers the University's objective of excellence in research, scholarship,
and education by publishing worldwide in

Oxford New York

Auckland Cape Town Dar es Salaam Hong Kong Karachi
Kuala Lumpur Madrid Melbourne Mexico City Nairobi
New Delhi Shanghai Taipei Toronto

With offices in

Argentina Austria Brazil Chile Czech Republic France Greece
Guatemala Hungary Italy Japan Poland Portugal Singapore
South Korea Switzerland Thailand Turkey Ukraine Vietnam

Oxford is a registered trade mark of Oxford University Press
in the UK and in certain other countries

Published in the United States
by Oxford University Press Inc., New York

First edition published 1998
Second edition published 2002
Third edition published 2007

British Library Cataloguing in Publication Data

Data available

Library of Congress Cataloging in Publication Data

Data available

Typeset by Graphicraft Limited, Hong Kong
Printed in Great Britain
on acid-free paper by
CPI Bath Ltd, Bath

ISBN 978-0-19-929097-0

1 3 5 7 9 10 8 6 4 2

Preface

Several excellent textbooks of human nutrition are available. We have attempted to produce a book that differs from most of them by asking our contributors to describe what they regard as those aspects of their topics that are essential to the understanding and practice of human nutrition. Most of the authors are international authorities on the subjects on which they have written and all are very experienced teachers. We were initially reluctant to accept the offer of the publishers to produce yet another textbook of human nutrition. We were persuaded to do so because we felt there was a need for a book that described the essential information required by students embarking on a University course in human nutrition, and by those in training in the health and food science professions where the importance of nutrition is being increasingly recognized. Many of our clinical colleagues in medicine, dentistry, nursing and physiotherapy, and school teachers, provided strong encouragement for this project since they too required a simple reference volume, having themselves received little formal training in nutrition. An increasingly informed public expects its health providers to have knowledge of one of the most important determinants of individual and public health. Health professionals and food scientists need to be able to disentangle scientifically established nutrition principles from the morass of misinformation available in the public domain. The book may also be of value to those in the fitness industry and last but not least individual members of the public who have sufficient knowledge of biology and chemistry and who wish to be informed of the essentials of human nutrition. The book is not intended to be a detailed reference volume and each chapter contains further reading for those wishing to extend the information provided in the text.

We have tried to emphasize that nutritional science encompasses a spectrum of disciplines and involves the use of many methodologies. In the past, the major advances in nutrition were made at the level of organs and organisms, many from studies of experimental animals. Most present advances have been at the population level and, even more recently, at the molecular level. The discovery that dietary alteration can modify gene expression suggests that what we eat has even more profound implications than had previously been believed. These disciplines now need to be integrated at the human level to promote the practical application of nutritional science in metabolic, clinical and public health nutrition.

This medium-sized textbook has become popular especially in universities in Europe and the Southern Hemisphere. Human nutrition science has continued to evolve since our second edition in 2002 and Oxford University Press asked us to prepare this third edition.

Eighteen new writers have joined the authorship of the book. Some are very well-known nutritional scientists. Fourteen of the 40 chapters are completely rewritten and all the others have been revised and updated. We are very grateful to our chapter writers for their expert and well-described material—and also for their tolerance of our editing of what they wrote. We have been somewhat interventionist editors in our attempt to keep the writing simple and readable and the different chapters fairly consistent.

We thought it important not to let 'Essentials' get too wordy, too long, heavy and costly.

Although we two editors live and work in two separate countries, it has been an enjoyable and creative task to work together, with the help of many emails and teleconferences.

We hope that readers will find our book useful in their study of human nutrition. For those who would like more detail, each chapter has a list of suggestions for further reading. These references are not comprehensive but selected, and most of them should be accessible.

We have arranged to participate in an Editors' Forum via OUP's Online Resource Centre. Twice a year, we will send notes on new developments in the whole area of human nutrition. In addition, we would welcome comments from students, lecturers or general readers.

Prof Jim Mann <jim.mann@stonebow.otago.ac.nz>

Prof Stewart Truswell <s.truswell@mmb.usyd.edu.au>

 To see topical and scientifically robust updates on nutrition associated with this textbook, and active web links to many of the journal articles in the Reference areas, please see the dedicated Online Resource Centre at www.oxfordtextbooks.co.uk/orc/mann3e/.

Acknowledgements

The editors are very pleased that so many leading nutrition scientists have been prepared to contribute and have tolerated our editing. Our knowledge of nutrition has been moulded by many discussions with many colleagues over several years. Lesley Day has been the main editorial assistant for the book in Otago. She assisted with the revision of many of the chapters following the editorial process and ensured the standardized format required by the publishers. We are grateful to her for playing a very key role in the production of the book.

Marianne Alexander has been Professor Truswell's secretary in Sydney for all three editions. Beth Gray was editorial assistant for the first two editions and has played an important role, especially with regard to obtaining permissions for reproducing published work and the preparation of all figures.

Contents

Abbreviations

AA	arachidonic acid
AAS	atomic absorption spectrophotometry
ACE	angiotensin-converting enzyme
ACP	acyl carrier protein
ADH	alcohol dehydrogenase; antidiuretic hormone
ADI	acceptable daily intake
AGP	α1-acid glycoprotein
AGRP	agouti-related proteins
AI	adequate intake
AIDS	acquired immunodeficiency syndrome
ALDH	aldehyde dehydrogenases
AN	anorexia nervosa
AOAC	Association of Official Analytical Chemists
ATP	adenosine triphosphate
BMD	bone mineral density
BMI	body mass index
BMR	basal metabolic rate
BN	bulimia nervosa
BSE	bovine spongiform encephalopathy
BST	bovine somatotrophin
CAP	Common Agricultural Policy
CBT	cognitive behavioural therapy
CHD	coronary heart disease
CCK	cholecystokinin
CoA	co-enzyme A
COMA	Committee on Medical Aspects of Food Policy
CPAP	continuous positive airways pressure
CRP	C-reactive protein
CSA	childhood sexual abuse
CT	computerized tomography
DASH	Dietary Approaches to Stop Hypertension
DE	digestible energy
DEXA	dual energy X-ray absorptiometry
DFEs	dietary folate equivalents
DGGs	dietary goals and guidelines
DHA	docosahexaenoic acid
DIT	diet-induced thermogenesis
DLW	doubly labelled water
DP	degree of polymerization
DRI	dietary reference intakes

DRV	dietary reference values
DV	daily value
EAR	estimated average requirement
EASD	European Association for the Study of Diabetes
ECF	extracellular fluid
EDNOS	eating disorder not otherwise specified
EFA	essential fatty acids
EFSA	European Food Safety Authority
EGRA	erythrocyte glutathione reductase activity
EPA	eicosapentaenoic acid
FAD	flavin adenine dinucleotide
FAO	Food and Agriculture Organization
FDA	Food and Drug Administration
FEP	free erythrocyte protoporphyrin
FFM	fat-free mass
FFQ	food frequency questionnaires
FG	fasting glucose
FIVE	familial isolated vitamin E deficiency
FMN	flavin mononucleotide
FSA	Food Standards Agency
FSANZ	Food Standards of Australia and New Zealand
GABA	γ-amino butyric acid
GE	gross energy
GFR	glomerular filtration rate
GI	glycaemic index
GL	glycaemic load
GLC	gas–liquid chromatography
GM	genetically modified
GPx	glutathione peroxidase
GRAS	generally regarded as safe
GST	glutathione S-transferase
GTP	guanosine triphosphate
HAART	highly active antiretroviral therapy
HACCP	hazard analysis of critical control points
HCP	haem carrier protein
HDL	high-density lipoprotein
HERP	human exposure/rodent potency index
HG	hyperemesis gravidarum
HIV	human immunodeficiency virus
HPLC	high-performance liquid chromatography
ICF	intracellular fluid
ICCIDD	International Council for the Control of Iodine Deficiency Disorders
IDA	iron deficiency anaemia
IDD	iodine-deficiency disorders
IDDM	insulin-dependent diabetes

IF	intrinsic factor
IFG	impaired fasting glucose
IGF	insulin-like growth factor
IGT	impaired glucose tolerance
IHD	ischaemic heart disease
IL	interleukin
IOTF	International Obesity Taskforce
IPT	interpersonal psychotherapy
IRBP	interstitial retinoid binding protein
IRP	iron-responsive protein
IU	international units
JEFCA	joint expert committee on food additives
KKP	key kitchen person
LBM	lean body mass
LBW	low birth weight
LCP	long-chain ω-3 polyunsaturated
LDL	low-density lipoprotein
ME	metabolizable energy
MPOD	macular pigment optical density
MRDR	modified relative dose–response
MSG	monosodium glutamate
MTHFR	methylene tetrahydrofolate reductase
MUAC	mid-upper arm circumference
MUFA	monounsaturated fatty avids
MZ	meso-zeaxanthin
NAD	nicotinamide-adenine-dinucleotide
NADP	nicotinamide-adenine-dinucleotide phosphate
NASH	non-alcoholic steatohepatitis
NDO	non-digestible oligosaccharides
NE	niacin equivalents
NIDDM	non-insulin-dependent diabetes
NMES	non-milk extrinsic sugar
NOEL	no observed effect level
NPRQ	non-protein respiratory quotient
NPY	neuropeptide Y
NRV	nutrient reference values
NSP	non-starch polysaccharide
NTD	neural tube defects
p.p.m.	parts per million
PAF	platelet-activating agent
PAL	physical activity level
PBM	peak bone mass
PCB	polychlorinated biphenyls
PCV	packed cell volume
PEM	protein-energy malnutrition

PIVKA	protein induced by vitamin K absence
PLP	pyridoxal 5′-phosphate
PTH	parathyroid hormone
PUFA	polyunsaturated fatty acids
PVC	polyvinyl chloride
PYY	peptide YY
RBP	retinol binding protein
RDA	recommended dietary allowance
RDI	recommended dietary intake
RDS	rapidly digestible starch
RE	retinol equivalents
RES	reticuloendothelial system
RMR	resting metabolic rate
RNI	recommended nutrient intake
RS	resistant starch
SCFA	short-chain fatty acids
SHP	starch hydrolysis product
SNRI	selective norepinephrine reuptake inhibitor
SSRI	selective serotonin reuptake inhibitor
TBW	total body water
TEE	total energy expenditure
TfR	transferrin receptor
THF	tetrahydrofolate reductase
TIBC	total iron binding capacity
TNF	tumour necrosis factor
TPP	thiamin pyrophosphate
TTR	transthyretin
UDP	uridine diphosphate
UIL	upper intake level
UNAIDS	United Nations Programme on HIV/AIDS
USI	universal salt iodization
UV	ultraviolet
vCJD	variant Creutzfeldt–Jakob disease
VDR	vitamin D receptor
VLCD	very-low-calorie diets
VLDL	very-low-density lipoprotein
WHO	World Health Organization

Contributors

Margaret Allman-Farinelli, PhD, MPhilPH, Dip Nutr Diet
Research Fellow
NSW Centre for Overweight and Obesity
Medical Foundation Building, K25
University of Sydney
NSW 2006
Australia

Soumela Amanatidis, BSc, Dip Nutr Diet
Community Nutritionist
Central Sydney Area Health Service
Queen Mary Building
Grose Street, Camperdown
NSW 2050
Australia

Annie Anderson, PhD, SRD
Professor and Director for Centre for Public Health
    Nutrition Research
Ninewells Hospital & Medical School
University of Dundee
Dundee, DD1 9SY
Scotland, UK

Katrine Baghurst, PhD
Nutrition Consultant
82, Cave Avenue
Bridgewater, 5155
South Australia

Ron Bowrey, BE, PhD
Former Research Director
Meadow Lea Foods
Macquarie Park
NSW 2113
Australia

Kim Bell Anderson, PhD
Human Nutrition Unit, Building G08
University of Sydney
NSW 2006
Australia

Sheila Bingham, MA, PhD
Deputy Director
MRC Dunn Human Nutrition Unit
Welcome Trust/MRC Building
Hills Road
Cambridge, CB2 2DH
UK

Colin W. Binns, MB, BS, MPH, PhD, FRACGP,
    FAFOM, FAFPHM
Professor of Public Health
School of Public Health
Curtin University
Perth
WA 6845
Australia

Louise Burke, PhD, Grad Dip Diet, FACSM
Head of Department of Sports Nutrition
Australian Institute of Sport
Bruce
ACT 2617
Australia

Ian D. Caterson, AM, MB, BS, PhD, FRACP
Boden Professor of Human Nutrition
Human Nutrition Unit, Building G08
University of Sydney
NSW 2006
Australia

Alexandra Chisholm, PhD
Senior Lecturer/Research Dietitian
Department of Human Nutrition
University of Otago
Dunedin
New Zealand

John Cummings, MB, ChB, MSc, MA, FRCP (Lond)
    FRCP (Edin)
Professor of Experimental Gastroenterology
Department of Pathology and Neuroscience
Ninewells Hospital and Medical School
Dundee, DD1 9SY
Scotland, UK

Ailsa Goulding, PhD, FACN
Professorial Fellow
Department of Medicine
Otago Medical School
University of Otago
Dunedin
New Zealand

Andrea Grant, MSc
Assistant Research Fellow
Department of Medical and Surgical Sciences
University of Otago

Dunedin
New Zealand

Trish Griffiths, BSc, Dip Nutr Diet, MPH, Grad Dip
    Comm M
Manager, Nutrition Services
Bread Research Institute Australia
North Ryde
NSW 2113
Australia

Caroline Horwath, PhD
Senior Lecturer in Human Nutrition
Department of Human Nutrition
University of Otago
Dunedin
New Zealand

Paula Hunt, BSc (Hons), RD
Nutrition Works
Westwood Lodge
Wells Road
Ilkley
West Yorkshire, LS29 9F
UK

Alan A. Jackson, CBE, MA, MD, FRCP, MRCPCH
Professor of Human Nutrition
University of Southampton
Southampton General Hospital
Tremona Road
Southampton, SP16 6YD
UK

W. Philip T. James, CBE, MD, DSc, FRCP (Edin), FRSE
Chairman, International Obesity Task Force
231, North Gower Street
London, NW1 2NR
UK

Martijn B. Katan, PhD
Professor of Nutrition
Institute of Health Sciences
Vrije Universiteit Amsterdam
De Boelelaan 1085
1081 HV
Amsterdam

Anita Lawrence, M. MedSci, PhD
Nutrition Manager
Dairy Australia
60, City Road
Southbank
Victoria 3006
Australia

Helen M. Leach, MA (Hons), PhD, FRSNZ
Professor in Anthropology
Department of Anthropology
University of Otago
Dunedin
New Zealand

Claus Leitzmann, BSc, MSc, PhD
Professor of Human Nutrition
Institut fur Ernährungswissenschaft
Justus-Liebig Universität Giessen
Wilhelmstrasse 20
Germany

Philippa Lyons-Wall, PhD, Dip Nutr Diet
Senior Lecturer in Nutrition and Dietetics
School of Public Health
Queensland University of Technology
Victoria Park Road
Queensland 4059
Australia

Professor Patrick MacPhail, MB, BCh, PhD, FCP(SA),
    FRCP
Professor Emeritus
Department of Medicine
University of the Witwatersrand
Helen Joseph Hospital
Perth Road
Westdene, 2092
Johannesburg
South Africa

Jim I. Mann, CNZM, MA, DM, PhD, FRACP,
    FRSNZ
Professor in Human Nutrition and Medicine
Department of Human Nutrition
University of Otago
Dunedin
New Zealand

Jennifer McMahon, MBE, FN, PhD, MBA
Department of Human Nutrition
University of Otago
Dunedin
New Zealand

M. Alain Mourey, MSc
Nutritionist
Economic Security Unit
International Committee of the Red Cross
19, Ave de la Paix
1202 Geneva
Switzerland

Sue Monro, BSc, Dip Nutr Diet
Dietitian
Wentworthville NSW 2145
Australia

Abdullah Omari, MB, BS, MMed
Human Nutrition Unit, Building G08
University of Sydney
NSW 2006
Australia

Winsome R. Parnell, BHSc, MSc, PhD, NZRD
Associate Professor in Human Nutrition
Department of Human Nutrition
University of Otago
Dunedin
New Zealand

Robert Peveler, BM BCh, MA, DPhil, FRCPsych
Professor of Liaison Psychiatry
Clinical Neurosciences Division
University of Southampton,
and
Hon Consultant Psychiatrist
Hampshire Partnership NHS Trust
Royal South Hants Hospital
UK

Andrew Prentice, PhD
Professor of International Nutrition
London School of Hygiene & Tropical Medicine
Keppel Street
London, WC1E 7HT
UK

Neville Rigby
Director of Policy and Public Affairs
IASO International Obesity Task Force
231, North Gower Street
London NW1 2NR
UK

James Robinson, MD, ScD, FRACP, FRSNZ
Emeritus Professor in Physiology
Department of Physiology
Otago Medical School
Dunedin
New Zealand

Samir Samman, PhD
Associate Professor
Human Nutrition Unit, Building G08
University of Sydney
Sydney, NSW 2006
Australia

Donna Secker, MSc, PhD, RD
Clinical Dietitian
The Hospital for Sick Children
555, University Avenue
Toronto, Ontario
Canada

C. Murray Skeaff, PhD
Professor in Human Nutrition
Department of Human Nutrition
University of Otago
Dunedin
New Zealand

Ross Smith, MD, BS, FRACS
Professor of Surgery
University Department of Surgery
Royal North Shore Hospital
St Leonards
NSW 2065
Australia

Christine D. Thomson, MHSc, PhD
Professor in Human Nutrition
Department of Human Nutrition
University of Otago
Dunedin
New Zealand

David Thurnham, PhD
Emeritus Professor of Human Nutrition
Northern Ireland Centre for Food and Nutrition
University of Ulster
Cromore Road
Coleraine, BT52 1SWA
UK

Stewart Truswell, AO, MD, DSc, FRCP, FFPH, FIUNS
Emeritus Professor of Human Nutrition
Human Nutrition Unit, Building G08
University of Sydney
NSW 2006
Australia

Hannah Turner, BSc, DClinPsych
Clinical Psychologist
University of Southampton Mental Health Clinical
    Group
Royal South Hants Hospital
Southampton, SO14 0YG
UK

Wija A. van Staveren, MSc, PhD, RD
Emeritus Professor, Nutrition and Gerontology
Division of Human Nutrition

Wageningen University
Wageningen
The Netherlands

H.H. (Este) Vorster, DSc
Professor and Director of Research
Faculty of Health Sciences
North-West University
Potchefstroom, 2520
South Africa

Bernhard Watzl, PhD
Acting Head, Institute of Nutritional Physiology
Federal Research Centre for Nutrition and Food
Haid-und-Neu-Str. 9
76131 Karlsruhe
Germany

Peter Williams, PhD, Dip Nutr Diet, MHP, FDAA
Associate Professor in Nutrition and Dietetics
School of Health Sciences
University of Wollongong

NSW 2522
Australia

Martin Wiseman, MB, BS, FRCP, FRCPath
Medical & Scientific Adviser
World Cancer Research Fund International
19, Harley Street
London, W1 9QJ
UK
(and Visiting Professor in Human Nutrition
Institute of Human Nutrition
University of Southampton
UK)

Stanley H. Zlotkin, MD, PhD, FRCPC
Professor
Department of Gastroenterology and Nutrition
The Hospital for Sick Children
555, University Avenue
Toronto, Ontario
Canada

Permissions

Copyright Acknowledgements

The editors and publishers would like to express their thanks to those who have granted permission for reproduction of original material either unmodified, or in modified form. This acknowledgement extends to copyright holders including publishers, institutions, organizations and individuals who have cleared items for inclusion in this publication, as listed below.

Tables

2.2 and 2.3 FAO/WHO Expert Consultation on Carbohydrates in Human Nutrition, with permission. 6.2 With permission from Lippincott, Williams and Wilkins. 8.1 With permission from National Academy Press (for the Institute of Medicine), Washington DC, USA. 8.2 With permission from New Zealand Institute for Crop and Food Research, Palmerston North, NZ. 9.2 With permission from the Food and Agriculture Organisation of the United Nations. 10.1, 10.2, 10.3, 22.1, and 22.2 With permission from the World Health Organisation.

Boxes

24.2 and 24.5 Copyright of the Commonwealth of Australia, Food Standards Australia New Zealand and Adjunct Professor H Greenfield and others at the University of South Wales. Certain Material used in this product has been reproduced with the permission of the Commonwealth of Australia, Food Standards Australia New Zealand, Professor H Greenfield and others at the University of New South Wales and other researchers. 24.3, 24.4, 24.7, 24.8, and 24.14 Composition of Foods–Food Standards Agency, © Crown copyright material is reproduced with the permission of the Controller of HMSO and Queen's Printer for Scotland. 24.6 With permission from the Australian Dairy Corporation. 24.9 With permission from the Australian Egg Corporation. 25.4 and 25.5 With permission from Journal of Food Protection, via the Copyright Clearance Centre, Inc.

Figures

5.1 Reprinted from *Human Nutrition and Dietetics, 9th Edition*, Eds Garrow and James, 1993, Churchill Livingstone, Edinburgh with permission from Elsevier. 5.2, 5.3, 10.7, and 15.2 With permission from Nature Publishing Group.

6.2 Brit Med J, Sought from BMJ Publishing Group. 10.2 With permission from Cambridge University Press. 10.3 and 34.4 With permission from the International Life

Sciences Institute. 10.5 With permission from the Nutrition Society. 15.1 *The American Journal of Clinical Nutrition* 2004; 79; 727–47, Adapted with permission by *The American Journal of Clinical Nutrition.* © Am J Clin Nutr. American Society of Nutrition. 17.1, 17.2, 34.1, and 34.2 With permission from the World Health Organisation. 17.4 Adapted by permission from Macmillan Publishers Ltd, *European Journal of Clinical Nutrition* 1996; 50: 277–283. 20.4 Reprinted by permission of the publisher from Seven Countries: A Multivariate Analysis of Death and Coronary Heart Disease by Ancel Keys, p. 253, Cambridge, MA: Harvard University Press, Copyright © 1980 by the President and Fellows of Harvard College. 20.5 With permission from Elsevier. 20.6 *Brit Med J* With permission from the BMJ Publishing Group. 20.7 *The Lancet* With permission from Elsevier.

20.8 *The New England Journal of Medicine* With permission from the Publishing Division of the Massachusetts Medical Society. 21.1 Cancer Incidence in Five Continents, Sought from IARC Press. 21.3 Permission sought. 21.4 Reprinted from Cell, 100: Hanahan & Weinerg, The Hallmarks of Cancer, p. 57, Copyright 2000, with permission from Elsevier. 22.1 With permission from Nature Publishing Group, via the Copyright Clearance Centre Inc. 22.2 With permission from the *American Medical Association*, all rights reserved, in respect of *Arch Intern Med*. 22.3 With permission from the *American Medical Association*, all rights reserved, in respect of JAMA. 22.4 © 2001 Massachusetts Medical Society in respect of *The New England Journal of Medicine*. 22.5 Copyright © 2002 American Diabetes Association from *Diabetes*, Vol 51, 2002, 3353–3361 Reprinted with permission from *The American Diabetes Association*. 22.6 and 34.3 With kind permission of Springer Science and Business Media. 29.1 Permission sought. 29.2 With permission of Blackwell Publishing. 29.3 Robbins GE & Trowbridge FL, Nutrition Assessment: A Comprehensive Guide for Planning Intervention, © 1984, Jones and Bartlett Publishers, Sudbury, MA www.jbpub.com Reprinted with permission. 29.4 With permission from Elsevier. 29.6 With permission from Blackwell Publishing. 33.1 With permission from McGraw Hill Australia. 34.5 Reprinted from *Clinics in Geriatric Medicine*, 18: 699–708, de Groot and van Staveren: 'Undernutrition in the European SENECA studies' © 2002, with permission from Elsevier. 34.6 Reprinted from Journal of Clinical Nutrition, 60: 619–630, Holick M *et al.*: "Vitamin D—new horizons for the 21st century" © 1994, with permission from Elsevier. 34.7 With permission from Oxford University Press. 36.3 The US Guide, MyPyramid.gov With permission from the U.S. Department of Agriculture, Centre for Nutrition Policy and Promotion. 36.3 Australian Guide to Healthy Eating, Copyright Commonwealth of Australia reproduced by permission.

1 Introduction

Stewart Truswell and Jim Mann

1.1 Definition

This book is about what we consider the essentials of human nutrition.

The science of human nutrition deals with all the effects on people of any component found in food. This starts with the physiological and biochemical processes involved in nourishment—how substances in food provide energy or are converted into body tissues, and the diseases that result from insufficiency or excess of essential nutrients (malnutrition). The role of food components in the development of chronic degenerative diseases, like coronary heart disease, cancer, dental caries, and so on, are major targets of research activity nowadays. The scope of nutrition extends to any effect of food on human function: fetal health and development, resistance to infection, mental function and athletic performance. There is growing interaction between nutritional science and molecular biology, which may help to explain the action of food components at the cellular level and the diversity of human biochemical responses.

Nutrition is also about why people choose to eat the foods they do, even if they have been advised that doing so may be unhealthy. The study of food habits thus overlaps with the social sciences of psychology, anthropology, sociology and economics. Dietetics and community nutrition are the application of nutritional knowledge to promote health and wellbeing.

Dietitians advise people how to modify what they eat in order to maintain or restore optimum health, and to help in the treatment of disease. People expect to enjoy eating the foods that promote these things; and the production, preparation and distribution of foods provides many people with employment.

A healthy diet means different things to different people. Those concerned with children's nutrition—parents, teachers and paediatricians—aim to promote healthy growth and development. For adults in affluent communities, nutrition research has become focused on attaining optimal health and 'preventing' (which mostly means 'delaying') chronic degenerative diseases of complex causation, especially obesity (Chapter 16), cardiovascular diseases (Chapter 20), cancer (Chapter 21) and diabetes (Chapter 22). These chronic diseases have also become major causes of ill health and premature death in many developing countries (Chapter 17) where they may coexist with chronic malnutrition (Chapter 18) and even periods of famine (Chapter 19).

Apart from behavioural and sociological aspects of eating there are two broad groups of questions in human nutrition, with appropriate methods for answering them:

First, what are the essential nutrients, the substances that are needed in the diet for normal function of the human body? How do they work in the body and from which foods can we obtain each of them? Many of the answers to these questions have been established.

Second, can we delay or even prevent the chronic degenerative diseases by modifying what we usually eat? These diseases, like coronary heart disease, have multiple causes, so nutrition can only be expected to make a contribution—causative or protective. The answers to these questions are at best provisional; much still has to be disentangled and confirmed.

1.2 Essential nutrients

Essential nutrients have been defined as chemical substances found in food that cannot be synthesized at all or in sufficient amounts in the body, and are necessary for life, growth and tissue repair. Water is the most important nutrient for survival. By the end of the nineteenth century the essential amino acids in proteins had been mostly identified, as well as the major inorganic nutrients such as calcium, potassium, iodine and iron.

The period 1890 to 1940 saw the discovery of 13 vitamins, organic compounds that are essential in small amounts. Each discovery was quite different; several involve fascinating stories. The research methods have comprised observations in poorly nourished humans, animal experiments, chemical fractionation of foods, biochemical research with tissues in the laboratory, and human trials.

Animal experiments played major roles in discovering which fraction of a curative diet was the missing essential food factor and how this fraction functions biochemically inside the body. The white laboratory rat is widely used, but it is not suitable for experimental deficiency of all nutrients; the right animal model has to be found. Lind demonstrated as early as 1747, in a controlled trial on board *HMS Salisbury*, that scurvy could be cured by a few oranges and lemons, but progress towards identifying *vitamin C* had to wait until 1907 when the guinea-pig was found to be susceptible to an illness like scurvy. Rats and other laboratory animals do not become ill on a diet lacking fruit and vegetables; they make their own vitamin C in the liver from glucose.

For *thiamin* (vitamin B$_1$) deficiency, birds provide good experimental models. The first step in the discovery of this vitamin was the chance observation in 1890 by Eijkman in Java (while looking for what was expected to be a bacterial cause of beri-beri) that chickens became ill with polyneuritis on a diet of cooked polished rice but stayed well if they were fed cheap unhusked rice. Human trials in Java, Malaysia and the Philippines showed that beri-beri could be prevented or cured with rice bran (or 'polish'). A bird that is unusually sensitive to thiamin deficiency, a type of rice bird, was used by Dutch workers in Java to test the different fractions in rice bran. The anti-beri-beri vitamin was first isolated in crystalline form in 1926. It took another 10 years of work before two teams of chemists in the USA and Germany were able to synthesize vitamin B$_1$, which was given the chemical name thiamin.

To find the cause of *pellagra*, which was endemic among the rural poor in the south-eastern states of the USA at the beginning of this century, Goldberger gave restricted maize diets to healthy volunteers, some of whom developed early signs of the disease. But the missing substance, niacin, could not be identified until there was an animal model—in this case 'black tongue' in dogs.

In the 1920s linoleic and linolenic acids were identified as essential fatty acids. Then came the development of analytical techniques for determining micro amounts of trace elements in foods and tissues. In this way the other group of essential micronutrients emerged, the trace elements copper, zinc, manganese, selenium, molybdenum, fluoride and chromium.

There is an additional group of food components such as dietary fibre and some carotenoids that are not considered to be essential but which are important for maintenance of health and possibly also for reducing the risk of chronic disease.

1.3 Relation of diet to chronic diseases

More recent is the realization that environmental factors, including dietary factors, are of importance in many of the chronic degenerative diseases that are major causes of ill health and death in affluent societies. The nutritional component of these is more difficult to study than is usually the case with classical nutritional deficiency diseases because these diseases have multiple causes and take years to develop. The dietary factor may be a 'risk factor' rather than a direct cause, but for some of these diseases there is sufficient evidence to show that dietary change can appreciably reduce the risk of developing the condition. The scientific methods for investigating these conditions, their causes, and treatment and prevention differ appreciably from those used for studying adequacy of nutrient intakes.

Very often the first clue to the association between a food or nutrient and a disease comes from observing striking differences in incidence of that disease between countries (or groups within a country); these differences correlate with differences in intake of dietary components. Sometimes dietary changes over time in a single country have been found to coincide with changes in disease rates. Such observations give rise to hypotheses (theories) about possible diet–disease links rather than proof of causation because many potential causative factors may change in parallel with dietary change and it is impossible to disentangle the separate effects.

Animal experiments, because they are usually short term, are not as useful for investigating diet and chronic diseases, and can be misleading. More information has come, and continues to come, from well-designed (human) *epidemiological* studies that record the relationship between dietary intake, or variables known to be related to diet, and the chronic disease under question. Studies can either investigate subjects after diagnosis of the disease (retrospective studies) or before diagnosis (prospective studies).

Retrospective or *case–control studies* are quicker and less expensive to carry out, but are less reliable than prospective studies. A series of people who have been diagnosed with cancer of the large bowel, for example, will be asked what they usually eat, or what they ate before they became ill. These are the 'cases'. They are compared with at least an equal number of 'controls' who are people without bowel cancer but of the same age and gender and, if possible, social conditions. Weaknesses of the method include: the possibility that the disease may affect food habits; that the cases cannot recall their diet accurately before the cancer really started; that the controls may have some other disease (known or latent) that affects their dietary habits; and that food intakes are recorded by cases and controls in a different way (bias).

Prospective or *cohort studies* avoid the biases involved in asking people to recall past eating habits. Information about food intake and other characteristics are collected well before onset of the disease. Large numbers of people must therefore be interviewed and examined; they must be of an age at which bowel cancer (for example) starts to be fairly common (in the middle aged) and in a population that has a fairly high rate of this disease. The healthy cohort thus examined and recorded is then followed up for 5 years or more. Eventually, a proportion will be diagnosed with bowel cancer and the original dietary details of those who develop cancer can be compared with the diets of the majority who have not developed the disease. Usually a number of dietary and other environmental factors are found to be more (or less) frequent in those who develop the disease. These, then, are apparent risk factors, or protective factors. But they are not necessarily the operative factors. Fruit consumption may appear to be protective but perhaps in this cohort, smokers eat less fruit and smoking may be more directly related. This 'confounding' must be analysed, in effect, by analysing the data to see the relationship of fruit to the disease at different levels of smoking.

Prospective studies usually provide stronger evidence of a diet–disease association than case–control studies, and where several prospective studies produce similar findings from different parts of the world this is impressive evidence of association (positive or negative) but it is still not final proof of causation. If an association is deemed not due to bias or confounding, is qualitatively strong, biologically credible, follows a plausible time sequence, and especially if there is evidence of a dose–response relationship, it is likely that the association is causal. However, there are some negative issues with regard to cohort studies. The prospective follow-up of large numbers of people (usually thousands or tens of thousands) is a complicated and costly exercise. Furthermore, assessing dietary intake at one point in time may not provide a true reflection of usual intake. It is also conceivable that a dietary factor operating before the study has started, perhaps even in childhood, may be responsible for promoting a disease.

Definitive proof that a dietary characteristic is a direct causative or protective factor requires one or more *randomized controlled prevention trials*. These involve either the addition of a nutrient or other food component as a supplement to those in the experimental group, and a placebo (dummy) capsule or tablet taken by the control group, or the prescription of a dietary regimen to the experimental group while the controls continue to follow their usual diet. Disease (and death) outcomes in the two groups are compared. Such trials have the advantage of being able to prove causality as well as the potential cost–benefit of the dietary change. However, they are costly to carry out because, as with prospective studies, it is usually necessary to study large numbers of people over a prolonged period of time. Quite often a single trial or a single prospective study does not in itself produce a definitive answer, but by combining the results of all completed investigations in a *meta-analysis* more meaningful answers are obtained. For example, a much clearer picture has emerged regarding the role of dietary factors in the aetiology of coronary heart disease from meta-analyses of both prospective studies and clinical trials.

In addition to epidemiological studies and trials, much research involving the role of diet in chronic degenerative disease has centred around the effects of diet on modifying risk factors rather than the disease itself. For many chronic diseases there are biochem-ical markers of risk. High plasma cholesterol, for example, is an important risk factor for coronary heart disease. Innumerable studies have examined the role of different nutrients and foods on plasma cholesterol or other risk factors. Such studies are cheaper and easier to undertake than epidemiological studies and randomized controlled trials with disease outcome because far fewer people can be studied over a relatively short period of time. They have helped to find which foods lower cholesterol and so should help protect against coronary heart disease. It is this information that has formed the basis of the public health messages that have undoubtedly contributed to the decline in the incidence of coronary disease in most affluent societies over the last 40 years.

Several international organizations, including the World Health Organization and the World Cancer Research Fund, have attempted to establish clear guidelines regarding the degree of confidence that can be placed on observed associations between dietary factors and chronic diseases. An association is described as 'convincingly causal' when randomized controlled trials show that modifying the factor can influence disease outcome, or when several cohort (prospective) studies show consistent associations that cannot be explained by chance or confounding. For an association to be regarded as convincing there should also be confirmatory evidence from experimental studies in humans or animals, and there should be a biological gradient or dose–response between the degree or level of exposure to the dietary factor and the disease risk—meaning the greater the exposure to the food or nutrient, the greater the risk. Associations may be defined as 'probably causal' if several cohort and/or case–control studies consistently demonstrate biologically plausible associations that cannot be explained by chance, bias or confounding. Associations that are based on lesser degrees of evidence are described as 'possible' or 'suggestive' and are generally regarded as insufficient to warrant recommendations for dietary change. We should be sure of our ground before we advise individuals or populations to change a diet to which they are accustomed. Food habits have strong cultural values.

1.4 Tools of the trade

As with any other science or profession, nutrition has its specialized techniques and technical terms. Those that are frequently used in research and professional work are introduced here. They are described in more detail further on in the book.

1.4.1 Measuring food and drink intake

Which foods (and drinks) does a person or a group of people usually eat (and drink) and how many grams of each per day? Unless the subject is confined within a special research facility under constant observation the answer can never be 100% accurate. Information about food intake is subjective and depends on memory; people do not always notice, or know, the exact description of the foods they are given to eat (especially in mixed dishes). When asked to record what they eat they may alter their diet. People do not eat the same every day so it is difficult to obtain a profile of their usual diet.

The different techniques used are described in Chapter 28. One set of methods estimates the amounts of food produced and sold in a whole country and divides these by the estimated population. This is 'food disappearance' or food moving into consumption. Obviously some of this food is wasted and some is eaten by tourists and pets. The main value of the data is for following national trends and for seeing if people appear to be eating too little or too much of some foods.

Other methods capture the particular foods and amounts of them that individuals say they actually ate. These methods rely either on the subjects' memories or on asking them to write down everything they eat or drink for (usually) several days.

1.4.2 Food composition tables (see Chapter 27)

Ideally food tables would contain all the usual foods eaten in a country and give average numbers for the calories (food energy), the major essential nutrients and other important food components (e.g. dietary fibre) of each food, measured by chemical analysis. In many smaller less-affluent countries there is no complete set of food composition data, so 'borrowed' data are used from one of the 'big' Western countries (e.g. the UK, USA, or Germany). Food tables are used to calculate people's nutrient intakes from their food intake estimates. Most food tables are also available as computer software, which greatly speeds up the computations (for 20 subjects $\times$ 4 days $\times$ 80 foods or drinks $\times$ 35 nutrients, that is 224 000 computations).

1.4.3 Dietary reference values and guidelines (see Chapter 36)

Computer software packages for dietary analyses generate printouts that show what a subject or groups of individuals have eaten in terms of nutrients. This does not mean anything unless comparison is made with normative dietary reference values. Two sets are used, but they differ somewhat from country to country. For essential nutrients (protein, vitamins, minerals) the reference is in a table of *recommended nutrient intakes* (*dietary reference intakes* in the USA). For some nutrients that are not essential but which may be related to disease risk (e.g. saturated fat, which is related to risk of coronary heart disease) advice regarding intake is in recommendations called *dietary guidelines*.

1.4.4 Biomarkers: biochemical tests

If an individual (or group) is found to eat less than the recommended intake of nutrient 'A' then they may not have any features of 'A' deficiency. The food intake may have been under-reported or only temporarily less than usual, and there are large body stores for some nutrients. Some people may have lower requirements than average. On the other hand, individuals can suffer deficiency of nutrient 'A' despite an acceptable intake if they have an unusually high requirement, perhaps because of increased losses from disease. For many nutrients, biochemical tests using blood or urine are available to help estimate the amount of the nutrient functioning inside the body (see Chapter 29). Furthermore, *biomarkers* provide a more objective and often more economical method for estimating intake of some food components (e.g. urinary sodium for salt) than food intake measurement, and they can also be used to check the reliability of subject histories or records of food intake.

1.4.5 Human studies and trials

Most of the detailed knowledge in human nutrition comes from a range of different types of human experiments. They may last from hours to years and may include just two or three subjects or thousands of subjects. The following are examples:

- Absorption studies. Some nutrients are poorly absorbed, and absorption of nutrients is better from some foods than from others. Many studies have been done to measure bioavailability—that is, the percentage of the nutrient intake that is available to be used inside the body. After a test meal, the increase in some nutrients can be measured in blood samples. Isotopes may be needed to label the nutrient.

- Metabolic studies. The diet is usually changed in one way only, and the result is measured in a change in blood or excreta (urine and/or faeces). One type is the *balance experiment*. This may measure, for example, the intake of calcium and its excretion in urine and faeces. Because of the minor variability of urine production and the major variability of defecation these measurements have to be made for a metabolic period of several days every time any dietary change is made.

- Another example is the effect of a controlled (usually single) change of diet on blood plasma cholesterol, a risk factor for coronary heart disease (see Chapter 20). Such an effect is known to take 10–14 days if it is going to appear and the experiment should include control periods before and after the dietary change being examined.

Interpreting the results of such studies is a complex matter. There is individual variation in the way people absorb and metabolize nutrients (see Box 1.1). There is also the possibility that changes observed over a short time period may not persist indefinitely because humans may adapt to dietary change. Furthermore, when one component is added or removed from the diet there are usually consequential changes to the

---

BOX 1.1 Nutrition and genes

Some nutrients or their active metabolites affect the functioning of some genes.

- Firstly, for example, some forms of vitamin A, retinoic acids, affect transcription of genes for cellular differentiation (Chapter 11). Likewise 1,25 di-OH vitamin D switches on the gene for calcium transport—and possibly other genes (Chapter 14).

- Secondly, variations of some genes (polymorphism) affects the function of some nutrients. Examples include alcohol metabolism (Chapter 6), haemochromatosis (Chapter 9), folate metabolism (Chapter 12), familial hypercholesterolaemia (Chapter 20), lipoprotein apo-E types (Chapter 20), genes and cancer (Chapter 21) and lactase insufficiency (Chapter 24).

- Thirdly, in some of the plants that provide our food, a gene from another species has been inserted or an endogenous gene has been inactivated to produce a crop that is easier to grow (e.g. GM maize) or has an improved nutritional profile (e.g. golden rice) (Chapter 25). Some nutrition research departments are now giving priority to *nutrigenomics*, the application of genomics technologies in nutrition sciences and food technology.

rest of the diet as some other food is put in its place. An apparent effect of removing one food may at least in part be due to the effect of its replacement or to the energy deficit that will result if it is not replaced. Before recommending dietary change it is imperative that nutritionists consider not only the role of individual nutrients as determinants of health and disease, but also diet as a whole and the complex dynamics of dietary change, in order to ensure that overall benefit will accrue from any changes that are made.

FURTHER READING

1. **Truswell, A.S**. (2001) Levels and kinds of evidence for public health nutrition. *Lancet*, **357**, 1061–2.

 To see topical and scientifically robust updates on nutrition associated with this textbook, and active web links to many of the journal articles in the Reference areas, please see the dedicated Online Resource Centre at www.oxfordtextbooks.co.uk/orc/mann3e/.

PART 1

Energy and macronutrients

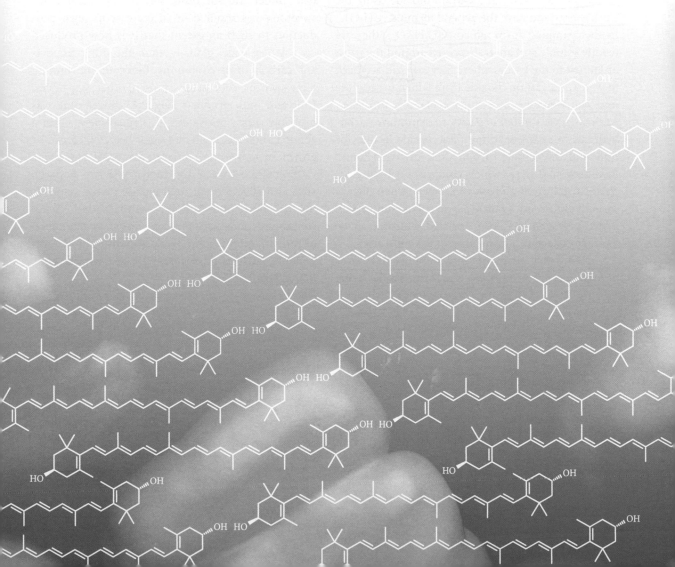

2 Carbohydrates

John Cummings and Jim Mann

broken down?
converted?

Carbohydrates are stored energy. They are synthesized by plants from water and carbon dioxide using the sun's energy and have the general formula $(CH_2O)_N$. In their simplest form, glucose $(C_6H_{12}O_6)$, they are readily soluble and are transported around the plant or animal to the tissues where they are oxidized back to water and carbon dioxide from which process the host gains energy for cellular metabolic processes. Animals have limited capacity to synthesize carbohydrates but can make the disaccharide lactose for milk and the storage carbohydrate glycogen found in muscle and liver, which comprises a branched-chain structure of glucose molecules. When dietary carbohydrate is not available as an energy source, and stored glycogen has been depleted, glucose can be made from lactate, glyerol and some amino acids.

Carbohydrates are the most important source of food energy in the world, the major staples being cereals, such as rice, wheat, maize, barley, rye, oats, millet and sorghum. The human passion for sweetness has resulted in an increase in sugar production to such an extent that it is now produced on a larger scale, globally, than the other important carbohydrate-containing foods in the human diet, such as root crops, pulses, other vegetables, fruit and milk products (Fig. 2.1). Sugar cane was probably first cultivated in Papua New Guinea about 10 000 years ago and sugar beet, which can be grown in temperate climates, some 250 years ago. Carbohydrate-containing foods provide between 40% and 80% of total food energy intake, depending on culture and economic status. Carbohydrate-containing foods also contribute important amounts of protein, vitamins, minerals and other food components, such as phytochemicals and antioxidants, to the diet.

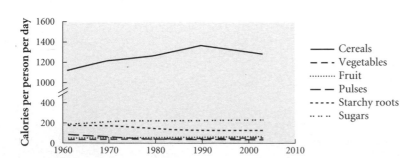

Fig. 2.1 World sources of food energy (cals/person/day) from major carbohydrate sources (1961–2003).

Source: FAOSTAT data 2006.

2.1 Classification of dietary carbohydrates

Despite being principally a source of energy, carbohydrates are a diverse group of substances with varied chemical and physiological properties with differing importance to health. They may be grouped or classified in various ways but as chemistry ultimately determines function, classification according to molecular size—characterized by the degree of polymerization (DP), the type of linkage (α or non-α linked) and the individual monomers present—is the only approach that has stood the test of time (Table 2.1). This classification is analogous to that used for dietary fat, which is based on the chain length of the fatty acids, the number and position of the double bonds, and their conformation as *cis* or *trans*.

2.1.1 Sugars

The three principal monosaccharides are glucose, fructose and galactose (Fig. 2.2) and they are the building blocks of naturally occurring di-, oligo- and polysaccharides. Free glucose and fructose occur in honey and cooked or dried fruit (invert sugar) and in small amounts in raw fruit, berries and vegetables, especially carrots, onions, swede, turnip and tomatoes. Corn syrup (a glucose syrup produced by the hydrolysis of corn starch) and high-fructose corn syrup (which contains glucose and fructose) are increasingly being used by the food industry. Fructose is the sweetest of all the food carbohydrates.

The polyols, such as sorbitol, are alcohols of glucose and other sugars. They are found naturally in some fruits and made commercially by using aldose reductase to convert the aldehyde group of the glucose molecule to the alcohol. Sorbitol is used as a replacement for sucrose in the diet of people with diabetes but confers little benefit.

The principal disaccharides are sucrose (α-Glc$(1\rightarrow2)\beta$-Fru) and lactose (β-Gal$(1\rightarrow4)\beta$Glc) (Fig. 2.2). Sucrose is found very widely in fruit, berries and vegetables, and can be extracted from sugar cane or beet. Lactose is the main sugar in milk. Maltose, a disaccharide derived from starch, occurs in sprouted wheat and barley. Trehalose (α-Glc$(1\rightarrow4)\alpha$-Glc) is

Table 2.1 The major dietary carbohydrates

Class (DP*)	Sub-group	Principal components
Sugars (1–2)	i Monosaccharides	Glucose, fructose, galactose
	ii Disaccharides	Sucrose, lactose, maltose, trehalose
	iii Polyols (sugar alcohols)	Sorbitol, mannitol, lactitol, xylitol, erythritol
Oligosaccharides (3–9)** (short-chain carbohydrates)	i Malto-oligosaccharides (α-glucans)	Maltodextrins
	ii Non α-glucan oligosaccharides	Raffinose, stachyose, fructo- and galacto-oligosaccharides, polydextrose, inulin
Polysaccharides (≥10)	i Starch (α-glucans)	Amylose, amylopectin, modified starches
	ii Non-starch polysaccharides (NSPs)	Cellulose, hemicellulose, pectin, arabinoxylans, glucomannans, plant gums and mucilages, hydrocolloids

*Degree of polymerization or number of monomeric (single sugar) units.
**See IUB-IUPAC definition and Cummings *et al.* (1997).

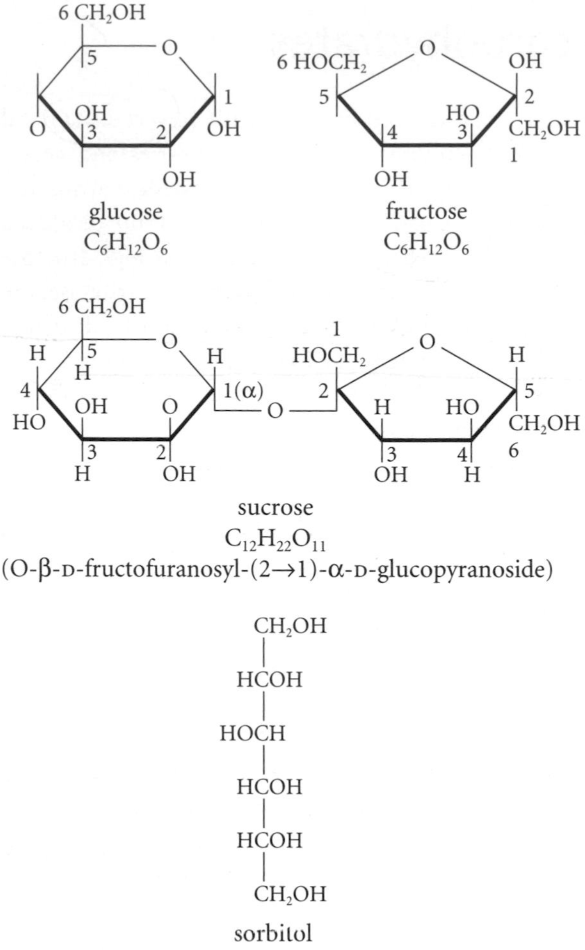

glucose
$C_6H_{12}O_6$

fructose
$C_6H_{12}O_6$

sucrose
$C_{12}H_{22}O_{11}$
(O-β-D-fructofuranosyl-(2→1)-α-D-glucopyranoside)

CH_2OH
|
HCOH
|
HOCH
|
HCOH
|
HCOH
|
CH_2OH

sorbitol

Fig. 2.2 The structure of mono- and disaccharides.

found in yeast, fungi (mushrooms) and in small amounts in bread and honey. It is used by the food industry as a replacement for sucrose where a less sweet taste is desired but with similar technological properties.

2.1.2 Oligosaccharides (short-chain carbohydrates)

Oligosaccharides are not clearly defined but, according to convention, they are carbohydrates with a DP of 2–10. However, nutritionists consider the disaccharides (DP 2) to be sugars. The division between oligosaccharides and polysaccharides at DP 10 is somewhat arbitrary as there is a continuum of molecular

size from single sugars to complex polymers of DP 100 000 or more. In reality, the division is made analytically by defining oligosaccharides as carbohydrates other than mono- and disaccharides that remain in solution in 80% (w/v) ethanol. A better term is 'short-chain carbohydrates'. Food oligosaccharides fall into two groups. First, the maltodextrins, which are mostly derived from starch and include maltotriose and α-limit dextrins that have both α-1,4 and α-1,6 bonds and are on average DP 8. Maltodextrins are widely used in the food industry as sweeteners, as fat substitutes and to modify the texture of food products. They are digested and absorbed like other α-glucans. Second are the oligosaccharides that are not α-glucans. The other oligosaccharides include raffinose (α-Gal(1→6)α-Glc(1→2)β-Fru), stachyose ((Gal)$_2$ 1:6 Glu 1:2 Fru) and verbascose ((Gal)$_3$ 1:6 Glu 1:2 Fru). They are, in effect, sucrose joined to varying numbers of galactose molecules and they are found in a variety of plant seeds such as peas, beans and lentils. Also important in this group are inulin and fructo-oligosaccharides (α-Glc(1→2)β-Fru(2→1)β-Fru$_{(N)}$ or β-Fru(2→1)β-Fru$_{(N)}$). They are fructans and are the storage carbohydrates in artichokes with small amounts of the lower-molecular-weight varieties found in wheat, rye, asparagus and members of the onion, leek and garlic families. They may also be produced industrially. The chemical bonds linking these oligosaccharides are not α-1,4 or 1,6 glucans and, therefore, they are not susceptible to pancreatic or brush-border enzyme breakdown. They have become known as 'non-digestible oligosaccharides' or NDO. Some of them, mainly the fructans and galactans, have unique properties in the gut and are known as prebiotics (see section 2.10.5).

2.1.3 Polysaccharides

These divide into α-glucans (starch) and non-α-glucans (non-starch polysaccharides).

Starch Starch is the storage carbohydrate of plants such as cereals, root vegetables and legumes and consists only of glucose molecules. It occurs in a partially

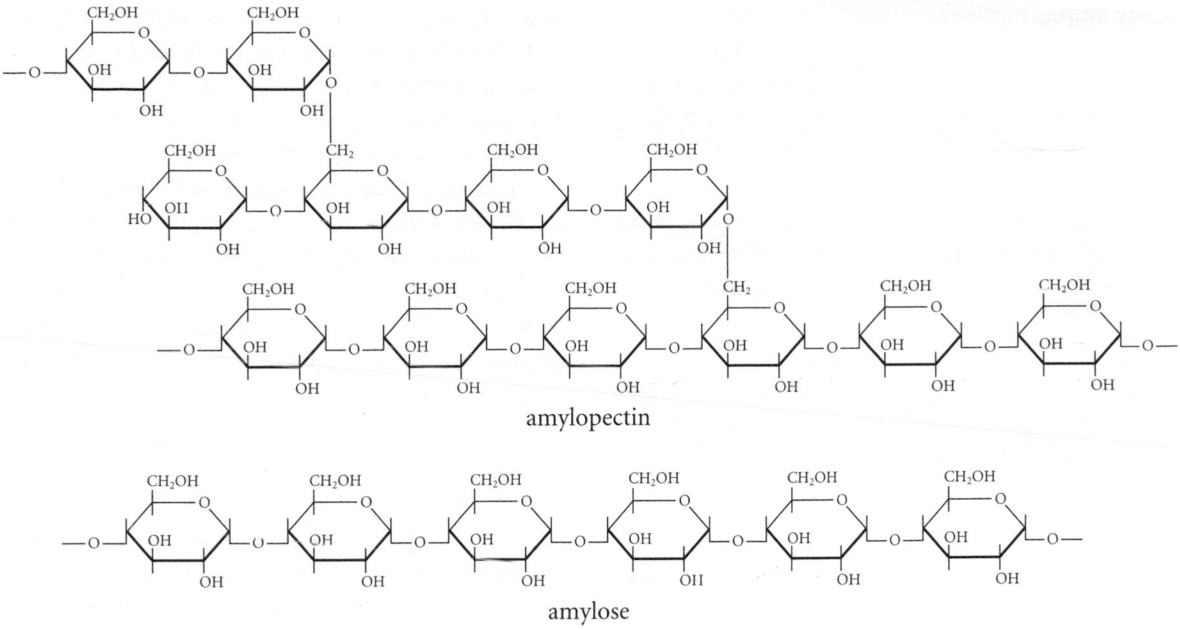

Fig. 2.3 The structure of amylose and amylopectin.

crystalline form in granules and comprises two polymers: amylose (DP ~ 10^3) and amylopectin (DP ~ 10^4–10^5). Most common cereal starches contain 15–30% amylose, which is a non-branching helical chain of glucose residues linked by α-1,4 glucosidic bonds (Fig. 2.3). Amylopectin is a high-molecular-weight, highly branched polymer containing both α-1,4 and α-1,6 linkages (Fig. 2.3). Some waxy starches (maize, rice, sorghum, barley) contain largely amylopectin. In animals and humans, carbohydrate is stored in the liver and muscle in limited amounts as glycogen, which has a structure similar to amylopectin but is even more highly branched. The crystalline form of the amylose and amylopectin in starch granules confers on them distinct X-ray diffraction patterns (A, B and C). The A type is characteristic of cereals (rice, wheat, maize) and the B type of potato, banana and high-amylose starches, while the C type is intermediate between A and B, as found in legumes. In their native (raw) form the B starches are resistant to digestion by pancreatic amylase. Starch, which is not digested in the small bowel, is known as 'resistant starch' (see section 2.5.1). The crystalline structure is

lost when starch is heated in water (gelatinization), thus permitting digestion to take place. Recrystallization (retrogradation) takes place to a variable extent after cooking and is in the B form.

Modified starch   Because many starches do not have the functional properties needed to impart or maintain desired qualities in food products, some have been modified, by either chemical processing or plant breeding techniques, to obtain these properties. Various processes are used to modify starch, the two most important being substitution and cross-linking. Substitution involves etherification or esterification of a relatively small number of hydroxyl groups on the glucose units of amylose and amylopectin. This reduces retrogradation, which is part of the process of staling of bread for example. Substitution also lowers gelatinization temperature, provides freeze–thaw stability and increases viscosity. Cross-linking involves the introduction of a limited number of linkages between the chains of amylose and amylopectin. The process reinforces the hydrogen bonding that occurs within the granule. Cross-linking increases gelatinization temperature, improves acid and heat stabilities, inhibits gel formation and controls viscosity during processing. Techniques of plant breeding, including genetic modification, can also be used to alter the proportions of amylose and amylopectin in starchy foods. For example, high-amylose corn starch requires higher temperatures for gelatinization and is more prone to retrogradation. Varying the composition of starchy foods may alter nutritional properties as well as conferring different functional properties.

Non-starch polysaccharides (NSPs) Non-starch polysaccharides are principally the polysaccharides of the plant cell wall. They comprise a mixture of many molecular forms of which cellulose, a straight-chain β-1,4-linked glucan (DP 10^3–10^6) is the most widely distributed. Because of its linear, unbranched nature, cellulose molecules are able to pack closely together in a three-dimensional lattice work, forming microfibrils. These form the basis of cellulose fibres, which are woven into the plant cell wall and give it structure. Cellulose comprises 10–30% of the NSPs in foods.

By contrast, the hemicelluloses are a diverse group of polysaccharide polymers that contain a mixture of hexose (6C) and pentose (5C) sugars, often in highly branched chains. Mostly they comprise a backbone of xylose sugars with branches of arabinose, mannose, galactose and glucose, and have a DP of 150–200. Typical of the hemicelluloses are the arabinoxylans found in cereals. About half the hemicelluloses contain uronic acids, which are carboxylated derivatives of glucose and galactose. They are important in determining the properties of hemicelluloses, behaving as carboxylic acids, and are able to form salts with metal ions such as calcium and zinc.

Common to all cell walls are pectins, which are primarily β-1,4-D-galacturonic acid polymers, although they usually contain 10–25% other sugars such as rhamnose, galactose and arabinose, as side chains. Some 3–11% of the uronic acids have methyl substitutions, which improve the gel-forming properties of pectin, as used in jam making. Some residues are acetylated. Calcium and magnesium salts of uronic acids are characteristic of pectins.

Chemically related to the cell wall NSPs—but not strictly cell wall components—are the plant gums and mucilages. Plant gums are sticky exudates that form at the sites of injuries to plants. They are mostly highly branched, complex uronic acid-containing polymers. Gum Arabic, named after the Arabian port from which it was originally exported to Europe, comes from the acacia tree and is one of the better-known plant gums. It is sold commercially as an adhesive and used in the food industry as a thickener and to retard sugar crystallization. Other plant gums include karaya (sterculia) and tragacanth, which are licensed food additives.

Plant mucilages are botanically very different in that they are usually mixed with the endosperm of the storage carbohydrates of seeds. Their role is to retain water and prevent desiccation. They are neutral polysaccharides like the hemicelluloses, of which guar gum, from the cluster bean, and carob gum are similar β-1,4-D-galactomannans with α-1,6-galactose single-unit side chains. Again, they are widely used in the pharmaceutical and food industries as thickeners and stabilizers in salad creams, soups and toothpastes.

The algal polysaccharides, which include carageenan, agar and alginate, are all NSPs, extracted from seaweeds or algae. They replace cellulose in the cell wall and have gel-forming properties. Carageenan and agar are highly sulphated and the ability of carageenan to react with milk protein has led to its use in dairy products and chocolate.

Because of the nature of the chemical bonds in NSPs they are not digested by the normal enzymes in the gut. They are extensively degraded by bacteria in the lower bowel through a process known as fermentation (see section 2.5.4).

2.2 Measurement of dietary carbohydrate

In North America, total carbohydrate in the diet has traditionally been estimated by measuring moisture, fat, protein, and ash, subtracting the sum from the total dry weight of the food. The remainder is considered to be carbohydrate 'by difference'. In Europe and Australasia, measurement is based on the sum of individual carbohydrates. The consultation by the Food and Agriculture Organization (FAO) and the World Health Organization (WHO) strongly advised use of the latter approach because the figure arrived at by difference includes non-carbohydrate components (lignin, tannins, waxes and some organic acids) and this compounds the analytical errors of all the other determinations and does not allow a detailed characterization of dietary carbohydrate, which is necessary for understanding the relationship between carbohydrates and health.

A single comprehensive system to measure all the carbohydrate fractions in the diet does not exist, although one is urgently needed. Hence, food tables will often give only a figure for total carbohydrate, starch and sometimes NSPs. What is always missing at the present time are data on oligosaccharides and resistant starch.

After homogenization of a diet or food, and lipid extraction if necessary, free sugars (mono- and disaccharides) can be extracted into aqueous solutions and measured by gas–liquid chromatography (GLC) or high-performance liquid chromatography (HPLC).

Enzymic methods also exist for individual sugars. Oligosaccharides or short-chain carbohydrates are more difficult to determine and are measured as those carbohydrates other than free sugars that are soluble in 80% ethanol and not susceptible to pancreatic amylase. Starch and maltodextrins are hydrolyzed and NSPs precipitated with ethanol. Fructans are hydrolyzed enzymatically and the monosaccharide constituents reduced to acid-stable alditol derivatives, while the remaining oligosaccharides are hydrolyzed with sulphuric acid and measured as alditol acetates by GLC.

Starch is solubilized and then hydrolyzed with a combination of amylolytic enzymes, and the increase in glucose is measured either enzymatically/calorimetrically or by GLC. Starch can be subdivided analytically into rapid digestible (RDS), slowly digestible (SDS) and resistant starch (RS). RDS and SDS relate to the rate of release of glucose from starch and are relevant to the concept of the glycaemic index (see section 2.6).

After starch has been hydrolyzed enzymatically, NSPs can be precipitated with 80% ethanol, hydrolyzed with sulphuric acid, and the released sugars measured calorimetrically, by GLC or HPLC. Techniques exist for separate measurement of cellulose in the process. The division of NSPs into soluble and insoluble is method (pH) dependent and is not recommended.

2.3 Other terms used to describe carbohydrates

A classification based purely on chemistry has the advantage of defining carbohydrate comprehensively and precisely, and allows an accurate methodology for measurement. However, chemistry does not always translate directly into physiology because each of the major classes of carbohydrate has a variety of overlapping physiological effects. A classification based on physiological properties alone creates a number of problems as it requires that a single effect be considered overridingly important and used as the basis of the classification and makes measurement difficult. This dichotomy has led to the introduction of a number of terms to describe various fractions and subfractions of carbohydrate.

2.3.1 Extrinsic and intrinsic sugars

Intrinsic sugars are those incorporated within the cell walls of plants, that is, they are naturally occurring and are always accompanied by other important nutrients. Extrinsic sugars are those added to foods. Lactose in milk does not fall readily into either category but milk has important nutritional properties, so the term non-milk extrinsic sugar (NMES) was introduced in the UK to indicate the group of sugars other than intrinsic and milk sugars that should be restricted in the diet. This terminology has not gained widespread use. The WHO/FAO Expert Consultation on *Diet, Nutrition and the Prevention of Chronic Diseases* (WHO Technical Report Series 916) confirmed the use of the term 'free sugars', which refers to all 'monosaccharides and disaccharides added to foods by the manufacturer, cook and consumer, plus sugars naturally present in honey, syrups and fruit juices'. The Expert Consultation suggested that free sugars should contribute less than 10% of total energy.

2.3.2 Total sugars

Dividing sugars into intrinsic and extrinsic creates problems for the analyst and, therefore, for food labelling. Analytically, it is not readily possible to distinguish in a processed food which sugars might have been added and which are naturally present in say, fruit, in that food. Moreover, there is probably little difference physiologically between the way the body absorbs and metabolizes the sucrose present in a banana and that in a sugary drink, for example. Of course the nutritional profile of these two foods will be very different. For labelling purposes, therefore, the category of 'total sugars' has been developed, which includes all sugars from whatever source in a food, and is defined as all monosaccharides and disaccharides other than polyols. This term is now accepted by the European Union, Australia and New Zealand and may yet be adopted by other countries. Other terms in use include 'sugars', used mainly in the USA and Canada, and added sugars, refined sugars, saccharose and free sugars.

2.3.3 Complex carbohydrate

The term complex carbohydrate was first introduced in 1977 in *Dietary goals for the United States* to encourage consumption of what were considered 'healthy foods' such as wholegrain cereals, fruit and vegetables. Subsequently, the term came to be used to distinguish between sugar and polysaccharides (Table 2.1). Complex carbohydrate has, however, never been formally defined and eventually it became equated with starch. It has not proved useful to distinguish 'healthy' food because many fruit and vegetables are low in poly-saccharides and starch. Moreover, starch can have many forms, each with contrasting metabolic properties. RDS derived from most cooked starchy cereals or warm potatoes is almost as rapidly absorbed as many sugars. On the other hand, some starch (such as that found in unripe bananas, partly milled grains and seeds) is fairly resistant to digestion in the small intestine of humans and from a physiological perspective is digested and metabolized more like NSPs. The term complex carbohydrate, therefore, is not useful in the context of a chemically based approach to carbohydrates or in nutritional recommendations.

2.3.4 Glycaemic carbohydrate

Perhaps the most useful distinction with regard to human health is whether or not the carbohydrate source does or does not directly provide glucose as an energy source following the process of digestion and absorption in the small intestine. Carbohydrate that provides glucose for metabolism is referred to as 'glycaemic carbohydrate', whereas carbohydrate that passes to the large intestine prior to being fermented is referred to as 'non-glycaemic carbohydrate'. Most mono- and disaccharides, some oligosaccharides (maltodextrins) and RDS may be classed as glycaemic carbohydrate. SDS are also considered to be glycaemic carbohydrate, though glucose is less rapidly generated. The remaining oligosaccharides, non-starch polysaccharides and RS are considered to be non-glycaemic carbohydrates. Some carbohydrate-containing foods contain both glycaemic and non-glycaemic carbohydrate. The extent to which carbohydrate in foods raises blood glucose concentrations compared with an equivalent amount of reference carbohydrate has also been used as a means of classifying dietary carbohydrate; it is known as the glycaemic index (see section 2.6).

Analogous to the concept of glycaemic carbohydrate are the terms 'available and unavailable carbohydrate'. These were introduced by McCance and Lawrence in 1921 while preparing food tables for diabetic diets. Available carbohydrate was defined as 'starch and soluble sugars' and unavailable carbohydrate as 'mainly hemicellulose and fibre (cellulose)'. The terms glycaemic and non-glycaemic are probably more useful and followed on from McCance and Lawrence's original ideas.

2.3.5 Dietary fibre

There is no internationally agreed definition of dietary fibre. The original definition of dietary fibre in 1972 by Trowell was 'the proportion of food which is derived from the cellular walls of plants which is digested very poorly in human beings'. This, however, is not a clear description of a component of the diet but more a physiological concept of non-digestibility. Allied to (and the progenitor of) this concept were the epidemiological observations of Burkitt and others in the early 1960s, which led to the proposal that diets that are low in fibre are associated with the occurrence of many non-communicable Western diseases such as bowel cancer, diverticular disease, coronary heart disease and gallstones. What Burkitt correctly observed in Africa was a type of diet high in vegetables and unprocessed cereals but low in meat and fat. Today we know that fibre is only one component of the diet that is important in this context and that other aspects of lifestyle such as exercise, smoking and obesity also contribute.

The principal component of dietary fibre by any definition is NSPs and measurement of NSPs provides a useful surrogate marker for a healthy diet. The idea of non-digestible material leads to complicated and unmeasurable groupings of dietary components, which will differ from person to person. Physiology is a bad basis for defining food components. Apart from NSPs, many things have been suggested to be included as dietary fibre, such as resistant starch, some oligosaccharides, lignin, and even indigestible protein. True lignin is very difficult to measure and forms only a very minor part of the plant cell wall, except in wholegrain cereals. Its physiology and health effects have not been determined.

The terms soluble and insoluble fibre developed out of the early chemistry of NSPs. However, this separation is not chemically distinct, it can be changed by simply altering the pH of the extraction, and the physiological roles of soluble and insoluble NSPs in foods are not clear. Much of the early work on soluble fibre, which suggested that it had good cholesterol-lowering properties, was from studies using pure polysaccharides such as pectin, guar, psyllium and milling fractions like oat bran. All plant cell wall/NSP complexes, as they exist in foods, contain a 'soluble' fraction and ascribing specific physiological properties to, or making dietary recommendations for distinct subfractions of NSP is not justified at present.

2.4 Availability and consumption

The major sources of carbohydrate worldwide are cereals (wheat, rice, maize, barley, oats, rye, millet and sorghum), root crops (potatoes, cassava (manioc), yams, sweet potatoes and taro), sugar cane and beet, pulses, vegetables, fruit, and milk products. World production of cereals, sugar cane, vegetables and fruits has increased over the last 20–30 years. Production of root crops, pulses and sugar beet, however, has changed little on a worldwide basis; pulse production has decreased in some Asian countries and root crop production has fallen in Europe. At first glance these data suggest that overall food production is keeping pace with population growth, which has continued in most parts of the world. Increased production, however, is due largely to improved agricultural practices, principally the increased use of fertilizers, and there has been no appreciable increase in areas under cultivation for these crops. This suggests that the steady increase in production may not be sustained in all countries. Indeed, for the continent of Africa, cereal production is already inadequate and it seems conceivable—indeed likely—that there are major problems ahead. The proportional reduction of root crops and pulses may have nutritional consequences.

Fig. 2.1 shows the calories available per person per day from carbohydrate-containing foods available for consumption on a worldwide basis. These data differ from overall crop production statistics because much cereal production goes into animal feed (especially maize and barley) or is grown for seed, or is used in distilling (barley). In terms of agricultural production for food, in 2003 rice was the main cereal, followed by wheat, then maize. Fig. 2.1 shows clearly that cereal crops provide by far the biggest contribution to energy intake of any food—46% in 2003.

Notable, however, is the steady rise in energy from sugar, which was in 1961 very similar to that obtained from starchy roots (potatoes, sweet potato, yams, etc.) while by 2003 sugar had become the second source of energy from carbohydrate, providing 244 calories per person per day compared with 145 from starchy roots. Overall, including sugars, carbohydrate-containing foods provided 68% of food energy in 2003 worldwide.

Population surveys permit a broad overview of the carbohydrate consumption in different parts of the world (Table 2.2). As a percentage of total energy intake, the contribution from all carbohydrates ranges from about 40% to over 80% (representing about 250–400 g carbohydrate/day) with relatively more affluent countries such as those in North America, Europe and Australasia at the lower end of the range, and less affluent countries at the higher end. Starch accounts for 20–50% and sugars 9–27% of total energy, with low intakes of sugars generally associated with high total carbohydrate intakes. In Western

Table 2.2 Intake of carbohydrate and its components in adults in various countries since 1980 (abstracted from FAO/WHO Expert Consultation on Carbohydrates in Human Nutrition)

Country	Year	n	Energy (kcal)	Carbohydrate		Starch		Sugars	
				g	% energy	g	% energy	g	% energy
Malawi*	1997	141	1457	287	78.7	–	–	–	–
S Africa—coloured	1990	976	1981	224	45.2	147	29.7	77	15.6
China	1992	3682	2396	355	59.3	–	–	–	–
Vietnam	1988	7462	1998	407	81.5	–	–	–	–
Netherlands	1987–88	4134	2309	244	42.2	122	21.1	119	20.6
UK**	2001	1724	M 2313	M 275	M 47.6	M 157	M 27.3	M 118	M 20.4
			F 1632	F 203	F 49.7	F 110	F 26.9	F 88	F 21.6
Chile	1995	859	1981	287	58.0	–	–	–	–
USA	1988–91	7931	2109	244	46.3	–	–	–	–
Australia	1983	6255	2190	232	42.4	125	22.8	107	19.5
Papua New Guinea	1991	750	2628	406	61.8	349	53.1	57	8.7

*Gibson, R.S. (1997) Personal communication.
**National Diet and Nutrition Survey 2002. The Stationery Office London.

countries 20–25% of total energy is derived from sugars, about one-third from naturally occurring sources (vegetables, milk, fruits and juices) and two-thirds from added sugars, especially sucrose. In North America a relatively high proportion of free sugars comes from corn syrup solids or high-fructose corn syrups, so that sucrose intake—but not total sugar intake—is lower than in most European countries. Trends in total carbohydrate consumption suggest a falling intake in most relatively affluent countries, reflecting a progressive decline in overall energy intake.

2.5 Digestion and absorption of carbohydrate

2.5.1 Sugars and starch (Fig. 2.4)

Virtually all carbohydrates absorbed in the small intestine are hydrolyzed to their constituent monosaccharides before absorption. Some carbohydrates, such as lactose in many populations, most oligosaccharides except maltodextrins, some starches and all NSPs, resist digestion and pass into the large bowel where they are fermented (see section 2.5.4). Other carbohydrates are digested and absorbed largely from the upper part of the small bowel.

Carbohydrate digestion starts in the mouth where salivary α amylase is secreted. However, its activity is substantially inhibited by low pH when ingested food enters the stomach and so is relatively unimportant compared with that resulting from pancreatic amylase in the small intestine. Amylase is the only active carbohydrate-digesting enzyme produced by the pancreas. α-Amylase hydrolyzes the α-1,4 bonds but only those that are not at the ends of a molecule or next to α-1,6 branch points, so α-amylase produces a mixture of maltose, maltotriose and α-limit

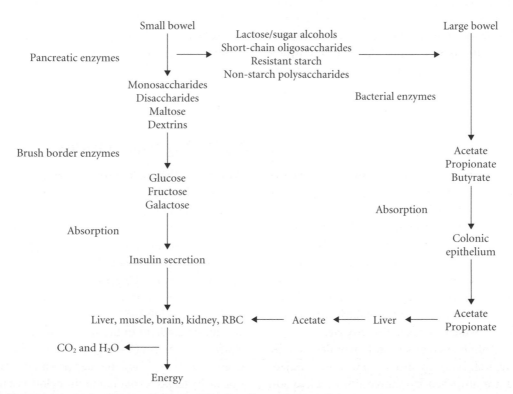

Fig. 2.4 The two principal pathways of carbohydrate digestion and absorption.

dextrins. Small bowel mucosa is, therefore, presented with a mixture of disaccharides, α-limit dextrins and a few monosaccharides. The surface of the small intestine is covered with microvilli, which give a total absorptive surface of up to 200 m², which is many times the area of the planar intestinal surface. The microvilli extend into the unstirred water-layer phase of the intestinal lumen. This microvillus membrane is known as the brush border and in it are the three principal enzymes that complete digestion to mono-saccharides: these are glucoamylase (α-glucosidase) and sucrose-isomaltase (which are able to reduce the products of starch digestion to glucose monomers and sucrase to glucose and fructose) and lactase (β-galactosidase, the expression of which is retained in the brush border after weaning in only a minority of world populations, mainly those in northern climates (it is able to hydrolyse lactose to glucose and galactose).

In close association with these enzymes are trans-porters that take these monosaccharides into the portal blood. Glucose and galactose are both absorbed into the enterocyte by a process of active transport facilitated by sodium glucose cotransporters (SGLT-1). Sodium is pumped from the cell to create a sodium gradient between the intestinal lumen and the interior of the cell. The resultant sodium gradient drives the cotransporter so that one molecule of sodium and one molecule of glucose or galactose are transported into the cytoplasm of the enterocyte against a concentration gradient. Glucose is pumped out of the enterocyte and into the intracellular space by glucose transporter 2 (GLUT 2). This is one of a large family of more than 12 facilitative glucose transporters that are found in tissues throughout the body, which transport D-glucose down its con-centration gradient (from high to low), a process described as facilitative diffusion. Fructose is taken up by a similar process of facilitated transport by the glucose transporter 5 (GLUT 5), which may also be the means by which it exits the enterocyte.

Sugar alcohols such as sorbitol, mannitol, xylotol and erythritol, have no specific transport mechan-ism and are absorbed by simple diffusion. At low doses this works well, but, as the amount ingested increases, so the transport capacity of the small bowel is overwhelmed and they partly pass into the large bowel. Because of their relatively low mole-cular weight, they retain considerable amounts of water within the bowel, which can lead to diarrhoea after excess consumption.

Any starch that escapes the normal small bowel digestive processes is called resistant starch. As already indicated (section 2.2), starch may resist digestion because it is enclosed in whole grains or is otherwise physically inaccessible (RS1), or because it is present in the B-type crystalline form (RS2) or because it has retrograded after cooking and cooling (RS3). Some modified starch (e.g. hydroxypropyl or acetylated starch) will also resist digestion (RS4). The amount of RS in the diet is not accurately known because measuring it is technically difficult. This is because almost any handling of starchy foods from diet collections (i.e. mixing with water, homogenization, freezing or cooling) will affect RS content. Present estimates for countries with westernized diets are in the range of 3–10 g/day. Clearly this is very diet dependent. A couple of relatively unripe bananas will readily provide 20 g RS. A biscuit made with potato flour would give 10 g. The amount of RS that cscapes digestion also varies among people, partly dependent on transit time through the small bowel.

2.5.2 Oligosaccharides

Aside from the maltodextrins, which are derived from starch, the oligosaccharides are a neglected group of carbohydrates from the point of view of their digestion. However, the nature of their bonds means they are not susceptible to either pancreatic or brush border hydrolysis and so they pass entirely into the large intestine. Oligosaccharides, therefore, are not glycaemic carbohydrates. The lower-molecular-weight species (DP 3–5) have the potential to provide an osmotic gradient in the small bowel, and if taken in large quantities (15–30 g) can cause disturbances in gut function. They are better known for their propensity to gas formation in the colon as a result of their rapid fermentation.

2.5.3 Non-starch polysaccharides (NSPs)

NSPs escape digestion in the small bowel and pass into the large bowel where they are fermented. The reason for their resistance to digestion is, again, partly because of their physical form. They are almost entirely found in plant cell walls and are, therefore, associated with wholegrain foods, fruit and vegetables. Equally importantly, the chemical bonds in these molecules are not susceptible to brush border or pancreatic digestive enzymes. For example, the bonds in cellulose are principally β-1,4 in contrast to α-1,4 in starch. This minor stereochemical difference is sufficient to prevent hydrolysis by pancreatic amylase. The amount of NSPs in the diet varies (12–36 g/day), with higher amounts being characteristic of vegetarian diets or populations with high fruit and vegetable intake, such as on some Pacific islands. High NSP intake is not characteristic of Third-World diets because rice and maize are low in NSPs and fruit and vegetables are in short supply, so intakes are more likely to be in the 16–25 g/day range.

2.5.4 Fermentation (Fig. 2.5)

Virtually all carbohydrate that enters the large bowel will be fermented by the commensal bacteria that live in the colon at densities of up to 10^{12} cells/g. Recovery

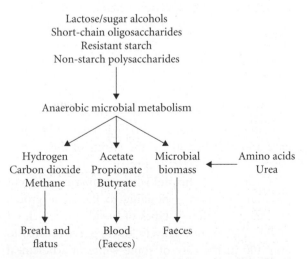

Fig. 2.5 Fermentation of carbohydrate in the large bowel.

of oligosaccharides in faeces is effectively nil, while RS and NSP excretion is rarely more than 2–4 g/day with intakes in the 20–40 g range. Only very resistant retrograded starches survive partly, again the amount depending on colonic transit time, although occasional individuals are unable to digest some RS fractions. Microcrystalline cellulose may resist fermentation because of its highly condensed structure, an observation that led to the belief that cellulose was not digested in the human gut. This is because microcrystalline cellulose was used in many early experiments of cellulose digestion. However, cellulose naturally present in the cell wall of food is completely fermented unless it is in association with large amounts of lignin. Other polysaccharides of the plant cell wall are also readily fermented, even when given in purified forms such as pectin or guar gum. This process is facilitated by the ability of these latter substances to form gels readily accessible to the microbiota.

Microbial fermentation is an anaerobic process and is, therefore, unique to the body and thus produces unique products. As Fig. 2.5 shows, these include principally the short-chain fatty acids (SCFAs), acetate, propionate and butyrate, which are the two-, three- and four-carbon fatty acids of the same series that include C12–C22 fatty acids known as the major lipids of the diet. The SCFAs are, however, much more water soluble. They are rapidly absorbed. Butyrate is the major energy source for the colonic epithelial cell, in contrast to glutamine for the small bowel and glucose for most other tissues. Butyrate also has differentiating properties in the cell, arresting cell division through its ability to regulate gene expression. This property provides a credible link between the dietary intake of fermented carbohydrates, such as NSPs, and protection against colorectal cancer.

Propionate is absorbed and passes to the liver where it is taken up and metabolized aerobically. This molecule is not seen as having significant regulatory properties in humans, although it may moderate hepatic lipid metabolism. However, in ruminant animals, propionate is crucial to life because it is used to synthesize glucose in the liver.

Acetate is the major SCFA produced in all types of fermentation and the molar ratio of acetate to propionate to butyrate is around 60:20:20. Acetate is rapidly absorbed, stimulating sodium absorption, and passes to the liver and then into the blood from where it is available as an energy source. Fasting blood acetate levels are about 50 µmol/L, rising 8–12 hours later to 100–300 µmol/L after meals containing fermentable carbohydrate. Acetate is rapidly cleared from the blood with a half-life of only a few minutes and is metabolized principally by skeletal and cardiac muscle and the brain. Acetate spares free fatty acid oxidation in humans and its absorption does not stimulate insulin release. Another precursor of blood acetate is alcohol.

Thus, fermentation is an integral part of digestion and provides energy, which is up to 70% of the available energy in equivalent monosaccharides. By convention, the energy value of oligosaccharides has been set as 2 kcal/g, although there has been a reluctance to set values for RS and NSPs. The total energy provided from fermentation in the human is probably only 5% of total energy requirements, although it could be more.

Fermentation of amino acids, derived from protein, also occurs in the large bowel and, in addition to SCFAs, yields ammonia, amines, phenols and sulphur compounds. Fermentation also gives rise to the gases hydrogen and carbon dioxide. Much of the hydrogen is converted to methane by bacteria, and both hydrogen and methane are excreted in breath and flatus. Gas production, especially if rapid, is one of the principal complaints of people unused to eating foods containing significant amounts of fermentable carbohydrate. Another product of fermentation is microbial biomass or microbial growth. These bacteria are excreted in faeces and this is one of the principal mechanisms of laxation by NSPs especially. Also produced from fermentation is lactate. This occurs usually during rapid fermentation of soluble carbohydrates such as oligosaccharides. Both D and L lactate are produced and both are absorbed. Ethyl alcohol is also produced during hind-gut fermentation, which is driven by bacteria, although it is more characteristic of fermentation due to yeasts as in brewing and wine making.

2.6 Glycaemic response to carbohydrate foods

Plasma glucose levels rise 5–45 minutes after any meal that contains sugars or digestible starch, and usually return to fasting levels 2–3 hours later. This rise in blood glucose is known as the glycaemic response and depends upon the rate and extent of digestion, absorption and clearance from the plasma. The glycaemic index of a carbohydrate-containing food is defined as the incremental area under the blood glucose response curve following a 50 g carbohydrate portion of a test food, expressed as a percentage of the response to the same amount of carbohydrate from a standard food (either glucose or white bread) taken by the same subject. The glycaemic index (GI) of a range of carbohydrate-containing foods derived from studies in humans is shown in Table 2.3.

GI is influenced by a number of attributes of foods (see Table 2.4). As a general rule, foods that are rich in

glucose and rapidly digested starches, such as white bread or cornflakes, will have a relatively large glycaemic response because they are rapidly digested and absorbed. On the other hand, foods that are rich in slowly digested and resistant starch, non-starch polysaccharides and some oligosaccharides, such as the pulses, will have a low GI. Foods containing fructose also have a relatively low GI because fructose is very rapidly absorbed and metabolized and contributes very little to blood glucose. Carbohydrate-containing foods that are also high in fat and protein have a low GI because of the effects of these other components on gastric emptying.

GI is especially helpful when comparing different variations of foods belonging to the same group, for example different types of breads for which GI might range from relatively low (e.g. rye breads) to over 100 in the case of some white or wholemeal

Table 2.3 Glycaemic index (GI) of a range of carbohydrate-containing foods (pp. 86 and 87, FAO/WHO Expert Consultation on Carbohydrates in Human Nutrition)

	GI		GI		GI
Baked Goods		**Grains**		**Pasta**	
Cakes	87	Pearled barley	36	Linguine	71
Cookies	90	Cracked barley	72	Macaroni	64
Crackers, wheat	99	Buckwheat	78	Spaghetti, white	59
Muffins	88	Bulgur	68	Spaghetti, durum	78
Rice cakes	123	Couscous	93	Spaghetti, brown	53
		Sweet corn	78		
Breads		Millet	101	**Potatoes**	
Barley kernel	49	Rice, white	81	Instant	118
Barley flour	95	Rice, low amylose	126	Baked	121
Rye flour	92	Rice, high amylose	83	New	81
Rye crispbread	93	Rice, brown	79	White, boiled	80
White bread	101	Rice, instant	128	White, mashed	100
Wholemeal flour	99	Rice, parboiled	68	French fries	107
		Speciality rices	78	Sweet potato	77
Breakfast cereals		Rye kernels	48	Yam	73
All Bran	60	Tapioca	115		
Cornflakes	119			**Snacks**	
Muesli	80	**Dairy products**		Jelly beans	114
Oat bran	78	Ice cream	84	Lifesavers	100
Porridge oats	87	Milk, whole	39	Chocolate	84
Puffed rice	123	Milk, skim	46	Popcorn	79
Puffed wheat	105	Yoghurt, with sugar	48	Corn chips	105
Shredded wheat	99	Yoghurt, with artificial		Potato chips	77
		sweetener	27	Peanuts	21
Fruit					
Apple	52	**Legumes**		**Soups**	
Apple juice	58	Baked beans	69	Bean soups	84
Apricots, dried	44	Black-eyed peas	59	Tomato	54
Apricots, canned	91	Butter beans	44		
Banana	83	Chickpeas	47	**Sugars**	
Banana, underripe	51	Canned chickpeas	59	Honey	104
Banana, overripe	82	Haricot beans	54	Fructose	32
Kiwifruit	75	Kidney beans	42	Glucose	138
Mango	80	Kidney beans, canned	74	Sucrose	87
Orange	62	Lentils	38	Lactose	65
Orange juice	74	Lentils, green	42		
Paw paw	83	Lentils, green canned	74		
Peach, canned	67	Lima beans	46		
Pear	54	Peas, dried green	56		
		Peas, green	68		
		Pinto beans	61		
		Soya beans	23		
		Split peas, yellow	45		

Table 2.4 Food factors influencing glycaemic response

Amount of carbohydrate
Nature of the monosaccharide components
Glucose
Fructose
Galactose
Nature of the starch
Amylose
Amylopectin
Crystalline form A, B or C
Starch–nutrient interaction
Resistant starch
Cooking/food processing
Degree of starch gelatinization/retrogradation
Particle size
Food form
Cellular structure
Other food components
Fat and protein
NSP (affects physical form and viscosity)

breads. While indices at the very high or very low extremes of the range are probably a true reflection of the glycaemic response, published figures in the mid-range are not particularly helpful in view of the inter- and intraindividual variability. It is often not appreciated that GI data are often based on the study of a relatively small number of healthy individuals.

The total glycaemic response to a food or meal is also determined by the amount of carbohydrate consumed as well as the GI. A product or food may have a high GI, but if only a small quantity is typically consumed, the total amount of glucose available as an immediate energy source or storage is limited. The concept of glycaemic load (GL) was introduced to quantify the overall glycaemic effect of a portion of food. GL is the product of the amount of available carbohydrate in a typical serving and the GI of the food divided by 100. While GL may be a more practical approach to determining the glycaemic response to food, this indicator is clearly dependent on GI and its pitfalls are therefore similar. The ranking of foods according to GL is in most instances similar to that for GI.

Along with the blood glucose response to carbohydrate meals there is an insulin response, which is also important in the control of metabolism. It often reflects the glycaemic response but can for some foods be more exaggerated, so the insulin response after apple juice is much greater than that after whole apples, while the glycaemic responses are similar. The presence of fat and protein in a meal increases insulin responses.

2.7 Carbohydrate metabolism

The concentration of glucose in the blood of adults is controlled within the range 4.0–5.5 mmol/L. However, when a carbohydrate-containing meal is ingested, the level may temporarily rise to as high as 7.5 mmol/L and fall to as low as 3.0–3.5 mmol/L during fasting. When levels are about 10 mmol/L, such as occurs in diabetes mellitus, or even at lower levels in some people, glucose spills into the urine (glycosuria). Close regulation of blood glucose is necessary, because the brain requires a continuous supply, although it can adapt to lower levels or even use ketone bodies from fat breakdown if adaptation occurs slowly.

Erythrocytes rely almost totally on glucose. Several metabolic pathways are involved in the utilization of glucose as an energy source and the maintenance of glucose homeostasis. The pathways are described in detail in textbooks of biochemistry and are summarized briefly here (Fig. 2.6).

2.7.1 Glycolysis

Following absorption, glucose, fructose and galactose are transported to the liver via the hepatic portal vein. Fructose and galactose are very rapidly converted

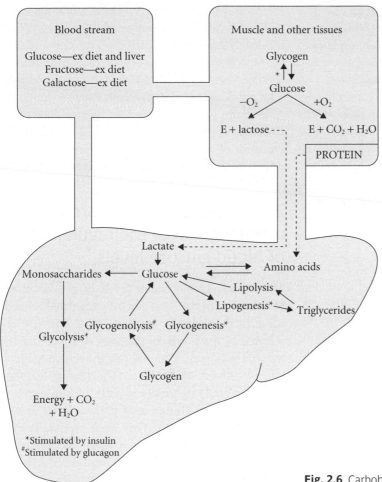

Fig. 2.6 Carbohydrate metabolism and its control.

to glucose. Fructose may also enter the glycolytic pathway directly. Very low concentrations of either of these sugars can be detected in the blood immediately after ingestion.

Glycolysis (the breakdown of glucose) occurs in the cytosol of all cells and may take place in the presence (aerobic) or absence (anaerobic) of oxygen. The pathway involves the metabolism of hexoses to pyruvate. Many reactions catalysed by different enzymes are involved but glycolysis is regulated by three enzymes that catalyse non-equilibrium reactions —namely, hexokinase (glycokinase), phosphofructokinase and pyruvate kinase. Under aerobic conditions, pyruvate is transported into the mitochondrion and is then oxidatively decarboxylated to acetyl coenzyme A (CoA), which enters the citric acid cycle.

Under anaerobic conditions (e.g. in exercising muscles or in red blood cells), pyruvate is converted to lactate, which is transported to the liver, where glucose is reformed via the process of gluconeogenesis (see below) and again becomes available via the circulation for oxidation in the tissues. This is known as the lactic acid cycle, or the Cori cycle.

2.7.2 Gluconeogenesis

Gluconeogenesis includes all mechanisms and pathways responsible for converting non-carbohydrates to glucose. In addition to lactate, the other major substrates are the glucogenic amino acids (especially glycine, alanine, glutamate and aspartate) and glycerol. In the liver, gluconeogenesis takes place in the cytosol, and this pathway involves the same enzymes as glycolysis except at three sites: glucose 6-phosphatase instead of hexokinase; fructose 1,6-biphosphatase instead of phosphofructokinase; and phosphoenolyruvate carboxykinase instead of pyruvate kinase.

Acylglycerols of adipose tissue are continuously undergoing hydrolysis to form free glycerol, which cannot be utilized by adipose tissue and therefore diffuses out into the blood and reaches the liver, where it is first converted to fructose 1,6-biphosphate before being converted to glucose.

Alanine is the main amino acid, which is transported from the muscle to the liver, where it may be converted to pyruvate.

2.7.3 Glycogenolysis

Glycogen represents the principal storage form of carbohydrate in animals and is present mainly in the liver and muscle. In the liver its major function is to service other tissues via formation of glucose when dietary sugars are not immediately available as an energy source between meals or while fasting. In muscle it serves only the needs of that organ by providing an immediate source of metabolic fuel. Glycogenolysis is the pathway by which the glycogen stores are converted via glucose 1-phosphate and glucose 6-phosphate to glucose. After 12–18 hours of fasting, the liver becomes totally depleted of glycogen, whereas muscle glycogen is depleted only after exercise.

2.7.4 Storage of carbohydrates as glycogen and triglyceride (glycogenesis and lipogenesis)

Glycogen is synthesized from glucose by glycogenesis. This is not the reverse of glycogenolysis but a completely separate pathway that usually operates for several hours after a carbohydrate-containing meal, when the amount of ingested carbohydrate far exceeds energy requirements for the tissues. Glycogen stores become saturated at around 1000 g. In some animal species, carbohydrates in excess of requirements are converted to fat via the pathway of lipogenesis: triose-phosphate provides the glycerol moiety of acylglycerol, and fatty acids may be synthesized from acetyl CoA ultimately derived from carbohydrate. Other than in the experimental situation of gross carbohydrate overfeeding, conversion of carbohydrate to stored lipid does not occur to any appreciable extent in humans.

Similarly, pyruvates, as well as intermediates of the citric acid cycle, provide the carbon skeletons for the synthesis of amino acids, but conversion to amino acids is an unimportant fate of ingested carbohydrate.

2.7.5 Metabolic and hormonal mechanisms for the regulation of blood glucose levels

The maintenance of stable levels of glucose in the blood is one of the most carefully regulated homeostatic mechanisms in the body (Fig. 2.6). Insulin, secreted by the β-cells of the islets of Langerhans in the pancreas, plays a central role in regulating blood glucose. About 40–50 units (15–20% of the total amount stored) are produced daily. Insulin secretion is stimulated by rising blood glucose levels as well as by amino acids, free fatty acids, ketone bodies, glucagon and secretin. Insulin lowers blood glucose by facilitating its entrance into insulin-sensitive tissues and the liver by enhancing the activity of glucose transporters. Insulin also stimulates the storage of glucose as glycogen (glycogenesis) and enhances the metabolism of glucose via the glycolytic pathway. The action of glucagon, secreted by the α-cells of the islets of Langerhans, opposes that of insulin. Secretion occurs in response to hypoglycaemia (low blood glucose levels). Glucagon stimulates glycogenolysis by activating the enzyme phosphorylase and enhances gluconeogenesis. Hypoglycaemia also stimulates the secretion of adrenaline by the chromaffin cells of the adrenal medulla and acts by stimulating the phosphorylase and hence glycogenolysis. Thyroid hormones, glucocorticoids and growth hormone have a smaller effect than insulin has on blood glucose, glucagon and adrenaline in healthy individuals. Resistance to the effects of insulin occurs in diabetes and in obesity.

2.8 Recommended intakes and energy value of carbohydrates

2.8.1 Recommended intakes of carbohydrates

The minimum amount of carbohydrate required to avoid ketosis is considered to be about 50 g/day. Glucose is an essential energy source for the brain, red blood cells and the renal medulla, the daily requirement being about 180 g/day. Approximately 130 g/day can be produced in the body from non-carbohydrate sources by gluconeogenesis, hence the amount of 50 g/day recommended intake. If this is not provided, these organs can adapt by utilizing ketones derived from fatty acid oxidation as a source of energy. A state of ketosis is undesirable because cognitive function may be impaired, and in pregnant women the fetus may be adversely affected. During pregnancy and lactation, the minimum required should probably be about 100 g/day.

Most people consume appreciably more than 100 g carbohydrate daily, with intakes ranging from 200 to 400 g/day (Table 2.2). The FAO/WHO Expert Consultation on carbohydrates (1998) suggested that at least 55% of total energy should be derived from carbohydrate obtained from a variety of food sources. A wide range, up to 75% of total energy, is regarded as acceptable. A significant adverse effect on health is possible with higher levels of intake because adequate amounts of protein, fat and other essential nutrients may be excluded. A comparable range was suggested by the WHO/FAO Expert Consultation on *Diet, Nutrition and the Prevention of Chronic Diseases* (2003) with a recommended restriction of free sugars to below 10% total energy. The level of intake of total carbohydrate in most Western countries is usually below 50% of food energy and many national bodies suggest lower population averages. British dietary reference values (DRVs) suggest a population average intake of 50% energy from total carbohydrate, which nevertheless represents an increase from current average intakes in that country of about 47%.

This recommendation is based on the proposal that starch, intrinsic sugars and milk should provide the balance of food energy not provided by fat (35%) and protein (15%), with a maximum of 10% for added or free sugars. No specific recommendation exists for component carbohydrates such as starch.

Recommendations for NSPs (dietary fibre intakes) are less easy to find because of lack of agreement as to what should be included and how to measure it. In the UK, a DRV of 18 g/day for NSPs was made, based on the relationship between NSP intake and bowel habit and bowel cancer risk. An increase from existing intakes of 12 g/day 'would be expected to increase average stool weight by 25%' and should reduce the risk of cancer. The joint WHO/FAO Expert Consultation (2003) recommended at least 20 g/day NSPs (25 g total dietary fibre), which should be provided by wholegrain cereals, fruit and vegetables. The recommendation is really to ensure a healthy intake of these foods, which for fruit and vegetables is five portions a day or 400 g/day.

2.8.2 Energy value of carbohydrates

Dietary carbohydrate has traditionally been assigned an energy value of 4 kcal/g (17 kJ/g), though when carbohydrates are expressed as monosaccharides the value of 3.75 kcal/g (15.7 kJ/g) is usually used. However, because RS and some oligosacchar-ides are not digested in the small intestine and the process of fermentation is less metabolically efficient than when digestion and absorption are completed in the small intestine, it is clear that these carbohydrates are providing the body with less energy. The energy value of all carbohydrate requires reassessment, but until this has been carried out, the FAO/WHO consultation recommends that the energy value of carbohydrates that reach the colon be set at 2 kcal/g (8 kJ/g).

2.9 Carbohydrates and diseases

2.9.1 Energy balance and obesity

The avoidance of obesity depends upon maintaining energy balance (see Chapters 5 and 16). However, the nature of dietary carbohydrate appears to influence energy balance. Diets rich in non-starch polysaccharides tend to be bulky, promote satiety and reduce the risks of excessive weight gain. Furthermore, randomized controlled trials have shown the potential of such diets to promote weight loss in those who have already become overweight or obese. Conversely, a high intake of energy-dense foods, whether they be high in fats or free sugars or both, increases the risk of excessive fat accumulation. There is particular concern around the potential of a high intake of free sugars in beverages and fruit juices to contribute to the increased risk of obesity in childhood. The physiological effects of energy intake on satiation and satiety appear to differ between solid foods and fluids. High-energy beverages (invariably high in free sugars) may be less 'sensed' than comparable energy intakes from solid foods, perhaps because of reduced gastric distension and more rapid transit times. As a result there may be a failure to adjust food intake to take into account the energy derived from beverages. This provides a major justification for recommending a restriction on intake of free sugars.

2.9.2 Carbohydrates and physical performance (see Chapter 33)

A high-carbohydrate diet in the day preceding endurance-type physical activity ('carbohydrate loading') enhances physical performance, as may a high carbohydrate pre-event meal and carbohydrate supplementation in the form of beverages containing free sugars. This is presumably achieved as a result of glycogenesis and accumulation of maximum glycogen stores. Similarly, carbohydrate intake after an event can aid recovery by replenishing depleted glycogen stores. Low-intensity recreational physical activity does not require carbohydrate supplementation. Some people may consume unnecessary extra energy in this way.

2.9.3 Carbohydrate through the life cycle

During the first 4–6 months of life, exclusive breast-feeding is recommended, with lactose being the major source of carbohydrate and accounting for about 40% of milk energy. The concentration of lactose is tailored to the needs of the maturing neonatal and infant gut, especially while colonic microflora and pancreatic amylase production are developing. For infants fed on formulae, the carbohydrate content should be as similar as possible to breast milk. Significant spill-over of carbohydrate into the neonatal colon occurs where, in breastfed infants, a largely saccharolytic flora dominated by bifidobacteria are responsible for fermentation and salvage of energy through SCFAs and lactate absorption. Bottle-fed babies, or those who are weaned early, develop a more diverse flora, which starts to resemble that of the adult much sooner.

Pre-school children can be fed the same foods as adults but, because of their rapid growth, they require a more energy-dense diet. Food should, therefore, provide more than 30% of energy from fat and less than 50% from carbohydrate. Thus, the change from breast milk, which provides more than 50% of the energy from fat, to an adult-type diet, should be gradual. The pre-school years are a particularly important time to teach the avoidance of sugary drinks and puddings, increased intake of which has been shown to be associated with the onset of obesity.

Early introduction of substantial amounts of carbohydrate from a single food source is a major determinant of malnutrition in developing countries because such foods may be deficient in some essential nutrients. In more affluent countries, sometimes vegetarian and vegan children tend to be fed diets that are high in non-glycaemic carbohydrate. Thus, they too may be at risk of insufficient energy for growth as well as nutrient deficiencies associated with a diet without meat or animal products.

Requirements for total energy and nutrients increase during pregnancy and lactation. The minimum requirement for carbohydrate is doubled to around 100 g/day but most women achieve adequate intakes by consuming a wide variety of carbohydrate-containing foods. Particular attention to carbohydrate intake may also be appropriate for some groups of older people—as with children, a diet with excessive intakes of non-glycaemic carbohydrate may be associated with a predisposition to undernutrition as a result of inadequate intake of total energy and some essential nutrients. While many will benefit from the satiety-promoting effects of diets rich in non-starch polysaccharides, for some an increase in sugars and rapidly digested starches may be necessary to ensure adequate energy intake.

2.9.4 Lipids and cardiovascular disease

For many adults, increasing the consumption of appropriate carbohydrate-containing foods will facilitate the reduction in saturated fatty acids that are causally linked to cardiovascular disease and increase the intake of antioxidants and other cardioprotective nutrients (see Chapter 20). High intake of wholegrain cereals and non-starch polysaccharides has been shown in prospective studies to be associated with reduced cardiovascular risk. However, high intakes of free sugars and rapidly digested starches may be associated with high triglycerides and very-low-density lipoproteins and reduced high-density lipoproteins. Large amounts of fructose or sucrose, especially when consumed in the context of relatively high fat intakes, may induce hypertriglyceridaemia. However, a high carbohydrate intake when derived from vegetables, intact fruits and wholegrain cereals does not appear to have long-term adverse effects on the overall lipoprotein profile.

2.9.5 Blood glucose and diabetes

Wholegrain carbohydrate-containing foods rich in non-starch polysaccharides and with a low glycaemic

response reduce the risk of developing type 2 diabetes. Diets high in sucrose may be associated with increased insulin resistance and, by contributing to the energy density of the diet, lead to the development of being overweight and obesity, the principal risk determinant of type 2 diabetes. Foods with a high content of non-starch polysaccharides and a low GI are associated with an improvement in glycaemic control in both type 1 and type 2 diabetes, as well as improvement in several other cardiovascular risk factors. The majority of patients with type 2 diabetes are overweight and restriction of free sugars along with other energy-dense foods will facilitate weight loss, a principal goal in the treatment of this condition since it is almost invariably associated with improved control of blood glucose and other clinical and metabolic abnormalities associated with diabetes (see also Chapter 22).

2.9.6 Dental caries

Dental diseases are a costly burden to healthcare services, accounting for between 5% and 10% of total healthcare expenditure. Dental caries rates appear to be declining in some relatively affluent countries but prevalence is increasing in many developing countries. Dental caries has a complex aetiology. The condition occurs because of demineralization of enamel and dentine by organic acids formed by bacteria in dental plaque through the anaerobic metabolism of sugars derived from the diet.

Free sugars and readily digestible starches appear to be involved, although lactose, sugar alcohols and oligosaccharides are less acidogenic than other carbohydrates. Dental caries occurs infrequently when the consumption of free sugars is below 15–20 kg per person per year, equivalent to a daily intake of 40–55 g per person or 6–8% of total energy intake. Frequency of consumption is also relevant, hence the recommendation that foods and drinks containing free sugars should be limited to a maximum of four times per day. Fluoride protects against dental caries, reducing rates by 20–40%, but it does not eliminate the condition.

2.10 Carbohydrate and gut disorders

2.10.1 Lactose malabsorption

The universal presence of lactose in milk means that all newborn mammalian species have the appropriate enzyme lactase (β1-4 galactosidase) in the brush border to deal with this sugar. However, after weaning, lactase activity declines rapidly in all species, including humans. Some human populations retain the ability to digest lactose. These are the traditional milk-drinking people who have their ancestors in the Aryan races of the Middle East and North India. In practice this means the majority of Northern Europeans and populations deriving from them including North American whites, and Australian and New Zealand whites. Individuals who do not have lactase can tolerate small amounts of milk in their diet, but large amounts lead to unabsorbed lactose, exerting an osmotic effect in the small bowel with fluid and sugar entering the large bowel. Here fermentation occurs and there is often rapid gas production producing abdominal pain together with an osmotic diarrhoea. The use of yoghurts and other fermented milk products, as well as the use of preparations of the enzyme lactase may foster lactose tolerance. Lactose intolerance is occasionally seen in adults of European descent.

2.10.2 Other carbohydrate intolerances

There are other less frequent clinical disorders in which digestion or absorption of sugar is disturbed, resulting in sugar intolerance with consequences similar to those of lactase deficiency. Most frequently they are seen in children secondary to underlying gastrointestinal disease, especially as a result of severe gastrointestinal infections, particularly in undernourished children. They may also be congenital and, although rare, such conditions may be life threatening in children. Three examples of these disorders are: sucrase-isomaltase deficiency, which is associated with watery diarrhoea following consumption of sucrose-containing foods; alactasia, or the total absence of lactase in infancy, which is accompanied by diarrhoea associated with milk (note the difference between this condition and lactose intolerance); and glucose–galactose malabsorption (diarrhoea from eating glucose, galactose or lactose). The diagnosis is usually suspected on the basis of clinical observations and is confirmed by sugar tolerance tests and measurement of breath hydrogen.

2.10.3 Large bowel function and its disorders

It is in the large bowel that dietary carbohydrates come to dominate the ambient physiology. NSPs are the principal dietary component to affect bowel habit. Other fermentable carbohydrates, such as RS and oligosaccharides, are mildly laxative but NSPs are the major controller of faecal bulk. NSPs from different sources have been shown to have contrasting effects on stool weight, with NSPs from wheat (particularly wheat bran) being the most potent laxative, increasing stool output by around 5 or 6 g/day per gram of NSPs fed from this source. Following close on the heels of wheat sources are NSPs from fruit and vegetables, which give around 4 g of stool per gram of NSPs fed, after which come the gums, oats and legumes and probably the least laxative of the NSPs sources, pectin. The effect of NSPs on bowel habit is modified principally by gut transit time, which is an innate control of large bowel function.

The mechanism whereby fermentable carbohydrates effect bowel habit is now well established. The notion that fibre acts like an inert sponge in the colon has now been superseded because we know that NSPs are extensively metabolized by colonic bacteria. Faecal weight, therefore, increases through a variety of mechanisms that include increased bacterial biomass (Fig. 2.5), increased hydration of stool mass associated with more rapid transit time and the presence of unmetabolized cell wall material, particularly lignified forms such as that present in bran.

It follows, because NSPs are such effective laxatives, that they have been used very widely in the management of constipation. There are many causes of constipation but the commonest one is low NSP-containing diets, often associated with a sedentary lifestyle, air travel and, sometimes, therapeutic diets, such as those used for weight reduction. Other physiological causes of low stool weight are pregnancy, some phases of the menstrual cycle and old age, where a combination of low food intake and lack of exercise are probably most important. Many drugs can also cause constipation and this symptom is a feature of irritable bowel syndrome. Diets high in NSPs are well established in the management of constipation. There is no universal prescription but the amount required is one that will produce a satisfactory bowel habit. The aim should be to increase the patient's NSP intake, which was likely to be around 12 g/day, to 18–24 g/day. Those who fail to respond to this sort of dietary change should be carefully screened for more serious causes of the problem. Easy ways of increasing NSP intake include:

• Increasing bread intake to 200 g/day and changing to 100% wholemeal

• Eating a whole wheat breakfast cereal

• Increasing fruit and vegetable intake to 400 g/day

• Eating more legumes such as beans and peas, although this may produce problems with gas due to oligosaccharide fermentation

• Use bulk laxatives such as ispagula and sterculia

Closely allied to constipation is irritable bowel syndrome (IBS), which is one of the commonest disorders seen in the gastroenterology clinic. It has two main presenting features, namely abdominal pain and altered bowel habit. It is, however, a very diverse disease with no clear aetiology. While the cause is unknown, NSPs have a significant role to play in the management of constipation-predominant IBS. However, wheat bran and its associated foods are not universally beneficial in this condition, possibly because it is thought that a significant number of IBS patients are wheat-intolerant without having the diagnostic features of coeliac disease. Furthermore, changing people onto significantly increased NSP intakes leads to excess gas production, and IBS patients may have a gut that is unusually sensitive to gas.

Colonic diverticular disease is another condition that benefits from carbohydrate in the diet, particularly NSPs. A diverticulum is a pouch that protrudes outwards from the wall of the bowel and is associated with hypertrophy of the muscle layers of the large intestine, particularly the sigmoid colon. Diverticular disease is very common in industrialized societies, the prevalence rising with age to about 30% of people over the age of 65. Many people with diverticula do not have symptoms, but those that do complain of lower abdominal pain and changes in bowel habit. High-NSP-containing diets were introduced in the 1960s and their use revolutionized the management of this condition. Wheat bran is thought to be more effective than other sources of NSPs or bulk laxatives, although bran is not a panacea and may aggravate gas production, feelings of abdominal distension and incomplete emptying of the rectum.

2.10.4 Cancer

Carbohydrates are not generally implicated either in the cause or prevention of the major cancers with the exception of colorectal cancer. In 1969, Burkitt pointed out that those countries where colorectal cancer risk was low, principally African countries, had high intakes of NSPs and large stool bulk. He suggested that lack of NSPs was the cause of large bowel cancer because it allowed slow transit time through the colon and cancer-forming chemicals to accumulate in the large bowel. We now know that there are other important contributors to colorectal cancer risk, in particular obesity, but nevertheless dietary fibre remains an important protective element of the diet. Not all epidemiological studies have shown a protective effect of fibre, probably because measuring dietary intake was not always done well and NSPs or fibre intakes were measured badly. However, in the recent European Prospective Investigation into Cancer (EPIC study) (Bingham et al., 2001) where dietary methodology and understanding of NSPs and their measurement were good, a clear inverse relationship was seen between the incidence of large bowel cancer and fibre intake. This is further discussed in Chapter 21.

2.10.5 Prebiotics

A prebiotic is a non-digestible food ingredient that beneficially affects the host by selectively stimulating the growth and/or activity of one of a limited number of bacteria in the colon, and thus improves host health.

Prebiotics are important because they can alter the balance of the gut microflora to achieve what is considered to be a healthy or balanced gut microbiota that is predominantly saccharolytic (i.e. breaks down carbohydrate). They are also an alternative to probiotics, which are difficult to handle in foodstuffs, but whose clear benefit to health in terms of diarrhoea prevention and immunomodulation are well established. The best-established prebiotics are fructo-oligosaccharides, inulin and galacto-oligosaccharides.

These have all clearly been shown to change the balance of the flora to one dominated by bifidobacteria and lactobacilli. These are primary carbohydrate-fermenting bacteria that do not contain pathogens and probably play a significant role in the maintenance of resistance to pathogen invasion through a variety of mechanisms. It is worth noting that the exclusively breast-fed baby has a microflora that is very similar to this pattern. Apart from altering the balance of the flora, prebiotics are also fermented producing SCFAs.

As already noted, prebiotic oligosaccharides are relatively poor laxatives and there are few published studies of their benefits in clinical studies. However, they have been shown to reduce recurrent episodes of *Clostridium difficile*-associated diarrhoea and animal studies have demonstrated clear anti-inflammatory properties in the gut. Perhaps most surprisingly, prebiotic carbohydrates increase calcium absorption and bone mineral density in adolescents. They might well prove to be designer carbohydrates of the future.

2.11 Other roles for carbohydrate and inborn errors of metabolism

Apart from their role in energy metabolism, carbohydrates are required for the synthesis of some larger complex molecules in the body, such as RNA and DNA which use the five-carbon sugars ribose and deoxyribose produced from glucose in the pentose phosphate pathway. Also synthesized from glucose by the oxidation of uridine diphosphate glucose is glucuronic acid, which is needed for the conjugation of sterols and foreign compounds like drugs to aid their water solubility and, thus, their excretion in bile and urine. Glucuronic acid is also a precursor of ascorbic acid (vitamin C) in species that can synthesize it, but humans lack the key enzymes for this reaction.

Glucose, galactose and fructose can undergo isomerization, epimerization and phosphorylation reactions, leading to the production of other sugars such as xylose, mannose, rhamnose and fucose.

Further transamidation leads to the formation of amino sugars such as glucosamine 6-phosphate which can be N-acetylated to N-acetyl glucosamine, which is an important precursor for glycoprotein synthesis. Glycoproteins are proteins conjugated to sugars and are essential constituents of mucus, which covers the epithelial surfaces of the body. Other glycoproteins include plasma proteins such as prothrombin, and immunoglobulins and peptide hormones such as follicle-stimulating hormone. Glycoproteins also occur at all surfaces and are important in cell recognition. The surface of the human erythrocyte is covered in a complex array of polysaccharides that are responsible for the determination of blood groups. In the gut lectins (proteins present in foods such as beans and peas) recognize cell-surface glycoproteins and bind to them and may cause acute reactions characteristic of food intolerance.

Proteoglycans are another class of molecule that have major carbohydrate content and include heparin, chondroitin sulphate and keratin. These carbohydrate chains are usually larger than glycoproteins and are called glucose aminoglycans or mucopolysaccharides.

A number of well-recognized inherited but rare disorders of carbohydrate metabolism are associated with these synthetic pathways. The mucopolysaccharidoses (e.g. Hunter syndrome) are characterized by accumulation and excretion of the oligosaccharides of proteoglycans resulting from deficiencies of enzymes that degrade dermatan or heparin. Clinically they are characterized by skeletal abnormalities and mental retardation. Abnormalities in the sulphation of glucose aminoglycans result in the chondrodystrophies, while there are a group of disorders (fucosidases, mucolipidoses and gangliosidoses) associated with reduced activity of lysozymal glycosidase activity, resulting in incomplete degradation of oligosaccharides and accumulation in tissues of products of glycoproteins and mucopolysaccharide breakdown. They give rise to skeletal abnormalities, enlargement of the liver and spleen, cataracts and mental retardation. Von Gierke disease is an example of the disorders of glycogen storage due to deficiency of glucose 6-phosphatase associated with hypoglycaemia during fasting, lactic acidaemia, hyperlipidaemia and hyperuricaemia.

Galactosaemia results from two inborn errors of galactose metabolism: deficiencies of the enzymes galactose 1-phosphate uridyl transferase and galactokinase. Galactosaemia may be associated with cataract formation and mental retardation if not recognized early and lactose withdrawn. Several genetically determined abnormalities of fructose metabolism occur and are associated with deficiencies of enzymes involved in the metabolism of fructose. In most of the conditions, avoidance of dietary fructose leads to a favourable outcome. For example, aldolase B deficiency (hereditary fructose intolerance) is associated with vomiting, failure to thrive and liver dysfunction. If the condition is recognized and dietary fructose withheld, infants with this deficiency are likely to thrive. Fructose 1-6-diphosphatase deficiency is associated with hypoglycaemia, acidosis, ketonuria and hyperventilation. Similarly, withdrawal of fructose leads to alleviation of the symptoms.

2.12 Future directions

There has been a considerable resurgence of interest in dietary carbohydrate recently with the advent of the role of GI as a means of determining optimum carbohydrate-containing foods for the maintenance of health and in a variety of disease states. Furthermore, the health-promoting qualities of carbohydrates that are not digested and absorbed in the small intestine are now being recognized. The prebiotic oligosaccharides, as components of functional foods, have potentially important health benefits. The extent to which sucrose and other sugars should be restricted or liberated will continue to be debated, as will the optimum contribution of total carbohydrate to the daily energy intake. Methodologies for the measurement of various dietary carbohydrates are likely to be refined, and given the advances in the field of molecular biology it seems highly likely that there will be further insights into the understanding of the molecular basis of many of the issues discussed in this chapter.

FURTHER READING

1. Asp, N.-G., van Amelsvoort, J.M.M., and Hautvast, J.G.A.J. (1996) Nutritional implications of resistant starch. *Nutr Res Rev*, **9**, 1–31 (final EURESTA report).

2. Burkitt, D.P. (1971) Epidemiology of cancer of the colon and rectum. *Cancer*, **28**, 3–13.

3. Bingham, S., Welch, A., McTaggart, A. *et al.* (2001) Nutritional Methods in the European Prospective Investigation of Cancer in Norfolk. *Public Health Nutr*, **4**, 847–858.

4. Cummings, J.H., Beatty, E.R., Kingman, S.M. *et al.* (1996) Digestion and physiological properties of

resistant starch in the human large bowel. *Br J Nutr*, **75**, 733–47.

5. **Cummings, J.H., Edmond, L.M., and Magee, E.A.** (2004) Dietary carbohydrates and health: do we still need the fibre concept? *Clin Nutr Suppl*, **1**, 5–17.

6. **Cummings, J.H., and Macfarlane, G.T.** (1991) The control and consequences of bacterial fermentation in the human colon. *J Appl Bacteriol*, **70**, 443–59.

7. **Cummings, J.H., Roberfroid, M.B., and Andersson, G.** *et al.* (1997) A new look at dietary carbohydrate: chemistry, physiology and health. *Eur J Clin Nutr*, **51**, 417–23.

8. **Department of Health** (1989) *Dietary sugars and human health*. London, HMSO.

9. **Department of Health** (1991) *Dietary reference values for food energy and nutrients for the UK*. No. 41. London, HMSO.

10. **Englyst, H.N., Kingman, S.M., and Cummings, J.H.** (1992) Classification and measurement of nutritionally important starch fractions. *Eur J Clin Nutr*, **46**, S33–S50.

11. **FAO/WHO** (1998) *Carbohydrates in human nutrition*. Report of a Joint FAO/WHO Expert Consultation. Paper 66. Rome, Food and Agricultural Organization.

12. **Foster-Powell, K., and Brand Miller, J.** (1995) International tables of glycaemic index. *Am J Clin Nutr*, **62**, 871S–893S.

13. **Jenkins, D.J.A., Wolever, T.M.S., Taylor, R.H.** *et al.* (1981) Glycemic index of foods: a physiological basis for carbohydrate exchange. *Am J Clin Nutr*, **34**, 362–6.

14. **Livesey, G.** (2001) Tolerance of low-digestible carbohydrates: a general view. *Br J Nutr*, **85**, S7–S16.

15. **Ludwig, D.S., and Eckel, R.H. (eds)** (2002) Is the glycaemic index important in human nutrition? *Am J Clin Nutr*, **76** (Suppl.), 261S–298S.

16. **Macfarlane, S., Macfarlane, G.T., and Cummings, J.H.** (2006) Prebiotics in the gastrointestinal tract. *Aliment Pharmacol Ther*, **24**, 701–14.

17. **Moynihan, P.** (2000) The British Nutrition Foundation Oral Task Force Report—issues relevant to dental health professionals. *Br Dental J*, **188**, 308–12.

18. **Trowell, H.** (1974) Definitions of fibre. *Lancet*, **1**, 503.

19. **WHO/FAO** (2003) *Diet, Nutrition and the Prevention of Chronic Diseases*. Report of a Joint WHO/FAO Expert Consultation. Geneva, World Health Organisation.

20. **Wolever, T.M.S., and Jenkins, D.J.A.** (1986) The use of the glycaemic index in predicting the blood glucose response to mixed meals. *Am J Clin Nutr*, **43**, 167–72.

To see topical and scientifically robust updates on nutrition associated with this textbook, and active web links to many of the journal articles in the Reference areas, please see the dedicated Online Resource Centre at www.oxfordtextbooks.co.uk/orc/mann3e/.

3 Lipids

Jim Mann and Murray Skeaff

Lipids are a group of compounds that dissolve in organic solvents such as petrol or chloroform, but are usually insoluble in water. The most obvious lipids are oils, which are liquid at room temperature, and fats, which are solid at room temperature. Many people in Western countries regard fats and oils as foods that should be avoided as far as possible because of their perceived role in the development of obesity and coronary heart disease. However, in addition to enhancing the flavour and palatability of food, lipids make an important contribution to adequate nutrition. They are major sources of energy; some are essential nutrients because they cannot be synthesized in the body, yet they are required for a range of metabolic and physiological processes and to maintain the structural and functional integrity of all cell membranes. Lipids are also the only form in which the body can store energy for a prolonged period of time. These stored lipids in adipose tissue also serve to provide insulation, help to control body temperature, and afford some physical protection to internal organs. Lipids include the fat-soluble vitamins. Triacylglycerols, usually referred to as triglycerides, make up the bulk of dietary lipid, with phospholipids and sterols making up nearly all the remainder.

3.1 Naturally occurring dietary lipids

Naturally occurring dietary lipids are derived from a wide variety of animal and plant sources including animal adipose tissue (the visible fat on meat, lard and suet); milk and products derived from milk fat (cream, butter, cheese and yoghurt); vegetable seeds, nuts, oils and products derived from them (e.g. margarines); eggs; fish oil; and plant leaves. Many sources of dietary lipid are visible and obvious, while others are less so, for example, those found in the muscle of lean meat, avocado, nuts and seeds, as well as those in processed or home-prepared foods such as pies, cakes, biscuits and chocolates. In most Western countries, dietary lipid provides 30–40% of total dietary energy. In Asian countries and throughout the developing world, the proportion of energy derived from dietary lipids is usually much lower.

3.1.1 Glycerides and fatty acids

Triglycerides make up about 95% of dietary lipids. A triglyceride molecule is formed from a molecule of glycerol (a three-carbon alcohol) with three fatty acids attached (Fig. 3.1). Fatty acids consist of an even-numbered chain of carbon atoms with hydrogens attached, a methyl group at one end and a carboxylic acid group at the other (Fig. 3.2). The carbon

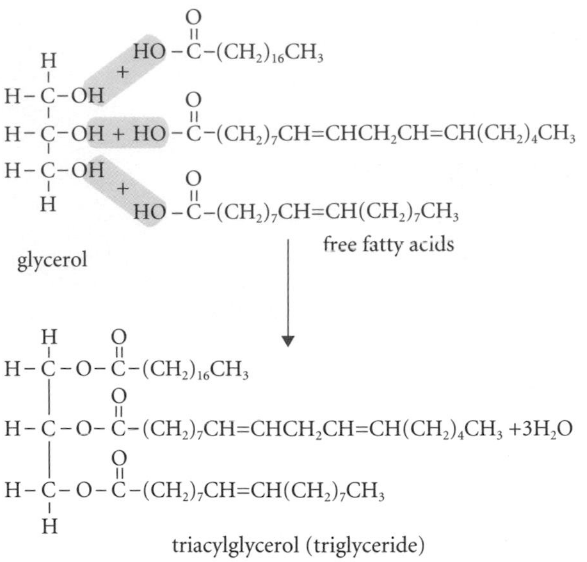

Fig. 3.1 Formation of a triglyceride molecule.

atoms were classically numbered from the carboxyl carbon (carbon number 1). The methyl end carbon is known as the n minus (n-) or omega (ω) carbon atom. The physical and biological properties of triglycerides are determined by the nature of the constituent fatty acids. They float on water and do not dissolve in it.

Saturated fatty acids are those in which carbon–carbon bonds are fully saturated with hydrogen atoms (i.e. four hydrogens per carbon–carbon bond). When two hydrogens are absent, the carbons form double bonds with each other and monounsaturated (a single double bond) or polyunsaturated (two or more double bonds) fatty acids result. Double bonds in polyunsaturated fatty acids are always separated by one CH_2 (methylene group). Fatty acids can be described by their common name, their chemical name, their full or simplified chemical structure, or a short-hand notation in which the first number indicates the number of carbon atoms and the second the number of double bonds (Fig. 3.2). For monounsaturated and polyunsaturated fatty acids, a third descriptor indicates the position of the first double bond relative to and including the methyl end. Inserting a double bond in a saturated fatty acid reduces its melting point. For this reason, fats (e.g. butter) containing a

predominance of saturated fatty acids are usually solid at room temperature while oils (e.g. soy bean oil) containing a predominance of polyunsaturated fatty acids are liquid at room temperature. The position of the unsaturated bonds in mono- and poly-unsaturated fatty acids has a profound influence on their health effects and nutritional properties. The position of the first double bond relative to the methyl end indicates the 'family' to which the unsaturated fatty acid belongs. Polyunsaturated fatty acids in which the first double bond is three carbon atoms from the methyl end of the carbon chain are called n-3 or ω-3 fatty acids, and those in which the first double bond is next to the sixth carbon atom are n-6 or ω-6 fatty acids. The third important family is the n-9 or ω-9 group in which the first double bond is next to the ninth carbon atom from the methyl end. Fatty acids are sometimes referred to as short-chain (i.e. fewer than 8 carbons), medium-chain (8–12 carbons), or long-chain (14 or more carbons) fatty acids. A list of the fatty acids of nutritional interest is given in Table 3.1.

A single triglyceride molecule may contain either three identical fatty acids or, more frequently, a combination of different fatty acids. It is important to appreciate that while one fatty acid, or class of fatty acids (e.g. saturated), might predominate in a particular food, most foods contain a wide range of fatty acids. Occasionally in naturally occurring glycerides, only one or two fatty acids are attached to a glycerol molecule. These are called monoacylglycerols (monoglycerides) and diacylglycerols (diglycerides). The major food sources of fatty acids and sources of triglycerides that contain them are shown in Table 3.2 and the detailed fatty acid composition of some fats and oils are given in Table 3.3.

3.1.2 Phospholipids

Phospholipids comprise a relatively small proportion of total dietary lipid. The four major phospholipids comprise a diglyceride in which the third position of the glycerol molecule is occupied by a phosphoric acid residue to which one of four different base groups is attached (choline, inositol, serine or ethanolamine).

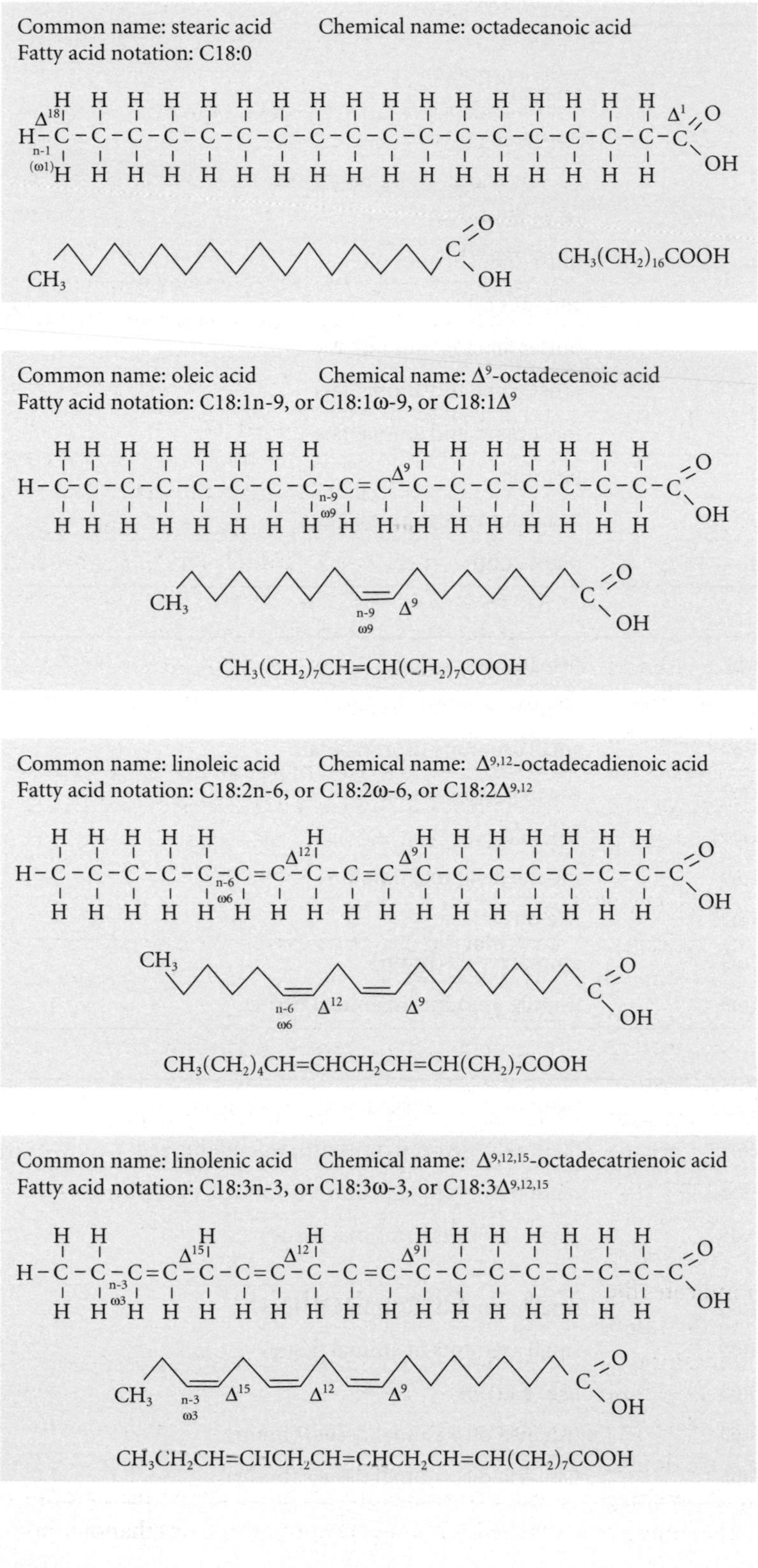

Common name: stearic acid   Chemical name: octadecanoic acid
Fatty acid notation: C18:0

$CH_3(CH_2)_{16}COOH$

Common name: oleic acid   Chemical name: Δ^9-octadecenoic acid
Fatty acid notation: C18:1n-9, or C18:1ω-9, or C18:1Δ^9

$CH_3(CH_2)_7CH=CH(CH_2)_7COOH$

Common name: linoleic acid   Chemical name: $\Delta^{9,12}$-octadecadienoic acid
Fatty acid notation: C18:2n-6, or C18:2ω-6, or C18:2$\Delta^{9,12}$

$CH_3(CH_2)_4CH=CHCH_2CH=CH(CH_2)_7COOH$

Common name: linolenic acid   Chemical name: $\Delta^{9,12,15}$-octadecatrienoic acid
Fatty acid notation: C18:3n-3, or C18:3ω-3, or C18:3$\Delta^{9,12,15}$

$CH_3CH_2CH=CHCH_2CH=CHCH_2CH=CH(CH_2)_7COOH$

Fig. 3.2 Names and structures of some common fatty acids.

Table 3.1 Fatty acid names and occurrence

Common Name	Nomenclature	Occurrence
Saturated		
Acetic	2:0	vinegar
Butyric	4:0	butter fat
Caproic	6:0	
Caprylic	8:0	palm kernel oil
Capric	10:0	butter fat, coconut oil
Lauric	12:0	coconut oil
Myristic	14:0	butter fat, coconut oil
Palmitic	16:0	most plant and animal fats
Stearic	18:0	most plant and animal fats
Arachidic	20:0	peanuts
Behenic	22:0	small amount in animal fats
Lignoceric	24:0	plant cutin
Monounsaturated		
Palmitoleic	16:1ω7	fish and animal fats
Oleic	18:1ω9	all plant and animal fats
cis-Vaccenic	18:1ω7	small amounts in animal fats
Eicosenoic	20:1ω9	rapeseed and animal fats
Gadoleic	20:1ω11	fish oils
Erucic	22:1ω9	rapeseed, animal tissue
Cetoleic	22:1ω13	fish oils
Nervonic	24:1ω9	animal tissue (brain)
Hexacosenoic	26:1ω9	minute amounts in animal tissues
Polyunsaturated		
Linoleic (LO)	18:2ω6	plant oils: cottonseed, sesame, soybean, corn, safflower
α-Linolenic (LN)	18:3ω3	plant oils: soybean, mustard, walnut, linseed
γ-Linolenic (GLA)	18:3ω6	plant oils: evening primrose, borrage, blackcurrant
Dihommo-γ linolenic acid (DGLA)	20:3ω6	small amounts in animal tissues
Arachidonic (AA)	20:4ω6	small amounts in animal tissues
Adrenic	22:4ω6	small amounts in animal tissues
Eicosapentaenoic acid (EPA)	20:5ω3	fish, fish oils
Docosapentaenoic (DPA)	22:5ω3	fish, fish oils, animal tissues (brain)
Docosahexaenoic(DHA)	22:6ω3	fish, fish oils, animal tissues (brain)

Table 3.2 Fat and cholesterol content of some common foods

Food item	Common serving size	Total fat (g)	SFA (g)	MFA (g)	PFA (g)	Chol (mg)
		per 100 g edible portion				
Skimmed milk	1 cup (260 g)	0.4	0.3	0.1	0.0	4
Yoghurt	1 pot (150 g)	2.4	1.5	0.6	0.1	8
Cottage cheese	1/2 cup (120 g)	3.5	2.2	0.9	0.1	9
Whole milk	1 cup (260 g)	4.0	2.4	1.1	0.1	12
Ice cream	1 cup (143 g)	10.8	6.5	2.3	0.3	30
Cheddar cheese	1 × 2 cm cube (22 g)	35.2	22.3	8.4	0.8	107
Cream	1 tbsp (15 g)	40.0	24.9	10.1	1.3	104
Wholemeal bread	1 slice (22 g)	1.7	0.4	0.4	0.6	1
Toasted muesli	1 cup (110 g)	16.6	7.7	5.0	2.9	0
Egg	1 medium (32 g)	11.6	3.4	4.6	1.2	412
Baked potato	1 potato (90 g)	0.2	0.0	0.0	0.1	0
Potato crisps	1 packet (50 g)	33.4	14.3	13.8	3.8	1
Cauliflower	1 stem + flower (90 g)	0.2	0.0	0.0	0.1	0
Lentils	1/2 cup (100 g)	0.5	0.1	0.1	0.2	0
Peanuts	1/3 cup (50 g)	49.0	9.2	23.4	13.9	0
Cashew nuts	18 cashews (28 g)	51.0	8.3	25.4	15.1	0
Sole	1 fillet (51 g)	1.2	0.3	0.4	0.3	53
Mackerel	1 fillet (89 g)	2.9	0.8	0.8	0.9	53
Salmon (tinned)	1/2 cup (120 g)	8.2	2.0	3.1	2.1	90
Sausage	1 serving (79 g)	25.2	11.3	10.8	1.2	48
Beef blade steak (lean)	1 steak (216 g)	5.0	2.2	1.9	0.2	60
Beef mince	1/2 cup (130 g)	13.8	5.7	5.4	0.5	68
Chicken breast (lean, no skin)	1 breast (192 g)	5.5	1.7	2.5	0.6	66
Fried chicken	1 wing (37 g)	28.4	8.7	13.4	2.7	116
Pork loin steak (lean)	1 fillet (98 g)	2.3	0.9	0.9	0.2	68
Lamb midloin chop	1 chop (50 g)	5.7	2.5	2.0	0.2	66
Pizza	1 slice (57 g)	10.5	4.5	3.3	1.8	13
Hamburger	1 burger (204 g)	15.6	5.7	5.4	2.4	22
Muesli bar	1 bar (32 g)	19.4	9.1	7.2	1.9	1
Biscuit	1 biscuit (12 g)	30.0	19.2	6.2	1.2	98
Salad dressing	1 tbsp (16 g)	48.3	7.0	11.1	28.1	0
Palm oil	1 tbsp (14 g)	98.7	44.7	41.1	8.2	0
Olive oil	1 tbsp (14 g)	99.6	16.6	65.3	11.8	0
Sunflower seed oil	1 tbsp (14 g)	99.7	11.7	21.1	61.9	0

SFA = saturated fatty acids; MFA = monounsaturated fatty acids; PFA = polyunsaturated fatty acids; Chol = cholesterol.

Table 3.3 Fatty acid composition of plant and animal fats

Food item	4:0	6:0	8:0	10:0	12:0	14:0	16:0	18:0	16:1	18:1	18:2ω6	18:3ω3	20:4ω6	20:5ω3	22:6ω3	20:1ω11	22:1ω13	22:5ω3
	Percentage of total acids																	
Plant fats																		
Olive	–	–	–	–	–	–	12	2	1	72	11	1	–	–	–	–	–	–
Palm	–	–	–	–	0	1	42	4	0	43	8	0	–	–	–	–	–	–
Canola	–	–	–	–	–	–	5	1	2	56	24	10	–	–	–	–	–	–
Safflower	–	–	–	–	–	–	8	3	0	13	76	0	–	–	–	–	–	–
Sunflower	–	–	–	–	–	0	6	6	0	33	53	0	–	–	–	–	–	–
Avocado	–	–	–	–	–	–	12	–	3	75	9	0	0	–	–	–	–	–
Soybean	–	–	–	–	0	0	10	4	0	25	52	7	–	–	–	–	–	–
Coconut	–	–	8	7	48	16	9	2	–	7	2	–	–	–	–	–	–	–
Animal fats																		
Butter	4	2	1	3	3	11	28	16	1	26	1	2	–	–	–	–	–	–
Beef	–	–	–	–	–	3	28	13	7	43	2	1	1	–	–	–	–	–
Chicken	–	–	–	–	–	1	27	7	7	41	14	1	1	–	–	–	–	–
Lamb	–	–	–	–	–	6	25	22	1	40	3	3	–	–	–	–	–	–
Pork	–	–	–	–	–	2	27	13	4	41	8	1	1	–	–	–	–	–
Salmon	–	–	–	–	–	5	19	4	6	23	1	1	1	8	11	8	5	3
Trout	–	–	–	–	–	2	37	13	5	17	1	–	–	3	11	2	2	2

Along with sphingomyelin, these four phospholipids make up more than 95% of the phospholipids found in the body and in foods. The structure of the most abundant phospholipid in nature, phosphatidylcholine (also known as lecithin), is shown in Fig. 3.3.

Phospholipids occur in virtually all animal and vegetable foods: liver, eggs, peanuts, soyabeans and wheatgerm are very rich sources. The base group endows the phospholipid with a polar region soluble in water, while the fatty acids constitute a non-polar region, insoluble in water. This amphipathic nature —having both polar and non-polar characteristics—

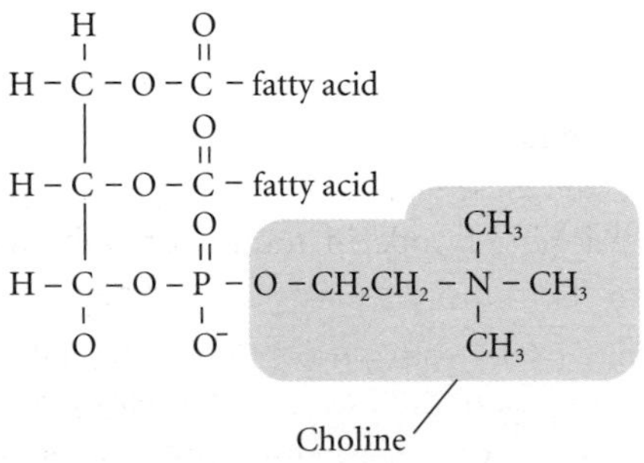

Fig. 3.3 Structure of phosphatidylcholine.

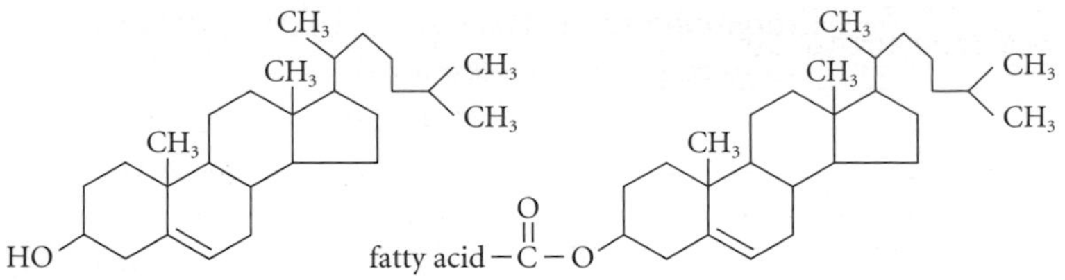

Fig. 3.4 Structure of cholesterol and cholesterol ester.

of the phospholipid enables it to act at the interface between aqueous and lipid media so they make excellent emulsifying agents. The structural integrity of all cell membranes and lipoproteins is dependent, among other factors, on the amphipathic nature of the constituent phospholipids. Phospholipids are also an important source of essential fatty acids.

3.1.3 Sterols

Sterols are also built up from carbon, hydrogen and oxygen, but in these lipid compounds (unlike triacylglycerols and phospholipids), the carbon, hydrogen and oxygen atoms are arranged in a series of four rings with a range of side chains. Cholesterol is the principal sterol of animal tissues and is found only in animal foods, especially eggs, meat, dairy products, fish and poultry. Cholesterol in food often has a fatty acid attached to it, so it is cholesterol ester (Fig. 3.4). Approximate quantities of cholesterol in some common foods are given in Table 3.2. The major sterols of plants (group name phytosterols) are β-sitosterol, campesterol and stigmasterol. Cholesterol plays an important structural role in membranes and lipoproteins, and functions as a precursor of bile acids, steroid hormones and vitamin D.

3.1.4 Other constituents of dietary fat

Dietary fats may also contain small quantities of other lipids including fatty alcohols, gangliosides, sulphatides and cerebrosides, as well as vitamin E (tocopherols, tocotrienols), carotenoids (α- and β-caroleve, lycopene and xanthophylls) and vitamins A and D (see Chapters 11, 13 and 14).

3.2 Dietary fats altered during food processing

The food industry incorporates fats and oils into margarines, biscuits, cakes, chocolates, pies, sauces and other manufactured food products. In addition to using naturally occurring lipids, food manufacturers use fats and oils that have been altered by the process of hydrogenation, adding hydrogen atoms to the double bonds in mono- or polyunsaturated fatty acids in order to increase the degree of saturation of the fatty acids in the oil (i.e. reduce the number of double bonds) and consequently increase the melting point of the fat. Through this process, a polyunsaturated oil that is liquid can be converted into a fat that is solid at room temperature. Hydrogenation of oils is used by manufacturers to produce a fat consistency appropriate to the texture of the desired food. Margarines usually contain hydrogenated fats. Hydrogenation also changes the configuration of some of the remaining double bonds from the natural *cis* configuration to a *trans* configuration. *Cis* mono- and polyunsaturated fatty acids have the two hydrogen atoms attached to the carbons on the same side of the double bond and the molecule bends at the double bond. In *trans* fatty acids, the hydrogens are placed on opposite sides of the double bond and the molecule stays straight at the double bond (Fig. 3.5). *Trans* unsaturated fatty acids behave biologically like saturated rather than like *cis* unsaturated fatty acids. The bulk of *trans* fatty acids in hydrogenated fats are

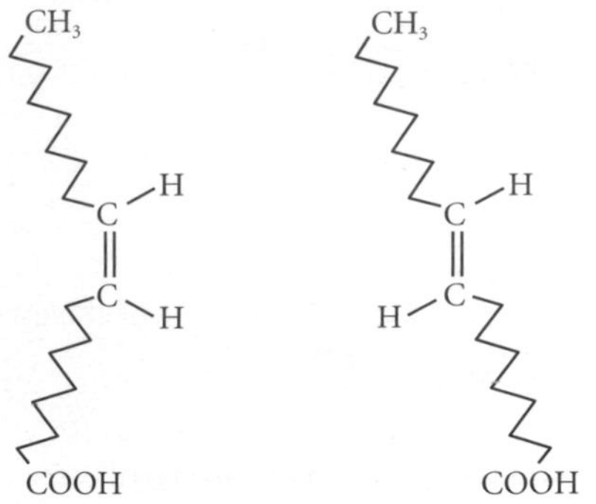

Oleic acid
(C18:1n-9 *cis*)

Elaidic acid
(C18:1n-9 *trans*)

Fig. 3.5 Structure of a *cis* and a *trans* monounsaturated fatty acid.

monounsaturated (elaidic acid, C18:1n-9 *trans*, is the *trans* equivalent of oleic acid).

Small quantities of *trans* fatty acids are found naturally in fats from ruminant animals (e.g. cows and sheep) but most of the dietary intake of *trans* fatty acids is derived from margarine and other manufactured foods containing hydrogenated fats. Unfortunately, information about the relative proportions of *cis* and *trans* fatty acids is not available for many foods, especially manufactured products, so it is not possible at present to quantify the total amount of *trans* unsaturated fatty acids in the diet. *Trans* fatty acids have in the past made up 5–10% of fatty acids in soft margarines and are now being reduced by manufacturers. Many soft margarines are now free of *trans* fatty acids whereas hard margarines contain up to 40–50% of fatty acids in the *trans* form.

3.3 Digestion, absorption and transport

3.3.1 Digestion (Fig. 3.6)

Triglycerides must be hydrolysed to fatty acids and monoglycerols before they can be absorbed. In children and adults, the process starts in the stomach where the churning action helps to create an emulsion. Fat entering the intestine is mixed with bile and further emulsified so that lipids are reduced to small bile acid-coated droplets that disperse in aqueous solutions and provide a sufficiently large surface area for the digestive enzymes to act. Bile acids facilitate the process of emulsification because they are amphipathic. Lipase enzymes secreted by the pancreas split by hydrolysis each triglyceride molecule, removing the two outer fatty acids, which can be absorbed with the remaining monoglyceride. Some monoglyceride (about 20%) is rearranged so that the lipase enzymes remove the third fatty acid. Phospholipids are hydrolysed by a phospholipase and cholesterol ester by cholesterol ester hydrolase. In the newborn, the pancreatic secretion of lipases is low, and fat digestion is augmented by lingual lipase secreted from the glands of the tongue and by a lipase present in human milk. The products of lipid digestion, along with other minor dietary lipids, such as fat-soluble vitamins, coalesce with bile acids into microscopic aggregates know as mixed micelles.

3.3.2 Absorption (Fig. 3.6)

Glycerol and fatty acids with a chain length of less than 12 carbon atoms can enter the portal vein system directly by diffusing across the enterocytes (cells lining the wall of the small intestine). On the other hand, monoglycerides, fatty acids, cholesterol, lysophospholipids and other dietary lipids diffuse from the mixed micelles into the enterocytes of the small intestine where they are resynthesized into triglycerides, phospholipids and cholesterol esters in preparation for their incorporation into chylomicrons. In general, absorption is efficient, with greater than 95% of dietary lipid absorbed (triglycerides, phospholipids and fat-soluble vitamins). Cholesterol, other sterols and β-caroleve are only partially absorbed (less than 30%).

Diseases that impair the secretion of bile (e.g. obstruction of the bile duct), that reduce secretion of lipase enzymes from the pancreas (e.g. pancreatitis

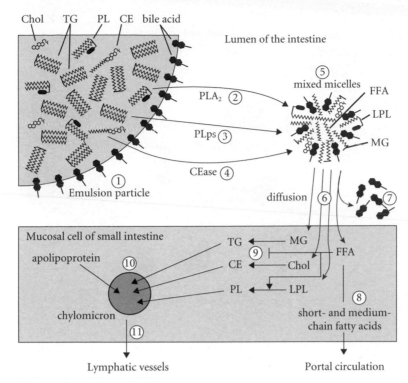

Fig. 3.6 Digestion and absorption of dietary lipids.
(1) Dietary lipid leaves the stomach and enters the upper region of the small intestine where bile acids, released from the gallbladder, surround and coat droplets of fat to form emulsion particles. The emulsion particles provide the surface area for the pancreatic enzymes to degrade the dietary lipids.
(2) Phospholipase A_2 (PLA$_2$) breaks down each phospholipid (PL) into a free fatty acid (FFA) and a lyso-phospholipid (LPL).
(3) Pancreatic lipase (PLps) converts triglyceride (TG) into a monoglyceride (MG) and two free fatty acids.
(4) Cholesterol esterase (CEase) splits cholesterol ester (CE) into free cholesterol (Chol) and a free fatty acid.
(5) The products of lipid digestion coalesce with bile acids into mixed micelles.
(6) The mixed micelles move close to the mucosal cell surface where the lipids diffuse down a concentration gradient into the mucosal cells.
(7) Bile acids are not absorbed.
(8) Short- and medium-chain fatty acids move immediately into the portal circulation where they are transported in the blood bound to albumin.
(9) To maintain the concentration gradient necessary for lipid diffusion, the breakdown products of lipid digestion are resynthesized into their parental lipids.
(10) The lipids are combined with apolipoproteins, synthesized in the mucosal cells, to form chylomicrons.
(11) Chylomicrons leave the mucosal cell via the lymphatic vessels.

or cystic fibrosis) or that damage the cell lining of the small intestine (e.g. coeliac disease) can lead to severe malabsorption of fat. Under such circumstances, medium-chain triglycerides can be better tolerated and are often used as part of the dietary treatment.

3.3.3 Lipid transport (Fig. 3.7)

Since lipids are not soluble in water, it is necessary for them to be associated with specific proteins, the apolipoproteins, to make water-miscible complexes. Free fatty acids make up only about 2% of total

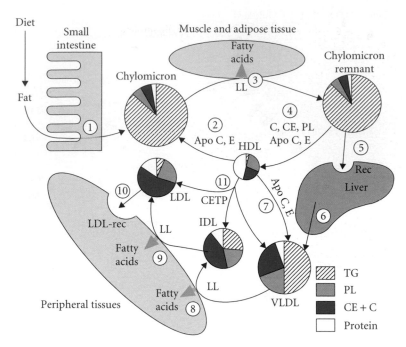

Fig. 3.7 Lipid transport and lipoprotein metabolism.
(1) Chylomicrons transport recently ingested fats into the blood
(2) Upon entering the blood, chylomicrons pick up apoliproteins C and E (apo C,E) from high-density lipoprotein (HDL).
(3) Apolipoprotein C activates lipoprotein lipase (LL) on the walls of the capillaries causing triglyceride to be broken down to glycerol and three fatty acids. The fatty acids are taken up primarily by adipose and muscle tissue.
(4) During breakdown of triglyceride (TG) some cholesterol (C), cholesterol ester (CE) and phospholipids (PL) along with apo C and E pinch off to form HDL.
(5) Following degradation of 70–80% of the chylomicron's TG, the resulting chylomicron remnant binds to receptors (rec) on the liver cells and is removed from the circulation.
(6) Lipids synthesized in the liver and those delivered to the liver by chylomicron remnants are packaged into very-low-density lipoproteins (VLDL) and secreted into the blood.
(7) VLDL picks up apo C and E from HDL.
(8) LL, activated by apo C, breaks down VLDL TG and the fatty acids are transferred to peripheral tissue (mainly muscle and adipose) resulting in the formation of intermediate-density lipoprotein (IDL).
(9) Nearly all of the TG is removed from IDL producing a cholesterol-rich LDL.
(10) Cholesterol is delivered to the cells when LDL binds to LDL-receptors (LDL-rec) and is taken up into the tissues.
(11) Cholesterol ester transfer protein redistributes cholesterol esters from HDL to VLDL, IDL and LDL.

plasma lipid and are transported in the blood as complexes with albumin. The remainder of lipid in the plasma is carried as lipoprotein complexes (lipid + protein = lipoprotein). The structure of a lipoprotein is given in Fig. 3.8. They consist of a core of neutral lipid (triglyceride and cholesterol esters) surrounded by a single surface layer of polar lipid (phospholipid and cholesterol). Coiled chains of apolipoproteins extend over the surface. There are five classes of lipoprotein, which are identified according to their density (Table 3.4) and five major groups of apolipoprotein (apo A, apo B, apo C, apo D and apo E), which play important roles in determining the functions of the lipoproteins. Each has a distinct physiological role (Table 3.5) and when present in inappropriate amounts (too high or too low) has different adverse health consequences.

Chylomicrons transport lipids of dietary origin, so they consist predominantly of triglycerides.

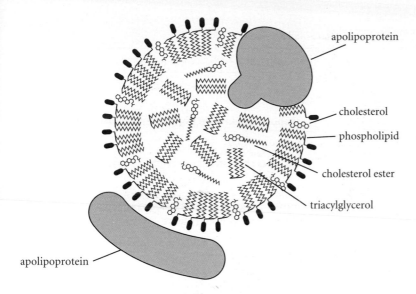

apolipoprotein

cholesterol

phospholipid

cholesterol ester

triacylglycerol

apolipoprotein

Fig. 3.8 Structure of a plasma lipoprotein.

Table 3.4 Composition of human plasma lipoproteins

Class	Density	Composition (weight %)		Percentage of total lipid (weight %)					Major apoproteins
		Protein	Lipid	TAG	PL	CE	Chol	FFA	
Chylomicrons[a]	<0.95	2	98	88	8	3	1	–	AI, AIV, B-48, Cs and E from HDL
Very-low-density lipoprotein (VLDL)[b]	0.95–1.006	10	90	56	20	15	8	1	B-100, Cs and E from HDL
Intermediate-density lipoprotein (IDL)[c]	1.006–1.019	11	89	29	26	34	9	1	B-100, E
Low-density lipoprotein (LDL)[c]	1.019–1.063	21	79	13	28	48	10	1	B-100
Lipoprotein(a) [Lp(a)][b]	1.05–1.12	31	69	11	29	48	11	1	B-100, apo(a)
High-density lipoprotein HDL$_2$[a]	1.063–1.125	33	68	16	43	31	10	–	As, Cs, E
High-density lipoprotein HDL$_3$[bc]	1.125–1.210	57	43	13	46	29	6	6	As, Cs, E
Albumin[b]	>1.281	99	1	–	–	–	–	100	Albumin

[a] Origin: intestine.
[b] Origin: liver.
[c] Origin: VLDL.
TAG = triacylglycerol (triglycerol); PL = phospholipid; CE = cholesterol ester; chol = cholesterol; FFA = free fatty acids.

Table 3.5 Functions of human plasma lipoproteins

Class	Function
Chylomicrons[a]	Transport dietary lipids from intestine to peripheral tissues and liver
Very-low-density lipoprotein (VLDL)[b]	Transports lipids from liver to peripheral tissues
Intermediate-density lipoprotein (IDL)[c]	Precursor of LDL
Low-density lipoprotein (LDL)[c]	Transports cholesterol to peripheral tissues and liver
Lipoprotein(a) (Lp(a))[b]	?
High-density lipoprotein HDL$_2$[a] High-density lipoprotein HDL$_3$[bc]	Removes cholesterol from tissues and transfers it to the liver or other lipoproteins
Albumin[b]	Transports free fatty acids from adipose tissue to peripheral tissues

[a] Origin: intestine.
[b] Origin: liver.
[c] Origin: VLDL.

Chylomicrons are abundant in the blood after eating food, particularly fatty food, but are scarce in fasting blood. The fatty acid composition of the lipids in chylomicrons is largely determined by the composition of the meal just eaten. Chylomicrons leave the enterocytes of the small intestine and enter the blood stream via lymph vessels. The enzyme lipoprotein lipase, located on the walls of capillary blood vessels, hydrolyses the triglycerides, allowing the free fatty acids to move into muscle or heart tissue where they can be used for energy, or into adipose tissue where they can be stored. During a short life in the circulation (15–30 minutes) more than 90% of the triglyceride in the chylomicron is removed. The resulting chylomicron remnant is cleared from the circulation by the liver. The fat-soluble vitamins (A, D, E and K) are delivered to the liver as part of the chylomicron remnant.

Very-low-density lipoproteins (VLDLs) are large triglyceride-rich particles made in the liver. They function as a vehicle for delivery of fatty acids to the heart, muscles and adipose tissue, lipoprotein lipase again being needed for their liberation. Lipoprotein lipase in the heart has a much stronger affinity for triglyceride than that in the adipose tissue or muscle, so when triglyceride concentration is low, triglyceride is preferentially taken up by heart tissue. Following removal of much of the triglyceride from VLDL, the remaining remnant particles are intermediate-density lipoproteins (IDL), which are the precursors of low-density lipoprotein.

Low-density lipoprotein (LDL) is the end product of VLDL metabolism and its lipid consists largely of cholesterol ester and cholesterol. Its surface has only one type of apolipoprotein, apo B100. LDL carries about 70% of all cholesterol in the plasma. LDL is taken up by the liver and other tissues by LDL receptors.

High-density lipoprotein (HDL) is synthesized and secreted both by the liver and intestine. A major function of HDL is to transfer apolipoproteins C and E to chylomicrons so that lipoprotein lipase can break down the triglycerides in the lipoproteins. HDL also plays a key role in the reverse transport of cholesterol, i.e. the transfer of cholesterol back from the tissues to the liver. HDL can be divided into two subfractions of different densities: HDL$_2$ and HDL$_3$.

Lipoprotein (a) (Lp(a)) is a complex of LDL with apolipoprotein (a).

Table 3.6 Nutritional determinants of lipoprotein levels

Nutritional factor	VLDL	LDL	HDL	Notes
Obesity	↑	↑	↓	
Saturated fat				
Lauric (12:0)	–	↑	↑	
Myristic (14:0)	–	↑↑	↑	
Palmitic (16:0)	–	↑↑	↑	
Stearic (18:0)	–	–	–	
Monounsaturated fat				
Oleic (18:1cis)	–	↓	↑	
Elaidic (18:1trans)	–	↑↑	↓	
Polyunsaturated fat (ω-6)				HDL may ↓ if 18:2ω-6 is
Linoleic (18:2ω-6)	–	↓↓	(↑)	>10% of total energy
Polyunsaturated fat (ω-3)				↑ in LDL if initial LDL
α-Linolenic (18:3ω-3)	↓↓	(↑)	(↓)	is high
Eicosapentaenoic (20:5ω-3)	↓↓	(↑)	(↓)	↓ in HDL if fed in large
Docosahexaenoic (22:6ω-3)	↓↓	(↑)	(↓)	quantities

↑,↓ = increase or decrease.
↑↑, ↓↓ = appreciable increase or decrease.
VLDL = very low-density lipoproteins; LDL = low-density lipoproteins; HDL = high-density lipoproteins.

3.3.4 Nutritional determinants of lipid and lipoprotein levels in blood

The fact that plasma lipid and lipoprotein levels are important predictors of coronary heart disease risk (discussed in Chapter 20) has led to a great deal of research into nutritional and other lifestyle factors that interact with genetic factors to determine their concentration in the blood (Table 3.6).

The chylomicron count and the fatty acid composition of chylomicron lipid are principally determined by the amount and type of fat eaten in the preceding meal. VLDL levels tend to be low in lean individuals and those who have regular physical activity. Obesity and an excessive intake of alcohol are associated with higher than average VLDL levels. An increased intake of carbohydrate (especially sugars and starches) is generally associated with an increase in VLDL as a result of increased hepatic synthesis of triglycerides, though adaptation may occur if the high carbohydrate intake is sustained over a prolonged period. Populations with habitual high carbohydrate intakes (e.g. Asians or African people who consume their traditional diets) do not have particularly high plasma VLDL concentrations. Consumption of eicosapentaenoic (20:5ω3) and docosahexaenoic (22:6ω3) acids as fish or fish oils lowers plasma VLDL levels. In routine clinical work, plasma triglyceride rather than VLDL is measured because the bulk of triglyceride levels in blood taken from fasting (10–12 hours) individuals tend to parallel levels of VLDL.

Levels of LDL and total plasma cholesterol are determined by an interaction of genetic factors and dietary characteristics. High intakes of saturated fatty acids, especially myristic and palmitic acids, and *trans* fatty acids (e.g. elaidic acid) are associated with raised LDL-cholesterol, while high intakes of linoleic acid, the major polyunsaturated acid in foods, and to a lesser extent *cis* monounsaturated fatty acids, tend to reduce cholesterol levels. The precise mechanism has not been established but high intakes of saturated fatty acids appear to decrease the removal of plasma LDL by LDL-receptors, whereas mono- and polyunsaturated fatty acids are associated with increased LDL receptor activity. Dietary cholesterol seems to be an important determinant of plasma total and LDL-cholesterol only when saturated fatty acids comprise a high proportion of dietary lipid (greater than 15% of energy) and cholesterol intake exceeds 300 mg/day. It is less clear whether dietary cholesterol plays a major role over the relatively low range of intakes now seen in many countries and when saturated fatty acid intake is reduced. Plant sterols (e.g. β-sitosterol) are very poorly absorbed and interfere with the absorption of cholesterol. This property of plant sterols has been utilized by incorporating them into margarines. Consumption of these margarines (25 g/day containing roughly 2 g plant sterols) can lower plasma total and LDL-cholesterol concentrations.

The ability of soluble forms of dietary fibre to reduce total and LDL-cholesterol is small compared with the effect of altering the nature of dietary fat. Dietary protein may also influence plasma lipids and lipo-proteins: soybean protein particularly has some cholesterol-lowering properties. Vegetarians have lower levels of total and LDL-cholesterol in general than non-vegetarians, but it is not clear which characteristic of the vegetarian diet principally accounts for this effect.

Debate centres around whether saturated fatty acids should be replaced by carbohydrate-containing foods or by fats and oils with a more favourable fatty acid profile (i.e. monounsaturated or polyunsaturated fatty acids with a *cis* configuration). However, provided energy balance is taken into account, it probably matters little whether appropriate carbohydrate-containing foods (see Chapter 2) or more acceptable fats and oils or indeed a combination of both provide replacement energy for saturated fats.

Dietary factors do not have much effect on HDL-cholesterol concentration. However, HDL-cholesterol can be slightly reduced by very high intakes of polyunsaturated fatty acids (e.g. when the dietary polyunsaturated fat to saturated fat ratio is greater than 1), or by increasing carbohydrate from more usual levels consumed (less than 45% of energy) in affluent societies to 60% or more of total energy, or by increasing *trans* unsaturated fatty acids. The HDL-lowering effect of a high-carbohydrate diet may be reduced or prevented if the carbohydrate is high in soluble forms of non-starch polysaccharide. HDL levels tend to be raised by diets relatively high in dietary cholesterol and saturated fatty acids, although this 'positive' effect is offset by the larger increases in LDL-cholesterol caused by such diets. Increasing *cis* forms of monounsaturated fatty acids appears to be a dictary means of maintaining HDL levels when reducing saturated fat consumption. Most dietary studies have not included measurements of the subfractions of HDL. HDL-cholesterol is raised in people who take substantial amounts of alcohol (see Chapter 6).

3.4 Essentials of lipid metabolism

3.4.1 Biosynthesis of fatty acids

Saturated and monounsaturated fatty acids can be synthesized in the body from carbohydrate and protein. This process of lipogenesis occurs especially in a well-fed person whose diet contains a high proportion of carbohydrate in the presence of an adequate energy intake. Insulin stimulates the biosynthesis of fatty acids. Lipogenesis is reduced during energy restriction or when the diet is high in fat. Unsaturated fatty acids may be further elongated or desaturated by various enzyme systems (Fig. 3.9).

3.4.2 Essential fatty acids

Essential fatty acids are those that cannot be synthesized in the body and must be supplied in the diet to avoid deficiency symptoms. They include members of the ω-6 (linoleic acid) and ω-3 (α-linolenic acid) families of fatty acids. When the diet is deficient in

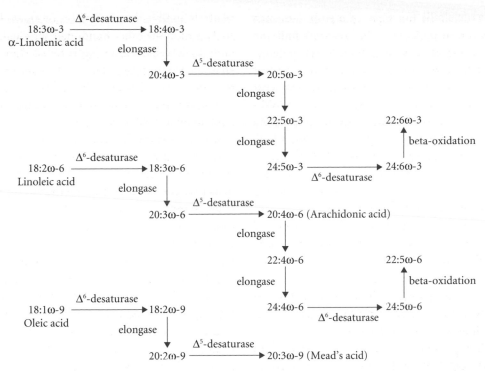

Fig. 3.9 Desaturation and elongation of polyunsaturated fatty acids.

linoleic acid, the most abundant unsaturated fatty acid in tissue, oleic acid, is desaturated and elongated to eicosatrienoic acid (20:3ω9), which is normally present in trace amounts. Increased plasma levels of this 20:3ω9 suggest a deficiency of essential fatty acids. Essential fatty acid deficiency is rare except in those with severe, untreated fat malabsorption or those suffering from famine. Symptoms include dry, cracked, scaly and bleeding skin, excessive thirst due to high water loss from the skin, and impaired liver function resulting from the accumulation of lipid in the liver (i.e. fatty liver).

Linoleic acid and α-linolenic acid are not only required for the structural integrity of all cell membranes, but they are also elongated and desaturated into longer chain, more polyunsaturated fatty acids that are the precursors to a group of hormone-like eicosanoid compounds, prostaglandins and leukotrienes (see section 3.4.4). Linoleic acid (18:2ω-6) is converted to arachidonic acid (20:4ω-6) while α-linolenic acid (18:3ω-3) is converted to eicosapentaenoic (20:5ω-3) and docosahexaenoic (22:6ω-3)

acids. A high ratio of linoleic to α-linolenic acid in the diet tends to reduce the amount of α-linolenic acid converted to eicosapentaenoic and docosahexaenoic acids.

There is some question as to whether the arachidonic, eicosapentaenoic and docosahexaenoic acids incorporated into the body's tissues come predominantly from endogenous desaturation and elongation of dietary essential fatty acids or are obtained from the diet as preformed fatty acids. Whatever the answer, the body appears to have a capacity to desaturate and elongate essential fatty acids, because individuals following strict vegan diets (no animal foods) ingest plenty of linoleic and α-linolenic acids but only negligible amounts of arachidonic, eicosapentaenoic and docosahexaenoic acids, yet have normal levels of these latter fatty acids in their blood.

3.4.3 Membrane structure

Unsaturated fatty acids in membrane lipids play an important role in maintaining fluidity. The critically important metabolic functions of membranes such as nutrient transport, receptor function and ion channels are affected by interactions between proteins and lipids. For example, the phosphoinositide cycle, which determines the responses of many cells to hormones, neurotransmitters and cell growth factors and which controls processes of cell division, is influenced by the proportion of ω-6 to ω-3 fatty acids.

3.4.4 Eicosanoids

Eicosanoids are biologically active, oxygenated metabolites of arachidonic acid, eicosapentaenoic acid (EPA), or dihomo-γ-linolenic acid (C20:3ω-6). They are produced in virtually all cells in the body, act locally, have short life spans, and act as modulators of numerous physiological processes including reproduction, blood pressure, haemostasis and inflammation. Eicosanoids are further categorized into prostaglandins/thromboxanes and leukotrienes, which are produced via the cyclo-oxygenase and lipoxygenase pathways, respectively (Fig. 3.10). Considerable recent interest has centred around the cardiovascular effects of eicosanoids, in particular the role they play in thrombosis (i.e. vessel blockage). Thromboxane A_2 (TxA$_2$), synthesized in platelets from arachidonic acid, stimulates vasoconstriction and platelet aggregation (i.e. clumping), while prostacyclin I$_2$ (PGI$_2$), produced from arachidonic acid in the endothelial cells of the vessel wall, has the opposing effects of stimulating vasodilation and inhibiting platelet aggregation. The balance of these two counteracting eicosanoids helps to determine the overall thrombotic tendency.

Research, initially based on the observation that the Inuit (Eskimo) people of Greenland have very low rates of coronary heart disease, led to the demonstration that a high dietary intake of EPA (usually in fish oil) can profoundly influence the balance of thromboxanes and prostacyclins. Such diets lead to the substitution of EPA for arachidonic acid in platelet membranes. TxA$_2$ production decreases, not only because of lower levels of platelet arachidonic acid, but also because the increased levels of EPA in platelets inhibit the conversion of arachidonic acid to TxA$_2$. On the other hand, PGI$_2$ production in the endothelial cells is only slightly reduced and there is a sharp rise in the production of PGI$_3$ from EPA, which has equal vasodilatory and platelet-inhibiting properties. The overall changes in eicosanoid production contribute to reducing thrombotic risk.

Leukotrienes are believed to be important in several diseases involving inflammatory or hypersensitivity reactions including asthma, eczema and rheumatoid arthritis. The effect of EPA consumption on leukotriene synthesis is to shift production from the more inflammatory 4-series leukotrienes, synthesized from arachidonic acid, to the less inflammatory 5-series leukotrienes synthesized from EPA. This metabolic effect helps to explain the improvements in some of the clinical symptoms experienced by rheumatoid arthritis sufferers who consume significant quantities of fish (i.e. EPA).

3.4.5 Effects of fatty acids on other metabolic processes

Fatty acids influence a range of other metabolic processes that have been less well studied in humans. Hydrolysis of some phospholipids results in the formation of biologically active compounds such as the platelet activating agent (PAF) from 1-alkyl, 2-acyl phosphatidylcholine. Different polyunsaturated fatty acids in the precursor phospholipid can modify PAF formation. ω3 fatty acids influence the production of cytokines, including the interleukins and tumour necrosis factors, which are involved in regulation of the immune system. An exciting area of current research is the study of the effects of fatty acids on the expression of genes encoding enzymes that are involved in lipid metabolism, as well as the expression of genes involved in cell growth regulation.

3.4.6 Oxidation of fatty acids

Those fatty acids not incorporated into tissues or used for synthesis of eicosanoids are oxidized for

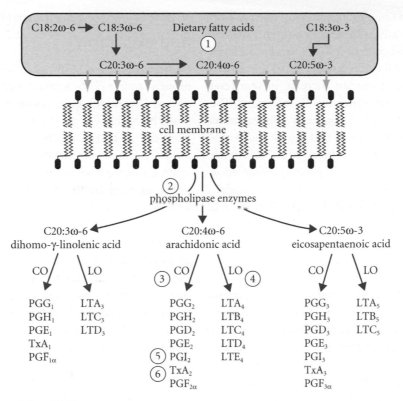

Fig. 3.10 Formation of eicosanoids
(1) Dihomo-γ-linolenic acid (DGLA), arachidonic acid (AA) and eicosapentaenoic (EPA) acid, obtained ready-made in the diet or via desaturation and elongation of their respective parent ω-6 (linolenic acid) or ω-3 (linolenic acid) essential fatty acids, are incorporated into the phospholipids of cell membranes.
(2) When cells are stimulated by hormones or activating substances, phospholipase enzymes release DGLA, AA and EPA into the interior of the cell.
(3) Once released from the cell membranes, DGLA, AA and EPA can be converted via the cyclo-oxygenase pathway (CO) into prostaglandins (PG) and thromboxanes (Tx) of the 1, 2 and 3 series, respectively;
(4) or via the lipoxygenase pathway (LO) to leukotrienes (LT) of the 3, 4 and 5 series, respectively.
(5) In platelets, AA is converted primarily to the 2 series thromboxane (TxA_2), which stimulates platelet clumping and increases blood pressure.
(6) In the endothelial cells lining arterial vessels, AA is converted into the 2 series prostacylin (PGI_2), which counters the action of TxA_2 by inhibiting platelet clumping and decreasing blood pressure.

energy. Oxidation of fatty acids occurs in the mitochondria of cells and involves a multiple-step process by which the fatty acid is gradually broken down to molecules of acetyl CoA, which are available to enter the tricarboxylic acid cycle and so to generate energy. The rate of oxidation of fatty acids is highest at times of low energy intake and particularly during starvation. As the acetyl CoA splits off, adenosine triphosphate (ATP) is generated, which is also a source of energy. Fatty acids of different chain lengths and degrees of saturation are oxidized via slightly different pathways but the ultimate purpose of each is the production of acetyl CoA and the generation of energy. Ketone bodies are produced during times of particularly rapid fatty acid oxidation during the process of ketogenesis. An absolute insulin deficiency such as is seen in severe uncontrolled insulin-dependent diabetes, results in a very high rate of production of ketones, and acidosis results because of accumulation of acetoacetic and β-hydroxybutyric acids. In healthy individuals with a functioning pancreas, the ingestion of glucose stimulates insulin secretion and thereby prevents or abolishes ketosis. This can be achieved by as little as 50–100 g of glucose daily. In the normal fasting individual, a modest increase in that level of ketone bodies stimulates insulin secretion. The insulin inhibits further ketogenesis and enhances peripheral ketone body use so that ketone body levels do not rise above 6–8 mol/L. (In severe diabetes, levels may be twice as high as this.) In prolonged starvation there is further ketone-body formation and a moderate degree of ketosis may result. However, ketoacidosis does not occur in the absence of insulin deficiency.

3.4.7 Lipid storage

Energy intake in excess of requirements is converted to fat for storage. Stored fat in adipose tissue provides the human body with a source of energy when energy supplies are not immediately available from ingested carbohydrate, fat or glycogen stores. Triacylglycerols are the main storage form of lipids and most stored lipids are found in adipose tissue. The lipid is stored as single droplets in cells called adipocytes, which can expand as more fat needs to be stored. Most of the lipid in adipose tissue is derived from dietary lipid and the stored lipid reflects the composition of dietary fat. The triacylglycerol stores of adipose tissue are not static but are continually undergoing lipolysis and re-esterification.

3.4.8 Cholesterol synthesis and excretion

Cholesterol is present in tissues and in plasma lipoproteins as free cholesterol or combined with a fatty acid as cholesterol ester. About half the cholesterol in the body comes from synthesis and the remainder from the diet. It is synthesized in the body from acetyl CoA via a long metabolic pathway. Cholesterol synthesis in the liver is regulated near the beginning of the pathway by the dietary cholesterol delivered by chylomicron remnants. In the tissues, a cholesterol balance is maintained between factors causing a gain of cholesterol (synthesis, uptake into cells, hydrolysis of stored cholesterol esters) and factors causing loss of cholesterol (steroid hormone synthesis, cholesterol ester formation, bile acid synthesis and reverse transport via HDL). The specific binding sites and receptors for LDL play a crucial role in cholesterol balance since they constitute the principal means by which LDL-cholesterol enters the cells. These receptors are defective in familial hypercholesterolaemia (see section 18.1.4). Excess cholesterol is excreted from the liver in the bile either unchanged as cholesterol or converted to bile salts. A large proportion of the bile salts that are excreted from the liver into the gastrointestinal tract are absorbed back into the portal circulation and returned to the liver as part of the enterohepatic circulation, but some pass on to the colon and are excreted as faecal bile acids.

3.5 Health effects of dietary lipids

Most fatty acids can be made in the body, except for the essential fatty acids (EFAs), linoleic and α-linolenic acids, which must be obtained from the diet (see section 3.4.2). The fact that specific deficiencies resulting from inadequate intakes of EFAs are very rare in adults, even in African and Asian countries where total dietary fat can provide as little as 10% of total energy, suggests that the minimum requirement is low. Amongst adults, EFA deficiency has only been reported when linoleic acid (18:2ω-6) intakes are less than 2–5 g/day or less than 1–2% of total energy. Most adult Western diets provide at least 10 g/day of EFA and healthy people have a substantial reserve in adipose tissues. Clinical manifestations of α-linolenic acid deficiency are rare in humans.

Amongst adults in Western countries, the major health issues concerning intake of fat centre around the role of excessive dietary fat in coronary heart disease (Chapter 20), obesity (Chapter 16) and certain cancers (Chapter 21). There is concern too regarding the optimal balance of ω-3 to ω-6 fatty acids with regard to risk of thrombosis and consequent coronary heart disease risk, as well as the effect this balance may have on inflammatory and immunological responses.

Human milk provides 6% of total energy as essential fatty acids (linoleic and α-linolenic acids); it also contains small amounts of longer chain, more polyunsaturated fatty acids such as arachidonic acid (AA; $C20:4\omega-6$) and docosahexaenoic acids (DHA; $22:6\omega-3$). Commercial baby milk formulae contain comparable amounts of essential fatty acids but only a few brands—in some countries—contain AA and DHA. Infants fed exclusively with formula without AA and DHA have lower levels of these fatty acids in their plasma and red blood cells in comparison with breast-fed infants. In premature infants, these reduced levels of DHA may be associated with impaired and delayed visual development since the retina and the brain have high contents of DHA (see Chapter 31).

Concern has been expressed that the desire to reduce total fat intake by some health-conscious parents in affluent societies might result in a diet high in complex carbohydrate and dietary fibre and containing insufficient energy for growth and development in childhood. These wide-ranging issues need to be taken into account when making nutritional and dietary recommendations.

3.6 Recommendations concerning fat intake

3.6.1 Minimum desirable intakes

In adults, it is necessary to ensure that dietary intake is adequate to meet energy needs and to meet the requirements for EFAs and fat-soluble vitamins. Adequate intakes are particular important during pregnancy and lactation. Thus, for most adults, dietary fat should provide at least 15% of total energy, and 20% for women of reproductive age. British recommendations suggest that at least 1% of total daily energy should be derived from linoleic acid and 0.2% energy from α-linolenic acid. This level is rather arbitrary and is based on the amounts required to cure EFA deficiency. In view of the divergent and often opposing effects of the various eicosanoids derived from ω-3 and ω-6 fatty acids, other recommendations have concentrated on the balance of the fatty acids in the diet. It has been suggested that the ratio of linoleic to α-linolenic should be between 5:1 and 10:1 (the range in human milk) and that those eating diets with a ratio greater than 10:1 should be encouraged to eat more ω-3-rich food such as green leafy vegetables, legumes and fish. Particular attention must be paid to promoting adequate maternal intakes of EFAs throughout pregnancy and lactation to meet the needs of the fetus and young infant in laying down lipids in their growing brains (which have a high content of DHA and AA).

For infants and young children, the amount and type of dietary fat are equally important. Breast milk fulfils all requirements (50–60% energy as fat, with appropriate balance of nutrients), and during weaning it is important to ensure that dietary fat intake does not fall too rapidly. At least until the age of 2 years, a child's diet should contain about 40% of energy from fat and provide similar levels of EFAs to breast milk. Infant formulae with AA and DHA in proportions similar to those found in breast milk are available in some countries.

It is necessary also to take into account associated substances, in particular several vitamins and antioxidants. These are considered in other chapters. In particular, vitamin E (Chapter 13) in edible oils is required to stabilize unsaturated fatty acids. Foods high in polyunsaturated fatty acids should contain at least 0.6 mg α-tocopherol equivalents per gram of polyunsaturated fatty acids. In countries where vitamin A deficiency is a public health problem, the use of red palm oil should be encouraged wherever it is available.

3.6.2 Upper limits of fat and oil intakes

In most Western countries, dietary recommendations concerning fat intake have focused primarily around desirable upper limits of intake. The strongest reason for reducing intake of total fat from the typical Western intake of about 35% or more total energy is the widespread problem of obesity and the expectation that reducing fat intake to 30% or less of total energy will help to reduce the near epidemic proportions of this global health problem (Chapter 16). Reducing total fat may also reduce the frequency of some cancers (Chapter 21) but the evidence here is more tenuous, and it may also be that the extent of fat reduction required to reduce cancer risk (to around 20% of total energy) is unlikely to be achievable in most Western countries in the foreseeable future. The case for reducing intake of saturated fatty acids from the typical Western intake of 12% or more of total energy to 10% or less of total energy is based on the expectation of reducing coronary heart disease rates. This remains a particularly important dietary recommendation since the use of high-fat (mostly saturated) convenience foods is increasing in many countries and powerful vested commercial interests are involved.

FURTHER READING

1. Clarke, R., Frost, C., Collins, R., Appleby, P., and Peto, R. (1997) Dietary lipids and blood cholesterol: quantitative meta-analysis of metabolic ward studies. *Br Med J*, **314**, 112–7.

2. Gurr, M.I., Harwood, J.L., and Frayn, K. (2001) *Lipid biochemistry*, 5th edition. London, Blackwell Science.

3. Tso, P. (1985) Gastrointestinal digestion and absorption of lipid. *Adv Lipid Res*, **21**, 143–86.

4. Vergroeson, A.J., and Crawford, M. (eds) (1989) *The role of fats in human nutrition*, 2nd edition. London, Academic Press.

To see topical and scientifically robust updates on nutrition associated with this textbook, and active web links to many of the journal articles in the Reference areas, please see the dedicated Online Resource Centre at www.oxfordtextbooks.co.uk/orc/mann3e/.

4 Protein

Alan A. Jackson

4.1 Normal growth and the maintenance of health

To maintain normal weight, function and health in adults and growth in childhood requires a constant intake of oxygen, water, energy and nutrients. In adults this intake is matched by an equivalent loss of elements as carbon dioxide, water and solutes in urine, or solids in stool. In this way, a balance is achieved and body weight and composition are maintained relatively constant over long periods of time. In childhood there is positive balance associated with the net deposition of new tissue. If intake is less than that needed for normal function then there is loss of weight and function is compromised to a point where it eventually impairs health: in childhood, growth is curtailed or stops.

Proteins are fundamental structural and functional elements within every cell and undergo extensive metabolic interaction. This widespread metabolic interaction is intimately linked to the metabolism of energy and other nutrients. Following water, protein is the next most abundant chemical compound in the body. All cells and tissues contain proteins. For an adult man who weighs 70 kg, about 16% will be protein, i.e. about 11 kg. A large proportion of this will be muscle (43%) with substantial proportions being present in skin (15%) and blood (16%). Half of the total is present in only four proteins: collagen, haemoglobin, myosin and actin, with collagen comprising about 25% of the overall total.

Proteins fulfil a range of functions and the amount of protein does not, in itself, provide any indication of the importance or relevance of the function. Indeed some of the most important functionally active proteins might only comprise a small proportion of the total present, e.g. peptide hormones such as insulin, growth factors or cytokines. The biochemical activity of proteins is an attribute of their individual structure, shape and size. This in turn is determined by the sequence of amino acids within the polypeptide chains, the characteristics of the individual amino acids (size, charge, hydrophobicity or hydrophilicity) and the environment, which together determine the primary, secondary and tertiary structure of the protein. The tertiary structure of the protein determines the nature of the biochemical reactions in which it will engage.

Proteins taken in the diet are broken down into amino acids in the processes of digestion and absorption. Absorbed amino acids contribute to the amino acid pool of the body, from which all proteins are synthesized. The proteins of the body exist in a 'dynamic state' as they are constantly turning over through the processes of protein synthesis and degradation (see Figs 4.1A and 4.1B). On average, the rates of synthesis and degradation are similar in adults, so that the amount of protein in the body remains more or less constant over long periods of time, and nitrogen

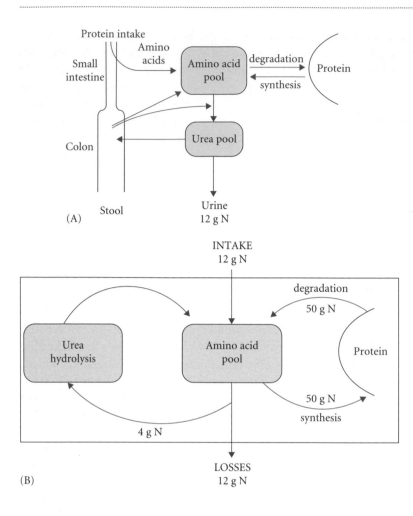

Fig. 4.1 (A) There is a dynamic interchange of protein, amino acids and nitrogen in the body, which conceptually takes place through an amino acid pool. Amino acids are added to the pool from the degradation of body proteins and also from dietary protein, following digestion and absorption. There is the continuous breakdown of amino acids, with energy being made available when the carbon skeleton is oxidized to water and CO_2. The amino group goes to the formation of urea. Although urea is an end product of mammalian metabolism, a significant proportion of the nitrogen is salvaged for further metabolic interaction following hydrolysis of urea by the flora resident in the colon. (B) The quantitative relations of these exchanges in normal adults expressed as grams of (amino) nitrogen (N) per day.

BOX 4.1 The pattern of amino acids that form proteins give them very different shapes, and chemical and physical properties, thereby enabling them to carry out a wide range of functions within the body

Structural		Transport/Communication	
Body:	skeleton and supporting tissues, skin and epithelia	Plasma proteins:	albumin, transferrin, apolipoproteins
Tissue:	connective tissues and ground substance	Hormones:	insulin, glucagon, growth hormone
Cell:	cellular architecture	Cell membrane and receptors:	intracellular communications/ second messenger
Protective		**Enzymatic**	
Barrier:	non-specific defences/turnover, keratins, skin, tears, mucin	Extracellular:	digestive, clotting; haemoglobin and O_2, CO_2 transport; acid base
Inflammation:	acute phase response	Metabolic pathways:	glycolysis, protein synthesis, citric acid cycle, urea cycle
Immune response:	cellular and humoral		

balance is achieved. During growth, protein synthesis exceeds protein degradation to enable net deposition of protein. The process of turnover is obvious for some proteins, e.g. enzymes, skin or mucosa, or digestive juices, but is also true for plasma proteins such as albumin or γ-globulins, and even structural proteins such as muscle and bone. There are many hundreds of proteins in the body, each of which is formed and degraded at a characteristic rate that may vary from minutes to days or even months. Each protein fulfils a specific function, which might be structural, protective, or enzymatic, or it might be involved in transport or an aspect of cellular communication (see Box 4.1).

4.2 Protein status of the body

There is no single way in which the protein status of an individual can be determined. Different approaches provide information on different aspects. The amount of protein contained in the body cannot be measured directly. However, most of the nitrogen in the body is present as amino acids in protein, and most protein is present as lean tissue. Thus, the nitrogen content of the body can be determined by *in vivo* neutron activation analysis (an expensive research procedure that requires special equipment and exposes the subject to radiation).

On the assumption that the protein content of tissues remains fairly constant, the determination of the lean body mass (which approximates the fat-free mass) also gives an index of the total protein content. Indirect measures of lean body mass include bioelectrical impedance, assessment of total body water, total body potassium, underwater weighing or fat-fold thickness (see Chapter 29). Organ and tissue size can be determined by imaging techniques. Muscle mass and changes in muscle content in clinical situations can be assessed from the urinary excretion of creatinine or the girth of limbs, such as the mid-upper arm circumference or thigh circumference. Determinations of the concentration of amino acids in plasma or the albumin concentration have been used as indirect indices of body protein status. However, each of these can be difficult to interpret (see below).

Assessment of the function of the metabolically active tissues has been used as an index of protein status, for example muscle function tests, liver function tests and tests of immune function. The content of the body is not static, and therefore measurements of the rates at which proteins are formed and degraded in the body and the rate at which nitrogen flows to the end products of metabolism provide one important approach to determining the mechanisms through which nitrogen equilibrium is maintained in health, positive balance is achieved during growth, or negative balance is brought about during wasting conditions.

4.3 Proteins, amino acids and other nitrogen-containing compounds

The structure and function of all proteins is related to their amino acid composition: the number and order of linkages, folding, intra-chain linkages, and the interaction with other groups to induce chemical change, e.g. phosphorylation/dephosphorylation, oxidation and reduction of sulphydral groups. The amino acids are linked in chains through peptide bonds. The structure of individual amino acids and the patterns of their linkages give the unique properties to an individual protein. Proteins may have critical requirements for either a tight or loose association with micronutrients and this is particularly likely for enzymes in

BOX 4.2 There are 20 amino acids that are found as the constituents of proteins. All are 'essential' for metabolism, but not all have to be provided preformed in the diet, because they can be made in sufficient amounts from other metabolic precursors. If the situation arises where the formation in the body is not adequate to satisfy the metabolic needs, the amino acids become conditionally essential

Indispensable (essential) amino acids	Conditionally indispensable (essential) amino acids	Dispensable (non-essential) amino acids
Leucine (Leu)	Tyrosine (Tyr)	Glutamic acid (Glu)
Isoleucine (Ile)	Glycine (Gly)	Alanine (Ala)
Valine (Val)	Serine (Ser)	Aspartic acid (Asp)
Phenylalanine (Phe)	Cysteine (Cys)	
Threonine (Thr)		
Methionine (Met)	Arginine (Arg)	
Tryptophan (Trp)	Glutamine (Gln)	
Lysine (Lys)	Asparagine (Asn)	
	Proline (Pro)	
	Histidine (His)	

which catalytic activity might require the presence of cofactors or prosthetic groups in close association with the active centres.

For each protein, the amino acid composition is characteristic. For a protein to be synthesized requires that all the amino acids needed are available at the point of synthesis. If one amino acid is in short supply, this will limit the process of protein synthesis; such an amino acid is defined as the 'limiting amino acid'. There is no dietary requirement for protein *per se*, but protein is important for the individual amino acids it contains. There are 20 amino acids required for protein synthesis and these are all 'metabolically essential' (see Box 4.2). Of the 20 amino acids found in protein, eight have to be provided preformed in the diet for adults and are identified as being 'indispensable' or 'essential' (isoleucine, leucine, lysine, methionine, phenylalanine, threonine, tryptophan and valine).

The other amino acids do not have to be provided preformed in the diet, provided that they can be

formed in the body from appropriate precursors in adequate amounts and are identified as being 'dispensable' or 'non-essential'. The non-essential amino acids are not necessarily of lesser biological importance. They have to be synthesized in adequate amounts endogenously. Their provision in the diet appears to spare additional quantities of other (essential) amino acids or sources of nitrogen that would be required for their synthesis.

In early childhood, a number of amino acids, which are not essential in adults, cannot be formed in adequate amounts, either because the demand is high, the pathways for their formation are not matured, or the rate of endogenous formation is not adequate (or some combination of these). These amino acids have been identified as being 'conditionally' essential, because of the limited ability of their endogenous formation relative to the magnitude of the demand (arginine, histidine, cysteine, glycine, tyrosine, glutamine and proline). There may be disease situations during adult life when for one reason or another a particular amino acid, or group of amino acids, becomes conditionally essential.

Although most of the amino acids are found in proteins, many amino acids also have metabolic activities that are not directly related to the formation of proteins, or act as the precursors for other important metabolically active compounds (see Box 4.3). Not all amino acids are found in proteins and there are a number of metabolically important amino acids that play no direct part in the formation of proteins (e.g. citrulline). There is a relatively small pool of free amino acids in all tissues. This is the pool from which amino acids for protein formation are derived, and to which amino acids coming from protein degradation contribute; therefore, the amino acid pools have a very high rate of turnover.

There are many other nitrogen-containing compounds that are not proteins, polypeptides or amino acids.

BOX 4.3 Amino acids are the precursors for many other metabolic intermediates and products with structural and functional roles

Product/Function	Examples
Nucleotides	Formation of DNA, RNA, ATP, NAD
Energy transduction	ATP, NAD, creatine
Neurotransmitters	Serotonin, adrenaline, noradrenaline, acetylcholine
Membrane structures	Head groups of phospholipids: choline, ethanolamine
Porphyrin	Haem compounds, cytochromes
Cellular replication	Polyamines
Fat digestion	Taurine, glycine-conjugated bile acids
Fat metabolism	Carnitine
Hormones	Thyroid, pituitary hormones

4.4 Dietary proteins, the amino acid pool and the dynamic state of body proteins

Before proteins taken in the diet can be utilized, they have to be broken down to the constituent amino acids through digestion. The catalytic breaking of the peptide bond is achieved through enzymes, which act initially in the acid environment of the stomach, and the process is completed in the alkaline environment of the small intestine. There is a series of proteolytic enzymes that selectively attack specific bonds (see Table 4.1). The products of digestion are presented for absorption as individual amino acids, dipeptides or small oligopeptides. Absorption takes place in the small intestine as an energy-dependent process through specific transporters. There is evidence for the absorption of small amounts of intact protein—it is unlikely to be of great nutritional significance, but may be of potential importance in the development of allergies. The extent of absorption of whole proteins is not clear, nor whether this can take place through intact bowel or requires mucosal lesions.

The absorptive capacity of the bowel for amino acids has to be greatly in excess of the dietary intake, because there is a considerable net daily secretion of proteins into the bowel. The protein is contained in secretions associated with digestion and the enzymes contained therein, mucins and sloughed cells. The amount varies, but estimates suggest a minimum of 70 g protein/day, and possibly up to 200–300 g protein/day—i.e. the amounts are at least as great as the dietary intake. Therefore, dietary amino acids mix with and are diluted by endogenous amino acids. These dietary and endogenous amino acids are taken up into the circulation and distributed to cells around the body.

Table 4.1 Human protein digestion

Organ	Activation	Enzyme	Substrate	Product
Stomach	pH < 4	Pepsin	Whole protein	Very large polypeptides with C-terminal Tyr, Phe, Trp, also Leu, Glu, Gln
Pancreas	pH 7.5 Enterokinase secreted by small intestinal mucosa	Endopeptidases	Bonds with peptide chain	
		Trypsin	Peptides	Peptide with basic amino acid at C terminus (arg, lys)
		Chymotrypsin	Peptides	Peptide with neutral amino acid at C terminus
		Exopeptidases	C-terminal bonds	
		Carboxypeptidase	Successive amino acids at C terminus	Amino acids
		Aminopeptidase	Successive amino acids at N terminus	Amino acids

Note: Enzymes that digest proteins are secreted as inactive precursors (e.g. pepsinogen, trypsinogen, chymotrypsinogen, etc.) and are activated under appropriate conditions by the removal of a small peptide from the parent molecule.

4.5 Protein turnover

When dietary amino acids are labelled with either stable or radioactive isotopes, their fate in the body can be determined. As a matter of course, there is retention of the labelled amino acids in the body, and the labelled amino acids can be recovered from the proteins of most tissues. This approach can be used as the basis for measuring the rate at which body proteins are synthesized and degraded. The relative rates of protein synthesis and degradation determine the overall nitrogen balance. For nitrogen balance to be achieved, the rates of protein synthesis and protein degradation have to be equal. If synthesis exceeds degradation then nitrogen balance is positive, and if degradation exceeds synthesis nitrogen balance is negative. Because overall balance is determined by the relative rates of synthesis and degradation, the achievement of balance itself provides no information on the absolute rates of either process. As shown in Fig. 4.2, negative nitrogen balance can result from a range of patterns of change in synthesis and degradation. As the factors that act on or control synthesis and degradation are different, interventions that are designed to modify balance or improve growth might act on one or the other process. On average, about 50% of protein synthesis takes place in the visceral tissues, with liver predominating (25%), and 50% takes place in the carcass, with muscle predominating (25%). Although the mass of liver is much less than the mass of muscle, the intensity of turnover in liver (fractional turnover, 100% per day) is much greater than that in muscle (fractional turnover, 18% per day).

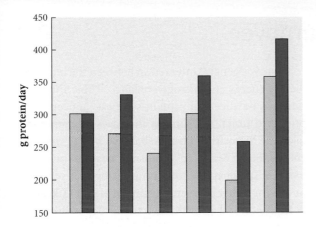

Fig. 4.2 Proteins in the body are constantly turning over (i.e. they are being syntheziised and degraded). The net amount of protein is determined by the relative rates of synthesis and degradation, not the absolute rate. When the rate of protein synthesis (▢) is equal to the rate of protein degradation (■), there is no change in the amount of protein (first column). Loss of protein and negative nitrogen balance will result when the relative rate of protein degradation exceeds the rate of protein synthesis. The five columns to the right show that this might be achieved either through a decrease in protein synthesis, an increase in protein degradation or any combination of the two, at either high or low absolute rates of protein synthesis and degradation.

4.6 Protein synthesis and degradation

The fact that the body constituents are in a dynamic state and that proteins are constantly being synthesized, and constantly being degraded, represents a major and fundamental aspect of the metabolic function of the body. Protein synthesis is an intracellular event, and the amount and pattern of proteins being formed in a cell at any point in time are determined by the factors that control genomic expression, the translation of the message, and the control exerted on the activity of the synthetic machinery on ribosomes. Protein degradation is also an intracellular event and is thought to take place through three major pathways —the calcium–protease, ATP–ubiquitin or lysozomal pathways.

In normal adults, about 4 g protein/kg body weight are synthesized each day: about 300 g protein/day in men and 250 g protein/day in women. In newborn infants, the rate is about 12 g protein/kg, falling to about 6 g/kg by 1 year of age. Basal metabolic rate is closely related to the size, shape and body composition of an individual, and the same is true for protein synthesis. In adults in a steady state, protein synthesis is matched by an equivalent rate of protein degradation, but in infancy and childhood, because of the net tissue and protein deposition associated with growth, protein synthesis exceeds protein degradation.

Dietary intake and the metabolic behaviour of the body show a diurnal rhythmicity. Food is normally ingested during the daytime. There is a diurnal pattern of nitrogen excretion in urine, which is more marked on higher protein intakes, with increased losses during the day and reduced losses during the night. On average over a 24-hour period, nitrogen equilibrium is maintained. However, as intake exceeds losses during the day and losses exceed intake during the night, there is a diurnal pattern of nitrogen balance, with balance being positive during the day and negative during the night. It is likely that nitrogen is retained in a number of forms during the day. There is evidence that protein deposition is most marked in the gastrointestinal tract, liver and other visceral tissues, with lesser deposition in muscle. There are equivalent losses of these relatively labile pools of protein during the night. In situations of fasting or longer-term undernutrition, the early losses of protein appear to be from the liver and gastrointestinal tract, but after a short time the majority of the losses are borne by peripheral tissues such as muscle and skin.

Despite the diurnal swings in protein turnover, the effect of protein intake on the average whole-body protein synthesis is relatively modest, provided the intake exceeds the minimal dietary requirement. Below the minimal dietary requirement (about 0.66 g/kg/day, there is a relative fall in protein synthesis during the fed period.

4.7 Energy cost of protein turnover

Both protein synthesis and protein degradation consume energy, 4 kJ/g of protein of average composition. Protein degradation takes place through ATP-dependent pathways, which are both lysozomal and non-lysozomal. At the level of the whole body, the biochemical cost of peptide bond formation is estimated to be about 15–20% of the resting energy expenditure. There are additional energy costs to the body if protein turnover is to be sustained, as processes such as transport of amino acids into cells requires energy, etc. If the full energy costs of maintaining the system are included, then the physiological cost is probably in the region of 33% of resting energy expenditure.

There is a general interaction between the intake of dietary energy and nitrogen balance. Thus, although nitrogen balance and protein synthesis appear to be protected functions, modest increases in energy intake lead to positive nitrogen balance, and decreasing energy intake results in a transient negative nitrogen balance. In general, about 2 mg nitrogen is retained or lost for a change in energy intake of 4 kJ (1 kcal).

In childhood growth, net tissue deposition is a normal feature. During adulthood, the demands for net tissue formation occurs under three important circumstances: in women during pregnancy, or during lactation, or during recovery from some wasting condition.

4.8 Growth

Growth consists of a complex of processes and changes in the body. There is an increase in stature and size and the proportions of the individual tissues change, resulting in changes in the composition of the body. These changes are related to the physiological maturation of function, which is an orderly series of changes in time. Maturation of function underlies development in general, and mental or intellectual development in particular. The orderly sequence of neurological maturation is directly linked into more complex behavioural changes, which under normal circumstances involve social interaction and the development of patterns of behaviour that are identified as social development.

At the level of cells and tissues, growth can be characterized as an increase in the number of cells (hypertrophy), an increase in the size of cells (hyperplasia), or a combination of the two processes (mixed hypertrophy and hyperplasia), which then leads to differentiation and specialization of function.

Net protein deposition is required for growth to take place and therefore protein synthesis must exceed protein degradation. There is an increase in protein synthesis, but there is also an increase in protein degradation, so that overall about 1.5–2.0 g protein are synthesized for every 1 g of net deposition. The apparent inefficiency of the system might be accounted for by:

1. a measure of flexibility to allow remodelling;
2. transcriptional and translational errors; and
3. wear and tear on the protein synthetic machinery.

4.9 Linear growth

Linear growth is a function of the growth and development of the long bones, and the deposition of a collagenous matrix (protein) within which the deposition of mineral crystals can take place. Ultimate adult height is determined by the genetic make-up of an individual, but at every stage of development there are factors that might operate to limit the extent to which this potential is achieved. Following an illness or deprivation, there may be recovery in height gain when the adverse influence is removed, but there may be a loss of some of the capacity for achieving the full genetic potential.

The hormones insulin, thyroid hormone, growth hormone and insulin-like growth factors (IGFs) have all been shown to modulate linear growth within physiological ranges. Calcification is directly related to vitamin D hormones, parathormone and osteocalcin.

An adequate intake of energy is an absolute requirement for growth, but is not in itself sufficient to achieve optimal growth in height—an adequate intake of protein and other nutrients is also required. Human and animal studies have identified a specific need for dietary protein, which is thought to have a direct effect on IGFs. Balance studies indicate the need for adequate calcium, phosphorus, zinc and other micronutrients.

Adverse influences, such as infection, inflammation and psychological and social factors may act either directly or indirectly, through nutritional considerations. Activity is an important trophic factor for the healthy development and calcification of bones.

Stunting, or linear growth retardation, is the major nutritional problem across the globe affecting socially and economically disadvantaged children within and between societies. There is clear evidence that stunted individuals have increased mortality from a variety of causes and an increased number of illnesses. Stunted individuals have a decrease in their physical work performance and impaired mental and intellectual function.

4.10 Protein turnover in muscle and its control

Muscle contains a large proportion of the protein in the body. Considerable interest has been shown in the growth of muscle, which is commercially important for the livestock industry. Muscle is one tissue most affected by wasting, and because it is relatively accessible it has been the subject of more detailed study *in vivo* in humans than any other tissue. Hormones, the availability of energy and nutrients, and muscle activity (stretch) all make a contribution to the rate of muscle tissue deposition.

Protein turnover in muscle is responsive to the hormonal state. Insulin, growth hormone and testosterone have overall anabolic effects, mainly by stimulating protein synthesis. Corticosteroids produce a decrease in synthesis and an increase in degradation. Thyroid hormones increase protein synthesis and degradation. However, at normal physiological levels they have a greater effect on synthesis than on degradation, thus exerting a net anabolic effect. At hyperthyroid levels, the increase in degradation exceeds the increase in synthesis and thus the hormone exerts an overall catabolic effect. β-Adrenergic anabolic agents such as clenbuterol promote muscle growth by decreasing protein degradation.

People on bed-rest go into negative nitrogen balance and lose weight through wasting of muscle. Activity is required to maintain muscle mass and the pull of contracting muscles on bone serves to promote bone growth. Mechanical signals exert an effect on cellular function through direct effect on the intracellular cytoskeleton, through activated ion channels and through second-messenger signal transduction processes. Prostaglandins (PGs) have a direct effect on muscle protein synthesis and degradation, with PGF_{2a} stimulating synthesis and PGE_2 stimulating degradation. The activity of phospholipase A2 makes arachidonic acid available for the synthesis of PGF_{2a} (blocked by indomethacin). The activity of phospholipase A2 is enhanced by stretch (activation of calcium) or insulin (cyclic AMP), and inhibited by glucocorticoids. Lipopolysaccharide exerts an influence on the release of arachidonic acid under the action of phospholipase A2, with the formation of PGE_2, which increases protein degradation through increased proteolysis within the lysozomes.

Stress, trauma and surgery have all been shown to induce a negative nitrogen balance in rats and humans. In wasted individuals or people on low-protein diets, a catabolic response, with negative nitrogen balance, may not be evident. Those who do not show this response are more likely to die, giving the impression that the negative response is purposive and that under these circumstances the catabolic response is more important than conserving body protein.

4.11 Injury and trauma

Injury and trauma are characterized by an inflammatory or acute-phase response. This is a coordinated metabolic response by the body that appears to be designed to limit damage, remove foreign material and repair damaged tissue. Under the influence of cytokines, there is a shift in the pattern of protein synthesis and degradation in the body. Substrate from endogenous sources is made available to support the activity of the immune system. In muscle, protein synthesis falls and protein degradation might increase, resulting in net loss of protein from muscle, with wasting. The amino acids made available by muscle wasting may provide substrate for protein synthesis in liver and the immune system. In the liver, there is a shift in the pattern of proteins synthesized, with a reduction in the formation of the usual secretory proteins, albumin, lipoproteins, transferrin,

retinol-binding protein, and so on, and an increase in the formation of the acute-phase reactants, such as C-reactive protein, α-1-acid glycoprotein, α-2-macroglobulin, etc. In combination with a loss of appetite, the changes in protein turnover in liver and muscle result in a negative nitrogen balance. There is usually an increase in protein degradation overall, and the intensity of the increase is determined by the magnitude of the trauma. At the lower end of the scale, uncomplicated elective surgery is characterized by losses of less than 5 g/day. At the upper end of the scale, burn injury can lead to losses in excess of 70 g/day. The dietary intake appears to have an important influence on the extent to which protein synthesis can be maintained, and therefore the magnitude of the negative nitrogen balance and the severity of the consequent wasting.

4.12 Amino acids

The habitual dietary intake of about 80 g protein/day in adults is only one-quarter of the protein being formed in the body each day. The minimal dietary requirement for protein, about 35–40 g protein in adult men, is approximately one-tenth of the protein being formed in the body each day.

The pattern and amounts of amino acids required to support protein synthesis are determined by the amount and pattern of proteins being formed. It has been presumed that the overall pattern is dominated by proteins of mixed composition similar to that seen in muscle, but this is not necessarily true for all situations, especially in some pathological states. For example, the amino acid profile of collagen is very rich in glycine and proline, but poor in leucine

and the branched-chain amino acids. During growth, where the demands for collagen formation are increased, the balance of amino acids needed is likely to be shifted towards a collagen pattern. During an inflammatory response, there is increased synthesis of the antioxidant glutathione and the zinc-binding protein metallothion, both of which are particularly rich in cysteine. The demand for the most appropriate pattern of amino acids might vary with different situations. The nature of the demand may change from one time to another, being determined by the physiological state, such as pregnancy, lactation or growth, or the pathological state, such as infection, the response to trauma or any other reason for an acute-phase response.

4.13 Amino acid turnover

The amino acid pool is the precursor pool from which all amino acids are drawn for protein synthesis and other pathways. It is helpful to identify the pool

for each amino acid individually and to consider the general factors that are of importance (see Fig. 4.3). For any amino acid, there are three inflows to the

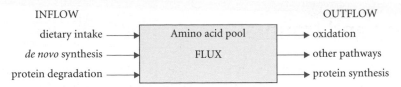

Fig. 4.3 The dynamic turnover of any amino acid in the body can be characterized by a model in which there is a single pool of an amino acid. Inflows to the pool are from three potential sources, protein degradation, the diet and *de novo* synthesis. There are three outflows from the pool, to protein synthesis, other metabolic pathways and to oxidation with the breakdown of the amino acid.

pool and three outflows. The flows from the pool to protein synthesis and other metabolic pathways represent the metabolic demand for the amino acid. Flow to amino acid oxidation is determined either by the need to use the amino acid as a source of energy, or as a degradative pathway for amino acids in excess of what can be used effectively at that point in time. This demand has to be satisfied from:

1. amino acids coming from protein degradation; or
2. *de novo* synthesis of amino acids; or
3. dietary amino acids.

It might be expected that in a steady state amino acids coming from protein degradation would represent a perfect fit for the proteins that are being synthesized, and hence there should be no general need for amino acids to be added to the system. However, this is not so. The amino acids released from protein degradation are different from those used in protein synthesis, because some amino acids are altered during the time they are part of a polypeptide chain. For example, amino acids might be methylated or carboxylated. These post-translational modifications relate to the structure and function of the mature protein. Lysine as part of a protein might be methylated to trimethyl lysine. When the protein is degraded, the released trimethyl lysine is of no value in future protein synthesis, but it can act as a metabolic precursor for the synthesis of carnitine. Carnitine plays a fundamental role in fatty acid metabolism. The endogenous formation of carnitine facilitates fatty acid oxidation and limits the need for a dietary source of carnitine, but an additional source of lysine is still needed for protein synthesis to be maintained. As lysine is an indispensable amino acid, and cannot be synthesized endogenously in quantities sufficient to satisfy the metabolic need, lysine has to be obtained preformed in the diet.

4.14 Amino acid formation and oxidation

The *de novo* synthesis of an amino acid requires that its carbon skeleton can be made available from endogenous sources, and this skeleton then has an amino group effectively added in the right position. The sulphur moiety has to be added for the sulphur amino acids. In mammalian metabolism, some amino acids are readily formed from other metabolic intermediates, for example transaminating amino acids, alanine, glutamic and aspartic acid, derived from intermediates of the citric acid cycle, pyruvate, α-ketoglutarate and oxaloacetate. These amino acids are important in the movement of amino groups around the body and also in gluconeogenesis (e.g. the glucose–alanine cycle between the liver and the periphery) or renal gluconeogenesis from glutamine during fasting. Some dispensable amino acids derive directly from an indispensable amino acid (e.g. tyrosine from phenylalanine) and the endogenous formation of the amino acid is determined by the availability of the indispensable amino acid. Methionine and cysteine are amino acids that contain a sulphydryl group, with considerable chemical activity. Although methionine can be formed in the body from homocysteine, this is part of a cycle (methionine cycle) that generates methyl groups for metabolism and in which there is no net gain of methionine (see Fig. 4.4). Homocysteine

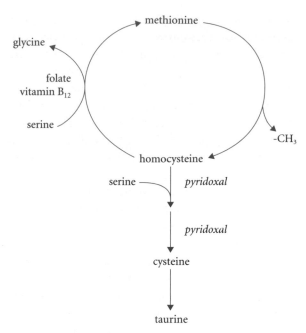

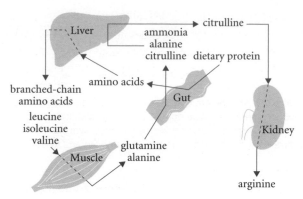

Fig. 4.4 The methionine cycle. Methionine has to be provided in the diet and like other amino acids is required for protein synthesis. In addition, it has a number of other important functions. Apart from acting as a signal for protein synthesis, it is the precursor for cysteine and other reactions in which methyl groups are made available to the metabolism. In donating its methyl group, methionine forms homocysteine, which can be reformed to methionine using a single carbon group, derived either from serine or betaine (a breakdown produce of choline). Homocysteine is a branch point in metabolism as it also has another important fate, the formation of cysteine and taurine. In these pathways, the sulphydryl group is transferred to the carbon skeleton of serine. Thus, serine is used for the further metabolism of homocysteine, down either pathway. Increased amounts of homocysteine in the circulation are associated with increased risk of cardiovascular disease.

Fig 4.5 There is a complex system of inter-organ co-operation for many aspects of amino acid metabolism and the partitioning of different functions between organs is of critical importance for effective metabolic control. Arginine is formed in significant amounts in both liver and kidney, but that formed in the liver goes to urea formation in general, whereas that formed in the kidney is exported and available for the needs of the rest of the body in, for example, the generation of nitric oxide. Arginine is formed from citrulline in the kidney, with the citrulline being derived from the gastrointestinal tract, where its formation is linked to the utilization of glutamine. Glutamine itself is formed in large amounts in muscle, in part from the breakdown of the branched-chain amino acids, leucine, isoleucine and valine. The branched-chain amino acids coming from dietary protein are, as a group, handled in a special way; following absorption they tend to pass through the liver without being metabolized and are preferentially taken up by the muscles.

has an alternative metabolic fate, towards the formation of cysteine. In this pathway, the sulfhydryl group derived from methionine is made available to a molecule of serine with the formation of cysteine; the carbon skeleton derived from methionine is subsequently oxidized. Cysteine is the precursor for taurine, which, with glycine, is required for the formation of bile salts from bile acids. Thus, cysteine can be formed in the body provided there is sufficient methionine and serine available. However, the pathway

for cysteine formation has not fully matured in the newborn, making cysteine a conditionally essential amino acid at this time.

For some amino acids, the pathway for their formation appears complex and tortuous, involving a complex pathway that is shared between a number of tissues. The renal formation of arginine is an example (see Fig. 4.5). Arginine is the precursor of nitric oxide, which has important metabolic functions as a neurotransmitter, in maintaining peripheral vascular tone and is one of several oxidative radicals formed during the oxidative burst of leukocytes. Arginine is also the direct precursor of urea, the main form in which nitrogen is excreted from the body. Arginine is formed in two main sites, the kidney and the liver. Arginine formed in the kidney is available for the rest of the body, whereas that formed in the liver is cleaved to urea and ornithine in the urea cycle. In both locations the arginine is made from citrulline, but whereas in liver the citrulline is generated locally in the mitochondria, in kidney it is imported. The imported citrulline has been formed in the gastrointestinal tract, one of the end products of the oxidation of glutamine. The glutamine itself has been generated in muscle from the branched-chain amino acids. During digestion and absorption of the amino acids taken in protein in a meal, most are first taken up by the liver, but more of the branched-chain amino acids pass directly through the liver and are taken up preferentially by muscle, where they give rise to glutamine. This complex pattern of metabolic interchange enables control to be exerted, and in particular creates a mechanism through which two important sets of metabolic interaction of arginine are separated, and therefore can be controlled independently.

Other amino acids, such as glycine, are required as the building blocks for more complex compounds in relatively large amounts (haemoglobin and other porphyrins, creatine, bile salts and glutathione), but the pathways that enable the formation of large quantities of the amino acid are not clear.

It has generally been considered that the carbon skeleton of the indispensable amino acids cannot be formed at all in the body. However, recent evidence shows that colonic bacteria synthesize these amino acids for their own use, with some being available to the host in amounts that may be physiologically useful.

In a number of inborn errors of metabolism, the enzymes involved in the oxidation of amino acids do not function normally, and there is considerable accumulation of an amino acid or its breakdown products. The extent to which the body can tolerate an excess of any single amino acid might vary, but almost always sustained, high, increased levels of amino acids in the body exert toxic effects. Therefore, the body goes to some lengths to maintain very low levels. The catabolic pathways for individual amino acids are active, although the activity may decrease on very low protein intakes. For the indispensable amino acids in particular, the amounts of individual amino acids usually found in diets are in excess of the usual requirements. This may be the reason why the body has not selected to maintain the pathways for their formation. The dietary requirement for the indispensable amino acids determines the minimal physiological requirement for protein and has been used for defining protein quality, protein requirements and the recommendations for protein for populations. For the dispensable amino acids, the body is able to tolerate larger amounts of the amino acid, but also control can be exerted at two levels—the rate of formation and the rate of oxidation—and therefore toxicity may be less likely. On a daily basis, for a person in balance, an equivalent amount of protein or amino acids is oxidized as it is taken in the diet. Therefore, for a person consuming 80 g protein each day, the equivalent of 80 g of amino acids will be oxidized to provide energy, with the amino group going to the formation of urea. Thus, the proportion of total energy derived from protein each day is similar to the relative contribution of protein to the energy in the diet.

4.15 Nitrogen balance

On average, about 16% of protein is nitrogen, and therefore by measuring the nitrogen (e.g. by the Kjeldahl method) and multiplying it by 6.25, the approximate protein content of a food or tissue can be obtained. Nitrogen balance identifies the overall relationship between the nitrogen removed from the environment for the body and the nitrogen returned to the environment. The intake is almost completely dietary, mainly as protein, but also in part as other nitrogen-containing compounds, such as nucleic acids, and creatine in meat. Nitrogen can be lost from the body through a number of routes, but 85–90% is lost in urine and 5–10% in stool, with skin and hair or other losses making up the remainder. Nitrogen is lost as soluble molecules in urine as urea (85%), ammonia (5%), creatinine (5%), uric acids (2–5%), and traces of individual amino acids or proteins. There may be large losses of nitrogen through unusual routes in pathological situations (e.g. through the skin in burns, as haemorrhage or via fistulae).

$$B = I - (U + F + other) \text{ g nitrogen/day}$$

where B = nitrogen balance, I = nitrogen intake, U = urinary nitrogen and F = faecal nitrogen.

The achievement of nitrogen balance in response to a change in either intake or losses is brought about largely by a change in the rate at which urea is excreted in the urine. A reduction in the dietary intake of protein is matched by an equivalent reduction in the urinary excretion in urea, which returns nitrogen equilibrium within 3–5 days. Faecal losses of nitrogen on habitual intakes are usually 1–2 g nitrogen/day, or about one-tenth of the intake. However, faecal nitrogen may increase considerably on diets that are rich in non-starch polysaccharides or fibre. There is then a reduction in the excretion of urea in urine equivalent to the increase in faecal nitrogen. Increased cutaneous losses, through excessive sweating, exudation or burns, are associated with a proportionate decrease in urinary urea.

In a system that is constantly turning over, the retention of body protein is a necessary condition for maintaining the integrity of the tissues and tissue protein. Any limitation in the availability of energy or a specific nutrient will lead to a net loss of tissue and negative nitrogen balance through increased losses of nitrogen. Thus, the major control over the protein content of the body is established by modifications in the rate at which nitrogen is lost from the body. Balance is re-established by a change in the rate of nitrogen excretion, which for most part means a change in the rate at which urea is excreted. Therefore, it is important to consider in some detail factors that might exert control or influence over the formation and excretion of urea.

4.16 Urea metabolism and the salvage of urea nitrogen

Urea is formed in the liver in a cyclical process on a molecule of ornithine (see Fig. 4.6). Within the mitochondrion, carbamyl phosphate (from ammonia and carbon dioxide) condenses with ornithine to form citrulline. The citrulline passes to the cytosol where a further amino group is donated from aspartic acid, with the eventual formation of arginine (which has three amino groups). This is hydrolysed with the formation of urea and the regeneration of ornithine. Urea is lost to the body by excretion through the kidney. In the kidney, urea fulfils an important physiological role in helping to generate and maintain the concentrating mechanism in the countercurrent system of the loops of Henle. The rate of loss of urea through the kidney is influenced by the activity of the hormone vasopressin on the collecting ducts. Urea is reabsorbed from urine in the collecting duct, so nitrogen is potentially retained in the system. Under all normal circumstances, more urea is formed in the liver than is excreted in the kidney. About one-third of the urea formed passes to the colon where it is hydrolysed by the resident microflora. About one-third of the nitrogen from urea released in this way is returned directly to urea formation, but the other two-thirds are incorporated into the nitrogen pool of the body, presumably as amino acids. In other words, urea-nitrogen has been salvaged. There are specific urea transporters in the collecting duct that are up-regulated on low-protein diets. Similar transporters exist in the colonocyte leading to coordinated regulation of increased retention of urea in the kidney with increased movement of urea into the colon.

In situations where the body is trying to economise on nitrogen, the proportion of urea-nitrogen lost in the urine is decreased, and the proportion salvaged through the colon is increased. This happens when the demand for nitrogen for protein synthesis increases, as in growth, or when the supply of nitrogen

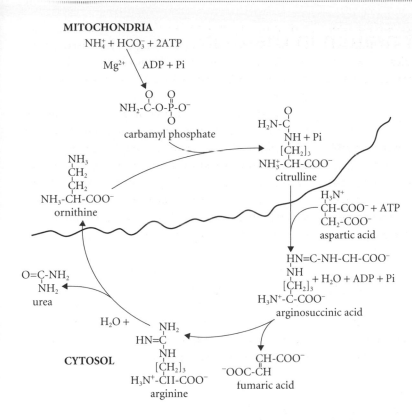

MITOCHONDRIA

$NH_4^+ + HCO_3^- + 2ATP$

Mg^{2+} \ $ADP + Pi$

carbamyl phosphate

ornithine

citrulline

aspartic acid

urea

arginosuccinic acid

CYTOSOL

arginine

fumaric acid

Fig. 4.6 The urea cycle. Urea is formed in the liver in a cyclical process between the mitochondria and the cytosol. A molecule of ornithine and the synthesis of a molecule of carbamyl phosphate from ammonia and CO_2 is the starting point with the ultimate formation of arginine, which is hydrolysed to reform ornithine and a molecule of urea. The cycle utilizes three molecules of ATP for each revolution.

is reduced, as on a low-protein diet. In situations of very rapid growth, in early infancy or during catch-up from wasting conditions, the salvage of urea-nitrogen may reach very high levels, compared with the dietary intake. In normal adults, increased salvage is seen as the intake falls from habitual levels of intake (around 75–80 g protein/day) to a protein intake around the minimum requirement (35–40 g/day). On the lower protein intake, balance is maintained by a reduction in the rate of urea excretion and an increase in urea-nitrogen salvage. Below this level of protein intake, nitrogen balance is not maintained, urea excretion increases and salvage falls. Thus, a central part of adapting to low-protein diets is an enhancement of the salvage of urea-nitrogen. In this way, nitrogen may be retained within the system in a functionally useful form.

The optimal intake of protein is likely to be that which provides appropriate amounts of the different amino acids to satisfy the needs of the system. There is no evidence that the ingestion of large amounts

of protein in itself confers any benefit. Indeed, the system may be stressed by the need to catabolize the excess amino acids that cannot be directed to synthetic pathways and have to be excreted as end products. High-protein intakes increase renal blood flow and glomerular filtration rate. In individuals with compromised renal function, this may increase the risk of further damage.

4.16.1 Low-protein therapeutic diets

The two clinical situations in which control of protein intake and metabolism are of considerable potential importance are renal failure and hepatic failure. In hepatic failure, there is a limitation in the liver's ability to detoxify ammonia through the formation of urea. In renal failure, the ability to excrete the urea is impaired. In each situation, reduction of the intake or modification the metabolism of protein or amino acids is an important part of treatment.

4.17 The nature of protein in the diet

The majority of foods are made of cellular material and therefore in the natural state contain protein. Processing of foods may alter the amounts and relative proportions of some amino acids, for example the Maillard reaction and browning reduces the available lysine (its ε-amino group forms a bond with sugars that cannot be digested). The pattern of amino acids in animal cells is similar to the pattern in human cells and therefore the match for animal protein foods is good; plant materials may have very different patterns of amino acids. This difference has in the past lead to the concept of first-class and second-class proteins, for animal and plant foods, respectively. However, diets are hardly ever made up of single foods. In most diets, different foods tend to complement each other in their amino acid pattern, so any potential imbalance is likely to be more apparent than real for most situations. Thus, the mixture of amino acids provided in most diets matches the dietary requirements for normal humans fairly well.

4.18 How much protein do we need?

4.18.1 From obligatory losses

One approach is to measure the losses of nitrogen on a protein-free diet adequate in energy. Urinary nitrogen (mostly urea) decreases rapidly for the first 5 days and then settles at a new low level. For adults, the 1973 committee of the Food and Agriculture Organization (FAO) and World Health Organization (WHO) estimated:

- urine loss: 37 mg/kg
- faecal loss: 12 mg/kg
- skin loss: 3 mg/kg
- miscellaneous loss: 2 mg/kg.

This gives a total of 54 mg × 6.25, which is 0.34 g protein/kg/day.

This is an average requirement, so the recommended daily intake (RDI) (+2 standard deviations) should be 0.44 g protein/kg or 29 g protein for a 65 kg adult.

However, this assumes an impossible 100% efficiency of metabolizing dietary protein and empirically it is not possible to achieve equilibrium nitrogen balance on 29 g protein/day. When protein intake is reduced, the many enzymes of amino acid catabolism rapidly decline in activity. Metabolic conditions for absorbed amino acids are far from normal in protein starvation. However on an ordinary diet they are actively oxidizing and transaminating the amino acids. Thus, although the factorial method using obligatory losses is useful for some other essential nutrients with simple metabolism, it cannot provide us realistic requirement numbers for protein.

4.18.2 From nitrogen balance

International and national recommendations for protein intake are based on this method. If protein intake is insufficient, the nitrogen balance is negative (below zero or equilibrium balance). However, above an adequate protein intake the balance becomes negative for a few days, if protein intake is changed from high-adequate to moderate-adequate. This has to be allowed for by testing at intakes near the expected requirement and allowing about 5 days for adjustment at each intake level. Nitrogen balance experiments need much attention to detail. Nitrogen intakes tend to be overestimated (people do not swallow every last crumb) and nitrogen losses tend to be under-estimated (some urine may be spilt; skin losses are very difficult to measure). The energy intake must neither be too much nor too little because any deviation moves the balance more positive or more negative, respectively.

Rand *et al.* (2003) selected well-designed balance experiments in healthy adults in several different countries. The protein intake was at two or more levels and near the expected requirement; each intake was for 10–14 days and only the last 5 days were used for calculating the balance. Energy intake was based on the subjects' usual diets. The subjects needed to have a quiet and unvarying life during the experiments and they lived in a special metabolic unit.

The amount of protein for nitrogen equilibrium in 235 subjects in ten studies was estimated by meta-analysis to be 105 mg nitrogen/kg/day ($\times$ 6.25 = 0.65 g protein/kg/day). However, this is an estimated average requirement (EAR). For the RDI, 2 standard deviations were added (and here the numbers were available, not estimated) giving 132 mg nitrogen/kg or ($\times$ 6.25) 0.83 g protein/kg. For someone who weighs, say, 65 kg this is 54 g protein per day. The protein should be of good quality, that is not too low in any of the indispensable amino acids.

4.18.3 Amino acid requirements

The indispensable (or essential) amino acids are not all present in the same amounts in body tissues; individual tissues differ in amino acid pattern and in turnover rates (which also affect requirements). Our foods also have different amino acid patterns and those near to the pattern of human requirements of indispensable amino acids have the best nutritive or biological value.

The first estimates of amino acid requirements by W.C. Rose (in men) (1957), R.M. Leverton and others (in women) and S.E. Snyderman (in infants) in the 1950s used nitrogen balances. The adult subjects were usually college graduate students in the USA. They had to eat a diet of pure corn starch and sugar and syrup, butter and oil, made into wafers or pudding, plus vitamin tablets and mineral salts. Instead of dietary protein they were given a mixture of pure L-amino acids. They were also allowed a little apple or grape juice (very low in protein), and lettuce

Table 4.2 Early and recent estimates of essential amino acid requirements of healthy human adults (mg/kg/day)

	N balance method (1)	^{13}C amino acid oxidation method (2)
Isoleucine	10	19
Leucine	14	42
Lysine	12	38
S-amino acids	13	19
Phenylalanine	14	33
Threonine	7	20
Tryptophan	3.5	5
Valine	10	24
	83.5	200

(1) Joint FAO/WHO (1973) Energy and Protein Requirements.
(2) Food & Nutrition Board, Institute of Medicine (2002).

and carrot. Average adult requirements from nitrogen balances are in Table 4.2.

In subsequent years researchers have reasoned that these requirements (from Rose, 1957) are too low. They add up to only 5.5 g, yet essential amino acids make up one-third to half the total amino acids in dietary proteins and 11–17 g protein would be quite inadequate. There were technical problems with the experiments. Rose's subjects received more dietary energy than expected. In the women's experiments, balance did not always reach equilibrium and nitrogen losses in skin were not taken into account.

Young and collaborators (1999) estimated essential amino acid requirements by an ingenious approach —biochemical evidence of increased oxidation of an indictor amino acid, labelled with the stable isotope ^{13}C, when intake of the test amino acid is below requirement (the indicator amino acid oxidation method; see Table 4.2).

When one essential amino acid is inadequate, protein synthesis using all the amino acids is impaired, so there is both increased oxidation of all amino acids and increased urea production, increased urinary nitrogen and negative nitrogen balance. In these stable isotope experiments, the diet also consists of protein-free starch and sugar, fat and oil in cookies with multivitamins and minerals. The L-amino acids are given in a mixture, providing the expected requirement of all essential amino acids and also non-essential amino acids. Only the intake of the test essential amino acid is varied. Typically each experiment lasts 7 days, each subject is tested at three levels of the test amino acid. On day 7, the ^{13}C-labelled indicator amino acid (e.g. leucine) is given by constant intravenous infusion over 24 hours and ^{13}CO$_2$ is collected and measured to indicate oxidation of the indicator amino acid. These experiments are very expensive and require gas chromatography mass spectrometry.

The Institute of Medicine (2002) has accepted the amino acids in the right-hand column of Table 4.2 in its dietary reference intake report for macronutrients. To grade the amino acid pattern of dietary proteins, either this pattern can be used or the amino acid pattern of whole hen's egg (which has the highest biological value of all the dietary proteins). These two amino acid patterns are similar when compared at the same total of essential amino acids.

4.19 How much protein do we eat?

The amount of protein eaten each day is determined by the total food intake and the protein content of the food. In general the proportion of energy derived from protein is between 11% and 15% of the total energy of the diet, which is generous for all normal purposes.

Fig. 4.7 shows the estimated amount of food available to different populations around the world on average. There is a twofold difference overall between the technologically developed countries and the underdeveloped countries. The protein available from non-meat sources is very similar for all countries, around 50 g protein/head/day, varying by less than ±10% for the extremes. In contrast, the protein available from meat sources varied tenfold between the extremes. Virtually all of the variation in protein availability between different countries was determined by the availability of meat protein. Within a population there are differences among individuals in the amount of protein taken. To a large extent this will be determined by the total food intake. Fig. 4.8 shows the relationship between protein intake and energy intake amongst a group of young women vegetarians. The proportion of energy derived from protein was similar for each woman. Those who were most active had the greatest intake of energy and the highest protein intake. Those who were relatively sedentary had a protein intake that approached the maintenance level.

In young children, energy expenditure per unit body weight is high, and therefore energy intake per unit body weight is high. In consequence, as a proportion of total energy, the dietary protein requirement for normal growth is relatively low. For example, for an infant weighing 10 kg at 1 year of age and growing at a normal rate, for an energy intake of 95 kcal/kg/day and a protein requirement of 1.5 g/kg/day, the proportion of total energy coming from protein would

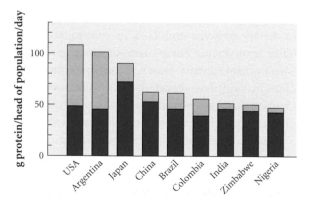

Fig. 4.7 The amount of protein available to the population can be assessed (g protein/head of population/day) and divided into meat protein (▨) and non-meat protein (■). For countries of widely different characteristics, the availability of non-meat protein falls within a narrow range (within ±10%) whereas the availability of meat protein varies widely, over a tenfold range.

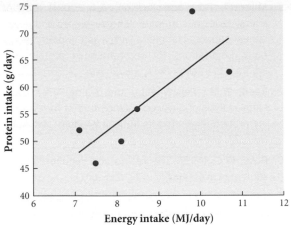

Fig. 4.8 Under most normal circumstances, the total food intake of a person is determined by their energy expenditure, which sets their energy requirement. The energy requirement consists of a reasonably fixed component, basal metabolic rate (BMR), and a variable component, which is determined primarily by the level of physical activity. The protein content of most diets provides between 10% and 15% of dietary energy and therefore the total protein intake is closely related to the total energy intake and hence the level of physical activity. MJ, megajoules.

be 6.3%. The highest relative requirement for protein is in sedentary individuals. For example, for a 70-year-old woman who weighs 80 kg, who is lying relatively immobile in bed, the proportion of total energy coming from protein would have to be 20%, which is not readily achievable on a normal diet.

4.20 Dietary protein deficiency and protein-deficient states

For the diets consumed by most populations, the intake of protein is adequate, provided that the overall intake of food is not limited (e.g. by inactivity or unavailability). However, for some diets in which the density of protein to energy is low, and/or where the quality of amino acids is low, there may be situations related to relative inactivity when the ability to satisfy the protein intake is marginal.

Protein-deficient states, where the content of protein in the body is reduced, are most likely to be the result of:

- an increase in demand (e.g. in infection or stress);
- an increase in losses (e.g. with haemorrhage, burns or diarrhoea); or
- a failure of the conservation systems (e.g. with impairment of urea salvage in the colon).

In correcting the deficient state, it is as important to remove the underlying cause as it is to provide adequate amounts of protein or amino acids in the diet. For the effects of protein-energy malnutrition in children, see Chapter 18.

4.21 Imbalance

In the midst of famine, severely undernourished people have a poorer appetite, take longer to mobilize oedema fluid, and are more likely to die when the protein content of their diet is similar to that consumed in western Europe or North America than when they are given a diet that is unusually low in protein (Collins *et al.*, 1998). In seriously shocked and traumatized individuals, intravenous protein in the form of albumin is associated with higher mortality (Cochrane Injuries Group Albumin Reviewers, 1998). Pregnant women given protein-dense diets give birth to smaller babies, and pre-term infants provided with high-protein diets may have poor brain development. Proteins are consumed in the diet as a source of amino acids and nitrogen—essential for life—but when the pattern of consumption is only a poor fit for the needs of the body, the imbalance can lead to serious ill health.

FURTHER READING

1. **Borgonha, S., Regan, M., Oh, S.-H., Condon, M., and Young, V.R.** (2002) Threonine requirement of healthy adults, derived with a 24-hour indicator amino acid balance technique. *Am J Clin Nutr*, **75**, 698–704.

2. **Brosnan, J.T.** (2001) Amino acids, then and now—a reflection on Sir Hans Krebs' contribution to nitrogen metabolism. *IUBMB Life*, **52**, 265–70.

3. **Cochrane Injuries Group Albumin Reviewers** (1998) Human albumin administration in critically ill patients: systematic review of randomized controlled trials. *Br Med J*, **317**, 235–40.

4. **Collins, S., Myatt, M., and Golden, B.** (1998) Dietary treatment of severe malnutrition in adults. *Am J Clin Nutr*, **68**, 193–9.

5. **Food and Nutrition Board, Institute of Medicine** (2002) *Dietary reference intakes for energy, carbohydrate, fiber, fat, fatty acids, cholesterol, protein and amino acids (macronutrients)*. Washington, DC, National Academy Press.

6. **Jackson, A.A.** (1998) Salvage of urea nitrogen in the large bowel: functional significance in metabolic control and adaptation. *Biochem Soc Trans*, **26**, 231–6.

7. **Millward, D.J., and Jackson, A.A.** (2004) Protein/energy ratios of current diets in developed and developing countries compared with a safe protein/energy ratio: implications for recommended protein and amino acid intakes. *Public Health Nutr*, **7**, 387–405.

8. **Rand, W.M., Pellett, P.L., and Young, V.R.** (2003) Meta-analysis of nitrogen balance studies for estimating protein requirements in healthy adults. *Am J Clin Nutr*, **77**, 109–27.

9. **Rose, W.C.** (1957) The amino acid requirements of adult man. *Nutr Abst Rev*, **27**, 631–647.

10. **Scrimshaw, N.S., Waterlow, J.C., and Schurch, B.** (1996) Energy and protein requirements. Proceedings of an IDECG workshop. *Eur J Clin Nutr*, **50**, S119–S185.

11. **Stewart, G., and Smith, C.P.** (2005) Urea nitrogen salvage mechanisms and their relevance to ruminants, non-ruminants and man. *Nutr Res Rev*, **18**, 49–62.

12. **Waterlow, J.C.** (1999) The mysteries of nitrogen balance. *Nutr Res Rev*, **12**, 25–54.

13. **Young, V.R., and Ajami, A.** (1999) The Rudolf Schoenheimer Centenary Lecture. Isotopes in nutrition research. *Proc Nutr Soc*, **58**, 15–32.

 To see topical and scientifically robust updates on nutrition associated with this textbook, and active web links to many of the journal articles in the Reference areas, please see the dedicated Online Resource Centre at www.oxfordtextbooks.co.uk/orc/mann3e/.

Energy

Andrew M. Prentice

Energy is the primary currency of nutrition. Mammals require energy to stay warm, and to drive all the processes of life itself. All of this energy is derived from the chemical combustion of food, a process requiring oxygen and producing carbon dioxide and water. It is the need to maintain an adequate supply of energy that is the major stimulus of food intake, and this appetite drive has an important influence on the intake of all other nutrients.

In humans, dietary energy is derived from four major food types: carbohydrate, fat, protein and alcohol. These are termed macronutrients and each can be composed of numerous subtypes that have a slightly different energy content. Generation of energy from the various macronutrients requires different chemical processes, and for each of them there are optional pathways that can be used in different metabolic circumstances. For instance, glucose can initially be utilized by muscle without oxygen (anaerobically) when a short burst of movement is required, or with oxygen (aerobically) for longer periods of activity. Ultimately all energy is derived through the process of oxidative phosphorylation that occurs in mitochondria. The biochemical pathways involved in these processes are summarized elsewhere (e.g. Cox, 2005). This chapter outlines the energy value of foods and how they may be calculated, and summarizes human energy needs and how these can be measured. It concludes by briefly summarizing the mechanisms by which energy balance is regulated.

5.1 The energy value of food

5.1.1 Chemical energy

The chemical energy of food is simply the total amount of energy that would be liberated by the food if it were combusted in oxygen (i.e. its heat of combustion). This can be measured directly in a bomb calorimeter whereby the heat liberated by burning a small sample of the food is accurately recorded. This total chemical energy of food is also referred to as its *gross energy* (GE).

5.1.2 Metabolizable energy

A portion of the GE of food is unavailable for human metabolism for a variety of reasons. First, not all of it can be digested and absorbed by the body (e.g. some components of dietary fibre, or the central parts of hard grains and nuts) and the energy will be lost in faeces. The proportion of GE that is actually absorbed across the digestive tract is termed *digestible energy* (DE). Secondly, even this DE is not fully available to

Table 5.1 Example of measuring the metabolizable energy of a diet

Subjects	
• Young women	
Methods	
• Provision of a diet of known composition over 7 days in a metabolic suite	
• Bomb calorimetry of duplicate portions of the diet and of all faeces and urine	
Measured values	
• Duplicate portions of diet	(a) 9900 kJ/day
• Faeces	(b) 710 kJ/day
• Urine	(c) 420 kJ/day
Derived values	
• Gross energy of food (a)	9900 kJ/day
• Digestible energy (a − b)	9190 kJ/day
• Digestibility coefficient [100(a − b)/a]	92.8%
Metabolizable energy (a − b − c)	8770 kJ/day

4.184 kJ = 1 kcal

the body because a number of the oxidative pathways are incapable of proceeding to completion. These are mostly confined to protein metabolism. For instance, amino acids are only oxidized as far as urea or ammonia. These compounds still contain energy, which is lost in the urine, and for which it is necessary to make a final adjustment in order to calculate the actual energy available for metabolism, known as *metabolizable energy* (ME).

5.1.3 Methods for assessing metabolizable energy intake

When very precise values are required in experimental studies of energy metabolism, it is possible to make direct measurements of ME, though this is extremely tiresome for the subjects and investigators alike. The method requires the accurate collection of duplicate portions of all foods consumed in proportion to the amount of each component of the diet that was eaten. Each food can then be analysed separately by bomb calorimetry or the whole diet can be homogenized together and a small aliquot of the homogenate measured. The same process must be performed for all the faeces and urine collected throughout

the period that the diet is eaten. Table 5.1 gives an example of the calculations used.

The ME of diets can also be calculated if the composition of the diet is accurately known. The

Table 5.2 Example of calculating the metabolizable energy of a diet

Subjects		
• Young women		
Methods		
• Weighed food records over 7 days		
• Food composition tables		
• Use of Atwater factors		
– carbohydrate	17 kJ/g	
– fat	37 kJ/g	
– protein	17 kJ/g	
– alcohol	29 kJ/g	
Derived values		
• Carbohydrate	245 g/day	4165 kJ/day
• Fat	90 g/day	3330 kJ/day
• Protein	75 g/day	1275 kJ/day
• Alcohol	0 g/day	0 kJ/day
Metabolizable energy		8770 kJ/day

composition can be obtained by chemical analysis of foods, or most frequently by reference to tables of food composition, which themselves have been derived from chemical analysis of a wide range of commonly consumed foods. Many countries have their own food tables reflecting their national diet. Once the macronutrient composition of a food or diet is known, the energy content is computed using standard conversion factors (see Table 5.2). These were first derived by W O. Atwater (and hence are frequently referred to as Atwater factors) in a series of experiments with human volunteers in which the conversion factors from GE to DE to ME were determined. It should be stressed that ME values of diets derived from food tables are somewhat imprecise since there may be variations in the actual composition of listed foods, and because the Atwater factors are approximate values derived from people consuming a 'standard' Western diet. It should be noted that the conversion factor for carbohydrates refers to the amount of carbohydrate in a food when expressed as available monosaccharides since dietary fibre and non-starch polysaccharides have a lower digestibility.

5.2 Measurement of energy expenditure

The ability to measure human energy expenditure has been important in many aspects of nutritional science, ranging from very precise studies into how energy balance is regulated, to large-scale estimations of the energy needs of populations. There are numerous techniques available each of which has advantages and disadvantages. It is important carefully to match the technique used to the situation at hand. Table 5.3 summarizes the major methods and lists their key features.

Table 5.3 Methods for measuring human energy expenditure

Method	Measurement principle	Advantages	Disadvantages	Applications
Direct calorimetry				
Whole-body chamber	Subject confined within a small-to-moderately sized chamber. Measures heat loss.	Historically had faster response time than indirect calorimetry (now no longer true). Good environment for strictly controlled studies.	Extreme technical complexity. Very high construction and running costs. Studies confined to small subject numbers. Artificial environment.	Initially used to validate the principle of indirect calorimetry. Some distinct applications in studying heat dynamics of exercise. Now largely obsolescent.
Body suit	Subject wears an insulated metabolic suit. Measures heat loss.	As above.	As above.	As above.

Table 5.3 (*cont'd*)

Method	Measurement principle	Advantages	Disadvantages	Applications
Indirect calorimetry				
Whole-body chamber	Subject confined within a small-to-moderately sized chamber. Measures oxygen consumption (and frequently also measures CO_2 production). Calculates EE from energy equivalence of oxygen consumed. Calculates macronutrient oxidation from RQ after adjustment for urinary nitrogen losses.	Very precise and repeatable. Provides minute-by-minute data. Measurements over 1–14 days. Good environment for strictly controlled studies. Measures macronutrient oxidation rates in addition to total EE. Represents gold standard.	Technically challenging. High production and running costs. Studies confined to relatively small subject numbers. Artificial environment.	Fundamental studies of the mechanisms regulating human energy balance. Includes effects of exercise, diet, physiological states such as pregnancy, and pharmacological effects of compounds intended to affect energy expenditure.
Bedside methods	Supine subject has Perspex hood placed over their head or entire bed covered with a plastic tent. Measures oxygen consumption (and frequently also measures CO_2 production). Calculations as for whole-body indirect calorimetry.	Accurate and reliable data. Commercially available versions with integrated gas meters, computers and display systems. User-friendly. Measurements possible over several hours. Good for measuring BMR. Can measure macronutrient oxidation rates in addition to total EE.	Relatively expensive. Requires periodic calibration.	Short-term studies of energy expenditure such as BMR or diet-induced thermogenesis. Can be used with hospital patients.
Ventilated hood methods	As for bedside methods but subjects can be standing (e.g. on cycle ergometer).	As above.	As above.	As above, and for exercise studies.
Douglas bag method	Subject wears mouthpiece with one-way valve and nose clip. Collects expired air directly into an impermeable 'Douglas' bag then measures volume and gas	Simple and robust. Provides reliable results. Inexpensive.	Prompt analysis required after gas collection to avoid gas leakages and diffusion. Only suitable for short periods of study.	Short-term studies of EE such as BMR or diet-induced thermogenesis. Can be used for ambulatory studies of

Table 5.3 (*cont'd*)

Method	Measurement principle	Advantages	Disadvantages	Applications
	concentrations of bag contents. Calculations as for whole-body indirect calorimetry.		Inconvenient and uncomfortable for subjects. Interferes with normal activity.	work and exercise. Can be used with hospital patients.
Ambulatory methods	Subject wears mouthpiece with one-way valve and nose clip, or ventilated mask, and carries gas analysis 'respirometer' strapped to their back. Measures oxygen consumption. Calculations as for whole-body indirect calorimetry but usually without CO_2 measurement and hence RQ.	Smaller and more compact than Douglas bag method. Relatively simple and robust. Yields reliable results.	Discomfort to subject after prolonged wearing of apparatus. Some versions require separate analysis of gas concentrations. Some versions are expensive.	Useful for studies of light to moderate physical activity in near-to-natural conditions.
Stable isotope methods				
Doubly labelled water	Assesses CO_2 turnover from differential rate of disappearance of ^2H and ^{18}O. Calculates EE from CO_2 production and an assumption about RQ.	Gold standard method for assessing habitual EE in free-living subjects. Measurements over 10–20 days.	^{18}O isotope is very expensive. High capital investment for mass spectrometer. Technically and mathematically challenging. Requires certain assumptions that can lead to errors if not correctly applied.	Studies of free-living EE in all subjects. Especially valuable for use in children as minimal subject cooperation is required.
Labelled bicarbonate	Assesses CO_2 turnover from rate of disappearance constantly infused ^{13}C bicarbonate. Calculates EE from CO_2 production and an assumption about RQ.	Requires no cumbersome apparatus except for a mini-pump to infuse the bicarbonate. Can assess expenditure over a shorter time frame than doubly labelled water.	High capital investment for mass spectrometer. Technically and mathematically challenging. Requires certain assumptions that can lead to errors if not correctly applied.	Especially applicable in clinical studies where a shorter time frame is required.

Table 5.3 (*cont'd*)

Method	Measurement principle	Advantages	Disadvantages	Applications
Heart-rate monitoring	Electrodes collect minute-by-minute heart-rate data and store on computer chip. EE can be calculated from individual calibration curves generated for each subject, or unconverted data can be used in a semi-quantitative manner.	Inexpensive and easy to use for both subject and investigator. Provides minute-by-minute data over periods of 7 days or greater.	Calibration of each subject is a cumbersome and time-consuming process. Can become tiresome to subjects if worn for long periods.	Generally used for large-scale epidemiological studies where comparative values are more important than absolute expenditure values (for instance in studies of activity levels and health).
Movement sensors	Sensors collect minute-by-minute movements of the body and store on computer chip. EE can be calculated from individual calibration curves generated for each subject, or unconverted data can be used in a semi-quantitative manner.	As above.	As above.	As above.
Time-and-motion studies and factorial method	Daily activities are recorded by subjects themselves or by an observer. EE calculated by reference to standard tables for the energy cost of activities.	Very inexpensive if subjects record their own activities. Provides good data on types of activities.	High subject burden if self-recording. May cause alteration in activity patterns to simplify recording.	Many applications. For instance, has frequently been used (with fieldworkers doing the recording) to study work and activity patterns among farmers etc. in developing countries.

EE = energy expenditure, RQ = respiratory quotient, BMR = basal metabolic rate.
Full details of all techniques can be found in: Murgatroyd *et al.* (1993).

5.2.1 Direct calorimetry

Principle Direct calorimetry, as the name implies, directly measures the *heat loss* from a subject. The first such study was conducted during a Parisian winter over two centuries ago by the father of energy metabolism, Antoine Lavoisier, when he measured the amount of water melted by a guinea pig kept in a small chamber surrounded by ice. By knowing the specific heat of melting ice, he was able to compute the heat liberated by all the metabolic processes within the animal.

Equipment Modern human direct calorimeters employ the same principle but use complex thermo-couple sensors and heat exchangers to measure the subject's radiative heat loss (heat lost through radia-tion as from any hot object), conductive heat loss (heat carried away by air passing over the skin and warming as it does so) and evaporative heat loss (heat lost as the specific heat of evaporation of perspira-tion). This can be achieved in a chamber ranging in size from just large enough to cover a man on a cycle ergometer to a moderately sized room. Attempts were also made to use an insulated body suit, but this proved too cumbersome. Direct calorimeters are extremely difficult and expensive to construct. Their main function has been to demonstrate that indirect calorimetry (which measures *heat production*; see below) gives precisely the same answers. There is a slight lag period between heat production and heat loss due to the temporary storage of heat in the body (for instance, when exercising a subject will become hot and some of the heat produced will take some minutes to exit the body as it cools down again). However, as long as time lag is accounted for, the two methods give precisely the same result. Because of the technical complexity of direct calorimeters, no more than a handful are still in commission worldwide.

5.2.2 Indirect calorimetry

Principle Indirect calorimetry measures *heat produc-tion* by assessing oxygen consumption and (option-ally) carbon dioxide production. Variations between different versions of the technique essentially come down to the method by which the exhaled respiratory gases are collected from the subject (see Table 5.3). In one form or another, indirect calorimetry is now the usual method for measuring human energy ex-penditure. It is much easier to perform than direct calorimetry and is less expensive. It can also be used to estimate the relative contribution of each of the macronutrients to the total energy expenditure—a major advantage over direct calorimetry.

Table 5.4 lists the basic constants used to calcul-ate energy expenditure by indirect calorimetry. The most important of these are the energy equivalence of each litre of oxygen consumed, which ranges between 19.48 kJ/L for protein and 21.12 kJ/L for carbohydrate —a difference of 8%. However, the body rarely com-busts single macronutrients and for most practical purposes it can be assumed that it is combusting a mixture of fuels, similar to the diet that a person

Table 5.4 Constants used in indirect calorimetry

	Fat	Carbohydrate[1]	Protein	Alcohol
Oxygen consumption (L/g)	2.101	0.746	0.952	1.461
Carbon dioxide production (L/g)	1.492	0.746	0.795	0.974
Respiratory quotient	0.710	1.000	0.835	0.667
Energy equivalence of oxygen (kJ/L)	19.61	21.12	19.48	20.33
Energy density (kJ/g)	39.40	15.76	18.55	29.68

[1]As monosaccharide equivalents.

is consuming, and therefore a generalized value of 20.3 kJ/L oxygen is frequently used. In most circumstances, this assumption will lead to an error of less than 3%. To achieve a greater accuracy, as would be required for detailed physiological studies of human energy regulation, it is necessary also to measure carbon dioxide production to calculate the *respiratory quotient* (RQ = carbon dioxide produced/oxygen consumed) and the urinary nitrogen output in order to estimate protein oxidation. If alcohol has been consumed, it is further necessary to estimate its contribution to energy expenditure by making separate measurements of the rate of decline of blood alcohol levels. Once all these variables are known, it is possible to use the precise values for the energy equivalence of oxygen.

Indirect calorimetry can be used to assess the mixture of fuels oxidized as follows. First, since protein and alcohol oxidation can be assessed as described above, it is possible to calculate their contributions to a subject's total oxygen consumption and carbon dioxide production using the values in Table 5.4. The remaining gas exchange is due to carbohydrate and fat oxidation and can be expressed as the non-protein, non-alcohol RQ (frequently termed the non-protein RQ (NPRQ) since most measurements are made in the absence of alcohol consumption). The following equation shows that the RQ for carbohydrate (glucose) oxidation is precisely 1.0 since 1 mole of carbon dioxide is liberated for each mole of oxygen consumed:

$$C_6H_{12}O_6 + 6O_2 = 6CO_2 + 6H_2O + heat$$

A similar calculation can be performed for fatty acid oxidation (e.g. palmitic acid, $C_{16}H_{34}O_2$) and reveals that the average for different fats yields an RQ of 0.701 (see Table 5.4). Thus, if the NPRQ is calculated to be 1.00, then only carbohydrate is being combusted, and if it is 0.701 then only fat is being combusted. Values between these indicate that a mixture of fat and carbohydrate is being combusted, the proportions of which can be calculated from nomograms or simultaneous equations. These are the basic principles. In practice there are many complexities to the calculations and many special circumstances

when adjustments must be made in order to obtain correct estimates. Readers interested in applying the techniques are referred to more advanced texts, such as that by Livesey and Elia (1988).

Equipment Table 5.3 lists the various types of equipment that can be used for indirect calorimetry, together with their major advantages and disadvantages.

The classic (now rarely used) method uses the Douglas bag (see Fig. 5.1). This is a large bag (usually with a 100-litre volume) that is impermeable to gases. The subject wears a nose clip and breathes through a mouthpiece connected to a one-way valve that allows them to inhale fresh air and exhale into the bag. At the end of the experiment—which has to be short (up to 15 minutes) because of limited capacity in the bag—the volume of expired air is measured with a gas meter. The oxygen and carbon dioxide contents are analysed. Oxygen consumption is calculated from the difference between oxygen in the ambient (inspired) and expired air, multiplied by the ventilation rate.

For short-term measurements during exercise, the Kofrani–Michaelis respirometer used to be used (see Fig. 5.1) because it measures expired air volume as it is produced, and therefore only a small sample of the expired air needs to be retained for subsequent gas analysis. New generations of these machines with similar working principles include the Oxylog and Cosmed K2. These portable respirometers were designed for short-term measurements at rest and during exercise in 'field' situations but can also be used in laboratory settings.

Ventilated hood systems (see Fig. 5.1) avoid the discomfort of a face mask. With this equipment, air flows over the subject's head (which is within a transparent Perspex or plastic hood) while they lie or sit quietly. The system is suited for situations in which the subject's gas exchange is measured in a laboratory or hospital setting for periods of between 30 minutes and several hours. There are a number of commercially available ventilated hood systems specially designed for use in a hospital setting.

Whole-body calorimeters (also called respiration chambers) represent the most sophisticated option and are chiefly used for detailed physiological

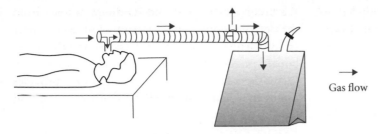

The Douglas bag

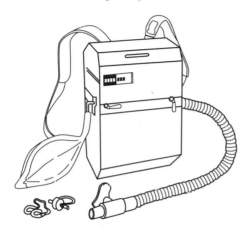

The Kofrani–Michaelis respirometer

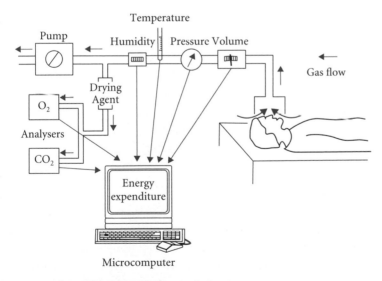

A ventilated-hood indirect calorimeter

Fig. 5.1 Most commonly used devices for indirect calorimetry.

Source: Garrow and James (1993)

experiments. Whole-body calorimeters are furnished airtight rooms (frequently about 10–15 m³) in which subjects can live for periods of 1–14 days. Respiratory gas exchange is measured continuously using small samples of air drawn from the inlet and outlet vents of the chamber. Subjects can carry out all the activities of a relatively sedentary life, as well as controlled exercise on a cycle ergometer or treadmill. Food and drink are passed in through one airlock and waste products out through another. Whole-body calorimeters are extremely accurate and precise.

5.2.3 Isotopic tracer methods

Doubly labelled water method

Principle The disadvantage of the methods described above is that none of them can capture information on the total habitual energy expenditure of someone living their normal life. In the mid-1980s it became possible to do this using the doubly labelled water ($^2H_2{}^{18}O$) method (see Speakman and Nagy 1997).

The principle of the method is illustrated in Fig. 5.2. The subject drinks an accurately weighed amount of water labelled with the harmless, non-radioactive isotopes of deuterium (^2H) and oxygen-18 (^{18}O) and then provides a series of saliva or urine samples for the next 10–20 days (the optimal duration depends on their activity level). These are analysed by mass spectrometry to assess the disappearance of the isotopes from the body (see Fig. 5.3). The ^2H labels

the body's water pool and its disappearance from the body (k_2) provides a measure of water turnover (rH_2O). The ^{18}O labels both the water and the bicarbonate pools, which are in rapid equilibrium with each other. The disappearance of ^{18}O (k_{18}) provides a measure of the combined turnover of water and

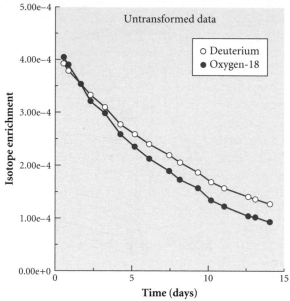

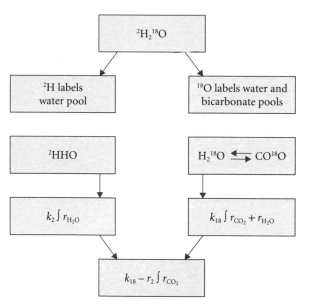

Fig. 5.2 Principle of the doubly labelled water. Production rates are represented by *r* and rate constants (calculated from the slope of the isotope disappearance curves shown in Fig. 5.3) are represented by *k*.

Source: Murgatroyd *et al.* (1993)

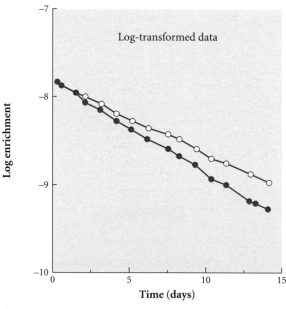

Fig. 5.3 Examples of isotope disappearance curves from the doubly labelled water method.

Source: Murgatroyd *et al.* (1993)

bicarbonate ($rH_2O + rCO_2$). Therefore, bicarbonate turnover can be calculated by difference ($k_{18} - k_2$) and is equivalent to the subject's carbon dioxide production rate. The value $k_{18} - k_2$ is represented by the difference in slope between the two isotope disappearance curves shown in Fig. 5.3. Carbon dioxide production can be converted to energy expenditure using classical indirect calorimetric calculations.

In practice, there are many theoretical and mathematical complications in the technique, but these can be overcome by using appropriate procedures and the method has been cross-validated against energy expenditure measured within a whole-body chamber. It is now recognized as the gold standard method for assessing total energy expenditure (TEE) in free-living people. By combining it with an assessment of basal metabolic rate (BMR), it becomes possible to estimate the energy costs of activity and thermogenesis (A&T = TEE – BMR) and as thermogenesis represents a small and rather constant proportion of A&T, in practice it provides a good measure of a person's activity level.

Equipment Doubly labelled water measurements require a mass spectrometer to analyse the levels of ^{2}H and ^{18}O. Because ^{18}O is so costly, it is necessary to use very small amounts that only raise the subject's levels a little above the natural background level. Hence, the mass spectrometer has to be extremely precise and the measurements are technically challenging. There are only a few specialist centres worldwide with the capacity to do the measurements and computations.

Labelled bicarbonate method

Principle The principle of the labelled bicarbonate method is similar to the doubly labelled water method insofar as it assesses carbon dioxide production from the rate of turnover of the body's bicarbonate pool. In the labelled bicarbonate method, this is achieved through a constant subcutaneous infusion of ^{13}C-labelled bicarbonate using a minipump strapped to the subject. As with doubly labelled water, samples of urine or saliva can be used to assess ^{13}C levels, which reach a steady state at a level proportional to the rate at which the subject's carbon dioxide production washes out the infused label. The method is suitable for relatively short-term assessments of up to about 24 hours and is ideally suited for use in hospitalized patients. In practice, however, this method has been rarely used.

Equipment The method requires a mass spectrometer capable of assessing ^{13}C enrichment.

5.2.4 Heart rate methods

Principle There is a linear relationship between energy expenditure and heart rate for all levels of expenditure above resting levels. The slope and intercept of this relationship vary among individuals according to age, sex and fitness levels, so must be determined in each person by a calibration experiment using a treadmill or cycle ergometer in which heart rate can be measured at different work rates. Once this is known, it is possible to convert records of a person's heart rate into an estimate of TEE. The method has been validated within whole-body calorimeters and shown to have little bias, and hence is excellent for assessing group values. However, its precision is limited to about ±1 MJ per day. It should be noted that heart rate traces can provide very reliable assessments of activity patterns and of inter-individual differences without actually having to convert the output into energy expenditure. This is true also of the actometers described below.

Equipment There are various commercially available ambulatory heart rate monitors that can be worn by a subject for long periods and that collect minute-by-minute data on a computer chip. These data can be uploaded straight into software that computes energy expenditure.

5.2.5 Movement sensors (actometers)

Principle The principle of actometers is very similar to that for heart rate but a measure of movement in three dimensions (so called 'tri-axial') is substituted for heart rate. Modern actometers are an advance over simple instruments such as pedometers because they can capture movement in all directions and can assess the intensity of movement. As with heart rate, it is necessary to calibrate each individual against an alternative indirect calorimetric procedure in order to calculate energy expenditure.

Equipment There are a number of commercially available ambulatory actometers that operate in a similar way to heart rate monitors by accumulating minute-by-minute data over periods of up to a week.

5.2.6 Time-and-motion studies

Principle Frequently it is desirable just to obtain a relatively rough-and-ready estimate of peoples' energy expenditure, for instance to estimate a population's average energy requirements. Time-and-motion studies (often called activity diaries) can be used for this purpose. If subjects are literate, they can be asked to record their own activity patterns over short intervals (e.g. 5 or 15 minutes) throughout the day. It is necessary to have illiterate subjects followed and observed by trained field workers. Each activity is then ascribed an energy cost from standard tables. It will be appreciated that there are many approximations involved in such a process and it also carries a high burden for the subjects that can lead to inaccurate record keeping. In its most approximate form, this sort of calculation is used by the World Health Organization (WHO) and Food and Agriculture Organization (FAO) in their system for calculating the estimated average requirements of a population (FAO/WHO/UNU, 2004; James and Schofield, 1990).

Equipment The method only requires record sheets, a watch and tables of the energy cost of different activities.

5.3 Human energy needs

The body's energy needs can be divided into three main components: basal metabolism, diet-induced thermogenesis and physical activity. Children, or adults recovering from illness and weight loss, require additional energy for the growth of new tissue, and pregnant and lactating women require additional energy to sustain the growth of their offspring.

5.3.1 Basal metabolism

Definition Basal metabolism represents the energy required to sustain the basic processes of life, which include breathing, circulation, tissue repair and renewal, and ionic pumping. In humans, basal metabolism generally produces enough heat to maintain thermoregulation without any need to specifically generate additional heat. In most people (except the very active), basal metabolism is the largest component of daily energy expenditure, representing up to 70% of all energy used.

Measurement BMR is a specific term that describes energy expenditure measured under the following highly standardized conditions: subjects should be lying completely still and should be emotionally relaxed immediately after waking in the morning; they must have fasted for the previous 12–14 hours and must not have performed heavy physical activity on the previous day; they must be healthy and free from fever; and the measurement must be made at thermoneutral temperature. The great advantage of applying such standardized conditions is that it permits comparisons among individuals and among different studies. Measurements made under similar conditions, but not quite meeting all of the above stipulations, are frequently referred to as resting metabolic rate. BMR is most frequently measured using a ventilated hood system but can also be assessed easily as part of a whole-body calorimetry protocol. The results as kJ/minute are frequently multiplied up over 24 hours and expressed as MJ/day. Because BMR is relatively predictable on the basis of a subject's age, sex, weight and height, a number of predictive equations are available from which a reasonable approximation on a person's BMR can be obtained without having to measure it

Table 5.5 Equations for estimating BMR from body weight*

Age Years	No.	BMR: MJ/day	SEE	BMR: kcal/day	SEE
Males					
<3	162	0.249 kg − 0.127	0.292	59.512 kg − 30.4	70
3–10	338	0.095 kg + 2.110	0.280	22.706 kg + 504.3	67
10–18	734	0.074 kg + 2.754	0.441	17.686 kg + 658.2	105
18–30	2879	0.063 kg + 2.896	0.641	15.057 kg + 692.2	153
30–60	646	0.048 kg + 3.653	0.700	11.472 kg + 873.1	167
≈ 60	50	0.049 kg + 2.459	0.686	11.711 kg + 587.7	164
Females					
<3	137	0.244 kg − 0.130	0.246	58.317 kg − 31.1	59
3–10	413	0.085 kg + 2.033	0.292	20.315 kg + 485.9	70
10–18	575	0.056 kg + 2.898	0.466	13.384 kg + 692.6	111
18–30	829	0.062 kg + 2.036	0.497	14.818 kg + 486.6	119
30–60	372	0.034 kg + 3.538	0.465	8.126 kg + 845.6	111
≈ 60	38	0.038 kg + 2.755	0.451	9.082 kg + 658.5	108

*Weight is expressed in kg.
SEE, standard error of the estimate.
Source: FAO/WHO/UNU (2004).

(Table 5.5) (FAO/WHO/UNU, 2004; James and Schofield, 1990).

Factors affecting basal metabolism An individual's BMR is largely determined by their body size and body composition, and differences in these variables can explain the fact that women have a lower BMR than men, and that BMR declines with age. The major determinant of BMR is the amount of lean tissue (often referred to as lean body mass (LBM) or fat-free mass since this is much more metabolically active than adipose tissue. BMR is therefore frequently expressed per kg LBM. Muscle is the major contributor to lean tissue, and in its resting basal state it has a moderately high energy expenditure. Visceral organs, especially the heart and liver, have an even higher metabolic rate, and hence the total basal metabolism is determined also by the composition of the lean tissue in terms of the proportion of muscle to visceral organ mass. On average, women have a lower BMR than men because they are smaller and, even if matched for weight, they have a lower proportion of lean tissue than men. Older people have a lower BMR because ageing is associated with a gradual substitution of lean tissue by fat. BMR is high in children largely because they have a higher proportion of visceral organ mass to total mass.

BMR declines when people are in negative energy balance. There are two components to this decline. The first is a decrease (of up to 20%) in the metabolic rate per kg LBM; this is an adaptive mechanism to spare energy in starvation and is mediated by alterations in thyroid status. The second is due to the fact that LBM itself declines with longer-term energy deficiency. There has been considerable controversy for over a century as to whether BMR is increased when people over-consume energy, and whether this constitutes a homeostatic mechanism ('adaptive thermogenesis') for stabilizing body weight. The current consensus, based on detailed whole-body calorimeter studies and doubly labelled water measurements is that such a mechanism does not exist, and that any increases in BMR can be accounted for by the increase in lean tissue mass that occurs with over-feeding.

BMR also changes as women pass through the various phases of reproduction and it even alters by a few per cent during the menstrual cycle. In pregnancy, BMR increases in proportion to the amount of new tissue accrued by the mother in the form of the fetus, placenta and uterus. In thin women and in those short of food in pregnancy, BMR is suppressed in the early stages of gestation; this appears to be an adaptation to help women reproduce in marginal conditions.

Certain stimulants (e.g. caffeine) and pharmacological agents (e.g. ephedrine) also affect BMR. Drug companies have been trying to develop compounds that will increase metabolic rate as possible anti-obesity agents (e.g. through stimulating the β3-adrenoreceptors) but so far they have either had minimal effects in humans or have had unacceptable side effects on heart rate or blood pressure.

Certain clinical conditions also affect BMR, especially fevers. Alterations in thyroid function can have a pronounced effect on BMR: hypothyroidism decreases BMR and hyperthyroidism increases it. Before specific hormone assays were available, measurements of BMR were widely used in the diagnosis of thyroid disorders.

5.3.2 Diet-induced thermogenesis

Definition Diet-induced thermogenesis (DIT), often also called the thermic effect of food, represents the additional energy required to absorb, digest, transport, interconvert and store the constituents of a meal. This is wasted energy that must be lost because no physiological process can be 100% efficient. It amounts to under 10% of total intake.

Experimental approach DIT is usually measured using a ventilated hood. With subjects resting, fasting energy expenditure is first measured for a short period in order to establish their baseline. Then they are fed a standard test meal and remain under the hood for a further 3–4 hours. Energy expenditure increases as the body processes the meal and then declines back to the initial baseline. DIT is assessed as the incremental area under the curve for energy expenditure.

Factors affecting diet-induced thermogenesis DIT is affected by the size and composition of the meal consumed. Protein tends to cause a higher DIT than fat and carbohydrate, though in practice these differences are trivial within the normal range of the mixed diets consumed by humans.

5.3.3 Physical activity

Definition Energy expenditure caused by movements or performing physical work is generally classified under the overall heading of physical activity. This includes both conscious movements and subconscious ones (fidgeting).

Experimental approach The energy expended on standardized activities, such as walking at a fixed pace on a treadmill or cycling on a cycle ergometer, can be measured by Douglas bag, or a portable respirometer or in a whole-body chamber. Everyday activities are usually measured using a portable respirometer and in the past these have been used for numerous studies of occupational physical activity, such as farming, factory work and coal mining. Tables have been compiled that summarize these values, together with values for the energy costs of the everyday activities of life, and these can be used to make an approximation of a person's total energy expenditure (FAO/WHO/UNU, 2004; Dunnin and Passmore, 1967). The energy cost of activities are usually expressed as kJ/minute, or as a multiple of BMR (termed the physical activity level (PAL)). The advantage of the latter is that it makes an automatic internal adjustment for differences between subjects of different weights, sexes and ages, since these variables are already factored into the BMR.

Factors affecting the energy costs of physical activity Clearly the total cost of physical activity is largely dependent on the amount of activity a person chooses to undertake. Within this, the specific cost of the individual activities will be influenced by the person's size, the speed of the activity, the times taken resting, the skill with which the activity is performed and the efficiency of the muscles. Perhaps surprisingly, the efficiency with which muscles can convert food energy (glucose and fatty acids) into useful work is very constant among individuals and averages only about 25%.

The energy cost of weight-bearing activities such as walking up stairs or uphill is directly proportional to a person's bodyweight, but in non-weight-bearing activities such as cycling a person's bodyweight has less influence on the overall energy cost.

Differences in physical activity represent the major source of variability in the energy needs of different people. At the lowest end of the range are the bed-bound sick and the very elderly. These will have a PAL of about $1.35 \times$ BMR. At the other end of the range are elite endurance athletes such as Tour de France cyclists who can sustain PAL values of almost $3 \times$ BMR. People in the developing world who are engaged in hard physical labour, for instance at the peak of the farming season, sustain activity levels equivalent to about $2 \times$ BMR. In modern society where sedentary occupations are combined with very inactive leisure time pursuits such as TV viewing, the average PAL is around $1.55 \times$ BMR. Children tend to have spontaneously high levels of energy expenditure (often up at about $1.8 \times$ BMR) that decline as they go through puberty, especially in girls.

5.3.4 Growth

Maintaining an adequate energy intake is essential at times of growth, and energy deficiency leads to stunting, wasting and ultimately to severe malnutrition (see Chapter 18). In fact, in humans the marginal energy costs of growth (i.e. over and above the other daily energy needs) are surprisingly small because human growth is extraordinarily slow—an evolutionary adaptation that allows plenty of time for the growth, organization and training of our large brain. Growth is fastest in the fetus, the very young neonate and during the adolescent growth spurt, but even at these periods the energy required for normal growth rarely exceeds 5% of the daily energy need.

Faster tissue deposition rates than these can occur in people recovering from a severe illness, from severe childhood malnutrition or from starvation. These very rapid rates are often accompanied by an inappropriate composition of new tissue with a higher proportion of fat tissue than is desirable. Generally these deviations in body composition are corrected naturally after several months of weight stability. Growing children may also show episodic growth, particularly those in developing countries who are frequently affected by infections. During the recovery phase after an illness, children can have very high energy needs. These are often not met by poor-energy and protein-deficient diets in developing countries, leading to a gradual falling away from optimal growth rates and nutritional status.

5.3.5 Pregnancy and lactation

The marginal extra energy costs of pregnancy and lactation are also quite low in humans due to the slow growth of the offspring. In pregnancy, a mother requires only around 10% extra energy, and in lactation only about 25% (see Chapter 30 for more detail). There is good evidence that when women are short of energy they display a range of energy-sparing mechanisms, both metabolic and behavioural, that can help ensure the success of reproduction.

5.4 Mechanisms for regulating energy balance

Energy balance is a dynamic state that constantly alters between positive deviations during meals and negative deviations during the intervals between meals. The challenge for the body is to ensure that these small deviations cancel out over time (except during periods of intentional growth when a slight positive energy balance is required). This regulation is achieved largely in the hypothalamus, which receives a wide range of neural and endocrine signals from the rest of the body; it integrates these through a complex network of interacting neural pathways. The hypothalamus then sends efferent neural signals to regulate appetite and energy expenditure. The short-term signals indicating energy sufficiency include blood glucose, amino acid and fatty acid levels, together with stomach- and gut-derived hormones, and vagal signals from the liver. The long-term signals consist of hormones secreted by adipose tissue in proportion to the amount of fat that is stored there. Primary among these is leptin. Plasma concentrations of leptin are directly proportional to fat stores, but are also strongly influenced by the direction of change in the fat stores. Leptin acts as the body's fuel gauge, allowing the brain to assess its energy reserves and their rate of change and hence it plays a vital role in regulating appetite and energy expenditure, tissue growth, reproduction and various other physiological processes.

It used to be thought that differences in energy expenditure were major determinants of a person's energy balance. For instance, over several decades there was a popular theory that obese people must have extraordinarily efficient metabolisms and low energy requirements. In the reverse direction, it was thought that many weight-losing clinical conditions such as AIDS and Alzheimer's disease were caused by a hypermetabolism that raised energy needs. Studies using the doubly labelled water method have now shown that there is little truth in these theories and that most deviations in energy balance can be traced to differences in food intake. Most differences in energy expenditure can be adequately explained by differences in age and reproductive state, body size, body composition and physical activity levels. There is, however, some flexibility in the efficiency of energy expenditure, particularly in times of weight loss or starvation when metabolic rate can decline by about 20%.

This realization that most of the regulation of energy balance is achieved on the intake side of the energy balance equation has had a profound impact on research in the field, and there has been astonishing progress over the past decade in understanding the neurohormonal regulation of appetite. There is still much to be learnt about how these longer-term regulatory mechanisms modulate the influence of short-term internal appetite cues (such as low glucose levels or surges in the appetite-stimulating hormone, ghrelin) and external appetite cues (such as the sight and smell of food or advertising). Nonetheless, these advances hold great promise for the development of therapeutic compounds to assist in the treatment of conditions such as obesity and anorexia nervosa.

FURTHER READING

1. **Blaxter, K.** (1989) *Energy metabolism in animals and man*. Cambridge, Cambridge University Press.

2. **Cox, S.** (2005) Energy: Metabolism. In: Caballero, B., Allen, L.H., and Prentice, A.M. (eds) *Encyclopedia of human nutrition*, 2nd edition. London, Elsevier, pp. 106–14.

3. **Durnin, J.V.G.A., and Passmore, R.** (1967) *Energy, work and leisure*. London, Heinemann.

4. **FAO/WHO/UNU** (2004) *Human energy requirements. FAO Technical Report Series 1*. Rome, Food and Agricultural Organization.

5. **Garrow, J.S., and James, W.P.T. (eds)** (1993) *Human nutrition and dietetics*, 9th edition. Edinburgh, Churchill Livingstone.

6. **James, W.P.T., and Schofield, E.C.** (1990) *Human energy requirements: A manual for planners and nutritionists*. Oxford, Oxford University Press.

7. **Livesey, G., and Elia, M.** (1988) Estimation of energy expenditure, net carbohydrate utilization, and fat oxidation and synthesis by indirect calorimetry: evaluation of errors with special reference to the detailed composition of fuels. *Am J Clin Nutr*, **47**, 608–28.

8. **Murgatroyd, P.R., Shetty, P.S., and Prentice, A.M.** (1993) Techniques for the measurement of human energy expenditure: a practical guide. *Int J Obesity*, **17**, 549–68.

9. **Speakman, J.R., and Nagy, K.** (1997) *Doubly-labelled water: Theory and practice*. Amsterdam, Kluwer Academic.

6 Alcohol

Stewart Truswell

Alcohol is the only substance that is both a nutrient and a drug that affects brain function. For chemists there are many alcohols, but in day-to-day parlance, in the pub or bar, and in this chapter, 'alcohol' is used to mean ethyl alcohol (ethanol), C_2H_5OH. Other nutrients can have minor and subtle effects on brain function. A hungry person's behaviour can change after a satisfying meal without alcohol. Coffee contains the nutrient niacin, but the mental stimulant in coffee is another substance, caffeine.

Alcohol is normally consumed not in a pure form (neat) but in aqueous solution, in alcoholic beverages that were first developed thousands of years ago. Beer was first drunk by the Sumerians and Babylonians, around 4000 BC, and has been brewed ever since. Wine is mentioned occasionally in the *Old Testament* (Genesis 9 in which Noah planted a vineyard and got drunk), and was important in the life of classical Greece and Rome. It featured in Jesus' first miracle at the marriage feast in Cana and at his last supper, and passed into the central part of the Christian mass. Alcoholic beverages were also developed in prehistoric times in East Asia (e.g. saké fermented from rice) and in Africa (beers from fermented millet or maize). Alcoholic beverages were thus independently discovered in different parts of the world by prehistoric sedentary agriculturalists who were growing barley, rice or grapes. However, the indigenous peoples of Oceania (the Polynesians and Australian Aborigines) and of America (American Indians) did not know about alcohol until the arrival of the Europeans, and had not established ways of using and controlling it.

From the basic fermented beverages, alcohol can be concentrated by the process of distillation (which was brought to Europe by the Arabs). Brandy and whisky first appeared in the fifteenth century.

6.1 Production of alcoholic beverages

Alcohol is produced by alcoholic fermentation of glucose. The specific enzymes are provided by certain yeasts, the Saccharomyces, which are unicellular fungi. The biochemical pathway first follows the usual ten steps of anaerobic glycolysis to pyruvate, as in animal metabolism (Chapter 2). Yeast contains the enzyme pyruvate decarboxylase, which is not present in animals. This converts pyruvate to acetaldehyde. Then alcohol dehydrogenase converts acetaldehyde to ethanol (the reverse of its role in humans). The overall reaction is:

$$C_6H_{12}O_6 + \text{cofactors} + ATP \rightarrow 2\ C_2H_5OH + 2CO_2$$

The cofactors include NADH, thiamin pyrophosphate and magnesium.

Grapes are unusual among fruits in containing a lot of sugar, nearly all glucose (around 16%), and so

Table 6.1 Successive stages of acute alcohol intoxication

Blood alcohol concentration (g/dL)	Stage	Effects
Up to 0.05	Feeling of well-being	Relaxed, talks a lot
0.05–0.08	Risky state	Judgement and finer movements affected
0.08–0.15	Dangerous state	Slow speech, balance affected, eyesight blurred, wants to fall asleep, likely to vomit, needs help to walk
0.2–0.4	Drunken stupor	Dead drunk, no bladder control, heavy breathing, unconscious (e.g. deep anaesthesia)
0.45–0.6	Death	Shock and death

provide an excellent substrate for alcoholic fermentation. Starch is a polymer of glucose. Before it can ferment to alcohol, it has to be hydrolysed to its constituent glucose units. Beers are made by malting the starch in barley. To do this, the barley is spread out, moist and warm, and allowed to germinate for several days. Enzymes are generated in the sprouting grain and these break down the stored starch into glucose. The barley is then heated and dried, which kills the embryo, which stops using sugar. For saké, a different process is used to break down the rice starch. It is first treated with a mould, *Aspergillus oryzae*, that grows on the rice and secretes an amylase to hydrolyse the starch.

Beer contains around 5% alcohol (unless it is alcohol-reduced), wines contain around 10% alcohol (unless they are fortified) and spirits are about 30% alcohol. Alcoholic beverages also contain variable amounts of unfermented sugars and dextrins (in beers), small amounts of alcohols other than ethyl (e.g. propyl alcohol), moderate amounts of potassium, almost no sodium, small amounts of riboflavin and niacin, but no thiamin, and sometimes vitamin C. They also contain a complex array of flavour compounds, colours (e.g. in red wines), phenolic compounds, a preservative such as sodium metabisulphite, and sometimes additives. A standard drink, such as one pint of beer (see Table 6.1), provides 10 g of ethanol.

6.2 Metabolism of alcohol

Ethanol is readily absorbed unchanged from the jejunum. It is one of the few substances that is also absorbed from the stomach. It is distributed throughout the total body water (moving easily through cell membranes), so that after having one drink its 10 g of alcohol is diluted in about 40 L of water in an adult, giving a peak concentration of 0.025 g/dL in the blood and in the rest of the body water. For comparison, the permitted limit of blood alcohol for driving in many countries is double this, 0.05 g/dL (11 mmol/L) and the driving limit varies from 0.02 g/dL in Sweden to 0.08 g/dL in the British Isles (Fig. 6.1). Alcohol is nearly all metabolized in the

liver, but a small amount is already metabolized as it passes through the stomach wall (first-pass metabolism). A small amount of alcohol passes unchanged into the urine, and an even smaller (but diagnostically useful) amount is excreted in the breath.

There are three possible pathways for alcohol metabolism in man. The major pathway in most people starts with alcohol dehydrogenase (ADH), a zinc-containing enzyme in the cytoplasm of the liver (Box 6.1). The ADH step is the rate-limiting step in alcohol metabolism. ADH occurs in slightly different forms, and some individuals have more active ADH than others. It seems a little surprising that humans

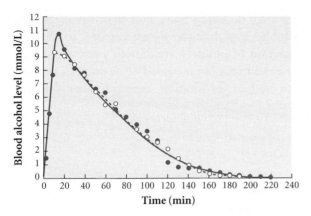

Fig. 6.1 Blood alcohol concentrations in a healthy young Caucasian man who took 0.3 g pure ethanol/kg body weight in orange juice, drunk rapidly and followed by a 4.4 MJ mixed meal (○ and ● are duplicate determinations). Ethanol was measured by gas chromatography.

BOX 6.1

$$CH_3CH_2OH + NAD \rightarrow CH_3CHO + NADH + H^+$$

Ethanol   ADH   Acetaldehyde

BOX 6.2

$$CH_3CH_2OH + NAD + H_2O \rightarrow CH_3COOH + NADH + H^+$$

Acetaldehyde   ALDH   Acetic acid

---

naturally possess this enzyme for dealing with beer and wine, to which our hunter–gatherer ancestors were not exposed. However, some alcohols are produced naturally inside the body by fermentation in the large intestine (e.g. small amounts of methyl alcohol from pectin) and they also occur in over-ripe fruits. The next step is conversion of acetaldehyde to acetate by aldehyde dehydrogenases (ALDHs), which are present in the cytoplasm, mitochondria and microsomes (Box 6.2). In most people, there is no build up of acetaldehyde, but nearly 50% of Chinese and Japanese people lack the mitochondrial ALDH, so after moderate intake of ethanol, their blood acetaldehyde increases. This causes facial flushing and headaches.

In long-term heavy drinkers, the microsomal ethanol-oxidizing system (MEOS) with cytochrome P450 becomes a second important route for alcohol metabolism. The microsomes proliferate (are induced) in heavy drinkers. As with ADH, ethanol is converted to acetaldehyde. A third minor pathway for conversion of ethanol to acetaldehyde is via catalase in peroxisomes.

On average, people can metabolize about 5 g of ethanol per hour (i.e. half a standard drink). The rate varies about twofold among individuals. Alcohol absorption can be slowed by having a meal (or even milk) in the stomach, but there is no agent that increases the rate of alcohol metabolism. Smaller people are likely to have smaller livers and therefore metabolize less alcohol per hour. Women on average have smaller livers than men, a lower percentage of total body water (in which to distribute the alcohol), and also have less first-pass gastric alcohol dehydrogenase, so that they are less tolerant of alcohol than men. East Asian people may suffer from headaches and flushing at quite low intakes of alcohol because of acetaldehyde accumulation. This may limit their intake.

A drug used to control alcohol addiction, disulfiram (Antabuse) antagonizes ALDH. People taking it experience unpleasant symptoms when they have a drink (such as headache, nausea and flushing) as a result of acetaldehyde accumulation.

6.3 Effect of alcohol on the brain

Pharmacologists classify ethanol as a central nervous system depressant, in the same group as general anaesthetics. With increasing levels of blood alcohol, people pass through successive stages of alcohol intoxication (Table 6.1).

At the biochemical level, alcohol affects a number of neurochemical processes simultaneously. The following have all been reported: decreased levels of cyclic AMP and cyclic GMP, inhibition of voltage-sensitive calcium channels, increased intracellular calcium, increased GABA (γ-aminobutyric acid) activity and decreased glutamate. Ethanol increases cell membrane fluidity.

Ingestion of alcohol has effects in other systems of the body. There is peripheral vasodilation and increased heart rate. The imbiber may feel warm but may be losing more heat than usual. Alcohol inhibits hypothalamic osmoreceptors, so there is secretion of pituitary antidiuretic hormone, which causes diuresis (an increased urine output), and this can lead to dehydration, especially after drinking spirits.

6.4 Energy value of ethanol

The gross chemical energy of ethanol can be measured outside the body in a bomb calorimeter, and the value is between the energy value of carbohydrates and that of fat, about 30 kJ or 7.1 kcal/g.

However, in a metabolic ward, with food intakes strictly controlled, Lieber (1992) replaced 50% of subjects' energy (calorie) intake by isocaloric amounts of ethanol (they had been accustomed to high alcohol intakes). Instead of gaining weight, they lost weight. Free-living heavy drinkers are not usually overweight. It appears that above a certain intake, ethanol provides less than 7 kcal/g. Alcohol increases the basal metabolic rate (thermogenesis) and it is thought that metabolism of alcohol by liver microsomes yields less energy than the ADH route.

In heavy drinkers, 10–30% (or more) of energy intake comes from alcohol, but alcoholic beverages contain no protein and very few micronutrients, so this nutrient-poor source of calories displaces other foods that normally provide essential nutrients. Appetite may be suppressed in heavy drinkers, either because of alcoholic gastritis or by associated smoking. Alcohol dependency is an important cause of conditioned (or secondary) nutritional deficiency—the drinker may have access to enough foods and their nutrients but is not eating them. Nutrients that are typically depleted in alcoholics include thiamin, folate, niacin and several inorganic nutrients (see below).

6.5 Direct consequences of alcohol intake

6.5.1 Acute intoxication

Acute intoxication can lead to road and other accidents, or domestic and other violence. Intoxicated people can suffer a range of injuries. Occasionally people consume such a large dose of alcohol that they die with lethal blood levels. The breathalyser was developed to reduce road traffic accidents. In many countries, a driver stopped at random by a police check who has a breathalyser reading corresponding to a blood level of 0.05 g/dL has his driver's licence suspended. This measure has reduced traffic accidents and contributed to the decline of alcohol consumption in a number of developed countries.

> **BOX 6.3 Different patterns of alcohol consumption**
>
> - The inexperienced drinker (e.g. an adolescent) who misjudges the dose and has an accident.
> - The person who doesn't drink during the week but drinks to excess and gets drunk on payday or Saturday night (one-night binge).
> - The person who enjoys a controlled one or two drinks most days.
> - The person who has too many drinks each day (most after work) or more or less maintains their (increasingly inefficient) usual life.
> - The person who drinks very heavily for weeks.

6.5.2 Hangovers

The excess intake of alcohol the night before may not yet have all been cleared from the blood. Dehydration may be present from diuresis and, with some drinks (e.g. brandy), toxic effects of higher alcohols contribute to the symptoms.

6.5.3 Chronic alcoholism

Some people become dependent or addicted to alcohol and cannot face the world unless they have some alcohol in their blood throughout the day. Thus, they maintain an intake of alcohol per day larger than their liver's capacity to metabolize it.

6.5.4 Alcohol withdrawal syndrome

Alcohol addicts who have maintained some alcohol in their blood continuously for weeks or even longer suffer withdrawal symptoms if an accident or illness abruptly removes them from their alcohol supply. There are tremors of the hands, anxiety, insomnia and tachycardia. Epileptic convulsions can occur and in severe cases there is agitation, mental confusion and hallucinations. This is delirium tremens, a severe illness.

6.5.5 Binge drinkers

One-night binge drinkers expect to get drunk. Men imbibe 80 g of alcohol (4 pints of beer) or more and women somewhat less.

The other pattern of alcohol excess is that a person starts drinking heavily and goes on for weeks. Consequently, as alcohol displaces much of the usual food intake, there can be an acute deficiency of micronutrients with the smallest reserve in the body, usually thiamin (see Wernicke–Korsakoff syndrome, p. 94).

6.6 Medical consequences of excess consumption

6.6.1 Liver disease

Alcohol causes three types of liver damage. The least severe is fatty liver. Metabolism of large amounts of ethanol in the liver produce an increased ratio of NADH/NAD, which depresses the citric acid cycle and oxidation of fatty acids, and favours triglyceride synthesis in the liver cells. It used to be thought that the fatty liver was due to an associated nutritional deficiency but fatty liver has been observed (using needle biopsy of the liver) in volunteers who took a moderately large intake of alcohol but with all nutrients provided under strictly controlled conditions in hospital. The symptoms of fatty liver are not striking; on abdominal examination a doctor can feel that the liver is somewhat enlarged.

Alcoholic hepatitis (inflammation of the liver) is more serious. This type is not caused by a virus but by prolonged excess alcohol intake. There is loss of appetite, fevers, tender liver, jaundice and elevation in the plasma of enzymes produced in the liver (e.g. aminotransferases (transaminases), γ-glutamyl transpeptidase and alkaline phosphatase).

Alcoholic cirrhosis may be associated with chronic alcoholism. When the liver has to metabolize large amounts of alcohol over a long time, membranes inside the cells become disordered and mitochondria show ballooning. In its fully developed form, irregular strands of fibrous tissue criss-cross the liver, replacing damaged liver parenchymal cells. These effects may be due to acetaldehyde or to free-radical generation by neutrophil polymorph white cells in the liver. Cirrhosis seems to occur in people who have managed to consume large amounts of alcohol over many years but carry on a reasonably regular life and were able to eat and to afford the alcohol. The amount of alcohol needed to cause cirrhosis is difficult to establish exactly because many people understate their alcohol consumption, especially heavy drinkers. It is greater than 40 g of ethanol/day in women and

50 g/day in men over years, usually much more. Not all cases of chronic hepatitis and cirrhosis are caused by alcohol excess. Some are caused by hepatitis viruses (B or C).

6.6.2 Metabolic effects

Moderate regular drinkers who are apparently well tend to have increased plasma triglycerides (an over-flow from the overproduction of fat in the liver). Plasma urate is raised because of reduced renal excretion, probably due to increased blood lactate, which follows alcohol ingestion.

6.6.3 Fetal alcohol syndrome

Women who drink alcohol heavily during pregnancy can give birth to a baby with an unusual facial appearance (small eyes, absent philtrum, thin upper lip), prenatal and postnatal growth impairment, central nervous system dysfunction and often other physical abnormalities. Mothers of children with the fetal alcohol syndrome were heavy drinkers during their pregnancy and most were socially deprived. More moderate drinkers may have babies that are small for dates but otherwise normal. Some authorities insist that pregnant women should avoid all alcohol, but in a careful prospective study in Dundee, Scotland, Sulaiman *et al.* (1988) found that, after adjustment for the effect of smoking, social class and mother's size, there was no detectable effect on pregnancy of alcohol consumption below 100 g/week (i.e. one standard drink a day).

6.6.4 Wernicke–Korsakoff syndrome

In binge drinkers who consume large amounts of alcohol and virtually stop eating for three or more weeks, brain function can be affected by acute thiamin deficiency. Ethanol uses up thiamin for its metabolism, yet alcoholic beverages provide no thiamin; there is no rich food source of thiamin and body stores are very small (Chapter 12). In Wernicke's encephalopathy, the patient is quietly confused—not an easy state to recognize in an alcoholic. The diagnostic feature, if the sufferer is brought to medical attention, is that the eyes cannot move properly (ophthalmoplegia). When Wernicke's encephalopathy is treated with thiamin, the ophthalmoplegia and confusion clear but the patient may be left with a memory disorder, the inability to recall what has happened recently (Korsakoff's psychosis). It has been suggested that when an alcoholic has a partner who provides food containing some thiamin, Wernicke's encephalopathy is less likely. The incidence has been high in Australia and as a preventive measure bread has been fortified with thiamin since 1991, as it already is in the USA, UK and most other developed countries. Korsakoff's psychosis can be permanent. It is one cause of alcohol-related brain damage. Wernicke's encephalopathy uncommonly occurs in people who have not taken alcohol, e.g. with persistent vomiting in pregnancy, hyperemesis gravidarum.

6.6.5 Other nutritional deficiencies in alcoholics

In societies with adequate food supply, vitamin deficiencies are rare but do occur in heavy drinkers. Chronic thiamin or other B-vitamin deficiency may be responsible for a peripheral neuropathy in the legs, with reduced function of the motor and sensory nerves and diminished ankle jerks. Folate metabolism is commonly impaired in alcoholics and megaloblastic anaemia may be seen. Vitamin A metabolism is abnormal where there is alcoholic liver disease: the liver does not store retinol normally or synthesize retinol-binding protein adequately. There can, consequently, be reduced plasma retinol and night blindness. Among inorganic nutrients, plasma magnesium and zinc can be subnormal in alcoholics.

6.6.6 Predisposition to some types of cancer

The risk of cancer of the mouth and pharynx is increased, especially when high alcohol intakes are combined with smoking. Other cancers associated with high alcohol consumption are those of the oesophagus or liver (primary cancer of the liver is a complication of cirrhosis), the rectum (in some beer drinkers) and possibly breast cancer.

6.6.7 Gastrointestinal complications

Chronic gastritis and gastric or duodenal ulcers may be associated with excessive alcohol consumption. Acute pancreatitis is a severe complication.

6.6.8 Hypertension

The prevalence of hypertension (raised arterial blood pressure) increases with usual alcohol intakes above three or four drinks per day. Prompt falls of moderately elevated blood pressures have been well documented in heavy drinkers admitted to hospital for detoxication. Increased prevalence of hypertension explains the greater risk of stroke from cerebral haemorrhage in heavy alcohol drinkers. The mechanism for the hypertensive effect of chronic alcoholism is not yet clear. Limiting alcohol consumption is a standard part of lifestyle modification recommended for people with hypertension.

6.7 Alcohol and coronary heart disease

Opposed to the deleterious effect of alcohol on blood pressure is its apparent effect in reducing the risk of coronary heart disease, the commonest single cause of death in many countries. Over 20 large population studies, undertaken by leading epidemiologists in several countries, have all found that light to moderate alcohol consumption appears to protect against coronary heart disease (CHD). At post-mortem examination, pathologists have long known to expect little or no atheroma in the arteries of people dying of alcoholic complications. However, the discovery that light to moderate drinking is negatively associated with CHD emerged only in the 1980s. It was surprising to find a major health benefit of drinking alcohol.

The longest established mechanism for this protective effect (known since 1969) is that alcohol consumption increases plasma high-density lipoprotein (HDL) cholesterol, which is a well-established protective factor for CHD (Chapter 18). This increase of HDL cholesterol in moderate drinkers is not sufficient to explain fully their lower risk of CHD.

Two other mechanisms have been proposed. It seems likely that alcohol reduces the tendency to thrombosis. It is not possible to test this directly but alcohol reduces the aggregation of platelets on glass in response to collagen and ADP. A third mechanism is that polyphenolic compounds (e.g. catechins) are present in wines, and they have antioxidant properties

Table 6.2 Relative risks of total mortality and mortality from coronary heart disease (CHD) in 276 802 men in the USA (aged 40–59 years at entry) in a 12-year follow-up

	Drinks per day							
	0	<1	1	2	3	4	5	6+
Total death rate	1.00	0.88	0.84	0.93	1.02	1.08	1.22	1.38
CHD death rate	1.00	0.86	0.79	0.80	0.83	0.74	0.85	0.92

Source: Boffetta P., and Garfinkel L. (1990) Alcohol drinking and mortality among men enrolled in an American Cancer Society Prospective Study. *Epidemiology*, 1, 342–8.

that may reduce oxidation of low-density lipoprotein (LDL) (Chapters 15 and 18). The evidence to support this is indirect. In one experiment, subjects consumed 400 mL red wine/day for 2 weeks: their blood was taken, LDL extracted and shown *in vitro* to be less susceptible to oxidation (by copper) than at the start of the experiment. It has been suggested that the antioxidants in wine, especially red wine, might explain the French paradox (Box 6.4).

The cardioprotective effect of regular light to moderate drinking does not apply to episodic heavy drinking, which increases the risk of sudden cardiac death. If there are more irregular heavy drinkers than regular light drinkers, the overall national heart disease relationship with alcohol is adverse, as in Russia at present.

6.7.1 Type 2 diabetes

In prospective cohort studies it appears that small intakes of alcohol may also reduce the risk of developing type 2 diabetes. In a meta-analysis of 15 studies in 369 000 individuals followed over 10 years, those who stated their daily alcohol consumption as 20–30 g had a relative risk of diabetes of around 0.70. Higher intakes were not protective. The mechanism could be by increased insulin sensitivity.

> **BOX 6.4 The French paradox**
>
> - The death rate from coronary heart disease in France is apparently lower than in any other developed country.
> - However, the French diet is considered to be rich in fat. National consumption of butter and cheese are both high, and plasma cholesterols measured with standardized techniques by WHO monitoring (MONICA) centres are much the same in Strasbourg and Lille (France) as in Glasgow (Scotland), a city with a high rate of CHD; percentages above 6.5 mmol/l are 46%, 49% and 43%, respectively.
> - It is suggested that France's high alcohol consumption (highest in the world) and antioxidants in vegetables and fruits or red wine might explain this French paradox.
> - Meanwhile, life expectancy at birth in 2000 was 79 years in Australia, Iceland, Italy, Sweden and Switzerland, the same as in France, and the French death rate from cirrhosis of the liver is about the highest in the world.

6.8 Alcohol and all-causes death rate: The J-shaped curve

Because of all the social and medical complications of excess alcohol intake we might expect a graph of total mortality against alcohol consumption to be a straight line upwards with the lowest rate in teetotallers. However, the results of at least 18 large prospective studies in seven different countries in men and women all show that the death rate in light to moderate drinkers is lower than in teetotallers.

This lower death rate at light to moderate intakes is due to protection from CHD, which is the commonest single cause of death. With higher intakes, the death rate climbs to exceed the teetotallers' rate due to increasing rates of accidents, cirrhosis, hyperten-

sion, strokes, some cancers, etc. However, note that nearly all prospective studies have studied people who were middle aged at entry (Table 6.3).

Whether moderate alcohol consumption is good for health overall depends on people's age and risk of CHD. For example, Scragg (1995) estimates that alcohol was responsible for 20% of all deaths in 15- to 34-year-olds in New Zealand, mostly from road injuries. In contrast, it is estimated to have prevented 0.5% of all deaths among 35- to 64-year-olds and prevented 3.4% of all deaths among people over 65 years of age. Since young people can expect to live longer than older people, the number of

Table 6.3 Volume of various alcoholic beverages providing approximately 10 g ethanol

Type of drink	Usual % ethanol[a] (by volume)	Vol. that provides approx. 10 g ethanol
Low-alcohol beer	2–3%	568 ml = 1 (UK) pint = 20 oz
Average beer	4–5%	285 ml = ½ (UK) pint = 10 oz
Average wine[b]	10%	120 ml = 4 oz
Fortified wine (e.g. sherry, port)	20%	60 ml = 2 oz
Spirits (e.g. whisky, gin, vodka, brandy)	40%	30 ml = 1 oz

Note: [a] (1) These are approximations. The exact percentage of alcohol should be on the label of the bottle. (2) The specific gravity of ethanol is 0.790. To convert to g/100 ml multiply by 0.79 (or 0.8).
[b] Wine bottles usually contain 750 ml = 6¼ standard drinks.

person-years lost among ages less than 35 years was greater than those saved in the older age group. Thus, advantageous effects of alcohol cannot be widely recommended as a beneficial public health measure. Room *et al.* (2005) quote WHO figures which indicate that alcohol is responsible for 6.8% of the burden of disease across North America, Western Europe, Japan and Australasia, but 12% of the burden in Russia and adjacent countries. The whole world estimate is 4%. This is because of lower national consumption of alcohol in Islamic countries and in the poorest countries.

6.9 Recognition of the problem drinker

There are different types of alcohol abuse. An 'alcoholic' is a group term for any person whose drinking is leading to harm. This harm may be alcohol dependence, physical disease or social harm.

People drinking more than others or more than they feel they should are very likely to underestimate their alcohol intake when asked. The spouse or other family member may give a very different answer. Doctors are trained to suspect when someone is drinking too much and researchers use tactfully drafted questionnaires. Alcohol can be smelt on the breath and measured quantitatively in the breath, blood or urine within hours of drinking. If a person has not been drinking recently, there are changes in the blood that are suggestive of long-term excessive alcohol intake:

1. Increased red cell volume (mean corpuscular volume).
2. Increased γ-glutamyl transpeptidase (GGT).
3. Increased plasma (fasting) triglycerides (i.e. very low-density lipoproteins).
4. Increased plasma urate.
5. Increased plasma aminotransferases (transaminases)
6. Increased plasma carbohydrate-deficient transferrin.

These vary in sensitivity and specificity. Enzymes (2) and (5) and proteins (3) and (6) are produced in the liver. Increased urate is a result of increased plasma lactate. Increased red cell volume is sometimes due to folate depletion; its cause in most cases is not yet clear.

6.10 Is alcoholism a disease or the top end of a normal distribution?

Alcoholism is a costly problem in most communities because of associated diseases, accidents, loss of earning, medical expenses and social misery. There are two philosophical approaches. One is the medical model, which sees alcoholism as a disease in individuals who should be treated by the health professions. The other is the society model: the more alcohol sold and consumed, the larger will be the number of alcoholics. There are sections of society (e.g. some occupations, deprived minorities) who are at increased risk and there are social practices that contribute to alcohol abuse.

Ledermann (1956) put forward the hypothesis that in a homogeneous population the distribution of alcohol consumption is a logarithmic normal curve and that the number of people who drink a certain amount can be calculated if the average consumption is known (Fig. 6.2). This theory predicts that major complications of alcoholism in a country will be related to average national consumption. Governments rely on this principle in maintaining substantial taxes on alcohol, restricted outlets and hours, lower age limits and other measures to reduce its free availability.

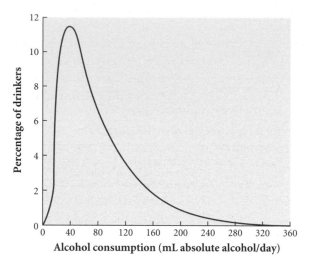

Fig. 6.2 Hypothetical curve proposed by Lederman (1956). In a homogeneous population, alcohol consumption is distributed in a logarithmic normal curve.

Source: Smith (1982).

6.11 Genetic liability to alcohol dependence?

Occurrence of alcoholism in families could be learnt rather than genetic. From comparing monozygotic with dizygotic twins, the heritability of amount and frequency of alcohol drinking appears to be about 0.36 (i.e. one-third of the way along the scale from purely environmental to purely genetic). However studies on twins cannot completely exclude environmental effects. Adoption studies have shown that the sons of alcoholic fathers are four times more likely to become alcoholics than the sons of fathers who were not alcoholics. The search is on to find one or more variations of brain metabolism that makes people more likely to become alcohol dependent. There have been several claims (e.g. abnormality of brain handling of dopamine or serotonin) but none has been convincingly confirmed.

6.12 Recommended intakes of alcohol

Nutritionists have been slow and reluctant to accept the accumulated evidence that there are some health benefits for older people of moderate alcohol intake, along with the undoubted costs of the many complications of excessive alcohol intake. The usual way in which alcohol is mentioned in national sets of dietary guidelines (see Chapter 35) is 'drink alcohol in moderation, if at all'.

Because women have lower rates of metabolizing alcohol, advice on safe drinking levels has to be different for men and women. Recommendations are expressed in standard drinks that contain 10 g of pure alcohol. Note that standard drinks are normally served in the pub but at home people tend to be more generous. In men, two to three standard drinks per day (20–30 g alcohol) (i.e. 140–210 g alcohol/week), are usually biologically safe, but no more than two drinks before driving, and a minority of men should not take this much, or even any alcohol (e.g. people with liver disease, taking other sedative drugs or with a history of alcohol dependence). In women, the biologically safe intake is one to two drinks (10–20 g alcohol) per day (i.e. 70 to 140 g alcohol/week). As well as the same contraindications as in men, intake should be one drink or less in pregnancy or if a woman thinks she might be pregnant. Children should not take alcohol but in some cultures they are offered a small glass of wine with the family's main meal and some believe this can be a good training in moderation in consumption of alcohol. The quantities of various alcoholic beverages providing 10 g of ethanol are shown in Table 6.3.

FURTHER READING

1. Doll, R., Peto, R., Hall, E. *et al.* (1994) Mortality in relation to consumption of alcohol: 13 years' observations on male British doctors. *Br Med J*, **309**, 911–18.

2. Feunekes, G.I.J., van't Veer, P., van Staveren, W.A. *et al.* (1999) Alcohol intake assessment: the sober facts. *Am J Epidemiol*, **150**, 105–12.

3. Frezza, M., di Padova, C., Pozzato, G. *et al.* (1990) High blood alcohol levels in women. The role of decreased gastric alcohol dehydrogenase activity and first-pass metabolism. *N Engl J Med*, **322**, 95–9.

4. Hall, W., and Zador, D. (1997) The alcohol withdrawal syndrome. *Lancet*, **349**, 1897–900.

5. Holman, C.D.J., English, D.R., Milne, E., and Winter, M.G. (1996) Meta-analysis of alcohol and all-cause mortality: a validation of NH and MRC recommendations. *Med J Aust*, **164**, 141–5.

6. Ledermann, S. (1956) *Alcool, alcoolisme, alcoolisation*. Paris, Presse Universitaires de France.

7. Lieber, L.S. (ed.) (1992) *Medical and nutritional complications of ulcoholism. Mechanisms and management.* New York & London, Plenum.

8. Koppes, L.L.J., Dekker, J.M., Hendricks, H.F.J., *et al.* (2005) Moderate alcohol consumption lowers the risk of type 2 diabetes. *Diabetes Care*, **28**, 719–25.

9. Norton, R., Batey, R., Dwyer, T., and MacMahon, S. (1987) Alcohol consumption and the risk of alcohol related cirrhosis in women. *Br Med J*, **295**, 80–2.

10. Pincock, S. (2003) Binge drinking on rise in UK and elsewhere. *Lancet*, **365**, 1126–7.

11. Rimm, E.B., Klasky, A., Grobbee, D., and Stampfer, M.J. (1996) Review of moderate alcohol consumption and reduced risk of coronary heart disease: is the effect due to beer, wine, or spirits? *Br Med J*, **312**, 731–6.

12. Rimm, E.B., Williams P., Fosher K., *et al.* (1999) Moderate alcohol intake and lower risk of coronary heart disease: meta-analysis of effects on lipids and haemostatic factors. *Br Med J*, **319**, 1523–8.

13. Room, R., Babor, T., and Rehm, J. (2005) Alcohol and public health. *Lancet*, **365**, 519–30.

14. Scragg, R. (1995) A quantification of alcohol-related mortality in New Zealand. *Aust NZ J Med*, **25**, 5–11.

15. Smith, R. (1982) In *Alcohol problems: ABC of alcohol. Alcohol and alcoholism*, p. 29. London, BMJ.

16. Sulaiman, N.D., Florey, C., Taylor, D.J. *et al.* (1988) Alcohol consumption in Dundee primigravidas and its effects on outcome of pregnancy. *Br Med J*, **296**, 1500–3.

PART 2

Organic and inorganic essential nutrients

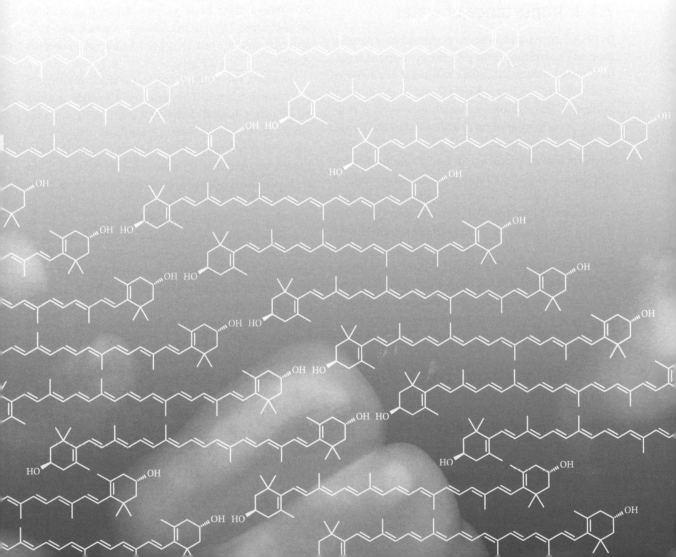

7 Water, electrolytes and acid–base balance

James Robinson

7.1 Body water

7.1.1 Importance of water

In 1913, Lawrence Henderson explained how peculiar properties resulting from a hydrogen-bonded structure make water an essential constituent of all known forms of life. It is, remarkably, liquid in the range of 'ordinary' temperatures at which biochemical reactions can occur in solution or at active sites of enzymes in contact with water. Its high specific heat moderates temperature gradients; its high latent heats allow efficient cooling by evaporation and protects against damage by frost. A dielectric constant that is large enough to reduce by 80 times the forces between charges immersed in it makes water a superb solvent for ionic compounds. It is also a good solvent for most organic compounds (apart from fats and hydrocarbons) and, even when the active sites of enzymes are in clefts that exclude water molecules, most reactants must arrive and most products move away in aqueous solution.

7.1.2 Amount and distribution in the body

The extent to which freely diffusible substances (e.g. ethanol, urea, isotopic forms of water) are diluted after being ingested or injected shows that adult persons contain about 35–45 L of water, which makes up 50–70% of their body weight, depending on how fat they are. The fat-free tissues contain 60–80% water by weight, but fat stored in fat cells contains none.

However, the body is not just a tracksuit-shaped bag, two-thirds full. The water is in a large number of smaller compartments—in cells, body cavities, blood vessels, etc. Dilution of solutes that do not cross cell membrancs gives volumes outside the cells (in the extracellular fluid, ECF) of between 12 and 20 L, the higher estimates being better than older ones, which were based on test solutes that failed to diffuse completely into dense tissues. The volumes quoted are approximate. No two people are identical; different observers and methods yield results that are similar but not the same. Hence, the books do not all agree, but 42 L for total body water (TBW), 23 L for intracellular water, and 19 L for extracellular water per 70 kg body weight are reasonable estimates. Of the ECF, 3.5 L is plasma circulating in the blood vessels. The rest bathes the cells—an overcrowded and somewhat salty pond we carry with us for them to live in. In 1878, Claude Bernard called the ECF the 'internal environment' of the cells; it nourishes them, supplies their needs and takes away their waste products. The circulating blood keeps it stirred so that it can transport heat and substances in solution from one cell to other cells, and between cells inside the

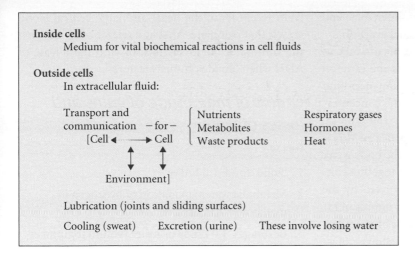

Fig. 7.1 Principal functions of water in the body.

body and the external environment. The principal functions of water in the body are summarized in Fig. 7.1.

7.1.3 Body fluids

The fluids in the body are not pure water. Intracellular fluid (ICF) and ECF are distinct solutions, with different things dissolved in them. The ECF is like diluted sea water, containing mainly sodium salts (chiefly chloride), some bicarbonate, and small but important concentrations of potassium, calcium and magnesium. The ICF contains mainly potassium salts (mostly organic phosphate and proteinate), small amounts of sodium, magnesium and bicarbonate, a little chloride, and a very little calcium (see Table 7.1). The cell membranes are somewhat permeable to sodium and potassium, hence cells must use a large part of the energy from their metabolism to pump out sodium that diffuses in and to get back potassium that leaks out. Even at rest the cells are very busy! They use about 40 kg adenosine triphosphate (ATP)

Table 7.1 Muscle cell fluid and blood plasma as typical intracellular fluid (ICF) and extracellular fluid (ECF)

Muscle cell fluid (mmol/L water)				Plasma (mmol/L water)			
K^+	150	Org P^-	130	Na^+	150	Cl^-	110
Na^+	10	HCO_3^-	10	K^+	5	HCO_3^-	27
Mg^{2+}	10	Cl^-	5	Ca^{2+}	2	Org^-	5
Ca^{2+}	10^{-4}	$Prot^{17-}$	2	Mg^{2+}	1	$H_2PO_4^-$	2
						$Prot^{17-}$	1
Reaction:	pH 7.1			pH 7.4			
Osmolarity:	285 mosmol/L cell water			285 mosmol/L plasma water			

Note: Because only about 95% of plasma is water, laboratory results per litre of plasma are lower than these. Average cell fluid is only about 80% water.
Source: Modified with permission from Bray, J.J., Cragg, P.A., Macknight, A.D.C., Mills, R.G., and Taylor, D.W. (1994) *Lecture notes on human physiology*, 3rd edition. Oxford, Blackwell.

each day to supply the energy for maintenance; and up to 0.5 kg per minute during maximal exertion!

The cell membranes are also permeable to water, so the total concentration (osmolarity) is the same in the cells and in the ECF. The concentration of sodium in the ECF is about 150 mmol/L, and the concentration of potassium in the cells is about 150 mmol/L cell water. A very important consequence of this is that so long as osmolarity throughout the body water is kept constant (the kidneys and thirst together control this), then the volume of ECF is fixed by the amount of sodium in it (litres of ECF = mmols of EC sodium ÷ 150 mmol/L), and the volume of the cells is likewise fixed by the amount of intracellular potassium (mmols cell potassium ÷ 150 mmol/L).

Note that the kidneys, by adjusting the excretion of water to keep osmolarity constant in the body fluids, set the stage both for the amount of sodium in the ECF to determine its volume, and for the cells to determine their own volume by regulating the amount of potassium they contain. This assumes an adequate supply of water; the kidneys cannot make water, only regulate its loss.

7.1.4 Water balance

The fact that people keep very much the same weight implies that the amount of water in the body is kept constant, gains being balanced against losses. Weighing is therefore the best way to measure day-to-day changes in the amount of water in the body.

Regulation of water balance Loss of water makes body fluids more concentrated. All the cells lose water and shrink as the osmotic pressure of the ECF rises. Special cells in the hypothalamus at the base of the brain respond to shrinking in two ways: (1) by sending messages that excite the sensation of thirst, and (2) by releasing into the blood an antidiuretic hormone (ADH) that allows the renal tubules to reabsorb water from dilute urine and return it to the blood. If the gains of water exceed the losses, cells swell, the thirst message is switched off, no more ADH is released and a flow of dilute urine ('water diuresis') quickly gets rid of excess water. There are also nervous paths from receptors in the heart and large central blood vessels that stimulate thirst and release of ADH when the volume of blood shrinks, or stop the release of ADH when blood volume is restored.

Orders of magnitude of gains and losses of water

Intake

1. 'Solid' food: 1.0 L/day.

2. Metabolic water (oxidation of hydrogen in metabolites): 0.3 L/day.

3. Beverages: 1.0 L/day or more (voluntary intakes may be much more!)

Output (Note: most of these are unavoidable losses from the body.)

1. *Evaporation* of vapour from skin and lung surfaces, which must be moist to remain flexible and to allow exchange of gases in solution. About 1.0 L/day at rest. Much more from the lungs with increased ventilation during exercise, especially at high altitudes. More than 2.0 L/day above 6000 m. The first successful ascent of Mount Everest depended partly on allowing for the magnitude of this loss.

2. *Sweat*: up to 15 L/day may be secreted by sweat glands to get rid of heat (normally much less).

3. *Faeces*: normally 0.1 L/day; with choleric diarrhoeas, this may reach 10 or 12 L/day.

4. *Urine*: at least as much water as can carry the day's soluble waste products in the most concentrated urine the kidneys can make. With normal kidneys, and urine four times as concentrated as plasma, this is about 0.6 L; it becomes 2.4 L if kidneys cannot make urine more concentrated than plasma, and may be more than 10 L in patients with diabetes insipidus who fail to produce ADH, or whose kidneys do not respond to it.

Wild animals (that are at greater risk from predators when they stand still to drink or urinate) often seem to drink only enough to replace unavoidable losses. Many people drink more and rely on water diuresis to match output to their voluntary intake.

Both excesses and deficiencies of body water can occur, and both may threaten life.

7.1.5 Deficiency of body water

Simple dehydration from loss of water may be caused by reduced intake or increased losses, or by a combination of both. Even when intake is zero, unavoidable losses continue, and they may be increased, for example, from the skin and lungs by activity and fever, or from the gut by diarrhoea or vomiting. The continuous aspiration of stomach contents to prevent vomiting can also make the mouth a channel of loss instead of intake.

If water is lost, first from the ECF, which is in contact with the external environment, and is not replaced, then the osmolarity of all the body fluids and the concentration of sodium in the plasma increase. Osmotic pressure could be corrected by excreting sodium, but this does not happen in man. Instead, sodium disappears from the urine and is avidly retained in the body. Its concentration in sweat, intestinal and other secretions is also reduced as more aldosterone is secreted from the adrenal cortex in response to the lower volumes of plasma and ECF. This 'dehydration reaction' has survival value—the high osmotic pressure maintains thirst and the output of ADH, minimizing urinary loss and keeping up the search for water. Increased osmolarity also withdraws water from cells and helps to sustain the volumes of ECF and circulating blood, which are essential to the search for water and which take precedence over the regulation of osmolarity. In rats, rabbits, sheep and dogs, an initial increase in the excretion of sodium may precede the onset of this dehydration reaction.

Symptoms The cardinal manifestation of primary deficiency of water is thirst, which can dominate what remains of a disordered consciousness ('My thirst was the tallest tree in a forest of pain' said Admiral Byrd). Loss of 20% or more by American men in the desert may have left their dry skin cracking and oozing blood ('blood sweat') as the men became senseless automata, scratching in the sand for water until they died from respiratory failure. See Box 7.1 for information on effects of water loss in open country in New Zealand.

> **BOX 7.1** Survival without water in New Zealand
>
> Amount of body water lost:
>
> - 1–5% of body weight: thirst; vague discomfort; economy of movement; no appetite; flushed skin; impatience; increased pulse rate; nausea.
> - 6–10% of body weight: dizziness; headache; laboured breathing; tingling in limbs; absence of saliva; blue body (cyanosis); indistinct speech; inability to walk.
> - 11–12% of body weight: delirium; twitching; swollen tongue; inability to swallow; deafness; dim vision; shrivelled skin; numb skin.
>
> 'A man can exist for days without food, but only for 2–5 days without water.'
>
> *Source*: Hildreth (1979).

Fresh water may be as unavailable at sea as it is in deserts. The dry mouth, swollen tongue and delirium with hallucinations are admirably described by Samuel Taylor Coleridge in *The Rime of the Ancient Mariner* (1798).

> And every tongue through utter drought,
> Was withered at the root;
> We could not speak, no more than if
> We had been choked with soot.
> With throats unslaked, with black lips baked,
> We could not laugh nor wail;
> Through utter drought all dumb we stood!
> I bit my arm, I suck'd the blood,
> And cried, 'A sail! a sail!'

During World War II, R.A. McCance (Professor of Experimental Medicine at Cambridge in England) was chairman of a subcommittee of the British Admiralty that was concerned with safeguarding the lives of hundreds of men cast adrift in lifeboats or rafts after their ships were sunk by enemy action. He studied volunteers in life rafts in temperate, arctic and tropical seas, and came to the firm conclusion that sea water could not be used to supplement limited supplies of fresh water. Reports of survivors showed that those who drank sea water became more delirious and were liable to disappear over the side. Sea water has a higher salt concentration than human kidneys can achieve; hence drinking it actually removes water from the body and makes dehydration worse. Any temporary improvement in circulation and feeling when water is withdrawn from cells is overshadowed by shortened survival. It is of no ultimate advantage to feel better on Monday and die on Tuesday if it happens that your party is not going to be rescued until Wednesday.

Treatment The remedy for primary water deficiency is water—as the predominant symptom of thirst indicates. It is important to realize that this kind of dehydration is not confined to oceans and deserts; it can even turn up in hospital wards if thirst fails or cannot be satisfied. Unconscious patients do not experience thirst; others may be too confused or too weak to drink water set beside them. Alexander Leaf once remarked: 'These people are in great danger, for their osmostat is in their physician's head.' A full jug and a glass on the bedside locker does not guarantee there is enough water in the patient.

Summing up In primary dehydration from simple lack of water, the cells share the loss with the ECF; and hence they arouse thirst, which normally indicates what is needed for treatment. Old people and their caregivers need to bear in mind that thirst, water diuresis and the response to ADH tend to become attenuated with advancing years; hence these people are increasingly at risk of dehydration, with the possibility of a vicious circle if chronically high osmolarity further impairs their awareness of thirst and their need for water.

7.1.6 Excess of body water

An excessive amount of water in the body is rarer than deficiency, because water diuresis protects against excess, and normal kidneys can excrete water as fast as the gut can absorb it. However, water diuresis can fail:

1. *In anuria* (no production of urine): with absence of renal function the kidneys cannot respond to absence of ADH.
2. *With inappropriate release of ADH*: e.g. after trauma, including surgery, head injury, or antidiuretic substances from some tumours.

If patients in these conditions are given much more than about 1 L per day, which they need to replace unavoidable losses, EC osmolarity and sodium concentration fall, so that water goes into cells, which swell. Weakness and cramps appear. Swelling of brain cells leads to water intoxication in which disturbances of consciousness and behaviour may progress to convulsions and death.

Low osmolarity and low plasma sodium concentration (hyponatraemia) can occur without an excess of total body water (e.g. if the water, but not the salt, lost in profuse sweating is replaced). Muscle cramps are then the chief feature—once known as miners' cramps and stokers' cramps, which were common in English coal mines and ships. J.B.S. Haldane showed in 1928 that extra salt prevents or cures these cramps, and miners in hot mines commonly added salt to their beer.

7.2 Sodium and extracellular fluid

7.2.1 Significance and functions of sodium

Salt has long been a valuable commodity and part of the fabric of human life and culture. We pay salaries, the *salarium* being the allowance for a Roman soldier to buy salt. And we still question whether a man is worth his salt. Salt mines are traditional sites of strenuous, unpleasant, but essential labour. Some animals in arid regions trek vast distances to salt licks to get the sodium they need in order to excrete potassium from their high-potassium vegetable diet.

Common salt is sodium chloride (NaCl). Each gram contains 17.1 mmol of sodium, which is the principal cation in most extracellular fluids and is responsible for 95% of their osmolarity. Its concentration, regulated at 150 mmol/L in man and most animals, helps to stabilize the potassium to sodium ratio. This determines the membrane potentials of most cells, and the action potentials underlying the transmission of nerve impulses and the contraction of muscles. It is responsible for maintaining the volume (at 1 L for every 150 mmol, or 9 g of NaCl) of the extracellular fluids that the cells live in.

7.2.2 Amount and distribution of sodium in the body

Adults contain about 5600 mmol of sodium (325 g NaCl). About half of that (2800 mmol) is dissolved in the extracellular fluids, with 300 in cells and 2500 in bone mineral. Half of the sodium in the bones is exchangeable with isotopically labelled Na, the rest is deeper and less accessible; hence in classical analyses of dissolved bodies, more sodium was found than with modern measurements, which are based on isotopic dilution during life.

7.2.3 Sodium balance

Intake

Diet: 70–250 mmol/day. Very variable with habit, taste and custom.

1. Natural foods contain 0.1–3.0 mmol sodium per 100 g: fruits 0.1 mmol/g; vegetables 0.3 mmol/g; meat, fish and eggs about 3.0 mmol/100 g.

2. Processed foods contain far more: bread around 20 mmol/100 g; cheese 30 mmol/100 g; salted butter 40 mmol/100 g; raw lean bacon as much as 80 mmol/100 g.

People add widely varying amounts of salt to their cooking or at the table. Nevertheless, discretionary salt intake is usually much lower than that obtained from manufactured and processed food products.

Output

1. *Faeces*: normally 5–10 mmol/day.

2. *Sweat*: 20–80 mmol/day. Extremely variable (see section 7.2.4 below).

3. *Urine*: variable. Normally somewhat less than dietary intake.

The kidneys are capable of excreting between 1 and 500 mmol/day. They normally keep the amount in the body constant by excreting the excess of intake over the sum of other losses. Homer Smith's one-time remark that the composition of the body depends 'not on what the mouth takes in but on what the kidneys keep' aptly sums up their control of sodium balance.

The rate of excretion of sodium depends on the balance between glomerular filtration rate (GFR × sodium concentration) and tubular reabsorption. When blood and ECF volumes fall, GFR is reduced by constriction of glomerular vessels, and reabsorption is increased by several factors. A major factor is aldosterone, secreted from the adrenal cortex. When blood pressure or volume is reduced and sympathetic nerves are activated, renin is released from the kidney; this is an enzyme that forms angiotensin I from a precursor in the plasma. Another enzyme in blood and some tissues converts this to angiotensin II, which stimulates the adrenal cortex. When blood volume increases, these conserving mechanisms are turned off, GFR increases and renal nerves inhibit instead of promote tubular reabsorption; reabsorption is also inhibited by a natriuretic peptide from the heart, and by other hormones that keep being discovered!

7.2.4 Sodium depletion

Deficiency of sodium is not caused simply by a deficient intake, for the kidneys can make the urine almost salt-free. Abnormal losses causing depletion may be in:

1. *Sweat*: Up to as much as 15 L/day. Sweat is hypotonic, but its sodium concentration of 50 mmol/L takes as much salt as there is in 5 L of normal ECF, so that even after osmolarity is corrected by replacing water, the volume of the ECF will be reduced by 5 L.

2. *Intestinal fluid*: 10 L/day of intestinal secretions are normally reabsorbed. However, with diarrhoea absorption is depressed and intestinal fluid secretion often increased; losses may reach 18 L/day in cholera, and the fluid lost is almost isotonic, equivalent to its own volume of ECF.

3. *Urine*: The kidneys normally act to guard the body's stores of sodium, but in Addison's disease the adrenal cortex fails to produce aldosterone, and the kidneys fail to conserve sodium. The kidneys may also lose sodium in some types of renal failure. Diuretic drugs and osmotic diuresis (e.g. with the load of glucose and ketone acids in diabetes) may remove large amounts of sodium in the urine.

Provided that osmolarity is maintained, 1 L of water is lost with every 150 mmol of sodium; the result used to be called 'dehydration secondary to loss of salt' but 'saline depletion' is a better description. It is important to realize that all the water that is lost comes from the ECF, which bears the brunt of the dehydration. Without loss from the cells, there are only weaker, non-osmotic stimuli to release ADH, so that the urine may not be extremely scanty and concentrated; thirst is also less pronounced than after the loss of a similar amount of water without salt, but the threat to survival through the reductions in the volumes of blood and ECF is much more severe.

Symptoms The cardinal manifestation is peripheral circulatory failure, which may be sudden and un-expected if premonitory signs are missed: dry mouth and tongue, shrunken skin that lacks turgor, sunken eyes with low pressure, a rapid weak pulse, and low blood pressure. Packed cell volume, and the concentrations of haemoglobin and plasma albumin, and blood viscosity all increase as the volume of plasma falls along with that of the ECF. When oxygen transport to tissues is badly impaired, cells swell taking up sodium and water; this further reduces the volume of ECF and may set up a vicious circle leading rapidly to a disastrous collapse of the circulation—a short of 'medical shock'.

Treatment Salt as well as water is required to treat this desperate state. Water given alone or by infusing glucose solutions will disappear into the cells with the risk of water intoxication. Isotonic saline supplies sodium and water in the proportions in which they are deficient.

7.2.5 Experimental human salt deficiency

R.A. McCance subjected himself, and a few other healthy people, to forced sweating for 2 hours each day while they ate a low-salt diet and drank only distilled water. They lost about 1 kg/day for 3 or 4 days, while plasma sodium concentrations remained normal. After that, the loss of sodium continued, but not the loss of weight; plasma sodium concentration fell and water moved into the cells. Their faces shrank, they lost their appetite and sense of taste, and they became very weak, weary and muddleheaded, with a general sense of exhaustion, little initiative, delayed excretion of water loads, and almost continuous muscle cramps. Many of McCance's symptoms resembled those of severe Addison's disease, although the adrenal glands were presumably overactive! They endured these miseries for a week or two, and then enjoyed a rapid cure by eating salty fried herrings and licking the salt out of the pan! McCance's fascinating description in the third of his Goulstonian lectures (McCance, 1936) is a precious medical and nutritional classic.

7.2.6 Excess of body sodium

An increased intake of salt does not usually increase the amount in the body, because the kidneys normally excrete the extra sodium and keep the volume of ECF constant. However they can be misdirected or malfunction, and retain too much sodium. Examples (with some contributory factors) include:

1. Congestive heart failure, whereby raised capillary pressure displaces fluid from the plasma to interstitial spaces and the congested liver fails to destroy aldosterone normally.

2. Deficiency of plasma albumin, e.g. from loss in the urine in nephrotic syndromes, or from failure of production in hepatic failure, or severe malnutrition,

Table 7.2 Summary of disturbances in the amount of water in the body

Disturbance	Cause	Osmotic pressure (plasma [Na])	Volume change	Manifestation
Excess water	Water only	Reduced	ICF↑ ECF↑	Water intoxication
	Excess Na	Normal	ECF↑	
Dehydration	Water loss	Increased	ICF↓ ECF↓	Thirst
	Na loss	Normal	ECF↓	Circulatory failure

famine oedema. The lowered plasma volume reduces GFR and releases renin, which stimulates secretion of aldosterone. However, the plasma volume is not always low, indicating that there are other factors involved; these are incompletely understood.

3. Failure of the kidneys to respond to natriuretic hormones (hormones stimulating sodium loss) that are released when plasma volume increases.

Retained sodium first increases osmolarity in the ECF, provoking thirst and release of ADH. Water is taken in, and retained to accompany the retained salt. With normal osmoregulation, 1 L of water is retained with each 150 mmol of sodium (9 g NaCl). If the extra saline is not held in the capillaries (e.g. if capillary pressure is raised or colloid osmotic pressure is low from lack of albumin), then it escapes into the tissues; hence, blood volume is not expanded and signals to retain sodium are not turned off. The excess saline accumulates as ECF outside the circulation, body weight increases, and accumulation of more than 4 L shows up as oedema.

Treatment Extremely low salt diets are unpalatable, and attempts to restrict salt may be counterproductive by provoking increased secretion of aldosterone. Patients are more compliant when dietary salt intake is reduced less rigorously, and renal excretion is increased with diuretics, which inhibit reabsorption of sodium by the renal tubules. See Table 7.2 for a summary of disturbances in the water content of the body.

7.3 Potassium

7.3.1 Significance and functions of potassium

According to a luminous phrase: 'Potassium is of the soil and not of the sea; it is of the cell and not of the sap' (attributed to Wallace Fenn). Just as sodium belongs typically to seas and extracellular fluids, potassium is the predominant cation in the cells of both animals and plants. Its salts, mainly organic, are responsible for most of the osmolarity of animal cells and they determine their volume. The cells' enzymes have evolved to require an environment rich in potassium. The hydrated potassium ion is smaller than that of sodium, and the cell membranes are much more permeable to it. Hence, the ratio of the IC concentration to the EC concentration of potassium largely determines the resting potentials of cells and the transient action potentials, which transmit messages and activate nerve cells and muscle fibres.

An increase in the small EC concentration of potassium lowers the concentration ratio of IC potassium to EC potassium; this depolarizes membranes and blocks transmission, whereas a decrease in EC potassium concentration increases the ratio, hyperpolarizes membranes and raises the threshold for excitation. Consequently, the small concentration of potassium in the ECF is critically important—large increases or decreases (twofold to threefold) can paralyse muscles and stop the heart.

The larger concentration of potassium in the cells is not so critical. Up to a third of body potassium can be lost without dramatic symptoms. A colleague in McCance's laboratory (Paul Fourman) depleted himself experimentally by ingesting ion-exchange resins, which prevented the absorption of potassium from his alimentary tract. He delayed analysing his stools until after a walking holiday, and then found that he had gone away without a fifth of his body's store of potassium. Presumably the IC and EC concentrations had been reduced without dangerously disturbing the critical ratio. Had the cells suddenly recovered their lost potassium, the EC concentration would have fallen to zero and he would have died.

7.3.2 Amount and distribution in the body

An average adult human's body contains about 3800 mmol of potassium; most of this (about 3200 mmol) is in the cells. Indeed, a total body count of the natural isotope, potassium-40, can yield an estimate of cell mass. About 300 mmol is contained in the skeleton, and only 80 mmol is in solution in the EC fluids. Hence, if the cells increased their content by only 1.25% (40 mmol) at the expense of the ECF, the external concentration would be halved, with potentially serious consequences for neuromuscular and cardiac function.

7.3.3 Potassium balance

Intake

Diet: around 100 mmol/day.

1. Meat is animal muscle and vegetables contain plant cells, hence all foods contain potassium. No foods are exceptionally rich or poor, and there are no large differences between natural and processed foods, as there are for sodium.
2. Wholemeal flour, meats and fish: 7–9 mmol/100 g.
3. Common vegetables: 5–9 mmol/100 g.
4. Milk, eggs and cheese: 4–6 mmol/100 g.
5. Fruit: 5–8 mmol/100 g (oranges have 5 mmol/100 g so orange juice is a useful source of potassium).

The lowest values are for salted butter at 0.5 mmol/100 g and eating apples at 0.3 mmol/100 g. Hence, ordinary mixed and vegetarian diets contain adequate amounts of potassium. It is difficult to devise a diet that is deficient.

Output

1. *Faeces*: about 10 mmol/day.
2. *Urine*: 90 mmol/day.

This can be varied widely to match alterations in intake. The kidneys hold the balance by adjusting the amount in the urine. They can excrete potassium rapidly if EC potassium concentration rises, and can conserve it when scarce, though not as avidly or as briskly as sodium. Their priority seems to be to keep the critically important concentration of potassium in the ECF within its normal range of 4–5 mmol/L.

7.3.4 Regulation of extracellular concentration

The most important factors are:

1. *Active uptake by cells*. This is maintained by ongoing metabolism and is promoted by insulin. Potassium must be supplied to prevent a lethal fall in EC potassium concentration when patients with diabetic ketoacidosis treated with insulin and glucose begin to rebuild the severely depleted stores of glycogen and potassium in their muscles.

2. *Excretion by the kidneys*. The bulk of the potassium in the glomerular filtrate is reabsorbed from proximal tubules; what appears in the urine is mostly secreted by distal tubules. The rate of tubular secretion is increased by:

• Increased EC potassium concentration: this helps to avoid a dangerous increase in EC concentration when potassium escapes from cells; but the potassium is lost from the body in the process.

- Aldosterone.
- Faster flow through distal tubules: the secretory mechanism seems to set the concentration of potassium in the tubular fluid, so that the rate is proportional to the flow.
- An increased concentration of sodium in distal tubular fluid, for potassium is secreted partly in exchange for reabsorbed sodium.

7.3.5 Potassium depletion

This implies a lack of potassium that is out of proportion to other body constituents. Small children and adults who have lost weight are not considered potassium-depleted; their IC and EC concentrations are normal.

Deficiency of potassium is rarely caused by an inadequate intake alone; it requires also a failure of renal conservation, or abnormal losses, or both.

1. The alimentary tract can become a source of zero intake or even of loss through vomiting, aspiration of stomach contents or diarrhoea, when lost fluid often contains more potassium than normal intestinal secretions. Abuse of purgatives can cause potassium depletion.

2. The kidneys may excrete instead of conserving potassium under the influence of adrenal steroids, diuretic drugs or acidosis. In diabetic ketoacidosis, deranged metabolism leads to loss of potassium from cells to ECF; increased renal excretion is driven by the high EC concentration and the osmotic diuresis provoked by large amounts of ketone acids and sodium in distal tubular fluid.

3. Most disturbances of acid–base balance increase the rate of excretion of potassium. Acidosis brings potassium out of cells, raising EC concentrations, so potassium removed from cells is excreted and lost. Alkalosis promotes uptake of potassium from plasma into cells including renal tubular cells, which pass it on into the urine. Thus, alkalosis as well as acidosis can deplete the body of potassium. Paradoxically, potassium depletion ultimately leaves distal tubular cells low in potassium so that they tend to secrete hydrogen ions instead of potassium, make the urine acid and add extra bicarbonate to the plasma, thus creating a state of alkalosis in the plasma, while cells and urine are abnormally acidic.

Symptoms The symptoms of potassium deficiency are mild, vague and non-specific, and include fatigue and ill-defined malaise with weak skeletal, cardiac and intestinal muscles; the kidneys cannot concentrate the urine maximally. These are not obvious; there are no dramatic effects if cells and ECF lose potassium in proportion. Physicians must therefore anticipate when deficiency is likely to occur and test for it. The electrocardiogram offers a readily available biological assay and may give an early warning to seek laboratory confirmation of serum potassium levels.

Treatment After causes of loss have been removed, replacement is usually by mouth—best as food. Infusions, when needed, must be slow and not concentrated, to avoid the danger of high EC potassium concentrations.

7.3.6 Excess of body potassium

Potassium is not stored in the body; there is no overstocking of cells corresponding to oedema. Localized excesses in the form of high concentrations of potassium in ECF are dangerous, but these are rare in the absence of renal damage. The kidneys may fail to protect against excessive concentrations:

1. *In shock*, cells deprived of oxygen cannot retain potassium, and kidneys without adequate blood flow cannot excrete it.

2. *In crush injuries*, crushed muscles release potassium and also muscle haemoglobin, which damages the kidneys by blocking the tubules.

3. *In anuria* (from any cause), excretion is impossible, and an increasing concentration of potassium in the plasma as cells break down may be a more pressing indication of the need for dialysis than a rising concentration of blood urea.

4. *In Addison's disease*, when adrenal cortical secretion is lacking, EC potassium concentration may be moderately increased without an increase in body potassium because the kidneys fail to conserve sodium but retain potassium.

7.4 Acid–base balance

7.4.1 Regulation

The maintenance of acid–base balance implies keeping the body fluids 'blandly alkaline' (i.e. plasma and other ECFs at pH 7.35–7.45; cells about pH 7.1; note that pH 6.8 is neutral at body temperature). This alkalinity is essential for cells in 'irritable' tissues (nerves, muscles and heart). It is achieved by:

1. controlling excretion of weakly acid carbon dioxide by the lungs (about 13 000 mmol/day); and

2. excretion of smaller amounts of non-volatile acid (hydrogen ions) or alkali (bicarbonate) by the kidneys.

The kidneys control the numerator and lungs the denominator of the Henderson–Hasselbalch equation:

$$pH = 6.1 + \log \frac{[HCO_3^-]}{0.03 P_{CO_2}} \quad \begin{array}{l} \leftarrow \text{kidneys} \\ \leftarrow \text{lungs and} \\ \quad \text{respiratory system} \end{array}$$

Normally, bicarbonate (HCO_3) concentration is kept near 24 mmol/L and partial pressure of carbon dioxide near 40 mmHg; hence, pH must be:

$$6.1 + \log (24/(0.03 \times 40)) = 6.1 + \log (24/1.2)$$
$$= 6.1 + \log 20 = 6.1 + 1.3 = 7.4.$$

Respiratory and renal diseases can disturb acid–base balance. Considering only dietary factors, it has been known for more than 100 years that meat diets leave excess acid and vegetarian diets excess alkali in the body to be dealt with. Claude Bernard, in 1865, noticed that rabbits that happened to be starved produced acid urine instead of the usual alkaline urine characteristic of herbivorous animals. He deduced that starvation made them temporarily carnivorous, living on their own flesh, and found that he could make their urine alkaline or acid at will by giving them grass or meat to eat. He did the same with a horse.

7.4.2 Dietary considerations

Meat diets yield sulphuric acid from S-amino acids, and phosphoric acid from nucleoproteins and phospholipids. Mixed diets leave about 70 mmol/day of hydrogen ions to be excreted. Food faddists may label sour fruits as 'acid foods' but the organic acids they contain are either not absorbed or are mostly oxidized to water and carbon dioxide. Most of this is breathed out, although a little remains in the body as bicarbonate; hence, these acids, taken in as potassium salts, leave an excess of potassium bicarbonate, which tends to make the blood more alkaline! Table 7.3 gives examples of food acids and their metabolic fates.

Table 7.3 Acids in fruits and their metabolic fate

Food source	Acid	Fate
Citrus, pineapples, tomatoes, summer fruits	Citric	Oxidized to CO_2 and HO_2
Apples, plums, tomatoes	Malic	Oxidized to CO_2 and HO_2
Cranberries, bilberries	Benzoic	Excreted as hippuric acid
Grapes	Tartaric	Not absorbed
Strawberries, rhubarb, spinach	Oxalic	Not absorbed; forms calcium oxalate in the gut

Source: Modified from Passmore, R. and Eastwood, M.A. (1988) *Davidson and Passmore's human nutrition and dietetics*, 8th edition. Edinburgh, Churchill Livingstone.

Hence, these dietary acids pose no threat to the body's 'bland alkalinity'. Organic acids that can pose threats are:

1. Acetoacetic and other keto acids, particularly produced in diabetic ketoacidosis; smaller, less important amounts during fasting.

2. Lactic acid produced in severe muscular exercise or from tissues inadequately supplied with oxygen (e.g. in shock when blood pressure is very low).

7.4.3 The reaction of the urine

The reaction of the urine depends on the balance between the amounts of bicarbonate in the glomerular filtrate and hydrogen ion secreted by the renal tubules. Since bicarbonate is formed as a by-product of the generation of hydrogen ions in the tubular cells, 1 mmol of bicarbonate is added to the plasma for each 1 mmol of hydrogen ions secreted into the urine. The secreted hydrogen ion first destroys filtered bicarbonate, but effects its 'reabsorption' by replacing it mmol for mmol by new bicarbonate in the plasma. Further secreted hydrogen ions convert filtered buffers, especially phosphate, into their acid forms in acid urine. Hydrogen ions are also excreted as ammonium, and 1 mmol of additional bicarbonate is added to the plasma for every 1 mmol of hydrogen ion excreted as acid buffer or ammonium. In alkalosis, the concentration of bicarbonate in the plasma may be so high that there is more in the glomerular filtrate than the total rate of hydrogen ion secretion can cope with; the excess bicarbonate then escapes in alkaline urine and lowers the concentration in the plasma.

FURTHER READING

1. **Bray, J.J., Cragg, P.A., Macknight, A.D.C., and Mills, R.G.** (1999) *Lecture notes on human physiology*, 4th edition. Oxford, Blackwell Scientific Publications.

2. **Hildreth, B.** (1979) *How to survive in the bush, on the coast, in the mountains of New Zealand*. Wellington, Government Printer.

3. **McCance, R.A.** (1936) Medical problems in mineral metabolism. *Lancet*, **227**, 823–30.

4. **Passmore, R., and Eastwood, M.A.** (1988) *Davidson and Passmore's human nutrition and dietetics*, 8th edition. Edinburgh, Churchill Livingstone.

5. **Robinson, J.R.** (1988) *Reflections on renal function*, 2nd edition. Oxford, Blackwell Scientific Publications.

6. **Wrong, O.** (1993) Water and monovalent electrolytes. In: Garrow, J.S., and James, W.P.T. (eds) *Human nutrition and dietetics*, 9th edition. Edinburgh, Churchill Livingstone, pp. 146–61.

 To see topical and scientifically robust updates on nutrition associated with this textbook, and active web links to many of the journal articles in the Reference areas, please see the dedicated Online Resource Centre at www.oxfordtextbooks.co.uk/orc/mann3e/.

8 Major minerals: calcium and magnesium

Ailsa Goulding

8.1 Calcium

Calcium (Ca) is a remarkable and fascinating mineral. It is an essential constituent of all forms of life and is critically important for good health and human nutrition. The skeleton contains 99% of the body's calcium and we need adequate dietary calcium and vitamin D to grow and keep healthy bones and teeth (Box 8.1). Calcium is a divalent cation with an atomic weight of 40 (40 mg Ca = 1 mmol Ca). Calcium is the fifth most abundant element in our bodies. It is the main mineral in bone, being stored as hydroxyapatite, $Ca_{10}(OH)_2(PO_4)_6$. The skeleton protects the vital organs, and provides a 'bank' of minerals from which calcium and phosphorus may be continually withdrawn or deposited according to physiological need. The total body calcium content differs widely among individuals at all ages because some people grow better skeletons than others. This is partly due to genetic factors and partly to environmental and nutritional influences. In contrast, intracellular and extracellular calcium concentrations are tightly controlled within narrow limits. This is essential because interactions of calcium ions with proteins alter molecular activity. Ordered movement of ionic calcium plays a critical role in regulating muscle contraction, nerve conductivity, ion transport, enzyme activation, blood clotting, and the secretion of hormones and neurotransmitters.

Life without calcium is impossible and small variations in plasma calcium concentrations may have serious consequences. Hypocalcaemia and hypercalcaemia are common medical emergencies. Low blood calcium (hypocalcaemia) may cause seizures and tetany (musculoskeletal spasms and twitching, particularly in the fingers and face) and tingling and numbness due to increased neuromuscular activity. High blood calcium (hypercalcaemia) results in thirst, mild mental confusion and irritability, loss of appetite, and general fatigue and weakness. Polyuria and constipation are common. When concentrations of calcium are high, calcium salts may precipitate in soft tissues and kidney stones may form.

> **BOX 8.1 Calcium**
>
> Important for growth and maintenance of strong bones and teeth, healthy nerve and muscle function, blood clotting and hormone release. Intake is needed daily to offset obligatory losses in urine and stools. When dietary supply is insufficient, bone calcium stores are resorbed via parathyroid hormone. Food sources include dairy products, soy products, leafy green vegetables, bread, tap water in hard water areas, nuts and seeds, and dried fruits. Vitamin D improves alimentary calcium absorption. High calcium intakes are useful in slowing osteoporotic bone loss.

8.1.1 Bone metabolism

There are two types of bone: dense cortical bone (80% of the skeleton) and spongy trabecular bone (20% of the skeleton). The skeleton undergoes constant renovation, rather like a building site. Old worn bits are being chiselled out or resorbed by multinucleate cells called osteoclasts, while new teams of cells called osteoblasts busily rebuild excavation holes with strong new bone. Bone cell activity affects biochemical markers: blood levels of alkaline phosphatase and osteocalcin reflect formation; urinary hydroxyproline, deoxypyridinoline and pyridinoline indicate resorption. Osteoblasts buried deep in bone mineral are called osteocytes; they seem to sense weight-bearing and may help to regulate bone remodelling responses to exercise. The different bone cells communicate actively. A complex, exquisitely sensitive 'internet' of chemical messages appears to control their differentiation and activity, but we understand this bone language poorly. When the activity of the osteoblasts and osteoclasts is matched, or coupled, bone mass is stable. The amount of bone destroyed by osteoclasts is replaced by an equal amount of new bone. When bone remodelling becomes uncoupled, and resorption exceeds formation, bone is lost. Bone mass can be measured accurately *in vivo* using dual energy X-ray absorptiometry (DEXA scanning) or computerized tomography (CT scanning).

8.1.2 Bone disorders

Children with vitamin D deficiency develop rickets, and adults, osteomalacia (see section 14.1). They do not calcify bone normally and their bones contain osteoid (unmineralized bone). Because this bone is weak, children with rickets often show bowed limbs. Rickets is still seen in developing countries but rarely in more affluent societies.

In developed countries the bone disease seen most often is osteoporosis. This is caused by substantial loss of bone. Although there is too little bone, what remains is normally calcified. Osteoporotic bones are thin and break easily, especially in the wrist, spine and hip. The thinner the bone density, the higher the risk of fractures.

8.1.3 Calcium stores

Bone stores   When plump people are being weighed they sometimes say a little smugly 'I've got big bones'. However, bones are strong rather than weighty. The bones of an average adult constitute 14% of body weight, and bone mineral 4%. Men accumulate more skeletal calcium (1200 g) than women (1000 g). Approximately one-fifth of this (21%) is in the skull, half (51%) is in the arms and legs, and the remainder (28%) is in the trunk (ribs 9%; pelvis 8%; spine 11%).

Peak bone mass   The heaviest bone mass an individual achieves is called their peak bone mass (PBM). This is generally reached by 18–20 years of age. To achieve average PBM values, men require a positive daily calcium gain of 160 mg and women 130 mg for every single day of the first 20 years of their lives! Ethnic, family and twin studies show that there are strong genetic influences on PBM. These may account for 80% of the variability in adult bone density. The variance in PBM is wide, with values ranging between 20% higher and 20% lower than the average. The variance does not change in the third and fourth decades of life, indicating that young adults with low density do not catch up bone density over time. Thus, if a good PBM is not attained by the mid-20s, it is unlikely to be achieved at all.

Calcium in extraskeletal stores and body fluids
These stores are small (15 g), comprising teeth (7 g), soft tissues (7 g), and plasma and intracellular fluids (1 g). Cytoplasm concentrations are one thousand times lower than those in plasma. Breast milk contains a high level of calcium (350 mg/L or 8.8 mmol/L), and a lactating mother transfers around 260 mg daily to her baby. The plasma calcium concentration is 2.2–2.6 mmol/L (8.8–10.4 mg/dL): half of this is bound to protein (37% to albumin and 10% to globulin), 47% is free or ionized, and 6% is complexed to anions (phosphate, citrate, bicarbonate). The ionized calcium is biologically active: levels are regulated by the parathyroid vitamin D axis and calcitonin.

Control of plasma calcium   When ionized plasma calcium concentrations fall, parathyroid hormone

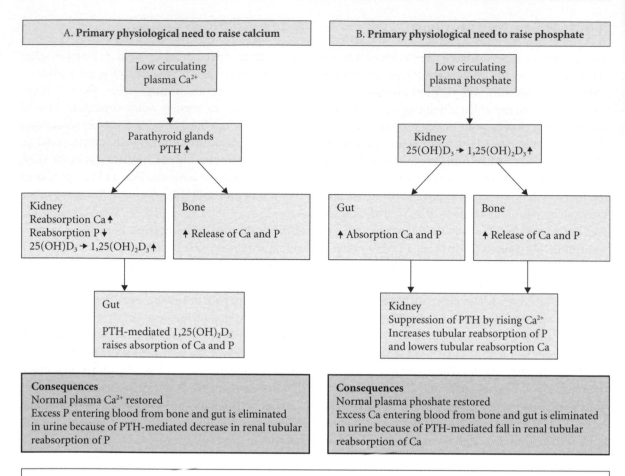

A. **Primary physiological need to raise calcium**

Low circulating plasma Ca^{2+}

Parathyroid glands
PTH ↑

Kidney
Reabsorption Ca ↑
Reabsorption P ↓
$25(OH)D_3 \rightarrow 1,25(OH)_2D_3$ ↑

Bone
↑ Release of Ca and P

Gut
PTH-mediated $1,25(OH)_2D_3$ raises absorption of Ca and P

Consequences
Normal plasma Ca^{2+} restored
Excess P entering blood from bone and gut is eliminated in urine because of PTH-mediated decrease in renal tubular reabsorption of P

B. **Primary physiological need to raise phosphate**

Low circulating plasma phosphate

Kidney
$25(OH)D_3 \rightarrow 1,25(OH)_2D_3$ ↑

Gut
↑ Absorption Ca and P

Bone
↑ Release of Ca and P

Kidney
Suppression of PTH by rising Ca^{2+}
Increases tubular reabsorption of P and lowers tubular reabsorption Ca

Consequences
Normal plasma phoshate restored
Excess Ca entering blood from bone and gut is eliminated in urine because of PTH-mediated fall in renal tubular reabsorption of Ca

Key: Ca^{2+} ionized calcium   PTH parathyroid hormone $25(OH)D_3$ 25-hydroxyvitamin D_3 (liver metabolite)
$1,25(OH)_2D_3$ 1,25-dihydrocholecalciferol or calcitriol (kidney metabolite)

Fig. 8.1 Coordinated actions of parathyroid hormone and calcitriol in target organs regulate levels of calcium and phosphate in plasma.

(PTH) is secreted to increase calcium input from kidney, bone and gut (Fig. 8.1). In the kidney, PTH augments the tubular reabsorption of calcium, decreases tubular reabsorption of phosphate and bicarbonate, and stimulates conversion of $25(OH)D_3$ to $1,25(OH)_2D_3$ (calcitriol). In bone, PTH promotes release of calcium and phosphate into blood. The effects of PTH on kidney and bone are direct and rapid and are assisted by $1,25(OH)_2D_3$; the ability of PTH to raise alimentary calcium and phosphate absorption is mediated solely by calcitriol. When normal plasma calcium concentrations are restored,

PTH secretion decreases, the flow of calcium from bone diminishes, urinary calcium rises and $1,25(OH)_2D_3$ synthesis is shut off. The system is robust and PTH and calcitriol influence each other's synthesis. The role of vitamin D is discussed in section 14.1.

Calcitonin, a hormone secreted by the thyroid gland, helps to fine-tune plasma calcium regulation. It lowers calcium by inhibiting bone resorption. It is secreted when ionized blood calcium levels rise above normal and probably helps to curb blood calcium fluctuations after meals. Calcitonin plays a smaller role in plasma calcium homeostasis than PTH and calcitriol, and patients who have had surgery on the thyroid gland maintain levels surprisingly well. In contrast, patients lacking either PTH or active vitamin D metabolites develop hypocalcaemia. Magnesium deficiency also causes hypocalcaemia because magnesium is a cofactor for PTH secretion. Restoring magnesium corrects the problem in alcoholics and patients with steatorrhoea. Total plasma calcium rarely falls below 1.25 mmol/L (5 mg/dL) because calcium ions from bone mineral constantly exchange with extracellular fluid.

Obligatory losses of calcium Significant amounts of calcium inevitably leak from the body. These are unavoidable dermal, faecal and renal losses of calcium, called obligatory losses. Dermal losses (epithelial cells and sweat) are generally less than 20 mg/day; faecal losses (unabsorbed digestive juice calcium) are 80–120 mg/day; while the obligatory urinary calcium loss varies between 40 and 200 mg/day, depending on how effectively calcium is reabsorbed from the glomerular filtrate. The tubules reabsorb more than 98% of the 10 000 mg calcium filtered daily by the glomeruli of the kidney. Dietary salt (NaCl), protein and caffeine aggravate obligatory urinary calcium loss.

8.1.4 Calcium balance and absorption

If more calcium is retained than excreted, a person is said to be in positive calcium balance. Negative calcium balance occurs if more calcium is excreted than ingested and zero calcium balance if the amount of calcium absorbed daily from food is matched exactly by the amounts of calcium lost in the faeces, urine and from the skin (Fig. 8.2).

Alimentary calcium absorption This is not as efficient as renal tubular calcium reabsorption. Absorption is normally less than 70% (and usually less than 30%) of the calcium entering the gut. Net calcium absorption (the difference between calcium ingested by mouth and calcium excreted in the faeces) can be determined by traditional metabolic balance techniques. To avoid negative calcium balance, net absorption must fully offset calcium losses

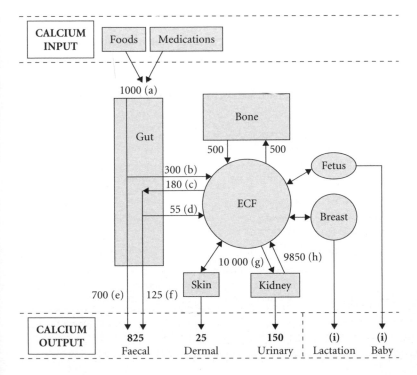

Fig. 8.2 Diagram of calcium influxes (mg/day) of subject in calcium balance (input = output). ECF, extracellular fluid; (a) total calcium ingested by mouth; (b) dietary calcium absorbed; (c) calcium in digestive secretions; (d) reabsorbed endogenous calcium; (e) unabsorbed dietary calcium; (f) endogenous faecal calcium excretion; (g) calcium load filtered at glomerulus; (h) calcium reabsorbed from glomerular filtrate (> 98%); (i) losses only incurred in pregnancy (full-term baby has 25–30 g calcium) or lactation (160–300 mg/day in breast milk).

from the urine and skin. However, measurement of net calcium absorption considerably underestimates the total calcium absorbed from the intestine into blood, because some faecal calcium (endogenous faecal) is derived from calcium resecreted into the intestine in the digestive juices, rather than from unabsorbed food calcium. True alimentary calcium absorption (amount actually absorbed from the gut) is measured with radioisotopes or stable isotopes, ^{42}Ca and ^{44}Ca.

Factors affecting the bioavailability of calcium in the intestine Variations in the efficiency of absorption are mainly determined by vitamin D metabolites and the rate of transit of gut contents through the intestine. Calcitriol improves calcium absorption (see Chapter 14). However, some is absorbed even in vitamin D-deficient states, because some calcium is absorbed by passive concentration-dependent diffusion. The duodenum absorbs calcium most avidly, but larger quantities of calcium are absorbed by the ileum and jejunum because food spends longer there. Some calcium is also absorbed from the colon, and surgical resection can impair absorption. Carbohydrates, such as lactose, improve calcium absorption by augmenting its passive diffusion across villous membranes. Diets rich in oxalate, fibre and phytic acid are reputed to depress alimentary absorption by complexing calcium in the gut. However, their overall effects seem small, possibly because bacterial breakdown of uronic acid and phytates in the colon frees calcium for absorption. Poor bioavailability of calcium from spinach is attributed to the high oxalate content. Dietary phosphorus increases the endogenous secretion of calcium into the gut. Lastly, calcium absorption diminishes in both sexes in the seventh decade of life because of lower renal synthesis of calcitriol and intestinal resistance to calcitriol, which contribute to the genesis of senile osteoporosis (see section 8.1.6).

Factors influencing urinary calcium loss Urinary excretion rises when the filtered load of calcium increases or the tubular reabsorption of calcium decreases. Acidifying agents, dietary sodium, protein and caffeine raise excretion. Phosphorus, alkaline agents (bicarbonate, citrate) and thiazide diuretics lower excretion. Variations in salt intake explain much of the day-to-day fluctuation in urinary calcium. One teaspoonful of salt (100 mmol NaCl) raises urinary calcium by 40 mg calcium/day, even on a low calcium intake. Purified sulphur-containing amino acids (methionine and cysteine) cause significant calciuria but phosphate in whole proteins mitigates their calciuric effect when consumed in foods. Vegetarians with an alkaline urine excrete less urinary calcium than meat-eaters, who have an acid urine.

8.1.5 Dietary calcium

Body calcium stores are built and maintained by extracting and retaining calcium from food. Dietary needs vary with gender, ethnicity, age and the magnitude of obligatory calcium loss (Table 8.1). It is critically important at all stages of life to consume and absorb enough dietary calcium to satisfy physiological calcium needs because some bone will be mobilized to maintain blood calcium levels whenever losses of calcium exceed alimentary calcium absorption (Fig. 8.3).

Threshold concepts Few people consume too much calcium from natural foods. However, many eat too

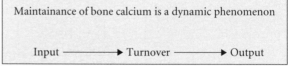

Maintainance of bone calcium is a dynamic phenomenon
Input ⟶ Turnover ⟶ Output

Dietary supply	Resorption/Formation	Urinary
		Faecal
Gastrointestinal		Dermal
absorption		Lactation

Loss of bone will ensue if:		
Ca input does not fully offset Ca output	Bone resorption is greater than bone formation	Obligatory Ca losses are not offset by a rise in Ca input

Fig. 8.3 Ways in which bone loss is caused.

little: this may affect their skeletons detrimentally, especially in childhood when skeletal needs are high, and in later life (> 65 years) when alimentary absorption of calcium deteriorates. There is a threshold intake for calcium below which skeletal calcium accumulation is a function of intake, and above which skeletal accumulation does not further increase, irrespective of further increases in intake. In other words, 'enough' calcium is good, but 'extra' calcium will not increase bone formation.

Recommended nutrient intake There is considerable controversy over the optimal daily dietary intake of calcium for individuals to achieve PBM, to maintain adult bone mass and to prevent loss of bone in later life. There may be ethnic and genetic differences in calcium requirements. Experts who argue for lower intakes point out that large sections of the population manage to grow and maintain bone on calcium intakes well below the current United States recommended dietary allowance (RDA) (Table 8.1).

Table 8.1 United States dietary recommendations for calcium and magnesium[a]

Life stage group		Calcium (mg/day)		Magnesium (mg/day)	
		RDA /AI*	UL	RDA/AI*	UL[b]
Infants	(0–6 m)	210*	ND	30*	ND
	(7–12 m)	270*	ND	75*	ND
Children	(1–3 y)	500*	2500	80	65
	(4–8 y)	800*	2500	130	110
Males	(9–13 y)	1300*	2500	240	350
	(14–18 y)	1300*	2500	410	350
	(19–30 y)	1000*	2500	400	350
	(31–50 y)	1000*	2500	420	350
	(>50 y)	1200*	2500	420	350
Females	(9–13 y)	1300*	2500	240	350
	(14–18 y)	1300*	2500	360	350
	(19–30 y)	1000*	2500	310	350
	(31–50 y)	1000*	2500	320	350
	(>50 y)	1200*	2500	320	350
Pregnancy	(≤18 y)	1300*	2500	400	350
	(19–30)	1000*	2500	350	350
	(31–50)	1000*	2500	360	350
Lactation	(≤18 y)	1300*	2500	360	350
	(19–30)	1000*	2500	310	350
	(31–50)	1000*	2500	320	350

[a] Food and Nutrition Board, Institute of Medicine (1997) *Dietary reference intakes for calcium, phosphorus, magnesium, vitamin* D *and fluoride*. National Academy Press, Washington DC.
RDA = recommended dietary allowance, AI = adequate intake, UL = tolerable upper intake level, ND = not determined.
[b]UL for magnesium represents intake from pharmacological agents only and does not include intake from food or water.

Many consider the even higher intakes recently advocated by the NIH Consensus Group in 1994 are extreme. It is disturbing to note that recommendations are continuing to climb. Many people find difficulty in consuming more than 1000 mg calcium daily from natural foods. Evidence of bone benefit from high dietary intakes in older adults seems insufficient to justify recommending calcium intakes exceeding the current United States RDA. Higher calcium intakes would require widespread use of food fortification or calcium supplementation by large sections of the population. A better way to boost the calcium economy would be to lower dietary salt intake. This will reduce obligatory loss of calcium and improve calcium balance. Moderate vitamin D supplementation may be useful in the housebound elderly.

Food sources of calcium Foods vary greatly in their calcium content (Table 8.2). Milk has an especially high calcium content, and in Western countries dairy products supply up to two-thirds of the total daily intake. Other excellent sources of calcium include cheeses, yoghurt and soymilk substitutes. Other good sources of calcium include nuts, canned fish with bones, leafy vegetables and dried fruit. In some countries, foods are fortified with mineral calcium salts.

Dietary advice to increase calcium intake while following nutritional guidelines for lowering fat intake includes:

- Have a serving of either yoghurt or milk daily for breakfast.
- Always have low-fat milk available in the fridge.
- Choose low-fat dairy products at the supermarket.
- Add cheese chunks or a sprinkling of nuts to salads/vegetables.
- Eat pieces of cheese, nuts or green vegetables as snacks.
- Add grated cheese or milk when serving soups and pasta.
- Use canned fish with bones in sandwich spreads.

Table 8.2 Calcium content of some common foods

Calcium sources	Serving size		mg Ca/ serving
Excellent sources			
Milk, whole	1 cup	250 ml	295
Trim[a], fat-reduced	1 cup	250 ml	375
Soymilk	1 cup	250 ml	255
Yoghurt	1 tub	150 g	180
Cheddar cheese	1 slice	20 g	150
Good sources			
Ice cream, vanilla	1 scoop	85 g	115
Cottage cheese	½ cup	120 g	75
Nuts, peanuts	½ cup	80 g	50
Almonds/walnuts	10 nuts	12 g/50 g	30
Canned sardines	½ cup	50 g	270
Canned salmon	½ cup	120 g	110
Leeks/broccoli	1 cup	150 g	100
Cabbage/spinach	1 cup	160 g	30–80
Dried apricots	½ cup	70 g	65
Dried figs	½ cup	100 g	290

[a]*Trim* milk is fat-reduced (0.4%) with added skimmed milk solids.
Source: Athar, N., McLaughlin, J., Taylor, G., and Suman, M. (2006) *The concise New Zealand food composition tables*, 7th edition. New Zealand Institute for Crop and Food Research, Palmerston North, New Zealand.

- Try tofu chunks with salads and casseroles.
- Add a little skimmed milk powder to recipes when baking.
- Serve vegetables in white sauces made with milk.
- Use yoghurt in place of cream with desserts.

Satisfactory intake of calcium may be sustained lifelong when individuals choose calcium-rich foods they like.

Calcium supplementation and food fortification
Individuals who find it difficult to eat enough calcium may benefit from mineral supplements. People
with very low calorie intakes, milk allergies or symptomatic lactose malabsorption may need to consume
foods fortified with calcium (soybean and citrus
drinks, breakfast cereals) or take supplements. These
are absorbed as well as food calcium.

Calcium intoxication Ingestion of large amounts
of alkaline calcium salts (more than 2.5 g Ca/day)
can override the ability of the kidney to excrete unwanted calcium, causing hypercalcaemia and meta-
static calcification of the cornea, kidneys and blood
vessels. People consuming huge quantities of calcium
carbonate in antacids are prone to this intoxication
(milk-alkali syndrome). Patients taking vitamin D,
or its metabolites, may suffer similar symptoms.
Large amounts of vitamin D are poisonous (see
section 14.1.10)

8.1.6 Factors affecting bone growth and attrition

Normal growth Both boys and girls display similar
linear gains in calcium up to the age of about 10 years
(Fig. 8.4). Their total body calcium then averages
400 g, indicating a daily increment of 110 mg over
this period. Skeletal growth accelerates at puberty.
Spinal density matures earlier in girls, who go through
puberty earlier than boys. Total body calcium doubles
in girls between the ages of 10 and 15 years (an average gain of 200 mg daily).

Boys have two extra years of prepubertal bone
gain before their pubertal growth spurt, when they
deposit over 400 mg calcium daily in bone. Children
do not have higher calcium absorption than adults.
Obligatory losses are also high and there are concerns
that many children consume too little calcium to
meet their skeletal needs. In teenagers, bone mass can
be increased by supplementation. However, the gain
may be temporary and catch-up may occur in children who consume less calcium. It may just take

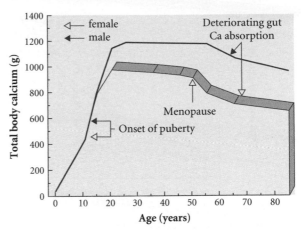

Fig. 8.4 Lifetime changes in total body calcium in men
(upper curve) and women (lower curve).

children longer to attain their skeletal potential on
moderate calcium intakes than on very high intakes.

Environmental factors such as calcium intake,
physical activity and sex steroid status influence bone
accrual. Cigarette smoking and excess alcohol affect
bone mass adversely whereas high physical activity,
adequate dietary calcium and sex steroids favour
bone accrual. Regular moderate exercise should be
recommended for youngsters. Children with good
lean body mass have the best bone mass (Fig. 8.5). In
teenagers with anorexia nervosa and athletic amenorrhoea, low oestrogen status causes poor PBM. Girls
who recover from these conditions continue to show
thin spinal bone years after plasma oestrogen levels
have returned to normal.

Bone attrition Bone density declines after middle
life. Falling levels of sex steroids cause trabecular loss,
while calcium deprivation speeds cortical loss. Effects
of oestrogen deprivation are particularly sharp at
menopause (Fig. 8.4). Bone losses are considerable:
from youth to old age, women lose half their trabecular bone and a third of their cortical bone, while men
lose a third of their trabecular bone and a fifth of their
cortical bone. Low bone mass in the elderly may be
due to poor PBM, to subsequent excessive loss of
bone, or to both of these factors. Bone density will

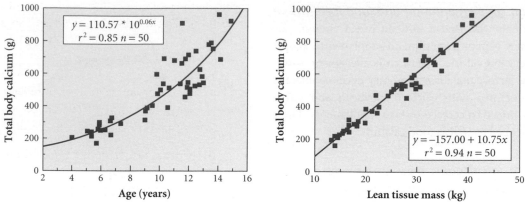

Fig. 8.5 Total body calcium changes in 50 growing girls aged 3 – 15 years, in relation to age ($r = 0.92$) and lean tissue mass ($r = 0.97$). Author's data.

fall below the fracture threshold at a younger age in people with low PBM than in those with high PBM. Variations in the genetic inheritance of factors affecting mineral metabolism and bone cells probably affect PBM, rate of bone loss and susceptibility to bone fracture importantly. People inheriting different polymorphisms of the vitamin D receptor gene may differ in their dietary requirements for calcium and vitamin D and in their bone density.

Bone fractures and osteoporosis Weak bones break more easily than strong ones. Thus, low bone density increases fracture risk, even in youth. In childhood, up to a third of all fractures affect the distal forearm.

Fractures at this site are particularly common in early puberty when bone is remodelling fast and calcium requirements are especially high. Children who break their wrists have lower bone density than those without fractures. Increasing calcium intake and physical activity during growth help to strengthen their skeletons and avoid fractures (see Box 8.2). Osteoporosis is a serious and expensive public health problem, particularly in women. It causes significant pain and morbidity among elderly people (see section 8.1.2). The incidence of osteoporotic fractures is expected to increase in future because people are living longer. In 1990, there were 1.66 million estimated hip fractures worldwide. By the year 2025, it is projected that there will be 1.16 million hip frac-

BOX 8.2

Case 1. A boy who habitually avoided milk products because he disliked the taste was seen at 6.5 years and 2 years later. At 7.8 years he broke his forearm falling less than standing height on carpet, playing with his sister. Although his total body calcium at 8.5 years was 582 g and his DXA bone mineral density (BMD) values were slightly above average (111% of expected values), he had experienced rapid, inappropriate weight gain, possibly because he ate almond croissants daily for breakfast and exercised little. In 2 years he had gained 14.1 kg (11.2 g fat per day) and his body mass index (BMI) had risen from the 75th to >95th percentile for age. At 8.5 years he had the average weight of a 12-year-old (41.2 kg) but ultradistal radius BMD suitable only for a 10-year-old. He thus fell heavily on insufficient bone. Obesity, milk avoidance and inactivity can increase fracture risk in growing children.

tures in men and 2.78 million in women due to osteoporosis. At present, the best way to avoid osteoporotic fractures in later life is to grow a good skeleton, to achieve optimal genetic skeletal mass and then to retain this as long as possible. Every effort should therefore be made to ensure life-long consumption absorption and retention of sufficient calcium to do this (see Box 8.3).

> **BOX 8.3**
>
> **Case 2.** A 73-year-old woman (ht 152 cm, wt 48 kg, BMI 20.8 kg/m²) referred for investigation had been diagnosed; lactose intolerant at age 7 years. She then avoided dairy products all her life without consuming other calcium-rich foods but was active and a keen gardener. DXA scans taken 65 years after diagnosis of lactose intolerance confirmed severe osteoporosis and a low total body calcium content of only 488 g (half the young adult value of 960 g). Her BMD T scores were: −5.63 (wrist); −3.10 (hip); −5.71 (spine); −3.89 (total body). She was promptly placed on bone-conserving medication to reduce fracture risk. This case shows that sustained dietary calcium deprivation is detrimental to bone health. T score compares BMD with normal young adult.

8.1.7 Other possible health effects of calcium

Hypertension and pre-eclampsia may be influenced by dietary calcium. High intakes are considered protective. However, the emphasis should be on maintaining good overall nutrition rather than on individual nutrients. Consumption of balanced meals that meet the recommendations of national health organizations and provide adequate calcium, potassium and magnesium are recommended. The novel Dietary Approaches to Stop Hypertension (DASH) trial (Doyle and Cashman, 2004) showed that this approach quickly lowered blood pressure. Bowel cancer risk may be lowered among subjects consuming a high calcium diet. More conclusive evidence is required to support this contention, which is based on epidemiological studies.

The consumption or absorption of other substances may be influenced by calcium intakes. Milk products contain considerable fat. However, fat-reduced dairy products are available for the cholesterol-conscious and those worried about obesity. There are concerns that high dietary calcium may lower iron absorption, but eating citrus fruit—with its high vitamin C content—can prevent this. High levels of calcium also aggravate the inhibitory effect of phytic acid on zinc absorption. Calcium binds gut oxalate so supplements do not induce kidney stones. Calcium may lower absorption of tetracyclines.

Population subgroups with special nutritional needs and who are vulnerable to calcium deprivation should be targeted to improve calcium economy and safeguard bone health. Such groups include:

- People with habitually low dietary calcium intakes.
- People with food allergies or lactose malabsorption.
- Adolescents building maximal bone.
- Girls with anorexia nervosa or athletic amenorrhoea.
- The calorie-conscious (slimmers often avoid dairy foods).
- People with very low dietary energy intakes.
- Pregnant women (last trimester) and lactating women.
- People with high intakes of common salt.
- People with heavy alcohol consumption.
- Patients with malabsorption syndromes.
- Patients taking corticosteroid medication.
- Patients with renal disease.
- Elderly people.
- People confined indoors who get no vitamin D from sunlight.

FURTHER READING

1. **Athar, N., McLaughlin, J., Taylor, G., and Suman, M.** (2006) *The concise New Zealand food composition tables*, 7th edition. New Zealand Institute for Crop and Food Research; Palmerston North.

2. **Doyle, L., and Cashman, K.D.** (2004) The DASH diet may have beneficial effects on bone health. *Nutr Rev*, **62**, 215–20.

3. **Goulding, A.** (2001) Bone mineral density and body composition in boys with distal forearm fractures: a dual

energy X-ray absorptiometry study. *J Pediatr*, **139**, 509–15.

4. **Matkovic, V.** (2005) Calcium supplementation and bone mineral density in females from childhood to young

adulthood: a randomized controlled trial. *Am J Clin Nutr*, **81**, 175–88.

5. **Nordin, B.E.C.** (1997) Calcium and osteoporosis. *Nutrition*, **13**, 664–86.

8.2 Magnesium

Andrea Grant

Ever since McCollum observed a deficiency of magnesium in both rats and dogs in the early 1930s, magnesium has been an intriguing mineral. It has both physiological and biochemical functions and important interrelationships, especially those with the cations calcium, potassium and sodium. Magnesium is also involved with second messengers, parathyroid hormone (PTH) secretion, vitamin D metabolism and bone functions.

8.2.1 Distribution and functions

About 60–65% of the body content, that is 1 mol (25 g) of magnesium in an adult person, is found in the skeleton. Like calcium, it is an integral part of the inorganic structure of bones and teeth. Unlike calcium, magnesium is the major divalent cation in the cells, accounting for most of the remaining magnesium, with 27% in the muscles and 7% in the other cells. Intracellular magnesium is involved in energy metabolism, acting mainly as a metal activator or cofactor for enzymes requiring adenosine triphosphate (ATP), in the replication of DNA and the synthesis of RNA and protein; it appears to be essential for all phosphate transferring systems. Several magnesium-activated enzymes are inhibited by calcium while in others magnesium can be replaced by manganese.

The remaining 1% of the body content of magnesium is in the extracellular fluids; the plasma concentration is about 1 mmol/L of which, as with calcium, about one-third is protein bound. Magnesium and calcium have somewhat similar effects on the excitability of muscle and nerve cells, but calcium has a further important function in signalling, which requires its concentration in the cells to be kept extremely low.

8.2.2 Metabolism

Magnesium is absorbed primarily from the small intestine, both by a facilitated process and by simple diffusion. Absorption can vary widely and on average about 40–60% of dietary intake is absorbed. Excretion is mainly through the kidneys, and increases with dietary intake. The kidney is extremely efficient in conserving magnesium; when the intake decreases, the urine can become almost magnesium-free. The intestinal and renal conservation and excretory mechanisms in normal individuals permit homeostasis over a wide range of intakes.

8.2.3 Dietary sources of magnesium

Magnesium is present like potassium in both animal and plant cells and is also the mineral in chlorophyll. Green vegetables, cereals, legumes and animal products are all good sources. In contrast to calcium, dairy products tend to be low in magnesium, with cow's milk containing 120 mg Mg/L (5 mmol/L) compared with 1200 mg Ca/L (30 mmol/L). The calcium, phosphate and protein in meat and other animal products reduce the bioavailability of magnesium from these sources. Average magnesium intake is about 320 mg/day (13 mmol/day) for males and 230 mg/day (10 mmol/day) for females.

8.2.4 Magnesium deficiency

Since magnesium is the second most abundant cation in cells after potassium, dietary deficiency is unlikely to occur in people eating a normal varied diet. Shils

Table 8.3 Magnesium depletion and accompanying changes

	Blood chemistry	Metabolic balances
Magnesium	Plasma Mg ↓	Mg negative
Potassium	Serum K ↓	K negative
Calcium	Serum Ca ↓	Ca positive
Sodium	Serum Na no change	Na positive

Table 8.4 Clinical conditions associated with occurrence of magnesium deficiency

- Habitual or sustained low dietary supply/intake (<250 mg/day)
- Poor alimentary absorption – malabsorption syndromes (such as Crohn's disease), short bowel syndrome, laxative abuse
- Excessive body losses – via sweat or urine (genetic disorders, diabetes, alcohol abuse, diuretics)
- Increased requirement – pregnancy or lactation
- Hospitalized patients – 65% of intensive care patients are hypomagnesaemic
- Endocrine disorders, such as parathyroid disorders and hyperaldosteronism

found it difficult to produce magnesium deficiency experimentally in his classical studies of the 1960s using human volunteers (Shils, 1969). These studies showed the interrelationships between magnesium and the other principal cations calcium, potassium and sodium. The plasma concentration of magnesium decreased progressively, as did serum potassium and calcium, whereas the serum sodium remained normal even though sodium was being retained (Table 8.3). Functional effects, including personality changes, abnormal neuromuscular function and gastrointestinal symptoms, were restored to normal only by repletion of magnesium. Hypomagnesaemia can precipitate hypocalcaemia because magnesium is required for the secretion of PTH.

Hypomagnesaemia is important clinically (Table 8.4) and is usually due to losses of magnesium from the kidney or gastrointestinal tract. Magnesium depletion induces neuromuscular excitability and may increase the risk of cardiac arrhythmias and cardiac arrest.

8.2.5 Magnesium excess

Large dietary intakes of magnesium appear unharmful to humans with normal renal function: hypermagnesaemia is uncommon and is almost impossible to achieve from food sources alone.

Magnesium supplementation is useful clinically to treat pregnancy-induced hypertension (pre-eclampsia and eclampsia). Many people also take oral magnesium supplements (such as Epsom salts) to prevent constipation, because they have a cathartic effect.

8.2.6 Magnesium status

Serum magnesium concentration is the most frequently used index of magnesium status. Plasma is not used because anticoagulants may be contaminated with magnesium.

8.2.7 Recommended nutrient intakes

The United States' recommended intakes of magnesium at different stages of life are shown in Table 8.1. The United Kingdom's are 300 mg/day for men and 270 mg/day for women.

Conclusion

The essential mineral magnesium is located intracellularly and in bone. It promotes enzyme actions and is needed for PTH secretion. It is widely distributed in foods. Severe deficiency is rare but mild hypomagnesaemia is common in ill patients, alcoholics and those with malabsorption syndromes.

Magnesium supplementation is used to prevent eclampsia and as a laxative.

Acknowledgement

The section on magnesium was originally written by the late Professor Marion Robinson. Andrea Grant helped to update it for the present edition.

FURTHER READING

1. Committee of Medical Aspects of Food Policy (COMA) (1991) Magnesium. In *Dietary reference values for food and energy and nutrients for the UK. Report 41*. London, HMSO, pp. 146–9.

2. **Fleet, J.E., and Cashman, K.D.** (2001) Magnesium. In: Bowman, B.A. and Russell, R.M. (eds) *Present knowledge in nutrition*, 8th edition. Washington, DC, ILSI, pp. 292–301.

3. **Food and Nutrition Board, Institute of Medicine** (1997) *Dietary reference intakes for calcium, phosphorus, magnesium, vitamin D and fluoride*. Washington, DC, National Academy Press.

4. **Knochel, J.P.** (1998) Disorders of magnesium metabolism. In: *Harrison's principles of internal medicine*, 14th edition. New York, McGraw Hill, pp. 2263–66.

5. **Shils, M.E.** (1969) Experimental production of magnesium deficiency in man. *Ann NY Acad Sci*, **162**, 847–55.

 To see topical and scientifically robust updates on nutrition associated with this textbook, and active web links to many of the journal articles in the Reference areas, please see the dedicated Online Resource Centre at www.oxfordtextbooks.co.uk/orc/mann3e/.

9 Iron

Patrick MacPhail

Iron deficiency is the most frequently encountered nutritional deficiency in man. It has been estimated that 500–600 million people suffer from iron-deficiency anaemia. Many more have depleted iron stores and are at risk for the development of anaemia. Paradoxically, iron overload is also a major clinical problem in some populations. Genetic haemochromatosis affects 1 in 300 people in populations of northern European origin. In rural sub-Saharan Africa, up to 25% of the adult population are iron overloaded, while in parts of Asia and the Mediterranean there is a high prevalence of iron overload secondary to thalassaemia major. Both iron deficiency and iron overload have serious consequences and are major causes of human morbidity.

Iron owes its importance in biology to its remarkable reactivity. Of paramount importance is the reversible one-electron oxidation–reduction reaction that allows iron to shuttle between ferrous (Fe^{2+}) and ferric (Fe^{3+}) forms. This reaction is exploited by most iron-dependent enzyme systems involving electron transport, oxygen carriage and iron transport across cell membranes. It is also responsible for the toxicity seen in acute and chronic iron overload. These contradictory properties are managed by highly specialized and conserved proteins involved in the storage and transport of iron and in regulating the concentration of intracellular iron.

In recent years there has been an explosion of knowledge about the proteins of iron metabolism, filling many gaps in our understanding and, at the same time, creating new questions that have still to be answered.

9.1 Basic iron metabolism

The total body iron content is about 50 mg/kg. Over 60% is in the haemoglobin of red blood cells and about 25% is in the form of stores, mainly in the liver. The remainder is distributed between myoglobin in muscles (8%) and in enzymes (5%). A small amount (about 3 mg) is in transit in the circulation bound to the plasma transport protein, transferrin.

9.1.1 Iron absorption

The mechanism by which iron is absorbed from the gut is not clearly understood, but recent work has uncovered the existence of a number of genes coding for proteins involved in the control of iron absorption and transport of iron across membranes. Four phases are recognized. In the *luminal phase*, food iron is solubilized, largely by acid secreted by the stomach, and is presented to the duodenum and upper jejunum where most iron absorption takes place. Factors that maintain the solubility of iron in the face of rising pH, such as valency (ferrous iron is better absorbed), mucin secreted by the cells lining the gut (mucosa) and chelators (ascorbic acid), appear to be important in this phase. The second phase, *mucosal uptake*, depends on iron binding to the brush border of the apical cells of the duodenal mucosa and transport of iron into the cell. In the third *intracellular phase*, iron either enters a storage compartment in the storage protein, ferritin, or is transported directly to the opposite side of the mucosal cell and released. In the *release phase*, iron is released from the mucosal cell into the portal circulation where it is bound to the transport protein, transferrin. Both iron uptake and particularly iron release by the mucosal cell are inversely related to the amount of iron stored in the body and directly related to the rate of erythropoiesis.

The recently discovered polypeptide, *hepcidin*, which is secreted by hepatocytes, plays a central role in the control of both iron absorption and the regulation of internal iron exchange. The mechanism whereby the body's iron status is sensed, and the secretion of hepcidin subsequently altered, involves a number of proteins expressed mainly in the liver (Fig. 9.1). The relationship between these proteins is uncertain since HFE and TfR1 (8 and 6 in Fig. 9.1) are expressed in Kupffer cells and somehow communicate with hepatocytes. Mutations of the genes coding for some of these proteins are responsible for the

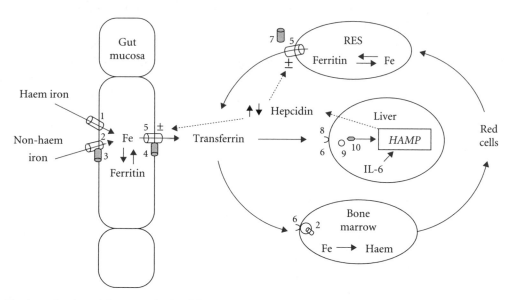

Fig. 9.1 The iron circuit and the central role of the liver. Iron, absorbed from the lumen of the small intestine (left), passes through the mucosal cell and enters the circulation where it is bound to transferrin and redistributed to tissues. Most goes to the bone marrow for the production of haemoglobin in red cells. After about 120 days, the red cells are engulfed by the reticuloendothelial system (RES) and the iron either stored in ferritin or redistributed back to transferrin. 1, Haem carrier protein (HCP1) transports haem into cells; 2, divalent metal transporter (DMT1) transports non-haem iron (Fe^{2+}) into cells; 3, duodenal cytochrome b (Dcytb), a ferrireductase, converts Fe^{3+} to Fe^{2+}; 4, hephaestin, a ferroxidase, converts Fe^{2+} to Fe^{3+}; 5, ferroportin 1 or IReg1 transports iron out of cells and is regulated by hepcidin; 6, transferrin receptor 1 (TfR1) binds with and transfers transferrin into cells and also forms a complex with HFE; 7, caeruloplasmin, a ferroxidase, converts Fe^{2+} to Fe^{3+}; 8, HFE (function unknown) binds to TfR1 on membrane and senses iron status; 9, transferrin receptor 2 (TfR2) (function unknown) senses iron status; 10, haemojuvelin (function unknown) senses iron status.

severe disturbances in iron metabolism that lead to iron overload (sections 9.1.3 and 9.7).

The gut mucosal cell (enterocyte) needs the ability to transport iron from the lumen into the cell, store the surplus iron and release it when required into the portal circulation. Two forms of dietary iron need to be accommodated, and specialized iron transporters are found on the luminal surface to cater for them. Haem iron, derived mainly from myoglobin and haemoglobin in food, is transported into the cell by *haem carrier protein 1* (HCP1) (1 in Fig. 9.1) where the haem molecule is 'opened' by the enzyme haemoxygenase and the iron released. Non-haem iron, derived from a wide variety of foods, has to be in the ferrous form before it can be transported across the cell membrane by the *divalent metal transporter* (DTM1 or NRAMP2) (2 in Fig. 9.1). The reduction from ferric to ferrous iron is achieved by a membrane-bound ferric reductase called *duodenal cytochrome b* (Dcytb) (3 in Fig. 9.1). Once in the cytoplasm, iron derived from these two iron sources is handled similarly, either being stored in *ferritin* or released into the portal circulation. The release of iron from all cells is mediated by a specialized transmembrane protein called *ferroportin* (5 in Fig. 9.1), the surface expression of which is controlled by *hepcidin*. In the case of the enterocyte, a copper-containing membrane-bound ferrioxidase, *hephaestin* (4 in Fig. 9.1), converts the iron to the ferric form to enable it to bind to the iron transporter, *transferrin*.

9.1.2 Internal iron exchange

Once released from the mucosal cell, iron enters the portal circulation and is bound to the transport protein, transferrin (Fig. 9.1). Normally, transferrin is about 30% saturated with iron and most of the absorbed iron is transported directly to the bone marrow where it is incorporated in haemoglobin. The mechanism of transferrin uptake by the young red cells, and all active cells, involves a specific *transferrin receptor* (TfR1) (6 in Fig. 9.1) expressed on the surface of the cell. The iron–transferrin receptor complex is taken into the cell contained within a vesicle. A fall in the pH within the vesicle causes the iron to be released from transferrin. The iron is then trans-

ported through the vesicle membrane into the cell by DMT1 (2 in Fig. 9.1). The transferrin-receptor complex, now devoid of iron, is cycled back to the cell surface where the transferrin is released back into the circulation. At the end of its lifespan, the red cell is engulfed by cells of the reticuloendothelial system (RES), located mainly in the liver, spleen and bone marrow. The iron is separated from haem and either stored in ferritin or as haemosiderin. Ferrous iron is released back into the circulation via ferroportin (5 in Fig. 9.1), again under the control of hepcidin, where it is converted to ferric iron by caeruloplasmin (7 in Fig. 9.1) and again picked up by transferrin.

It should be noted that most of the iron entering the circulation comes from recycled red cells via the RES and not from iron absorption (ratio about 20:1). There is normally only one way into the iron circuit and there is no way out except through blood loss or, in pregnancy, to the fetus. In reality, a small amount of iron is lost. In men, this amounts to about 1 mg/day, mainly through loss of blood and surface cells of the gut, urinary tract and skin. The loss is relatively easily balanced by iron absorption. In women, additional losses through menstruation (0.5 mg/day), and the cost of pregnancy (2 mg/day) and lactation (0.5 mg/day), make it more difficult to balance the loss through iron absorption.

9.1.3 The level of intracellular and circulating iron control the expression of important iron proteins

It has long been known that the body responds to changes in iron requirements by increasing or decreasing the release of iron from the gut and from the RES. The recent discovery of the iron transporter *ferroportin* and its regulator *hepcidin* has greatly enhanced our understanding of how this may be achieved (Fig. 9.1). Hepcidin, a small 25 amino acid peptide, is secreted by the liver under the influence of at least two known mechanisms. The first senses the demand for iron, possibly through the saturation of transferrin, and the second is part of the immunological response mediated by cytokines, particularly

IL-6. The proteins that sense iron requirements (6, 8, 9 and 10 in Fig. 9.1) work together but their relationship to each other is poorly understood. That mutations in any of these proteins may result in severe disturbances of iron metabolism attests to their central role in iron homeostasis. TfR1 and HFE (6 and 8) are present together on the cell surface and, through binding to circulating transferrin and in concert with two other proteins—*transferrin receptor 2* (TfR2) (9) and *haemojuvalin* (10)—appear to be able to sense the body's iron requirements. The result is a change in the rate of transcription of *HAMP*, the gene responsible for encoding hepcidin. Hepcidin in turn binds to ferroportin, causing the iron transporter to be internalized and degraded, thus inhibiting iron release. This feedback mechanism causes increased iron release when iron is scarce and switches off iron release when it is plentiful. The responsiveness of the system is enhanced by the fact that hepcidin, being a small polypeptide, is rapidly excreted by the kidney.

It has long been known that inflammation has a profound effect on iron metabolism. Pioneering work by Bothwell and Finch in the 1950s showed that inflammation induced by turpentine resulted in hypoferraemia, impaired iron absorption and impaired iron transport to the fetus. It is now understood that these effects are mediated through increased secretion of hepcidin, limiting iron release by ferroportin. IL-6, as part of the immune response, increases transcription of *HAMP*, bypassing the HFE-mediated effect. Injection of IL-6 results in a rapid rise in hepcidin and a profound fall in serum iron. If this is sustained, the resulting iron starvation inhibits haemopoiesis and leads to anaemia. While other factors such as shortened red cell survival and direct inhibition of the bone marrow contribute to the *anaemia of chronic disorders*, hepcidin-induced hypoferraemia is the central cause. The advantage to the body of the hypoferraemia induced by inflammation appears to be the limitation of iron supply to an invading organism.

While hepcidin controls the level of iron in the circulation, and hence its distribution, the level of intracellular iron within the cytosol of the cell controls the expression of some important proteins involved in the movement of iron in and out of cells. Control is at the level of the translation of messenger RNA (mRNA) to protein and is mediated by an iron–sulphur protein (iron-responsive protein or IRP), which binds to the mRNA. In the iron-deficient state, the IRP binds to the 5′ untranslated region of some mRNAs (e.g. ferritin) inhibiting translation and to the 3′ untranslated region of other mRNAs (e.g. transferrin receptor and DMT1) stabilizing the mRNA. In the presence of iron, the binding is lost and ferritin mRNA is translated while the mRNA of transferrin receptor and DMT1 becomes unstable. The result of this reciprocal arrangement is that ferritin mRNA is translated into protein when the level of iron in the cell rises and there is a need for iron storage while, when the level of iron is low, more transferrin receptor and more DMT1 is translated, facilitating the movement of iron into the cell.

9.2 Iron balance

Iron requirements must be balanced by iron supply if iron deficiency or iron overload are to be avoided. Several factors combine to influence iron balance (Fig. 9.2). Obligatory iron losses, the requirements of growth and pregnancy as well as pathological losses due to excessive menstrual and other bleeding must be balanced against iron supply. Iron supply is influenced by the amount and type of iron in food and the combination of various inhibitors and promoters of iron bioavailability. These requirements are buffered by iron, which can be mobilized from stores. In addition, the body has the ability to modulate iron absorption according to its needs. Iron absorption is inversely related to body iron stores with more iron being absorbed by iron-deficient individuals that by iron-replete and iron-overloaded individuals. In addition, an increased rate of blood formation (erythropoiesis) with increased demand for iron

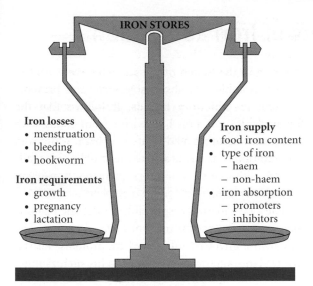

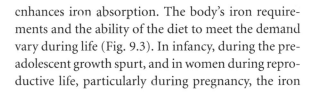

Fig. 9.2 Iron balance. Iron losses and requirements for growth (left) are balanced by iron supplied in the diet (right). Surplus iron is stored and can be drawn upon to supplement increased losses or requirements.

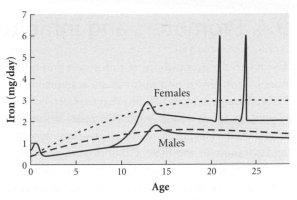

Fig. 9.3 Iron requirements for males and females vary during life. A Western diet, rich in meat and iron promoters (------) is able to meet iron requirements of the majority of females at all ages, except in infancy, at the peak of pubertal growth spurt, and at onset of menstruation and during pregnancies. In contrast, a cereal-based diet, without meat or iron promoters and with excess inhibitors of iron absorption (– – – –) is not able to meet the requirements of most childbearing women and some men.

enhances iron absorption. The body's iron requirements and the ability of the diet to meet the demand vary during life (Fig. 9.3). In infancy, during the pre-adolescent growth spurt, and in women during reproductive life, particularly during pregnancy, the iron requirements may exceed the iron supply, making iron deficiency more common during these periods. Individuals consuming a diet of low iron bioavailability are even more at risk.

9.3 Iron in food

Iron supply is greatly influenced by the composition of the diet. Two broad categories of iron are present in food: haem iron derived mainly from haemoglobin and myoglobin in meat, and non-haem iron in the form of iron salts, iron in other proteins and iron derived from processing or storage methods. Haem iron enters the mucosal cells by a different mechanism (see section 9.1.1) and is better absorbed than non-haem iron. It is also less influenced by the body's iron status and, because the iron is protected by the haem molecule, it is not affected by other constituents in the diet. Non-haem iron compounds are found in a wide variety of foods of both plant and animal origin. The iron is present in metalloproteins (e.g. ferritin, haemosiderin and lactoferrin), soluble iron, iron bound to phytates in plants, and contaminant iron such as ferric oxides and hydroxides introduced in the preparation and storage of food and by contamination from soil. The bioavailability of these forms of non-haem iron, unlike haem iron, is influenced by other constituents of the diet. Forms of iron that are similarly affected are said to enter a 'common pool'. The importance of this concept is that fortificant iron added to food will be subjected to the same inhibitory and promotive influences as the intrinsic food iron and will therefore have similar bioavailability. This concept, however, does not hold true for all forms of added iron. For example, most ferric salts, whether contaminant or added as fortificants, do not enter the common pool and have very low bioavailability.

9.4 Promoters and inhibitors of iron absorption

The relative concentrations of promoters and inhibitors of iron absorption in foods are responsible for the wide range of bioavailability that has been demonstrated in foods (Table 9.1). The most important *promoters* of non-haem iron absorption are ascorbic acid (vitamin C) and meat. Other organic acids (e.g. citric acid) and some spices have also been shown to enhance iron absorption. The major *inhibitors* of iron absorption are phytates and polyphenols, common constituents of cereals and many vegetables.

Ascorbic acid is thought to enhance iron absorption by converting ferric to ferrous iron and by chelating iron in the lumen of the gut. This keeps iron in a more soluble and absorbable form and prevents binding to inhibitory ligands. It follows that the bioavailability of non-haem iron from foods with significant ascorbic acid content is high. Moreover, the addition of ascorbic acid to meals of low bioavailability with potent inhibitors increases non-haem iron absorption.

The factor in meat responsible for enhancing non-haem iron absorption has not been identified. The enhancing effect is not shared by proteins derived from plants and other animal proteins such as milk,

Table 9.1 Relative bioavailability of non-haem iron in foods

Food	Bioavailability		
	Low	Intermediate	High
Cereals	Maize Oatmeal Rice Sorghum Whole wheat flour	Corn flour White flour	
Fruits	Apple Avocado Banana Grape Peach Pear Plum Rhubarb Strawberry	Cantaloupe Mango Pineapple	Guava Lemon Orange Pawpaw Tomato
Vegetables	Aubergine Legumes Soyflour	Carrot Potato	Beetroot Broccoli Cabbage Pumpkin
Beverages	Tea Coffee	Red wine	White wine
Nuts	All		
Animal proteins	Cheese Egg Milk		Fish Meat Poultry Breast milk

cheese and eggs. For example, substitution of beef for egg albumin as a source of protein in a test meal resulted in a fivefold increase in iron absorption. Present evidence suggests that peptides rich in the amino acid cysteine may play a role in the enhancement of non-haem iron absorption.

Polyphenols commonly found in many vegetables and in some grains are potent inhibitors of non-haem iron absorption. There is a strong inverse relationship between the concentration of polyphenols in foods and the absorption of iron from them. Many of the foods with low iron bioavailability listed in Table 9.1 are rich in polyphenols. Among the best-known polyphenols is tannin, found in tea and other beverages, which has a profound inhibitory effect on iron absorption. Polyphenols also form strongly coloured compounds with iron, which is a major problem in food fortification. This phenomenon can be illustrated by dropping a few crystals of ferrous sulphate into a cup of tea.

Phytates, found mainly in the husks of grains, are also major inhibitors of iron absorption. In this regard, iron absorption from unpolished rice is significantly worse than from polished rice, while increasing the bran content of a meal produces a dose-related depression in iron bioavailability. Both meat and ascorbic acid are able to overcome this inhibitory effect.

9.5 Recommended dietary intake

The concept of a recommended dietary intake of iron is difficult to reconcile with the wide range of bioavailability (Table 9.1). The total iron content of a diet is a meaningless, although commonly employed, measure of its nutritional adequacy and may provide a false sense of nutritional security. For example, foods with high iron content due to large quantities of contaminant iron, or inappropriate fortificant iron, may be nutritionally worthless because of the low bioavailability of the iron. On the other hand, haem iron, making up only 10–15% of the total ingested iron, may account for a third of the iron actually absorbed. Similarly, the iron absorbed from a meal containing non-haem iron may be doubled if the meal is taken with a glass of orange juice (30 mg ascorbic acid) or reduced to a third if taken with tea. However, it is possible to divide diets into ones of low, intermediate and high iron bioavailability. These correspond to iron absorption of about 5%, 10% and 15% in subjects with depleted iron stores.

A diet of low bioavailability (< 5%) with a high inhibitor content, negligible amounts of enhancers and little haem iron is based largely on unrefined cereals and legumes. Such diets are typical of many developing countries and supply about 0.7 mg of available iron daily, which is insufficient to meet the needs of most women, growing children and some men. A diet of intermediate bioavailability (about 10%) includes limited amounts of foods that promote iron absorption and supplies enough absorbed iron (about 1.5 mg) to meet the needs of 50% of women. A diet of high iron bioavailability (> 15%) contains generous amounts of food rich in promoters and haem iron. The inhibitor content is low as cereals are often highly refined. Such diets, typical of many developed countries, supply sufficient iron (> 2.1 mg daily) for most adults but still cannot match the daily amounts of absorbed iron required in the second half of pregnancy (5 mg daily).

The Food and Agriculture Organization/World Health Organization (FAO/WHO) recommendations (Table 9.2) based on estimates that apply to the 95th percentile of the population, are an attempt to take variations in bioavailability and requirements into account.

BOX 9.1

Although human milk contains less iron than cows milk, the iron in human milk is much more bioavailable (estimated absorption 45 to 100%). The US Institute of Medicine consider that the iron provided by exclusive breast feeding is adequate to meet the needs of infants up to the age of 6 months.

Table 9.2 FAO/WHO recommended daily iron intake for individuals consuming diets of low, intermediate and high iron bioavailability. Requirements are given for absorbed iron.

Group	Age (years)	Requirements of absorbed iron (µg/kg/day)	Recommended intake (mg/day)		
			Low (5%)	Intermediate (10%)	High (15%)
Children	0.25–1	120	21	11	7
	1–2	56	12	6	4
	2–6	44	14	7	5
	6–12	40	23	12	8
Boys	12–16	34	36	18	12
Girls	12–16	40	40	20	13
Adult men		18	23	11	8
Adult women					
Menstruating		43	48	24	16
Post-menopausal		18	19	9	6
Lactating		24	26	13	9

Source: FAO/WHO (1988).

9.6 Iron deficiency

In the past, iron deficiency was thought to be due largely to abnormal loss of iron rather than insufficient iron supply. Credence for this view was given by the obvious effects of pathological blood loss and the high prevalence of iron deficiency in the developing world where hookworm infestation is endemic. However, it is now apparent that the poor bioavailability of iron in largely unrefined cereal-based diets is the major cause of iron deficiency in most developing countries. The impact of such diets is obviously enhanced when pathological blood loss or increased physiological iron demand is also present. These factors explain the geographical and gender variation in the prevalence of iron-deficiency anaemia, which is most common in Asia where up to 60% of women and over 30% of men are anaemic. This should be compared with the prevalence in Europe and North America where less than 5% of females and 2% of

males are anaemic. The preponderance of females can be explained by increased physiological loss of iron in menstruation and pregnancy and to their lower food, and therefore iron, intake.

The development of iron deficiency is characterized by sequential changes in the amount of storage iron in the various iron compartments of the body (Fig. 9.4). In the first stage, iron stores become depleted, but there is enough iron to meet the needs of red cell production. When iron stores are exhausted, the amount of iron in the circulation starts to fall, and red cell production becomes compromised (iron-deficient erythropoiesis). In the final stage, iron stores are exhausted, the amount of iron in the circulation is very low, red cell production is drastically reduced and anaemia develops. The point at which the function of iron-containing enzymes becomes impaired is uncertain, but probably depends on the rate of

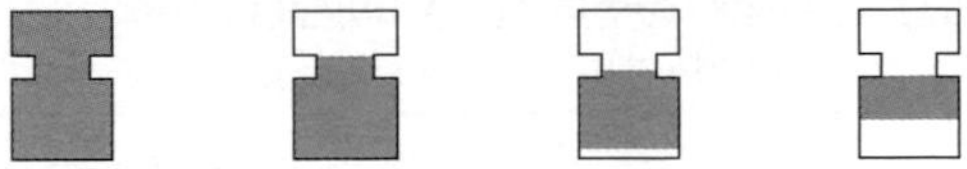

	Normal	Depleted stores	Iron-deficient erythropoiesis	Iron-deficiency anaemia	
IRON STORES RED CELLS					
Tissue iron	Normal	Depleted	Absent	Absent	
Serum ferritin	Normal	↓↓	↓↓↓	↓↓↓	
Serum iron	Normal	Normal	↓↓	↓↓↓	
Transferrin saturation	Normal	Normal	↓↓	↓↓↓	
Haemoglobin	Normal	Normal	Normal	↓↓	

Fig. 9.4 The measurement of iron status and the stages of iron depletion. As iron in each of the body compartments is depleted (moving from left to right), different measurements of iron status become abnormal. No single biochemical index can assess all stages.

renewal of the enzymes and the growth of the tissues involved.

Iron deficiency has been associated with a number of pathological consequences of which anaemia is the most obvious. Severe anaemia is associated with weakness, impaired effort tolerance and, eventually, heart failure. There is no doubt that even mild iron-deficiency anaemia limits work performance and studies in Indonesia and Sri Lanka have linked it to reduced productivity. There is evidence from animal experiments that both the anaemia and tissue iron depletion are important. In children, iron-deficiency anaemia is associated with impaired psychomotor development. In pregnancy, the weight of evidence suggests that iron-deficiency anaemia is associated with prematurity, low birth weight and increased perinatal mortality. Changes in the gastrointestinal tract (atrophy of the mucosa of the mouth, oesophagus and stomach) and the skin and nails (spoon-shaped nails), are well described but infrequent. Other less-well-recognized abnormalities include inability to adapt to cold and impaired immunity.

9.7 Iron overload

Excessive amounts of iron may accumulate in the body and result in organ damage. The *acute* ingestion of a large amount of bioavailable iron, usually in the form of ferrous sulphate tablets, will exceed both the ability of the mucosa to control iron absorption and the capacity of transferrin to bind iron in the circulation. The acute iron toxicity that results is thought to be due to the generation of free radicals by free iron, both in the gut and in the circulation. Most of the victims are children, who develop severe abdominal pain, vomiting, metabolic acidosis and cardiovascular collapse. Severe poisoning, requiring urgent chelation therapy, may follow ingestion of more than 30 mg of iron/kg.

Chronic iron overload develops insidiously and the recent discovery of novel genes coding for proteins involved in iron sensing and transport have greatly increased our understanding of iron overload. Iron overload, ranging from trivial to life threatening, is the end result of a large number of genetic abnormalities involving many of the proteins of iron metabolism. The types of *haemochromatosis*, in which hepcidin and its effect on ferroportin play a role, are listed in Table 9.3. Type 1 is the most common form and is found almost exclusively in people of north-western European origin, reaching a homozygous prevalence of 1.2 to 1.4% in Ireland and Denmark. Types 1 to 3 share common features but differ in severity and age of onset. In these types, iron floods the circulation and excessive iron is deposited over years in the liver, heart, pancreas and other organs. The damage to these organs is thought to be due to free radicals

Table 9.3 Classification of haemochromatosis

Type	Protein (see Fig. 9.1)	Gene (common mutation)	Clinical Picture
1 Classic (adult)	HFE (8)	*HFE* (C282Y in >80%)	Recessive inheritance. Severe iron overload with organ damage (liver, heart, pituitary). Type1 has variable expression. Parenchymal iron distribution (hepatocytes, cardiac muscle, endocrine tissues) with little or no iron in reticuloendothelial tissues (spleen, bone marrow). High transferrin saturation (> 50%), secondarily high serum ferritin. Low urinary hepcidin.
2 Juvenile	A Haemojuvelin (10) B Hepcidin	*HFE2* *HAMP*	
3 Non-HFE (adult)	Transferrin receptor 2 (9)	*TFR2*	
4 Dominant	Ferroportin (5)	*SLC40A1*	Dominant inheritance. Variable effects from severe to trivial. Reticuloendothelial iron distribution (spleen, Kupfer cells, bone marrow), parenchymal loading late and in severe cases. High serum ferritin, transferrin saturation normal, later high.

and can result in liver cirrhosis, liver cancer, heart failure, arthritis and endocrine disease (diabetes and impotence). Removal of iron by repeated bleeding is an effective treatment. Interestingly, recent epidemiological studies have shown that the majority of people homozygous for the common mutation of type 1 haemochromatosis (C282Y) do not go on to develop the full-blown clinical features.

Two other clinically important forms of iron overload, sometimes called secondary, should be mentioned. *African dietary iron* overload is caused by the ingestion, over many years, of large amounts of highly bioavailable iron in low-alcohol beer brewed in iron containers. Recent evidence suggests that there is also a genetic predisposition, possibly related to a muta-tion unique to Africans in the ferroportin gene, that may play a role. The distribution of iron is the same as that seen in haemochromatosis type 4 and, in severe cases, the toxic effects of iron are similar to those seen in the other forms of haemochromatosis. *Secondary iron overload* occurs in the so-called 'iron-loading anaemias' of which thalassaemia major is the most common. Excessive amounts of iron are absorbed over a relatively short period because of the increased turnover of red cells. In addition, repeated blood transfusions add to the iron burden. The iron overload occurs more rapidly and most victims die from iron-induced heart failure. A similar syndrome is seen in patients with bone marrow failure, kept alive by repeated blood transfusions.

9.8 Assessment of iron status

Iron-deficiency anaemia develops in three stages: (1) iron depletion, (2) iron-deficient erythropoiesis, and (3) iron-deficiency anaemia (Fig. 9.4). No single biochemical index can assess all three stages.

- During *iron depletion*, the amount of storage iron in the liver and in the reticuloendothelial cells of the spleen and bone marrow is progressively reduced and can be detected by a parallel fall in serum ferritin concentration. The serum ferritin concentration falls below 12 µg/L (12 ng/mL) when the iron stores are exhausted. Iron depletion is the only cause of a serum ferritin below this level. Other measurements of iron status are normal at this stage.

- In *iron-deficient erythropoiesis*, iron stores are exhausted (serum ferritin < 12 µg/L) and iron supply to the marrow is insufficient to meet the needs of haemoglobin production. This stage is detected by a low serum iron concentration and transferrin saturation below 16%, although the haemoglobin concentration is still within the normal range. Transferrin saturation is derived from the serum iron and the total iron binding capacity (TIBC) as shown below:

$$\text{Transferrin saturation (\%)}$$
$$= \frac{\text{Serum iron (µmol/L)}}{\text{Serum TIBC (µmol/L)}} \times 100$$

- In *iron-deficiency anaemia*, the supply of iron to the marrow is so reduced that the concentration of haemoglobin falls below normal. The 'cut-off' value below which anaemia is diagnosed varies according to age and gender (below 110 g/L in children younger than 6 years and in pregnant women; below 120 g/L in women and adolescents under 15 years and below 130 g/L in adult men). There are obviously many other causes of anaemia besides iron deficiency (e.g. vitamin B_{12} and folate deficiency, chronic infection and intrinsic diseases of the bone marrow). The diagnosis of anaemia due to iron deficiency therefore requires that other measurements of iron status are also in the iron-deficient range (serum ferritin < 12 µg/L and transferrin saturation < 16%). In addition, in established iron-deficiency anaemia, the red cells become small (microcytosis) and pale (hypochromia). These changes can be detected by examination of a blood film or by a fall in the mean cell volume (MCV) below 85 fl and in the mean cell haemoglobin concentration (MCHC) below 27 pg.

- Serum ferritin concentration and transferrin saturation are subject to variation due to causes other than iron status. For example, serum iron concentration and, hence, the transferrin saturation, exhibits marked diurnal (within-day) variation and is depressed in infection, while the serum ferritin concentration is elevated by inflammation and tissue damage. Other tests can be employed that circumvent these problems. The production of haem is dependent on the supply of iron to the marrow. When iron supply is restricted, protoporphyrin, a precursor of haem, accumulates in red cells. This *free erythrocyte protoporphyrin* (FEP) is not subject to diurnal variation and provides the same information as the transferrin saturation. In addition, the FEP can be measured very easily on a single drop of blood using a simple instrument called a haematofluorometer. A transferrin saturation lower than 16% is associated with an FEP greater than 70 µg/dL (1.24 µmol/L) red cells. The FEP is, however, also elevated in lead poisoning and in inflammation. In this situation, the serum ferritin concentration is usually elevated as well. Tissue iron depletion can also be measured by the concentration of *transferrin receptor* in plasma or serum. The expression of transferrin receptors on the surface of all cells is determined by the level of intracellular iron. In cellular iron depletion, the concentration of soluble transferrin receptor in the plasma rises but, unlike the serum ferritin concentration, the level is less affected by inflammation. Using these two measurements in the form of a ratio (serum transferrin receptor/log serum ferritin) has proved useful in distinguishing iron deficiency from inflammation as the cause of anaemia. However, no biochemical test currently available is able to unequivocally separate the two causes. Urinary hepcidin concentration, which is high in inflammation and low in iron deficiency, may prove helpful in this regard.

- The diagnosis of *iron overload* is also measured by a combination of measurements of iron status. A raised serum ferritin concentration (> 400 µg/L) and transferrin saturation greater than 60% are highly suggestive of types 1–3 haemochromatosis. However, high levels of serum ferritin may also be due to inflammation or tissue damage. The level of iron stored in the liver, previously determined on liver biopsy, can now be measured by magnetic resonance scanning.

9.9 Treatment and prevention of iron deficiency

Iron-deficiency anaemia is best treated by the oral administration of ferrous iron salts. The cheapest and most effective is ferrous sulphate, which is usually given in a dose of one tablet (65 mg of iron) two to three times a day. The increase in haemoglobin concentration that can be expected with optimal doses of ferrous sulphate is about 2 g/L/day. Gastrointestinal side effects of oral iron therapy are common, which has lead to a plethora of different oral iron compounds being available. Most differ in their formulation in an attempt to limit side effects, the most popular being slow-release preparations. None has been shown to be convincingly better than ferrous sulphate and all will correct iron deficiency in time. The addition of ascorbic acid, while enhancing food iron availability, does little to improve therapeutic efficacy and probably increases the side effects.

It has been argued that a better response to iron supplementation, particularly in pregnancy, would be obtained if iron was given weekly or twice weekly instead of daily. The argument is based on reduced side effects, easier monitoring and the supposed occurrence of a 'mucosal block' when iron is given daily. However, a 'mucosal block' has not been convincingly demonstrated in humans and, in practice, response to supplementation is dependent on the dose of iron administered, which makes weekly regimens less effective. In persons intolerant of oral iron therapy, it is possible to give iron by intramuscular or intravenous injection.

It is theoretically possible to prevent iron deficiency by manipulation of the diet. This is well illustrated by the low prevalence of iron deficiency in industrialized countries where the diet is rich in haem iron and in promoters of non-haem iron absorption. However, this approach is impractical and expensive in developing countries where the diets are cereal-based and the problem of iron deficiency is greatest.

The only alternative is to fortify foods with iron or with iron plus a promoter of iron absorption.

Unfortunately, the fortification of food with iron is fraught with practical difficulties. The major dilemma is the fact that the most bioavailable iron compounds are also the most soluble and the most reactive, leading to unacceptable changes in the taste and colour of the food vehicle. Insoluble salts, such as ferric orthophosphate and elemental iron powders, produce no changes in food but are poorly absorbed. The iron chelate, sodium ferric EDTA (Fe III EDTA) escapes the effects of inhibitors, particularly phytates, and, in this setting, the iron is two to three times better absorbed than ferrous sulphate. It also produces little change in the colour of the food vehicle. Field trials carried out systematically in iron-deficient populations have shown Fe III EDTA to be an effective fortificant. In one study, the prevalence of iron deficiency in women was reduced from 22% to 5% over a 2-year period. No harmful effects of the EDTA itself, which is widely used in the food industry as an antioxidant, have been detected and the Joint FAO/WHO Expert Committee on Food Additives (JECFA) considers Fe III EDTA safe for use in supervised fortification programmes. Similar claims have been made regarding the amino acid chelate ferrous bisglycinate. The use of either of these compounds has been limited because of cost in spite of their enhanced iron bioavailability. Fe III EDTA is about six times more expensive than ferrous sulphate, while ferrous bisglycinate is about 20 times more expensive.

Despite these limitations, fortification of food with iron is commonplace in the industrialized world. Paradoxically, these fortification programmes have often been carried out in a haphazard way with little attention being paid to the bioavailability of the fortificant or the efficacy of the programme. Iron used to fortify wheat flour contributes about 20% of the intake in the USA and 10% in the UK. Although there has been a decline in the prevalence of iron deficiency since iron fortification programmes were introduced, their efficacy remains uncertain. In particular, the value of elemental iron, widely used as a fortificant but thought to have very low bioavailability, has still to be proved. In contrast, iron fortification of infant formulas and infant cereals has been shown to be effective in combating iron deficiency in this target group. In 1999, the American Academy of Pediatrics recommended that all infant formulas should be fortified with iron. In most cases, ferrous sulphate has been used to fortify milk and soy-based products. The bio-availability of the iron in these preparations is greatly enhanced by the addition of ascorbic acid.

In the developing world, iron fortification programmes face additional problems. Foods are seldom centrally processed, making fortification a difficult logistical problem. Furthermore, the diets are largely cereal-based and lack natural promoters of iron absorption, which means that the added iron will be poorly absorbed. Methods of overcoming these problems were recently the subject of a SUSTAIN workshop, the proceedings of which were published in detail in the *International Journal for Vitamin and Nutrition Research*.

FURTHER READING

1. **FAO/WHO** (1988) *Requirements of vitamin A, iron, folate and vitamin B$_{12}$.* Report of a Joint Expert Consultation. FAO Food, and Nutrition Series, No. 23. Rome, Food and Agricultural Organization.

2. **Hershko, C.** (2005) Iron diseases. *Best Pract Res Clin Haematol*, **18**, 157–380.

3. **Hurrell, R., Bothwell, T., Cook, J.D.,** *et al.* (2002) The usefulness of elemental iron for cereal flour fortification. A SUSTAIN Task Force report. *Nutr Rev*, **60**, 391–406.

4. **SUSTAIN** (2004) Innovative ingredient technologies to enhance iron absorption. Proceedings of a SUSTAIN workshop. *Int J Vitam Nutr Res*, **74**, 385–475.

 To see topical and scientifically robust updates on nutrition associated with this textbook, and active web links to many of the journal articles in the Reference areas, please see the dedicated Online Resource Centre at www.oxfordtextbooks.co.uk/orc/mann3e/.

10 Trace elements

10.1 Zinc

Samir Samman

10.1.1 Historical perspective

The essentiality of zinc was first recognized in micro-organisms and plants in 1869 and 1926, respectively. Experimental deficiency was demonstrated in laboratory animals but the likelihood of deficiency in humans was considered remote because of the ubiquitous nature of zinc in the food supply and the relative difficulty in creating zinc-deficient animal models. Zinc deficiency was first recognized in humans in 1958.

10.1.2 Distribution and function

Zinc is one of the IIB series of metals with an atomic mass of 65.4 (Fig 10.1). It is the most common catalytic metal ion in the cytoplasm of cells. Adult humans contain between 1.2 and 2.3 g of zinc, which is distributed in all tissues. The highest concentrations of zinc are observed in the choroid of the eye and the prostate gland, but most of the body zinc is in bones and muscles. In liver cells, zinc is associated with all subcellular fractions. The plasma concentration of zinc is approximately 15 μmol/L, of which a third is bound to a_2-macroglobulin and the rest to albumin. However, only 10–20% of the zinc in blood is found in the plasma; the rest is in red blood cells associated mainly with carbonic anhydrase. The red cell membrane contains some zinc. Semen has 100 times the zinc concentration of plasma.

Molecular biological techniques (microarrays) have identified genes that are potential candidates for regulation by zinc and have highlighted the complexity of the effects of zinc status on gene expression: some genes are positively affected; others negatively; and some are affected only by extremes of zinc status (deficiency or excess). Some of the genes identified include those involved in the regulation of redox state, fatty acid synthesis and degradation, signal transduction, growth factor activity, platelet activation and the regulation of homocysteine concentrations. Zinc 'fingers' have been identified in the human genome. The proteins, which may contain up to 30 'fingers', have been identified as sequence-specific DNA-binding proteins that interact with DNA and act as transcriptional mediators. Zinc also plays a role in stabilizing macromolecules and cellular membranes and it can function as a site-specific antioxidant.

It can bind to or in close proximity to thiol groups of proteins and reduce their reactivity. Zinc is a constituent of a large number of mammalian enzymes (more than 150) where it functions at the active site or as a structural component or both. Carbonic anhydrase was the first discovered zinc metalloenzyme;

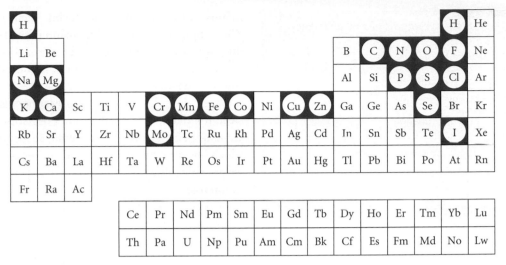

Fig. 10.1 Periodic table of the elements. Those essential for man are encircled in black. In addition, boron, silicon, nickel, arsenic and vanadium are still under consideration as ultratrace elements.

other enzymes include: carboxypeptidase, alkaline phosphatase, transferases, ligases, lyases, isomerases, DNA/RNA polymerase, reverse transcriptase and superoxide dismutase. Therefore, zinc is important in a number of major metabolic processes including protein and nucleic acid synthesis. Zinc is essential for the synthesis and action of insulin. It also helps to stabilize the proinsulin and insulin hexamers by forming complexes with them.

10.1.3 Absorption and excretion

Zinc is absorbed mainly from the duodenum but some is absorbed lower down the small intestine. The mode of absorption involves both saturable and passive mechanisms. The exact site of absorption depends on the form of zinc and the presence or absence of other nutrients, which may form complexes with zinc or impact on intestinal transit time. Once absorbed, zinc is transported to the liver bound to albumin.

The major route of zinc excretion is by the intestine followed by the kidneys and the skin. Faecal zinc originates from unabsorbed dietary sources, as well as zinc that is excreted into the intestine along with the digestive juices (endogenous excretion). Smaller amounts of zinc are excreted in the urine or shed

in skin cells. In addition, sexual activity in males contributes to zinc losses. In well-controlled metabolic ward studies, it has been shown that each ejaculate can contain up to 0.5 mg of zinc, which is thought to be derived from secretions of the prostate gland. Although conservation of zinc occurs during experimental zinc deficiency, the amount of zinc in ejaculates remains relatively high, thus representing a significant loss of zinc, particularly in people with low intakes. Hence, the role of zinc in men is analogous to iron in women in that it is lost as part of normal sexual function.

10.1.4 Deficiency

Zinc deficiency is estimated by the World Health Organization (WHO) to be one of the ten biggest factors that contribute to burden of disease in developing countries. Zinc deficiency was first observed in adolescents in Iran and Egypt. The first case was a 21-year-old man who resembled a 10-year-old boy. His main food was unleavened bread from unrefined wheat flour and he ate a considerable amount of clay. Other cases had hookworm infections and ate mostly unleavened wheat bread and beans. Unleavened bread prepared from unrefined wheat flour has a high

BOX 10.1 Some symptoms of zinc deficiency

Mild deficiency

- Stunted growth in children
- Decreased taste sensation
- Impaired immune function

Severe deficiency

- Dwarfism
- Hypogonadism and delayed sexual maturation
- Hypopigmented hair

phytate content, which interferes with zinc absorption. Further investigations identified zinc as the limiting nutrient responsible for numerous symptoms including growth retardation, hypogonadism and delayed sexual maturation. Other manifestations of zinc deficiency reported subsequently include diverse forms of skin lesions, impaired wound healing, loss of taste (hypogeusia), behavioural disturbances, night blindness and immune deficiency. These symptoms do not always occur together and seem to depend on the setting. For instance, in patients on total parenteral nutrition (if it lacks zinc), there is mental confusion, depression, eczema and alopecia. In young children, zinc deficiency is expressed as a reduction in appetite, poor taste acuity and poor growth.

Night blindness, a significant symptom of vitamin A deficiency in developing countries, can be due to deficiency of zinc, which is a coenzyme for the conversion of retinol to retinaldehyde by retinol dehydrogenase. Also, zinc deficiency may be partly responsible for the high rates of infection and diarrhoea in developing countries. Zinc supplementation of infants and young children has been shown in controlled trials to substantially reduce rates of diarrhoea and pneumonia. Despite these important findings in developing countries, there is no strong evidence that zinc lozenges are effective in treating symptoms of the common cold in developed countries.

Zinc deficiency is common in developing countries with high mortality. Deficiency has been observed in association with protein-energy malnutrition in infants with marasmus or during their recovery. Zinc supplements supplied to malnourished children during recovery promote weight gain and synthesis of lean tissue, and reduce common comorbidities. Anorexia nervosa in some ways resembles marasmus; however, the role of zinc in anorexia nervosa is unclear. It is likely that zinc deficiency develops in some anorexic patients through a generally inadequate diet, which sustains the disorder and prevents adequate weight gain. However, zinc does not appear to play a causal role.

In pregnancy, plasma zinc has been reported to be low and although this can be attributed partly to physiological changes unrelated to zinc depletion, the intakes of pregnant women are often below the recommendations. Adaptations in pregnancy such as increased absorption and reduced endogenous losses may help meet the requirement. Apart from possible reduction in induction of labour, caesarean section and preterm delivery and in some cases increases in birth weight and head circumference, zinc supplementation does not appear to have a significant or consistent effect on pregnancy outcome. Such inconsistencies may be related to small sample sizes, differing zinc status of pregnant women and inadequate study design.

Biochemical abnormalities of zinc deficiency include a reduction in plasma zinc concentrations, protein synthesis, activity of metalloproteins, resistance to infection, collagen synthesis and platelet aggregation. In view of the large number of zinc-finger proteins and the interaction between zinc and DNA, it has been hypothesized that zinc primarily restricts gene expression rather than the enzyme activities.

Conditions that predispose to deficiency are related to:

1. Decreased intake, possibly associated with an eating disorder.

2. Decreased absorption and/or bioavailability due to a high intake of an inhibitor (e.g. phytate) as noted in the first reported case of human zinc deficiency.

3. Decreased utilization secondary to other conditions such as alcoholism.

4. Increased losses in conditions such as diarrhoea and excessive vomiting, which may also be associated with an eating disorder.

5. Increased requirement associated with growth, pregnancy and lactation (the latter is recognized by a small increase in the recommended dietary intake for some countries).

10.1.5 Bioavailability and food sources

Zinc is available widely in the food supply but its bioavailability from different foods is highly variable. Zinc in animal products, crustacea and molluscs is more readily absorbed than from plant foods. Rich sources of zinc include oysters, red meat, lamb's liver and cheese. Cereal grains, legumes and nuts are rich in phytate, which reduces zinc absorption. The zinc content of refined cereals is lower than unrefined cereals but because the bran (which contains most of the phytate) has been removed, the bioavailability is greater. Although a number of factors are known to influence the bioavailability of zinc, a reliable algorithm to calculate available zinc remains to be worked out. The molar ratio of phytate:zinc has been proposed as a predictor of zinc bioavailability and ratios greater than 15 have been associated with suboptimal zinc status. The phytate × calcium:zinc in the diet has been suggested as a marker of zinc bioavailability; however, there is limited data on the phytate content of foods. WHO has put forward three categories of bioavailability (Table 10.1).

The extent of adaptation to foods with low bioavailability of zinc is not fully understood and is confounded by the interaction with other nutrients. Current methods used for studying zinc bioavailability in humans include metabolic balance studies and radioisotope and stable isotope techniques. The radioisotope techniques are limited by ethical considerations such as long radioactive half-lives and the amount of radiation exposure to subjects. Use of stable isotopes circumvents this issue but this technique requires costly instrumentation and demanding analytical procedures.

Table 10.1 Dietary determinants of zinc bioavailability

Estimated absorption	Type of diet
Low (< 15%)	Diets high in unrefined cereal grain
	Phytate:zinc molar ratio > 15
	Calcium > 1 g/day
Moderate (15–35%)	Mixed diet containing animal or fish protein
	Phytate:zinc molar ratio < 10
High (35–55%)	Refined diets, low in cereal fibre
	Phytate:zinc molar ratio < 5
	Dietary protein primarily from animal foods

Source: WHO (1996).

Absorption of zinc from breast milk is high even in cases of the inborn error of zinc absorption (acrodermatitis enteropathica). The fractional absorption is approximately 0.6 mg/day, while relatively little is excreted endogenously.

10.1.6 Nutrient reference values

The recommended dietary intake for zinc is 11–14 mg/day for men in different committee reports and 8 mg for women (3 mg and 4 mg extra for pregnancy and lactation, respectively). The upper intake level (UIL) is 40 mg/day.

10.1.7 Biochemical tests for status

The plasma zinc concentration represents less than 1% of the body pool of zinc and hence its measurement provides a limited amount of information about zinc status of individuals. Zinc from the plasma is taken up by the liver in response to cytokines released during stress and infection. In addition, plasma zinc concentrations fall in pregnancy, with injuries and in diseases such as liver cirrhosis and pernicious anaemia. Plasma zinc also undergoes diurnal variation, with a U-shaped curve over a 24-hour period. Peak concentrations are found in the mornings, and trough concentrations in the mid-evening. Despite its limitations, the concentration of zinc in plasma is the most commonly used diagnostic indicator, and the balance of evidence shows that the concentration falls in deficiency and rises in sufficiency (or with supplementation). The zinc concentration of other accessible tissues such as red blood cells and platelets remains unchanged during controlled zinc deficiency and supplementation trials. Leukocyte and neutrophil zinc concentrations have been shown to be affected by zinc status in some studies but not others. Low zinc concentrations in hair probably reflect chronic zinc deficiency and hence hair zinc analysis may be a good tool to determine zinc status in long-term studies.

Although urine is readily accessible, collection of a 24-hour urine sample is awkward, inconvenient and susceptible to environmental contamination by exogenous sources of metal, as well as endogenous sources such as seminal fluid. Well-controlled studies have indicated that urine is not a good biomarker because zinc excretion is only sensitive to extreme changes in zinc status.

The activity of some metalloenzymes is depressed during nutritional zinc deficiency whereas others remain unaffected. Alkaline phosphatase activity in erythrocyte membranes is sensitive to zinc depletion and repletion. It is postulated that the activity of this metalloenzyme may be a useful reflection of zinc status. This enzyme plus the metal binding protein metallothionein are potentially suitable markers that deserve further investigation.

Although frank deficiency can be identified, marginal status is difficult to measure. Despite extensive research in this field, little applied information has been obtained. It is recognized that the biochemical tests for status are not ideal. The only sure way to diagnose zinc deficiency is by response of clinical signs to zinc supplementation.

10.1.8 Toxicity

The ingestion of doses above 1 g results in a metallic taste in the mouth, nausea, fever, lethargy and gastric distress. This acute response occurs due to deliberate supplementation, occupational exposure, or by food poisoning. The rapid infusion of intravenous feeding solutions that contain zinc can cause similar symptoms. Very large doses have resulted in death.

Intervention studies have shown that high-dose zinc supplementation (50 mg/day) decreases plasma high-density lipoprotein c concentrations in males. The major effect, however, is due to the adverse interaction between zinc and copper absorption. Zinc induces the synthesis of metallothionein, a sulphur-rich protein, which binds copper with high affinity. In chronic toxicity, copper status is reduced, resulting in a decrease in copper-related functions including the reduction in copper metalloenzyme activity, copper deficiency and anaemia. The reduction of copper absorption is advantageous under some circumstances. It is required in the treatment of patients with (Kinnear) Wilson's disease and zinc supplementation is part of the management strategy. The UIL for zinc for adults is 40 mg/day.

FURTHER READING

1. **Abdullah Brooks, W., Yunus, M., Santosham, M., Wahed, M.A., Nahar, K., Yeasmin, S., and Black, R.E.** (2004) Zinc for severe pneumonia in very young children: double-blind placebo-controlled trial. *Lancet*, **363**, 1683–8.

2. **Gibson, R.S.** (2005) *Principles of nutritional assessment*, 2nd edition. Oxford, Oxford University Press.

3. **Mahomed, K.** (2006) Zinc supplementation in pregnancy. *Cochrane Database Syst Rev*, Issue 3.

4. **Marshall, I.** (2006) Zinc for the common cold. *Cochrane Database Syst Rev*, Issue 3.

5. **Prasad, A.S.** (1984) Discovery and importance of zinc in human nutrition. *Fed Proc*, **43**, 2829–34.

6. **Shrimpton, R., Gross, R., Darnton-Hill, I., and Young, M.** (2005) Zinc deficiency: what are the most appropriate interventions? *Br Med J*, **330**, 347–9.

7. **World Health Organization** (1996) *Trace elements in human nutrition and health*. Geneva, World Health Organization, pp. 72–104.

10.2 Copper

Samir Samman

10.2.1 Historical perspective

The essential role of copper was realised in 1926 and soon after it was shown that it is required for the synthesis of haemoglobin in rats. In 1962, copper deficiency was reported in humans.

10.2.2 Distribution and function

Copper is one of the IB series of metals with an atomic mass of 63.5. It is one of the most effective cations for binding to organic molecules. It is commonly used in biological reactions that involve electron transfer.

Adult humans contain about 100 mg copper, distributed in concentrations of about 1.5 mg/g in the skin, skeletal muscle, bone marrow, liver and brain. Studies in animals suggest that the copper content may decrease with age. The plasma concentration is 15 µmol/L (similar to zinc). Up to 90% of this is associated with caeruloplasmin. Other copper proteins include many of the oxidases, metallothionein, α-fetoglobulin, superoxide dismutase and transcuprein. A distinguishing feature of copper proteins and enzymes is that the majority are extracellular.

Copper has diverse functions including erythropoiesis, connective tissue synthesis (via lysyl oxidase), oxidative phosphorylation, thermogenesis and superoxide dismutation. As well as transporting copper, caeruloplasmin is one of the acute-phase proteins, and via its ferroxidase activity it catalyses the oxidation of ferrous iron. This latter reaction is essential for the mobilization of iron as a complex with transferrin. It is believed to be the mechanism by which copper is able to regulate the homeostasis of iron.

10.2.3 Absorption and excretion

Copper is absorbed by an active transport process initially, then mostly by carrier-mediated diffusion from the stomach and duodenum. As absorption has been shown to control homeostasis, the efficiency increases in cases of deficiency. Absorbed copper is transported to the liver by albumin, where it is transferred to caeruloplasmin. Copper is excreted mainly via the gastrointestinal tract. Less is excreted in the urine and from the skin.

10.2.4 Bioavailability and food sources

Copper has a wide distribution in the food supply but in particular it is found in foods of animal source, legumes, nuts and the water supply (copper pipes). The concentration in water tends to be variable and may contribute substantially to the overall intake. Absorption is enhanced by organic nutrients such as amino acids and, in particular, histidine. Conversely, absorption is inhibited by excesses of other divalent cations such as zinc and iron. Studies in animals suggest that vitamin C may have an adverse effect on copper absorption, but the results of trials in humans are not conclusive. Phytic acid and dietary fibre do not inhibit copper absorption.

10.2.5 Deficiency

Copper deficiency is relatively rare. It has been observed in protein-energy malnutrition, in patients on long-term copper-free total parenteral nutrition, and in premature infants fed cow's milk or unfortified formula. Symptoms include anaemia, neutropaenia, skeletal demineralization, decreased skin tone, connective tissue aneurysms, hypothermia, neurological symptoms and hair depigmentation. Conditions predisposing to deficiency are, in principle, similar to those described for zinc.

Defects in copper metabolism have been identified. Menkes' disease was established as a copper-related disorder following the recognition by Australian researchers that patients with the disease have kinks in their hair similar to those in the wool of sheep grazing on copper-deficient soils. The characteristics of the hair together with low concentrations of plasma copper and caeruloplasmin are features of the disease. Intestinal absorption of copper is defective.

Patients who lack plasma caeruloplasmin have been identified. Recent findings in patients with acaeruloplasminaemia have confirmed the essential role of this copper protein in iron metabolism. Symptoms associated with acaeruloplasminaemia include decreased copper and iron in plasma, increased iron concentrations in tissues and impaired copper absorption.

10.2.6 Nutrient reference values

No estimated average requirement (EAR) or recommended dietary intake (RDI) has been estimated for copper. An adequate intake for adults is approximately 1.2 mg/day, with another 0.3 mg recommended for lactation. The UIL should not exceed 10 mg/day.

10.2.7 Assessment of copper status

Frank copper deficiency can be determined by the measurement of plasma copper concentrations, or plasma caeruloplasmin (either as a concentration or an enzymatic activity) or by determination of the activities of copper-dependent enzymes such as superoxide dismutase. The haematocrit decreases and there is microcytic hypochromic anaemia. The assessment of marginal deficiency remains a challenge. However, it appears that the activity of serum diamine

oxidase responds to increases in dietary or supplemental copper and has the potential to reflect copper status.

10.2.8 Toxicity

Acute toxicity has been reported as a result of accidental ingestion of large doses of copper or in industrial accidents. The symptoms of small doses include vomiting and nausea, while large doses induce hepatic necrosis and haemolytic anaemia. Chronic toxicity is relatively rare.

Wilson's disease, Indian childhood cirrhosis and idiopathic copper toxicosis are disorders that predispose individuals to copper overload. Wilson's disease is a rare inborn error of metabolism with a reported incidence of 1 in 30 000. It is an autosomal recessive disease that gives rise to hepatolenticular degeneration. Less well quantified are the incidences of Indian childhood cirrhosis (reported initially in India but also in other parts of the world in non-Indian children) and idiopathic copper toxicity. There is little evidence to support the efficacy of copper restriction for the management of Wilson's disease and other diseases of copper storage. The primary intervention has to be pharmacological (chelation) therapy to increase urinary copper excretion.

FURTHER READING

1. **Danks, D.M., Campbell, P.E., Stevens, B.J., Mayne, V., and Cartwright, E.** (1972) Menke's kinky hair syndrome. An inherited defect in copper absorption with widespread effects. *Pediatrics*, **50**, 188–201.

2. **Gibson, R.S.** (2005) *Principles of nutritional assessment*, 2nd edition. Oxford, Oxford University Press.

3. **Roberts, E.A., and Schilsky, M.L.** (2003) A practice guideline on Wilson disease. *Hepatology*, **37**, 1475–92.

4. **Strain, J.J.** (1994) Newer aspects of micronutrients in chronic disease: copper. *Proc Nutr Soc*, **53**, 583–98.

5. **WHO** (1996) *Trace elements in human nutrition and health*. Geneva, World Health Organization, pp. 123–43.

10.3 Iodine

Christine Thomson

Iodine was one of the earliest trace elements to be identified as essential. As early as 2700 BC, the Chinese were treating goitre by feeding seaweed, marine animal preparations and burnt sponge (rich in iodine). In the first half of the nineteenth century, the incidence of goitre was linked with low iodine content of food and drinking water, and by the late nineteenth century the geographic distribution of endemic goitre and cretinism was recognized to extend around the world. In the 1920s, iodine was shown to be an integral component of the thyroid hormone thyroxine, which is required for normal growth and metabolism, and later, in 1952, of triiodothyronine.

10.3.1 Chemical structure and functions of iodine

Iodine functions as an integral part of the thyroid hormones, the prohormone thyroxine (T_4) and the more potent active form 3,5,3′-triiodothyronine (T_3), which is the key regulator of important cell processes. Selenium is essential for normal thyroid hormone metabolism as a component of the iodothyronine deiodinases that control the synthesis and degradation of the biologically active hormone, T_3. The thyroid hormones are required for normal growth and development of individual tissues such as the central nervous system, and for maturation of the whole body, and also for energy production and oxygen consumption in cells, thereby maintaining the body's metabolic rate.

If thyroid hormone secretion is inadequate, the basal metabolic rate is reduced and the general level of activity of the individual is decreased (hypothyroidism). Normal growth and development will also be impaired. The regulation of thyroid hormone synthesis, release and action is a complex process involving the thyroid, the pituitary, the brain and peripheral tissues. The hypothalamus regulates the plasma concentrations of the thyroid hormones by controlling the release from the pituitary of the thyroid-stimulating hormone (TSH) through a feedback mechanism related to the level of T_4 in the blood. If blood T_4 falls, the secretion of TSH is increased, which enhances both thyroid activities and the output of T_4 into the circulation. This fine control of T_4 secretion is important, as either an excess or a deficit in the hormone will be detrimental to normal function. If the level of circulating T_4 hormone is not maintained because of severe iodine deficiency, TSH remains elevated, and both these measures are used for diagnosis of hypothyroidism due to iodine deficiency.

10.3.2 Body content

Iodine occurs in the tissues in both inorganic (iodide) and organically bound forms. The adult human body contains about 15–50 mg iodine, of which 70–80% is in the thyroid gland (it has a remarkable concentrating power for iodine) and the remainder is mainly in the circulating blood.

10.3.3 Metabolism

The metabolism of iodine is closely linked to thyroid function, since the only known function for iodine is in the synthesis of thyroid hormones. Iodine is an anionic trace element that is rapidly absorbed in the form of iodide and taken up immediately by the thyroid gland. Iodide is converted to iodine in the thyroid gland, and bound to tyrosine residues from which the hormones T_3 and T_4 are formed. The thyroid gland needs to trap around 60 µg iodide per day to maintain an adequate supply of T_4. Excess inorganic iodine is readily excreted in the urine, with smaller amounts in faeces and sweat. Since faecal output and losses from the skin are small, 24-hour urinary excretion of iodine reflects the dietary intake and hence may be used for estimating the intake. Normally, urine contains more than 90% of all ingested iodine.

Table 10.2 Spectrum of the iodine-deficiency disorders (IDD)

Fetus	Abortions
	Stillbirths
	Congenital anomalies
	Increased perinatal mortality
	Increased infant mortality
	Neurological cretinism: mental deficiency, deaf mutism, spastic diplegia, squint
	Myxoedematous cretinism: mental deficiency, dwarfism, hypothyroidism
	Psychomotor defects
Neonate	Neonatal hypothyroidism
Child and adolescent	Retarded mental and physical development
Adult	Goitre and its complications
	Iodine-induced hyperthyroidism
All ages	Goitre
	Hypothyroidism
	Impaired mental function
	Increased susceptibility to nuclear radiation

Source: WHO/NHD (2001).

10.3.4 Deficiency

Iodine deficiency is recognized as a major international public health problem because of the large number of populations living in iodine-deficient environments, characterized primarily by iodine-deficient soils. WHO estimates indicate that 2 billion people have inadequate iodine nutrition; 285 million of these are school children. At least 20 million may suffer from mental defect that is preventable by correction of iodine deficiency. The term iodine-deficiency disorders (IDD) refers to the wide spectrum of effects of iodine deficiency on growth and development (Table 10.2). Goitre, a swelling of the thyroid gland (as shown in Fig. 10.2), is the most obvious and familiar feature of iodine deficiency. The swelling reflects an attempt by the thyroid to adapt to the increased need to produce hormones. Hyperplasia of the thyroid cells occurs and the thyroid gland increases in size. Other effects are seen at all stages of development, but especially during the fetal and neonatal periods.

The most damaging consequences of iodine deficiency are on fetal and infant development. Thyroid hormones and, therefore, iodine are essential for normal development of the brain, and insufficient levels may result in permanent mental retardation of the fetus or newborn child. Iodine deficiency is the world's greatest single cause of preventable brain damage and mental retardation. The most severe effect of fetal iodine deficiency is endemic cretinism, which affects up to 10% of populations living in severely iodine-deficient areas of the world. In general, those with cretinism are mentally defective, with other physical abnormalities. Clinical manifestations may differ with geographical location, and two quite distinct syndromes have been observed. In myxoedematous cretinism, hypothyroidism is present during fetal and early postnatal development and results in stunted growth and mental deficiency. In the nervous or neurological type of cretinism, mental retardation is present as well as hearing and speech defects and characteristic disorders of stance and gait, while hypothyroidism is absent. This syndrome appears to result from iodine deficiency of the mother during fetal development, emphasizing the importance of adequate iodine intake during pregnancy as well as early postnatal life.

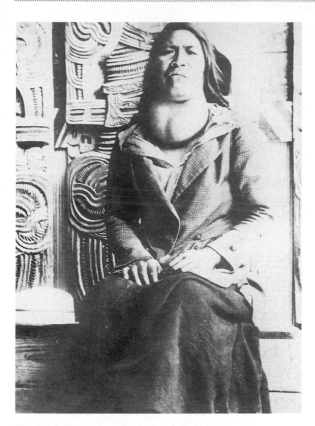

Fig. 10.2 Endemic goitre.

Source: Hercus, C.E., Benson, W.N., and Carter, C.L. (1925) Endemic goitre in New Zealand, and its relation to the soil iodine. *J Hygiene*, **2**, 321–402.

elevated hearing thresholds have been reported in school-age children with mild to moderate iodine deficiency (urinary iodine concentration of < 100 µg/L).

The major cause of IDD is inadequate dietary intake of iodine from foods grown in soils from which iodine has been leached by glaciation, high rainfall or flooding. Goitre is usually seen where the intake is less than 50 µg/day and cretinism where intake by the mother is 30 µg/day or less. However, thyroid function may also be impaired after exposure to antithyroid compounds in foods and drugs—called goitrogens—that prevent the uptake of iodine into the thyroid gland. Because selenium has an essential role in thyroid hormone metabolism, it has the potential to play a major part in the outcome of iodine deficiency through two aspects of its biological function. First, the selenium-containing iodothyronine 5′-deiodinases regulate the synthesis and degradation of T_3. Second, selenoperoxidases and possibly thioredoxin reductase protect the thyroid gland from hydrogen peroxide produced during the synthesis of thyroid hormones. Thus, selenium deficiency may exacerbate the hypothyroidism due to iodine deficiency and play a role in the aetiology of myxoedematous and nervous cretinism. In countries where iodine deficiency is not endemic, hypothyroidism is typically due to autoimmune disease.

10.3.5 Measures to prevent iodine deficiency

Iodization of salt has been the major method for combating iodine deficiency since the 1920s when it was first successfully used in Switzerland. Since then, introduction of iodized salt in a number of other countries including New Zealand has resulted in the elimination of goitre in these regions. Universal salt iodization is now the recommended strategy for prevention of IDD. However, the success of iodization depends on whether all salt is iodized, as acceptability of iodized salt may be a problem in some countries. In other countries such as those in Asia where millions of people are affected, there are major difficulties in producing, monitoring and distributing iodized

There are also detrimental effects of less obvious iodine deficiency on mental performance of school children, which may have considerable social consequences that are detrimental to national development. A meta-analysis of 18 studies in which comparisons were made between iodine-deficient populations and a control population revealed that mean IQ scores for the iodine-deficient and the non-iodine-deficient groups were 13.5 points apart, indicating the effect of iodine deficiency on neuropsychological development. Another meta-analysis of 37 studies in China confirmed this finding, and showed that adequate supplementation before and during pregnancy could prevent the IQ deficit, the effect evident in children born 3.5 years after the introduction of the iodine supplementation programme. The effects of less severe iodine deficiency are less clear, although salt. As a result of these difficulties, the United Nations Joint Committee on Health Policy in 1994 set a goal of achieving Universal Salt Iodization (USI) in all countries with an IDD problem recognized as being of public health significance. USI involves the iodization of all salt for human and livestock use, including salt used in the food industry.

Iodized oil by injection has been used in the prevention of endemic goitre in South America, Zaire and China. A single intramuscular injection of iodized oil given to girls and young women can correct severe iodine deficiency for a period of over 4 years. Because of hazards associated with injections, oral administration of iodized oil has been implemented with evidence of successful prevention of IDD.

Because the most damaging effects of iodine deficiency on mental and physical development of the fetus occur during early fetal developments, adequate iodine status of the mother is essential. In countries where iodine intakes are marginal or deficient, supplemental iodine for pregnant women and those planning pregnancy is recommended.

10.3.6 Towards elimination of iodine deficiency: Global Action

Iodine deficiency is recognized as a major international public health problem because of the large populations at risk due to their iodine-deficient environments, characterized primarily by iodine-deficient soil. An estimated 400 million people in Asia alone are affected by disorders resulting from severe iodine deficiency. Endemic cretinism affects up to 10% of the populations living in severely iodine-deficient areas in India, Indonesia and China. Cretinism is also prevalent in Papua New Guinea, Africa and South America. The International Council for the Control of Iodine Deficiency disorders (ICCIDD) formed in 1986 and is working closely with other international organizations to develop national programmes to prevent and control IDD. A Global Action Plan to eliminate IDD as a major public health problem by the year 2000 was adopted in 1990 by the United Nations system. Elimination of IDD by 2000 was also

the goal of the World Summit for Children in 1990, and this goal was reaffirmed in 1992 by delegates from 160 countries at the International Conference on Nutrition in Rome. Recent reports indicate that there has been substantial progress towards the elimination of iodine deficiency through the development of the WHO Global Database on Iodine Deficiency and the universal salt iodization policy in developing countries. However, in order to reach the goal of global elimination of IDD, continued efforts are needed to monitor at-risk populations and to strengthen and maintain salt iodization programmes.

10.3.7 Assessment of iodine status

The assessment of nutritional status of iodine is important in relation to a population or group living in an area or region that is suspected to be iodine deficient. The most important information comes from measurement of the urinary iodide in school children and pregnant women and blood TSH concentrations in neonates. The results of these two measurements indicate the severity of the problem, and can also be used to assess the effectiveness of remedial measures.

Urinary iodine excretion Approximately 90% of iodine intake is excreted in the urine and therefore 24-hour excretion of iodine reflects dietary intake and may be used for estimating the intake. However 24-hour urine samples are difficult to collect in the field situation, and non-fasting casual urine specimens are usually obtained in these situations. Urinary iodine concentration is the most practical biomarker for assessment of iodine nutrition. Optimal urinary iodine concentration is between 100 and 200 µg/L, corresponding to an intake of approximately 150–200 µg/day. Table 10.3 gives urinary concentrations associated with levels of iodine nutrition. Urinary iodine, however, is a sensitive indicator of recent iodine intake but not of thyroid function. Furthermore, where goitrogens are preventing the uptake of iodine into the thyroid gland and subsequent

Table 10.3 Epidemiological criteria for assessing iodine nutrition based on median urinary iodine concentrations in school-aged children

Median urinary iodine (µg/L)	Iodine intake	Iodine nutrition
< 20	Insufficient	Severe iodine deficiency
20–49	Insufficient	Moderate iodine deficiency
50–99	Insufficient	Mild iodine deficiency
100–199	Adequate	Optimal
200–299	More than adequate	Risk of iodine-induced hyperthyroidism within 5 10 years following introduction of iodized salt in susceptible groups
> 300	Excessive	Risk of adverse health consequences (iodine-induced hyperthyroidism, autoimmune thyroid diseases)

Source: WHO/NHD (2001).

synthesis of thyroid hormones, urinary iodine may be normal and therefore not a suitable marker for iodine status.

Assessment of thyroid size and goitre rate The prevalence of goitre reflects a population's history of iodine nutrition, but it does not properly reflect its present iodine status, because thyroid size decreases only slowly after iodine repletion. Goitre assessment is made by inspection, palpation, or more recently by ultrasonography. The recommended target group for monitoring goitre rate is school children. Normative values proposed by the WHO and the ICCIDD for thyroid volume by ultrasonography are based on data obtained from a large sample of iodine-replete school-age children. The percentage of children with thyroid glands greater than the 97th percentile of normative values characterizes mild (5–19%), moderate (20–29%) and severe (≥ 30%) deficiency.

Thyroid hormones The level of serum T_4 or TSH provides an indirect measure of iodine nutritional status. When iodine in the diet is limited, stimulation of the thyroid gland by increased plasma TSH may be enough to maintain circulating T_4 and T_3 con-

centrations. Therefore, plasma TSH concentrations are often elevated when T_4 and T_3 concentrations are within the normal range. In more severe deficiency (moderate deficiency), T_4 concentrations begin to decrease; and it is only in the severest of iodine deficiency, when median urinary iodine excretion is less than 20 µg/L, that plasma T_3 concentrations decline. TSH is not a particularly useful parameter to determine iodine status in adults, as it does not reflect recent dietary iodine intake and is not particularly sensitive to borderline deficiencies. However, neonates exhibit elevated serum TSH more frequently than adults, and therefore appear to be hypersensitive to the effects of iodine deficiency.

Serum thyroglobulin is a more sensitive indicator of mild iodine deficiency and iodine repletion than TSH or T_4 in children and adults, as levels are elevated in subjects with low iodine excretion, while TSH and T_4 levels remain within the normal range. For population studies, both TSH and thyroglobulin are recommended surveillance measures, and can be determined in blood spots on filter paper or serum samples. The percentage of neonates with TSH values greater than 5 µIU/mL whole blood defines the level of deficiency—mild (3–19%), moderate (20–39%)

and severe ($\geq 40\%$). Similarly, thyroglobulin values of 10–19, 20–39 or ≥ 40 ng/mL serum in school-age children represent mild, moderate and severe deficiency, respectively.

10.3.8 Dietary intakes of iodine

Iodine intakes vary considerably depending on geographical location, dietary habits and salt iodization. Adequate dietary intakes of iodine are around 100–150 µg/day. Intakes are usually assessed from urinary excretion, rather than direct measurement of food iodine, because of lack of good food composition data.

Foods of marine origin, such as sea fish and shellfish, seameal (custard made of ground seaweed) and seaweeds, are rich in iodine and reflect the greater iodine concentration of sea water compared with fresh water. The iodine content of plants and animals depends on the environment in which they grow, but generally, vegetables, fruit and cereals grown on soils with low iodine content are poor sources of iodine.

Because the mammary gland concentrates iodine, dairy products are usually a good source, but only if the cows get enough iodine. In recent years, iodine contamination in dairy products and bread has made a major contribution to the daily intake. The use of iodophors as sanitizers in the dairy industry has resulted in variable but considerable amounts of residual iodine in milk, cheese and other milk products. The use of these compounds, however, is declining in New Zealand and Australia, as it is in many other countries. Tasmania adopted the addition of iodate as a bread improver and as an iodine supplement, but iodates are not permitted in New Zealand. Other adventitious sources of iodine include kelp tablets and drugs, and beverages or foods containing the iodine-containing colouring erythrosine.

Iodized salt is another source of iodine and has been one of the most efficient means of improving iodine nutrition. The amount added varies widely in different regions. In Canada and the US, salt is iodized to a concentration of 77 p.p.m. iodine as potassium iodide, so that the daily recommended intake might be obtained from 2 g salt. Most other countries add 10–40 p.p.m. iodide to salt. However, in some countries both iodized salt and non-iodized salt is available. In developed countries, much of the salt intake now comes from processed foods; whether such foods contain iodized salt or not depends on local commercial practice.

10.3.9 Interactions

The utilization of absorbed iodine is influenced by goitrogens, which interfere with the biosynthesis of the hormones. Goitrogens are found in vegetables of the genus brassica: cabbage, turnip, swede, brussels sprouts and broccoli, and in some staple foods such as cassava, maize and lima beans that are used in developing countries. Goitrogens can become a problem where people whose iodine intake is only marginal eat these staple foods, particularly if they are not well cooked. Most goitrogens are inactivated by heat, but not when milk is pasteurized.

10.3.10 Requirement and recommended dietary intakes

Goitre occurs when iodine intakes are less than about 50 µg/day, and cretinism when maternal intake is 30 µg/day or less. Minimum requirement to prevent goitre, based on the urinary excretion associated with a high incidence of goitre in a population, is approximately 1 µg/kg body weight/day. However, recommended dietary intakes are based on physiological requirements, which are in turn based on a number of indicators, including thyroidal radioiodine accumulation and turnover, iodine balance studies, urinary iodide excretion, thyroid hormone measures and thyroid volume. From these data, a physiological requirement of around 100 µg/day is indicated, and a rather large safety margin is generally advised to ensure an adequate intake. In most countries, the recommended intake is in the range 150–200 µg/day. This level is adequate to maintain normal thyroid function that is essential for growth and development. Because of the increased requirements for thyroid hormones during pregnancy and the importance of adequate iodine for the fetus and neonate, recommended intakes for pregnant and lactating women are considerably higher at 200–230 µg/day for pregnancy and 200–290 µg/day for lactation. Requirements may also increase if the diets contain goitrogens. Table 36.2 gives recommended intakes for iodine.

10.3.11 Toxicity

Intakes between 50 and 1000 µg are considered safe. The effects of high iodine intake on thyroid function are variable and depend on the health of the thyroid gland. Dietary intakes of up 1000 µg/day have few long-term effects when the thyroid is healthy. Daily intakes of 2000 µg iodine should be regarded as excessive or potentially harmful. Such intakes are unlikely to be obtained from normal diets of natural foods except where they are exceptionally high in marine fish or seaweed, or where foods are contaminated with iodine from iodophors or other adventitious sources.

Excess intakes of iodide can cause enlargement of the thyroid gland, just as deficiency can, as well as hypothyroidism and elevated TSH, and increased incidence of autoimmune thyroid disease. People who have underlying autoimmune disease such as Grave's disease or Hashimoto's thyroiditis, or who have previously been iodine deficient, may be more sensitive to iodine. Iodine-induced thyrotoxicosis (Jod–Basedow syndrome) following the iodization programmes has been described, particularly in women over 40 years of age who had always been living in a low-iodine environment.

Iodine overload may occur in vegans when seaweed and iodine-containing dietary supplements are consumed. The use of kelp supplements is not recommended as these can contain very high but variable amounts of iodine.

FURTHER READING

1. **Hercus, C.E., Benson, W.N., and Carter, C.L.** (1925) Endemic goitre in New Zealand, and its relation to the soil iodine. *J Hygiene*, **24**, 321–402.

2. **Hetzel, B.S.** (1989) *The story of iodine deficiency: An international challenge in nutrition*. Oxford, Oxford University Press.

3. **Hetzel, B.S., Potter, B.J., and Dulberg, E.M.** (1990) The iodine deficiency disorders: nature, pathogenesis and epidemiology. *World Rev Nutr Diet*, **62**, 59–119.

4. **WHO** (2004) *Iodine status worldwide: WHO global database on iodine deficiency*. Geneva: World Health Organization. http://www3.who.int/whosis/menu.cfm

5. **WHO/NHD** (2001) *Assessment of iodine deficiency disorders and monitoring their elimination: A guide for programme managers*, 2nd edition. Geneva, World Health Organization.

6. **WHO/UNICEF/ICCIDD** (1993) *Global prevalence of iodine deficiency disorders. Micronutrient deficiency information systems (MDIS) working paper No. 1*. Geneva, World Health Organization.

10.4 Selenium
Christine Thomson

Selenium first attracted interest in the 1930s as a toxic trace element that caused loss of hair and blind staggers in livestock that consumed high-selenium plants in South Dakota. In 1957, selenium was shown to be essential for animals when traces of this mineral prevented liver necrosis in vitamin E-deficient rats, and later to prevent a variety of economically important diseases in domestic animals, such as white muscle disease in cattle and sheep, hepatosis dietetica in swine, and exudative diathesis in poultry. The demonstration in 1973 of a biochemical function for selenium as a constituent of the selenoenzyme glutathione peroxidase (GPx) helped to explain the interrelationship between selenium and vitamin E. The importance of selenium in human nutrition was highlighted in reports in 1979 of selenium deficiency in a patient in New Zealand on total parenteral nutrition and of the selenium-responsive condition Keshan disease in China. Considerable research during the last two decades has provided information on the metabolism and importance of selenium in human nutrition, leading to the establishment of recommended dietary intakes based on amounts required to maximize plasma selenoproteins. More recently, the focus on selenium has turned to possible benefits from higher levels of selenium intake in maintaining human health, by protecting against certain types of cancer and cardiovascular disease, and through the maintenance of a healthy immune system.

10.4.1 Functions of selenium

Selenium exerts its biological effects as a constituent of several selenoproteins of which there are 25 in humans. These selenoproteins are involved in a wide variety of processes in the body, including antioxidant defence and redox metabolism, thyroid metabolism, immune function, reproductive function and many others, with implications of clinical importance in many diseases such as cancer and autoimmune thyroid disease. The following have been purified and studied:

- Glutathione peroxidase (GPx)
  - Cytosolic, cellular (GPx1)
  - Gastrointestinal (GPx2)
  - Plasma (GPx3)
  - Phospholipid hydroperoxide (GPx4)
- Selenoprotein P
- Iodothyronine 5′-deiodinases (types I, II, III)
- Thioredoxin reductase (TR1, TR2, TR3)
- Selenophosphate synthetase 2
- Sep15 (15 kDa selenoprotein)
- Selenoprotein W
- Selenoprotein R (methionine-R-sulphoxide reductase; MsrB1)
- Selenoproteins H, I, K, M, N, O, P, S, T, V

The selenium is present in all selenoproteins as selenocysteine at the active site. Selenocysteine is inserted into proteins cotranslationally in response to the UGA codon, which, in addition to selenocysteine insertion, functions to terminate protein synthesis. These two functions are distinguished by the presence or absence of an RNA stem–loop structure, designated the selenocysteine insertion sequence (SECIS) element in the 3′ untranslated region of eukaryotic mRNAs.

The first of the selenoproteins to be characterized was GPx, which consists of four identical subunits, each containing one selenocysteine at the active site. Activity of this enzyme can be reduced to less than 1% in tissues of selenium-deficient animals. GPx is present in at least five different forms. In cells including erythrocytes (GPx1), the gastrointestinal tract (GPx2) and plasma (GPx3), this enzyme may function *in vivo* to remove hydrogen peroxide, thereby preventing the initiation of peroxidation of membranes and oxidative damage. However, the significance of this function in the body is uncertain, and it seems likely that the oxidant defence role for selenium is exerted more through other selenoproteins. GPx may have more specific functions in arachidonic acid metabolism in platelets, microbiocidal activity in leucocytes, and the immune response mechanism.

Another selenium-containing enzyme, phospholipid hydroperoxide GPx (GPx4), is different from the classic GPx in that it can metabolize fatty acid hydroperoxides that are esterified in phospholipids in cell membranes, and thus may play a role as an antioxidant in protecting biomembranes. This function is most likely the basis of the selenium/vitamin E interaction in the pathogenesis of several deficiency diseases in animals. GPx4 is also required for sperm fertilization and is involved in redox signalling and regulatory processes such as inhibition of lipoxygenases and apoptosis.

A plasma protein designated selenoprotein P, purified and characterized from rat and human plasma, is the major selenoprotein in plasma and provides more than 50% of total plasma selenium. It is therefore a useful biomarker of selenium status. Selenoprotein P is a glycoprotein containing selenium as selenocysteine, and its concentration in rat plasma falls to 10% in selenium deficiency. Its function is still unclear, but there is evidence for both an antioxidant role and a transport role in distributing selenium to peripheral tissues such as the brain.

The discovery that type I iodothyronine 5'-deiodinase—and more recently type II and type III deiodinases—are selenoproteins indicates a role for selenium in metabolism of thyroid hormones, which regulate most metabolic functions and are essential for growth and development. These enzymes catalyse the conversion of thyroxine (T_4) to its active metabolite triiodothyronine (T_3). Selenium deficiency results in an increase in levels of plasma T_4 and a corresponding decrease in levels of the more active T_3. GPx is also involved in the removal of excess hydrogen peroxide and reactive oxygen species formed during thyroid hormone metabolism. The interactions of selenium and iodine deficiencies have implications for both human health and livestock production. In humans, selenium deficiency may exacerbate effects of concurrent iodine deficiency.

Another family of selenoproteins is the thioredoxin reductases, NADPH-dependent flavoenzymes that reduce the disulphide of thioredoxin. The activity of thioredoxin reductase declines in selenium deficiency and selenium is present in the active site as selenocysteine. There are three distinct human thioredoxin reductases in humans, which are involved in a large number of cellular and intercellular processes.

Several selenium-containing enzymes have been identified in microorganisms and other selenoproteins have been found in animal tissues, suggesting further functions for selenium. Selenophosphate synthetase 2 is a selenoenzyme required for the formation of tRNA-bound selenocysteine during the synthesis of selenoproteins.

Selenoprotein W is found in muscle and other tissues and derived its name because it is one of the missing selenoproteins in lambs suffering from white muscle disease. Its concentration decreases during selenium deficiency, but it is retained in the brain. However, the function of selenoprotein W is still unknown.

Selenoprotein R is also referred to as methionine-R-sulfoxide reductase (MsrB1) and is involved in a number of processes including antioxidant functions, regulation of enzyme activity and cell signalling, and may protect the brain from oxidative damage.

Other selenoproteins include a 15 kDa selenoprotein and selenoproteins H, I, K, M, N, O, S, T and V, the functions of which are unknown. In addition, selenium has strong interactions with heavy metals such as cadmium, silver and mercury and may protect against toxic effects of these metals.

10.4.2 Metabolism of selenium

Selenoamino acids are the main dietary forms of selenium, with selenium replacing sulphur in selenomethionine in general proteins in plant and animal foods and selenocysteine in selenoenzymes in animal foods. Inorganic forms of selenium, such as selenite and selenate, are used in experimental diets and as supplements. The metabolism of selenium, including absorption, transport, distribution, excretion, retention and transformation to the active form, is dependent on the chemical form and amount ingested, and on interacting dietary factors. There is considerable species variation in selenium metabolism.

Absorption Selenium is absorbed mainly from the duodenum. Selenomethionine and methionine share the same active transport mechanism, but little is known about the transport of selenocysteine. Absorption of inorganic forms such as selenite and selenate is via a passive mechanism. Absorption of selenium is generally high in human subjects, probably about 80% from food; selenomethionine appears to be better absorbed than selenite. Absorption is unaffected by selenium status, suggesting that there is no homeostatic regulation of absorption.

Transport Little is known about the transport of selenium in the body, although it appears to be transported bound to plasma proteins. Selenoprotein P in plasma has been suggested as a transport protein, and plasma also contains extracellular GPx, but smaller molecular weight forms of selenium are more likely to act as transport proteins.

Metabolism and distribution An outline of selenium metabolism is shown in Fig. 10.3. Selenium in animal tissues occurs in association with protein, and

Dietary forms   **Tissue forms**

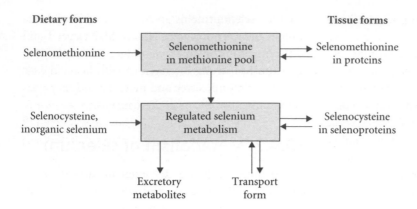

Fig. 10.3 Outline of selenium metabolism.

Source: Levander, O.A. and Burk, R.F. (1996) Selenium. In: Ziegler, E.E. and Filer, L.J. (eds). *Present Knowledge of Nutrition*, 7th edition. Washington, DC: ILSI Press, pp. 320–8.

is present in two main forms. The first is selenocysteine, which is present as the active form of selenium in selenoproteins. The second is selenomethionine, which is non-specifically incorporated in place of methionine in a variety of proteins, unregulated by the selenium status of the animal.

Selenium levels in tissues are influenced by dietary intake, as reflected in the wide variation in blood selenium concentrations of residents of countries with differing soil selenium levels (Fig. 10.4). The form administered also influences retention of selenium, with selenomethionine more effective in raising blood selenium levels than sodium selenite or selenate. Both inorganic and organic forms of selenium are transformed to selenide. Selenite and selenate are reduced to selenide, organic selenocysteine is directly lysed to selenide, and selenomethionine is transformed to selenocysteine and then lysed to selenide. Selenide (-2 oxidation state) is transformed to selenocysteine

on tRNA and the selenocysteinyl residue is incorporated into the active site of selenoproteins by the UGA codon, which is specific to selenocysteine. The non-specific incorporation of selenomethionine into protein contributes to tissue selenium, which is not immediately available for synthesis of functional forms of selenium, until it is catabolized.

Excretion Urine is the principal route of selenium excretion, followed by faeces in which it is mainly unabsorbed selenium. Homeostasis of selenium is achieved by regulation of its excretion. Daily urinary excretion is closely associated with plasma selenium and dietary intake. Balance studies show that over a wide range of intakes, urinary excretion accounts for 50–60% of the total amount excreted. Measurement of plasma renal clearance of selenium (which expresses its rate of excretion in the urine in terms of the amount contained per unit volume of plasma) shows

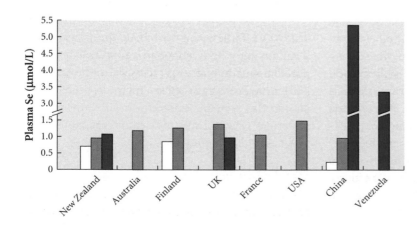

Fig. 10.4 Blood selenium values (µmol/L). New Zealand: pre-1990 (□), 1995–99 (■), post-2000 (■); Finland: pre-1984 (□), post-1984 (■); UK: pre-1990 (■), post-1990 (■); China: low Se (□), medium Se (■), high Se (■).

that kidneys of residents of the low-selenium country New Zealand excrete selenium more sparingly than those of North America, and Chinese from low selenium areas have even lower renal clearances. This indicates possible adaptation to low selenium status.

Surplus selenium is methylated to methylated selenium metabolites from the common intermediate selenide. 1 β-Methyl seleno-*N*-acetyl-D-galactosamine (selenosugar) is the major urinary metabolite. Trimethylselenonium ion is excreted in response to very high intakes of selenium and may be used as a biological marker for excessive doses. Excessive selenium is excreted not only in urine, but also in expired air as volatile dimethylselenide.

Bioavailability As well as absorption, utilization of a nutrient also includes transformation to a biochemically active form which for selenium is assessed by monitoring changes in tissue GPx. Animal studies show a wide variation in the bioavailability of selenium from different foods. In rats, the bioavailability from mushrooms, tuna, wheat, beef kidney and Brazil nuts is 5%, 57%, 83%, 97% and 124%, respectively, in comparison with sodium selenite. Human studies also show differences among various forms such as selenate, wheat and yeast.

10.4.3 Deficiency

Interaction between selenium and vitamin E is observed in the aetiology of many deficiency diseases in animals and pure selenium deficiency is in fact rare. Thus, selenium deficiency may only occur when a low selenium status is linked with an additional stress such as chemical exposure or increased oxidant stress due to vitamin E deficiency. Although residents in some low-selenium areas have low levels of blood selenium, GPx activity and selenoprotein, there is little evidence that these are suboptimal or have resulted in changes in other oxidative defence mechanisms. Moreover, people have not shown noticeably improved health when GPx activity is saturated by selenium supplementation. Whether any of the newer functions of selenium are suboptimal in persons with low selenium status is being investigated.

Selenium-responsive diseases in humans Keshan disease, an endemic cardiomyopathy occurring in low-selenium areas of China, was reported in 1979 to be responsive to supplementation with sodium selenite. The principal pathological finding is multifocal necrosis of the myocardium. The disease is associated with low selenium intake and low blood and hair levels, and affects mainly children and women of childbearing age. Because some features of Keshan disease (e.g. seasonal variation) cannot be explained solely on the basis of very low selenium status, Chinese researchers have suggested that some other factors may be involved such as a virus, mineral imbalance or environmental toxins. Recent research on coxsackievirus B-induced myocarditis in selenium-deficient mice supports a possible viral involvement. Another disease that has been associated with poor selenium status as well as iodine deficiency in China is Kashin–Beck disease, an endemic osteoarthritis that occurs during pre-adolescent or adolescent years, but other aetiological factors are probably involved.

Selenium deficiency has been associated with long-term intravenous nutrition, because of the low levels of selenium in the fluids. Clinical symptoms of cardiomyopathy, muscle pain and muscular weakness are responsive to selenium supplementation, but are not seen in all patients with extremely low selenium status, indicating that there may be other interacting factors. Furthermore, children on very low selenium synthetic diets for inborn errors of metabolism, such as phenylketonuria, do not develop clinical selenium-deficiency syndromes.

Anecdotal reports from New Zealand farmers in low-selenium areas where sheep have selenium-responsive muscular dystrophy indicate their conviction that selenium relieves their own muscular aches and pains, although double-blind trials have failed to give a clear-cut answer.

10.4.4 Selenium and human health

Selenium and immune function Recent work on host response to myocarditic and non-myocarditic strains of coxsackievirus B3 in mice showed that selenium deficiency and vitamin E deficiency potentiated cardiotoxicity of myocarditic strains, but in addition, the non-myocarditic strain caused heart lesions in selenium-deficient mice. This specific nutrient deficiency allowed a benign virus to become virulent, apparently as a result of a change in the viral genome. This observation may help to clarify the aetiology of Keshan disease and may also be applicable to other RNA viruses. Selenium and vitamin E deficiencies have also been shown to enhance the intensity of infection with influenza, the protozoan parasite *Trypanosoma cruzi* and *Heligmosomoides polyrus*. Selenium may also slow the progression of human immunodeficiency virus 1 disease.

Selenium is essential for optimal function of many aspects of the immune system, influencing both the innate and the acquired immune system, and has a role to play in the defence system of animals against bacteria and other infections including viral infection. The mechanisms for the involvement of selenium in the immune system are likely to be related to its antioxidant function through the antioxidant selenoproteins glutathione peroxidases, thioredoxin reductases or selenoprotein P.

Selenium and cancer Several lines of scientific enquiry suggest an association of cancer with low levels of selenium in the diet. Evidence for the role of selenium as an anticarcinogenic agent comes from *in vitro* and animal studies that suggest that selenium is protective against tumorigenesis at high levels of intake. Evidence from prospective studies linking low selenium status with increased incidence of cancer at various cancer sites has been conflicting, but the strongest evidence is available for prostate and breast cancer. There have been eight intervention trials in humans of the effect of selenium, alone or with other nutrients, on the incidence of cancer or concentrations of biomarkers. All have shown positive effects of selenium; however, five of these were carried out in China, where selenium and other nutrient deficiencies are common. The strongest evidence comes from The Nutritional Prevention of Cancer Trial which was a 10-year controlled clinical trial in the USA to test the efficacy of selenium in preventing skin cancer. There was no effect of daily supplementation with 200 µg selenium on skin cancer, but there was a statistically significant reduction in total cancer (50%), and cancer of the prostate, lung and colorectum. The effects were strongest in subjects with the lowest selenium status. Further studies are needed to confirm these observations and there are at present several selenium intervention studies in progress, particularly in relation to prostate cancer.

The level of selenium intake required for the protective effect appears to be higher than that required to maximize selenoproteins, suggesting that other processes, such as the involvement of anticarcinogenic methylated selenium metabolites, might be involved. However, the association of selenium with a reduction in DNA damage and oxidative stress and recent evidence of an effect of selenoprotein polymorphisms on cancer risk suggest that selenoproteins are also involved.

Selenium and cardiovascular disease Lack of dietary selenium has also been implicated in the aetiology of cardiovascular diseases, but the evidence is less convincing than for cancer. A large case–control study in Finland suggested selenium was an independent risk factor for myocardial infarction in a low-selenium population, with elevated risk below a threshold serum concentration. However, other prospective studies have not shown this correlation. On the other hand, a low level of erythrocyte GPx1 has been shown to be a predictor of cardiovascular events in patients with coronary artery disease. Selenium-dependent glutathione peroxidases have been shown to have protective effects against processes relevant to atherosclerosis, in particular in individuals, such as smokers, at risk from increased oxidant stress. These processes include the inhibition of low-density lipoprotein oxidation, the inhibition of pro-atherogenic 15-lipoxygenase by GPx4, and modification of expression of adhesion molecules induced by cytokines. Further evidence must come from controlled intervention trials.

10.4.5 Assessment of selenium status

Blood selenium concentration is a useful measure of selenium status and intake, but other tissues are often assessed as well. Plasma or serum selenium reflects short-term status and erythrocyte selenium reflects longer-term status. Toenail selenium is being used more frequently, as toenail concentrations provide a stable assessment of longer-term dietary intake, but selenium-containing shampoos restrict the use of hair. Urinary excretion can also be used to assess selenium status, and total dietary intake is estimated as twice the daily urinary excretion.

The close relationship between blood or red cell GPx activity and selenium concentrations (Fig. 10.5) is useful for assessment in people with relatively low status, but not once the saturating activity of the enzyme is reached at blood selenium concentrations above 100 µg/L (1.27 µmol/L). More recently, measurement of selenoprotein P has been used to assess selenium status and recent evidence suggests that it might be a better biomarker than GPx. There is

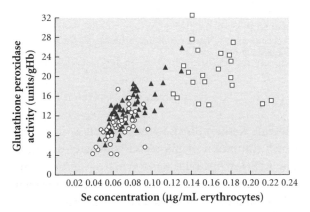

Fig. 10.5 Relationship between selenium concentration of erythrocytes (µg/mL erythrocytes) and glutathione peroxidase (GPx) activity for Otago patients (O), Otago blood donors (▲) and overseas subjects (□). (To convert µg selenium/mL to µmol/litre multiply by 12.66.)

Source: Rea, H.M., Thomson, C.D., Campbell, D.R., and Robinson, M.F. (1979) Relation between erythrocyte selenium concentrations and glutathione peroxidase (EC 1.11.1.9.) activities in New Zealand residents and visitors to New Zealand. *Br J Nutr*, **42**, 201–8.

also the potential for measurement of other enzymes as functional markers; however, their use is limited at present by the lack of simple assay techniques. Furthermore, the conclusions drawn from measurement of one selenoprotein may not apply to all biological functions of selenium because of differences in responses of tissues and these proteins to deficient, adequate or high levels of selenium. Therefore, there may be no single indicator of functional selenium status, but rather a series of markers that apply to specific problems associated with suboptimal selenium status.

10.4.6 Dietary intake

Food is the major source of selenium, with drinking water contributing little. Dietary intake varies with the geographic source of the foods and eating habits of the people. Plant food concentrations reflect selenium content of soils and availability for uptake, as plants generally do not require selenium for growth; the selenium content of cereals and grains grown in soils poor or rich in selenium may vary over 100-fold. However, some plants, such as garlic, mushrooms and broccoli, have developed the ability to accumulate selenium from the soil and therefore may contain high levels of selenium. Brazil nuts are also exceptionally good sources of selenium, but the content varies greatly depending on where they are grown. Animal foods vary less. Fish and organ meats are the richest sources, followed by muscle meats, cereals and grains, and dairy products, with fruits and vegetables mostly poor sources. Average daily dietary intakes vary considerably depending on the levels of selenium in soils (Table 10.4) ranging from about 10 µg selenium in the low-soil-selenium areas of China where Keshan disease is endemic, to median intakes in New Zealand of 56 and 39 µg/day for males and females, respectively, and up to over 200 µg in seleniferous areas in Venezuela. In 1985, selenium was added to fertilizers in Finland as a way of increasing selenium intake throughout the population, and the daily intake rose from 40 µg to close to 100 µg/day, resulting in an increase in serum selenium in a group of

Table 10.4 Daily dietary intakes and whole blood values of selenium

Country	Selenium intake (μg/day)	Plasma or serum selenium[a] (μmol/L)
China		
Keshan disease area	7–11	0.20–0.30
Non-Keshan disease area	40–120	0.49–1.41
Seleniferous area	750–4990	4.52–6.25
New Zealand		
Before 1990	28–32	0.56–0.87
After 1990	30–60	0.89–1.17
Finland		
Before 1984	25	0.70–1.05
After 1984	67–110	0.92–1.60
Great Britain		
Before 1990	60	1.25–1.52
After 1990	29–39	0.78–1.00
USA	60–220	1.11–1.88
Venezuela	200–350	2.73–3.99

[a]Mean values.

Source: Adapted from Thomson, C.D. (2004) Selenium and iodine intakes and status in New Zealand and Australia. *Br J Nutr*, **91**, 661–72; Combs, G.F. Jr (2001) Selenium in global food systems. *Br J Nutr*, **85**, 517–47.

healthy individuals of 0.82–0.89 μmol/L in 1985 to 1.52 μmol/L in 1989–91. In New Zealand, intakes are higher in the North Island due to importation of Australian wheat, but intakes in this country have also increased as a result of increases in selenium concentrations in animal foods due to supplementation of commercial fertilizers and animal feeds.

10.4.7 Requirements and recommended dietary intakes

Many countries have proposed recommended dietary intakes of selenium based on estimates of requirements from Chinese intakes for endemic and non-endemic Keshan disease areas, as well as intakes at which saturation of plasma GPx activity occurred. The RDI for Australia was the first set in the world in 1986 and may have been cautiously on the high side at 85 μg and 70 μg selenium/day for Australian men and women. Others, including recommended intakes of the USA and Canada, the UK and European countries, are summarized in Table 36.2.

Each set of recommended intakes can be met from habitual diets in each country. Whether optimal health depends upon saturation of GPx activity has yet to be resolved. The US/Canadian recommended dietary allowance is based on desirability of full activity of GPx, whereas a WHO group concluded that only two-thirds of the maximal activity was needed, based on the observation that abnormalities in metabolism of hydrogen peroxide in blood cells is apparent only when enzyme activity falls to one-quarter or less of normal. This led to a wide range of dietary recommendations, with the WHO recommendations of 40 µg/day approaching intakes in countries with naturally low selenium status such as New Zealand. As a result of more recent research in humans on selenium requirements for maximal levels of selenoproteins such as selenoprotein P as well as GPx, the new Australia/New Zealand nutrient reference values for selenium (EAR: 60 and 55 µg/day for males and females, respectively; RDI: 70 and 60 µg/day) are higher than the 2001 US/Canadian recommendations.

In the future, several of the other newly discovered selenoproteins might be used as endpoints for determining selenium requirements. However, maximal activity of some of these proteins occurs at dietary intakes of selenium less than those needed for maximal GPx activity.

10.4.8 Toxicity

The margin between an adequate and a toxic intake of selenium is quite narrow. Over-exposure or selenosis may occur from consuming high-selenium foods grown in seleniferous areas in Venezuela and some areas of China. The most common sign of poisoning is loss of hair and nails, but the skin, nervous system and teeth may also be involved. Garlic odour on the breath is an indication of excessive selenium exposure (from breathing out dimethylselenide). Sensitive biochemical techniques are lacking for selenium toxicity, which is at present diagnosed from hair loss and nail changes. Some effects of selenium toxicity are seen in individuals with dietary intakes as low as 900 µg, and the upper safe limit of dietary intake has been suggested as 400 µg per day.

FURTHER READING

1. **Combs, G.F. Jr** (2001) Selenium in global food systems. *Br J Nutr*, **85**, 517–47.

2. **NHMRC** (2006) *Nutrient reference values for Australia and New Zealand including recommended dietary intakes*. Canberra, NHMRC, Wellington, Ministry of Health.

3. **Rayman, M.P.** (2005) Selenium in cancer prevention: a review of the evidence and mechanism of action. *Proc Nutr Soc*, **64**, 527–54.

4. **Thomson, C.D.** (2004) Assessment of requirements for selenium and adequacy of selenium status: a review. *Eur J Clin Nutr*, **58**, 391–402.

5. **Thomson, C.D.** (2004) Selenium and iodine intakes and status in New Zealand and Australia. *Br J Nutr*, **91**, 661–72.

10.5 Fluoride
Stewart Truswell

The fluoride iron (F) is generally regarded as a beneficial nutrient because intakes of 1–4 mg/day reduce the prevalence of dental caries (decay). Nutritional authorities have until recently hesitated to classify fluoride as an essential nutrient. The dental benefit is not life-saving. However, many millions of people in the USA, Australia and New Zealand and parts of other countries—some 400 million worldwide—have fluoride added to their drinking water at the water works, at the controlled level of 1 mg/L (1 p.p.m.). As well as this, most toothpastes contain added fluoride and dentists periodically paint children's teeth with fluoride solution as a preventive measure against tooth decay.

However, the US Institute of Medicine, in collaboration with Canada, decided in 1997 to set a recommended intake for fluoride; Australia and New Zealand followed suit in 2005; and in Germany, Austria and Switzerland 'guiding values' for fluoride have been published (2001, 2002).

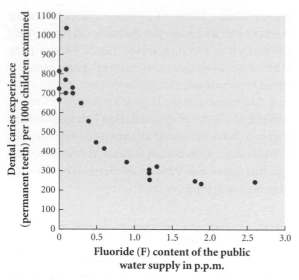

Fig. 10.6 Relation between the amount of dental caries (permanent teeth) observed in 7257 selected 12–14-year-old white schoolchildren from 21 US cities (in four states) and the fluoride content of the public water supply.

Source: Dean (1942).

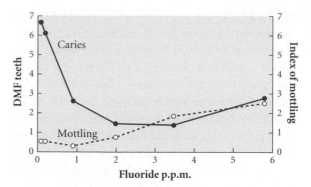

Fig. 10.7 Caries and enamel mottling according to fluoride level in drinking water for UK children aged 12–14 years. DMF, decayed, missing and filled teeth.

Source: Forrest (1956).

From many studies of United States children, Dean (1942) showed an inverse relation between the natural fluoride concentration of communal water supplies in the range of 0–2 p.p.m. (µg/g) fluoride and the prevalence of dental caries (Fig. 10.6). Natural water supplies commonly range from 0.1 to 5 p.p.m. in fluoride content and in some places (e.g. bore holes) the fluoride concentration is much higher. Earlier, a direct association had been found between the fluoride content of water supplies (0–6 p.p.m.) and the occurrence of enamel fluorosis (or mottled enamel) from barely noticeable white flecks affecting a small percentage of the enamel to brown-stained or pitted enamel, in the most severe cases (Fig. 10.7). This is a cosmetic effect and milder forms are not readily apparent to the affected individual or casual observer. Figs 10.6 and 10.7 show little increase in benefit with water containing fluoride above 1 p.p.m., while mottling only became apparent above 2 p.p.m. This concentration therefore offered maximal protection against dental caries with minimal risk of dental fluorosis. Moreover, in communities where the natural water supplies were unusually low in fluoride, less that 0.3 p.p.m., addition of fluoride or fluoridation of the water supply to achieve 1 p.p.m. has been followed by a remarkable decline in prevalence of dental decay in the children, of up to 60%. Indeed, the impact of fluoridation of water supplies and more recently of toothpastes containing fluoride has been a cost-effective triumph of public health.

10.5.1 Function

Fluoride acts to reduce dental caries in two ways:

1. When ingested by young children while the permanent (second set of) teeth are forming inside the jaw, before they erupt, the blood-borne fluoride combines in the calcium phosphate hydroxyapatite crystals of the enamel, making it more resistant to acid erosion. Erosion of dental enamel by acid, produced by mouth bacteria metabolizing sugars, is the cause of caries. For this fluoride action, young children should either be drinking water with adequate natural or added fluoride or be given fluoride tablets before their permanent teeth erupt.

2. Fluoride also has a post-eruptive action. In solution in the saliva or in contact with the teeth via toothpaste, it inhibits bacterial enzymes that produce acid in plaques on the teeth and it increases remineralization of incipient enamel lesions. This means that fluoride continues to have cariostatic action in adult life.

10.5.2 Metabolism of fluoride

The fluoride ion occurs in water, and both ionic and non-ionic or bound forms occur in food and beverages. Ionic fluoride is rapidly and almost completely absorbed, whereas organic or protein-bound forms are less well absorbed (about 75%), and inorganic bone fluoride as in bone meal even less (< 50%). There is a transitory rise in plasma fluoride following fluoride ingestion, after which it returns to about 0.1 p.p.m. Some fluoride is taken up by the bones and retained for a long time, but most is rapidly excreted in the urine, with small amounts in sweat and faeces. The urinary output gives a good indication of the daily fluoride intake, whereas the bone fluoride content reflects the long-term intake. There is minimal transfer of fluoride across the placenta. Fluoride content of breast milk is little affected by small supplements of fluoride, such as 1.5 mg/day.

10.5.3 Sources of fluoride

Dietary sources   Beverages are the principal sources of fluoride but their contribution depends on the fluoride concentration of the water supply. Tea leaves, and hence tea infusions, are also major sources (about 1–2 p.p.m.) depending on the water fluoride content and strength of the infusion. Thus, beverages can give as little as 0.2 mg/day for non-tea drinkers drinking unfluoridated or low fluoride water, and up to 2–4 mg/day or even more for liberal drinkers of strong tea prepared with fluoridated water.

Bottled water   The fluoride content of bottled water (and carbonated beverages) depends on that of its source, and it may well be absent. If people drink most of their day's water from bottles, they may be by-passing the dental benefit of tap water.

Foods contain traces of fluoride, contributing for an adult about 0.5 mg/day; plant foods (1 p.p.m.) generally contain more fluoride than animal foods (0.1 p.p.m.), apart from marine fish (2–5 p.p.m.). The fluoride content of processed food comes mainly from the fluoride content of the water used in processing or in the home. The fluoride content of infant formulas reflects the processing of the powdered formula and also the water used to make it up. Milk formulas usually contain more fluoride than human milk, and this needs to be monitored, as does the fluoride content of infants' solid foods.

Non-dietary sources   These include fluoride tablets or drops given mainly to children exposed to low-fluoride water during the formation and maturation of teeth, as well as fluoride toothpastes, and fluoride solutions painted on teeth by dentists.

10.5.4 Effects of high intakes

The cosmetic effect of enamel fluorosis occurs when too much is ingested while teeth are forming *during the first 8 years of life*; this can happen from too liberal use of fluoride tablets and/or fluoride toothpastes that can contain as much as 1000 p.p.m. fluoride. Young children are at risk if they regularly swallow large amounts, but toothpastes of lower fluoride content (400 p.p.m.) are now available for them.

The skeleton is affected by chronic high levels of fluoride intake as from long-term drinking water with 20 p.p.m. fluoride. This may cause dense bones and joint abnormalities; this skeletal fluorosis occurs in parts of India, China and South Africa.

The acute lethal dose of sodium fluoride is 5 g (i.e. 2300 mg). It would be impossible for water containing 1 mg/L to cause this.

Large doses of fluoride have been used in the treatment of osteoporosis, but the bone quality tends to be poor, fractures may increase, and there are doubts about the safety of such treatment.

10.5.5 Fluoride and dental health

There is evidence that dental health is improving, even in areas with low-fluoride water supplies, and the marked difference in caries prevalence between fluoridated and non-fluoridated (low-fluoride) areas has narrowed considerably. This most probably is related to the widespread introduction of fluoride toothpaste and other routine topical fluoride applications, as well as an increase in fluoride in the food chain. Some workers claim that much of the decline is independent of fluoride, but meta-analysis and other evidence strongly endorse the major role fluoride plays in preventing dental decay throughout life. The real issue has now become in what form fluoride is to be used in naturally low-fluoride areas. Water fluoridation has the great advantage of reaching all members of the community, particularly those with poor dental hygiene, whereas the use of fluoride toothpaste depends upon individual initiative. A combination of water and topical fluoride is probably desirable throughout life for optimal protection against caries. It is estimated that the lifetime benefit for the average New Zealander drinking fluoridated water is the prevention of a total of 2.4–12.0 decayed, missing or filled teeth.

10.5.6 Recommended dietary intake

Most national and international health organizations recommend a water supply in the range 0.7–1.0 p.p.m. fluoride for temperate climates, using the average local maximum temperature as a predictor of water intake; the lower concentrations are for warmer climates, where more beverages are drunk. The United States Institute of Medicine (1997) suggests 'adequate intakes' of fluoride are between 0.5 and 1.0 mg/day for young children from 6 months to 8 years of age, and in adults 4 mg/day in men and 3 mg/day in women. The same amounts are recommended for Australia and New Zealand.

10.5.7 Risks of water fluoridation?

It is widely agreed that fluoridation of drinking water to a level of 1 p.p.m. has no known adverse health effects. There is no good evidence that fluoridated water is associated with allergic reactions or hypersensitivity, sudden infant death syndrome, stomach or intestinal problems, birth defects, Down syndrome or genetic mutations. No association of cancer with exposure to fluoridated water has been found (see Doll and Kinlen, 1977; Smith, 1980).

FURTHER READING

1. **British Fluoridation Society** (2004) *One in a million: The facts about fluoridation*, 2nd edition. Liverpool UK, British Fluoridation Society.

2. **Dean, H.T., Arnold, F.A., and Elvove, E.** (1942) Domestic water and dental caries. V. Additional studies: experience in 4,425 white children, aged 12 to 14 years, of 13 cities in 4 states. *Pub Health Rep*, **57**, 1155–79.

3. **Doll, R., and Kinlen, L.** (1977) Fluoridation of water and cancer mortality in the USA. *Lancet*, **1**, 1300–2.

4. **Forrest, J.R.** (1956) Caries incidence and enamel defects in areas with different levels of fluoride in the drinking water. *Br Dental J*, **100**, 195–200.

5. **Institute of Medicine** (1997) *Dietary reference intakes for calcium, phosphorus, magnesium, vitamin D and fluoride*. Washington, DC, National Academy Press.

6. **McDonagh, M.S., Whiting, P.F., and Wilson, P.M.** (2000) Systematic review of water fluoridation. *Br Med J*, **321**, 855–9.

7. **Royal College of Physicians** (1976) *Fluoride, teeth and health*. London, Pitman Medical.

8. **Smith, A.H.** (1980) An examination of the relationship between fluoridation of water and cancer mortality in 20 large US cities. *NZ Med J*, **91**, 413–6.

 To see topical and scientifically robust updates on nutrition associated with this textbook, and active web links to many of the journal articles in the Reference areas, please see the dedicated Online Resource Centre at www.oxfordtextbooks.co.uk/orc/mann3e/.

11 Vitamin A and carotenoids

David I. Thurnham

11.1 History

Vitamin A deficiency has a long history—it was known to the ancient Egyptians and to Hippocrates. Liver was prescribed for night blindness. More recently, Snell demonstrated in 1880 that cod liver oil was effective in curing not only night blindness but also Bitôt's spots. Poor growth was a common feature of young rats fed on diets of pure protein, starch, sugar, lard and salts, and McCollum and Davis (1912) reported there was an essential fat-soluble factor in butter, egg yolk and cod liver oil that would overcome this growth inhibition. Osborn and Mendel reported similar results but it was McCollum and Davis who gave the name 'fat-soluble factor A' to the component in these foods to distinguish it from 'water-soluble factor B' they found in whey, yeast and rice polishings. Rosenheim and Drummond reported in 1920 that the vitamin A activity in plant foods was related to their content of carotene, a pigment isolated from carrots 100 years earlier. The ultimate confirmation that carotene is the source of plant vitamin A activity came from Thomas Moore in Cambridge, whose monograph on vitamin A is a classic (Moore, 1957).

nomenclature

11.2 Units, terminology, nomenclature and chemical structures

Vitamin A is the generic term used to include retinol and related structures with 20 carbon atoms and the pro-vitamin A carotenoids with 40 carbon atoms. The term 'retinoids' is used for the group of naturally occurring compounds that have a structure similar to retinol as well as others that have been synthesized in the search for new therapeutic compounds.

Pre-formed vitamin A structures include all-*trans* retinol (vitamin A_1, alcohol form), all-*trans* retinal (aldehyde form) and 3-dehydroretinol (vitamin A_2) (Fig. 11.1). In addition, there are various oxidized forms of retinol with vitamin A activity, namely all-*trans* retinoic acid and 9-*cis* retinoic acid, and so on, which are important in the genetic control of metabolic functions. The basic unit of activity of vitamin A is the retinol equivalent (RE) by which 1 µg RE is the same as 3.33 IU or 3.5 nmol. In foods and pharmaceutical preparations, vitamin A_1 occurs

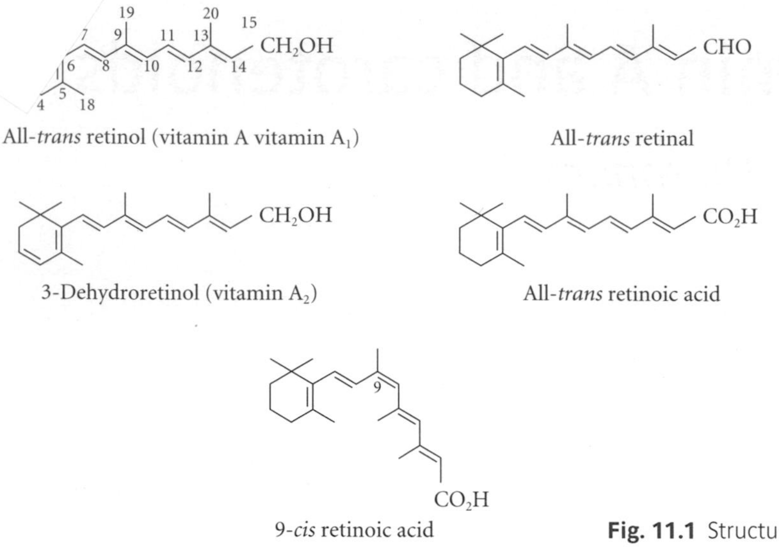

All-*trans* retinol (vitamin A vitamin A₁)

All-*trans* retinal

3-Dehydroretinol (vitamin A₂)

All-*trans* retinoic acid

9-*cis* retinoic acid

Fig. 11.1 Structures of the common retinoids.

mainly as vitamin A palmitate, although other esters can also occur. To overcome the need to use different weights if different esters are present, vitamin A activity is usually expressed as international units (IU).

The common carotenoids found in the blood are shown in Fig. 11.2. Of these only α-carotene, β-carotene and β-cryptoxanthin are pro-vitamin A carotenoids as they contain at least one β-ionone structure with no functional groups attached. The enzyme required to produce vitamin A₁ from pro-vitamin A carotenes is β-carotene-15,15'-dioxygenase (EC 1.13.11.21), which is predominantly found in the small intestine and the liver. The enzyme is believed to split carotene down the middle of the molecule (Fig. 11.3). β-Carotene has two β-ionone structures at each end of the molecule so theoretically should form two molecules of vitamin A₁ whereas all other carotenes have only one β-ionone structure and therefore can only form one molecule of vitamin A₁.

Units of β-carotene are determined by their bioequivalence to vitamin A₁. Thus, on the basis of the recommendations of FAO/WHO (1967), 1 μg RE is equivalent to 1 μg retinol, 6 μg of β-carotene or 12 μg of carotenoids containing only one β-ionone ring. More recently, the US Institute of Medicine (2000) revised the equivalencies of β-carotene and other pro-vitamin A carotenoids to 12 and 24 μg, respectively.

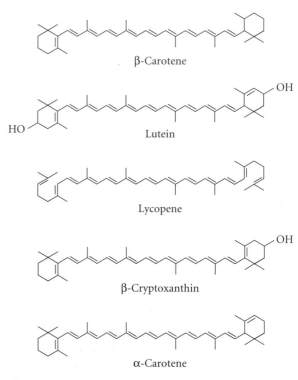

Fig. 11.2 Carotenoids found commonly in human blood.

IU are not used to quantify carotenes in current literature but older literature does sometime use them (when 1 μg β-carotene equals 1.67 IU or 1 μg retinol equals 10 IU β-carotene).

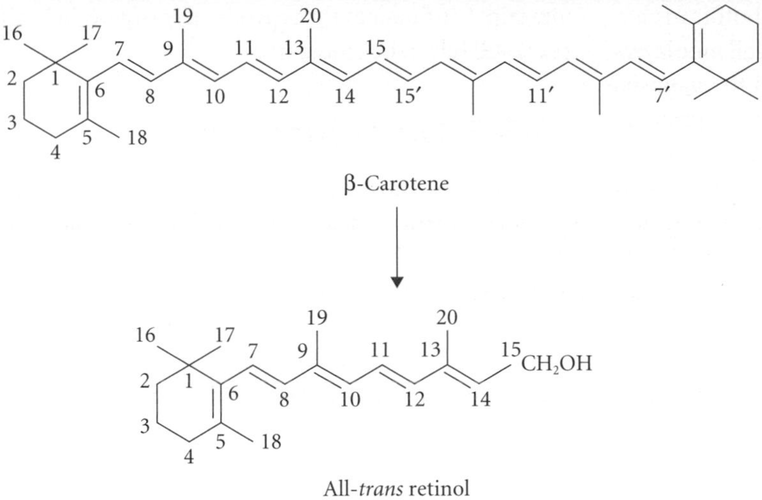

β-Carotene

All-*trans* retinol

Fig. 11.3 β-Carotene → retinol.

11.3 Functions of retinol: physiology, biochemistry and molecular biology

Retinoic acid supports many of the important functions of vitamin A (cellular differentiation, embryogenesis, synthesis of glycoproteins, immunity and growth) but it cannot be reduced back to retinol in the body; therefore an animal that is maintained only on retinoic acid will be blind and also fails to reproduce successfully. Only retinol can fully support vision and reproduction.

11.3.1 Vision

Both retinol and retinoic acid are needed to maintain a healthy eye. Retinol is needed for the visual process and one of the earliest signs of vitamin A deficiency is a failure to see in dim light, known as night blindness. Impairment of the surface of the eye in the form of xerosis or Bitôt's spots are also early signs of vitamin A deficiency and are likely to be due to inadequacy of retinoic acid. The latter is required to maintain the surface epithelium of the eye and in vitamin A deficiency, tear production is impaired, debris accumulates, and the eye is more vulnerable to bacterial attachment and disease.

The visual process is dependent on the ability to synthesize 11-*cis* retinal and its behaviour on exposure to light. There are two types of light receptor cell in the retina of the human eye—the rods and the cones. The rods are responsible for seeing at low light intensities, whereas the cones are used for light of higher intensities and colour vision. The chromophore (11-*cis* retinal) is the same in both but the proteins attached to it are different. In the rods, the chromophore is attached to rhodopsin, which is a G-protein (see below), while in the cones there is one of three very similar proteins known as iodopsin. Rhodopsin contains the protein opsin, ethanolamine-containing phospholipid, and the chromophore 11-*cis* retinal linked to interphotoreceptor-binding protein (IRBP). The basic mechanism of light excitation is common to both systems but it has been studied in far more detail in the rods as there are about a 100 million rods compared with 3 million cones in the human eye.

The retina of the mammalian eye comprises ten layers and the photoreceptors form the outermost of these, underneath the retinal pigment epithelium.

This means that before the process of phototransduction can begin, light has to pass through all nine layers. The chromophore receptors are linked to guanosine triphosphate (GTP)-binding proteins (G-proteins) and the latter regulate specific plasma membrane enzymes, or (in the case of rhodopsin) ion channels, in response to receptor binding. Before light excitation, the chromophore locks the receptor protein opsin by a Schiff-base linkage in its inactive form. The primary event in visual excitation is the photoisomerization of the 11-*cis* isomer of the Schiff-base of retinal to its all-*trans* form. The action of a photon of light is converted into the energy of atomic motion, and within a few picoseconds a series of intermediates of rhodopsin are formed. The activated rhodopsin is converted through prelumirhodopsin to metarhodopsin, and this interacts with transducin (a G-protein), which ultimately leads to the activation that cleaves cyclic guanosine monophosphate (c-GMP) to guanosine monophosphate (GMP). The changes in c-GMP and GMP lead to the closure of the sodium channel of the rod's outer membrane. Membrane hyperpolarization is then transmitted as an electrical signal to the optic nerve.

The action of light on rhodopsin is to alter its colour from magenta through orange to yellow and ultimately to white ('bleached'). In this form, it is opsin and unattached to all-*trans* retinal, although the latter is still bound to IRBP. The regeneration of 11-*cis* retinal takes place in the retinal pigment epithelium and its re-attachment to opsin generates rhodopsin to commence the cycle again.

11.3.2 Reproduction

Vitamin A deficiency results in infertility in males, while in females there are low rates of conception and high rates of stillbirths. Both retinol and retinoic acid are needed for successful reproduction, but the precise roles of the compounds are still not known for certain. β-Carotene may also function in reproduction because it is deposited in substantial amounts in the corpus luteum. As indicated below, the different retinoic acid isomers are important in the expression of many genes but the precise mechanisms by which vitamin A influences the reproductive organs in both sexes still has to be elucidated.

11.3.3 Other functions

Almost all the other functions of vitamin A are under genetic control and are mediated by retinoic acid derivatives. Retinoic acid binds to nuclear receptors and these bind to response elements on specific genes to increase or decrease the specific level of expression of the gene. There are two classes of nuclear retinoic acid receptors (RAR) and retinoid X receptors (RXR). Each family has three major subtypes, α, β and γ, and because the distribution of the different subtypes in cells is different, they are presumed to have different functions. The nuclear retinoid receptors generally act as heterodimers, of which the most common is RAR–RXR. To be active, RAR must bind to retinoic acid (either the 9-*cis* or all-*trans* isomer), whereas RXR need not. RXR can bind to 9-*cis* retinoic acid, a synthetic ligand, or it can also form heterodimers with nuclear receptors for triiodothyronine, 1,25-hydroxy vitamin D_3, the peroxisome proliferator-activated receptor, which is probably activated by an essential fatty acid metabolite, and so on. These other nuclear receptors are members of a super-family of nuclear receptors that include the receptors for oestrogen, progesterone, cortisol, testosterone and others. When activated, the dimeric nuclear receptors bind to 'response elements' in specific genes to increase or decrease the level of expression of that gene. In this way, vitamin A, through the actions of 9-*cis* and all-*trans* retinoic acid, is an important regulator of gene transcription, influencing a great many functions in the body.

Cellular differentiation Cellular differentiation is the series of morphological changes that take place to produce the mature epithelium. The outer skin is characterized by keratin-producing cells, whereas the gut is characterized by mucus-secreting tissue containing many goblet cells. Most of the functions of vitamin A in cell differentiation are regulated by retinoic acid because when vitamin A is lacking, keratin-producing cells replace mucus-secreting cells in the intestinal and respiratory tracts. The same process causes the xerosis and drying of the conjunctiva and cornea of the eye.

Embryogenesis Retinoic acid isomers play important roles in embryogenesis through their control of genes linked to development and growth (homeobox genes). Both deficiency and excess can have adverse effects. Implants containing all-*trans* retinoic acid placed in the anterior part of a developing chick limb bud mimic the activity of the naturally occurring zone of polarizing activity. Digit duplication depends on the concentration of all-*trans* retinoic acid. Experimental evidence and tragedies from over-exposure to synthetic retinoids highlight the particular importance of avoidance of excesses of vitamin A during pregnancy.

Active sulphate A key component in sulphate transfer reactions is adenosine 3′-phosphate-5′-phosphosulphate, and all-*trans* retinoic acid has been shown to induce several sulphotransferase enzymes in cellular and animal experiments. Sulphate transfer and incorporation is essential in the synthesis of mucopolysaccharides; hence, a lack of vitamin A may contribute to some or all of the features of vitamin A deficiency shown in Box 11.1.

Synthesis of glycoproteins and glycosaminoglycans
Glycoproteins are polypeptides with short chains of carbohydrates. They are important components in mucus. Many glycoproteins on the surface of the cell are receptors for other glycoproteins (e.g. growth factors). Glycosaminoglycans are long unbranched polysaccharide chains that provide a viscous extracellular matrix on the cell surface. They can provide a passageway for cell migration or lubrication between joints. Retinoids have been shown to be involved in the synthesis of some of these compounds.

Immunity and host defence Vitamin A is generally believed to be important for resistance to infections —hence the term 'anti-infective vitamin' was coined. Defining the precise role of vitamin A in immune mechanisms is more difficult. Mortality is higher in

> **BOX 11.1 Effects produced in vitamin A deficiency by impairment of mucopolysaccharide synthesis**
>
> - Reduced wettability of the eye surface
> - Reduced tear production contributing to the xerosis (dry and rough) of the eye surface
> - Reduced mucous production by mucous membranes with increased susceptibility to bacterial attachment and infection
> - Reduced ability to taste through changes in the tastebuds
> - Changes in the skin giving rise to follicular keratitis: seen more in adults than children
> - Changes in the ground substance of bone, cartilage and teeth resulting in defective formation of these substances during growth

communities where vitamin A deficiency is found, and vitamin A intervention reduces mortality. In vitamin A deficiency, epithelia lack their specialized functions like mucus production, which protect the respiratory tract and bowel from bacterial invasion. The protective effect of vitamin A in cell-mediated immunity is very clear in measles, which becomes a very serious infection in vitamin A-deficient children. Some evidence suggests that vitamin A helps maintain the lymphocyte pool, and that it functions in T-cell responses and may be involved in immunoglobulin production. It has been suggested that the metabolite 14-hydroxy-4,14-*retro*retinol is the active molecule in the immune system but its mechanism of action is not known.

Growth Vitamin A influences bone growth by modulating the growth of bones through remodelling. The vitamin is necessary for the normal cycle of growth, maturation and degeneration of cells in the epiphyseal cartilage. However, observations on the effect of vitamin A supplements on early child growth, in areas where vitamin A deficiency is a risk, are inconsistent. A study done in Indonesia where certain villages received extra vitamin A in the condiment monosodium glutamate showed that pre-school children had higher rates of growth in the treated compared with the control villages. Likewise Nepali pre-school children with and without xerophthalmia were given 120 000 RE or more at baseline, the children with xerophthalmia showed significantly higher rates of growth. However, within the same study, 3377 poorly growing children (12–60 months) without xerophthalmia, who were allocated to receive 120 000 or 300 RE at 3-month intervals, showed no differences in weight gain or linear growth.

The explanation for the inconsistencies in these studies is probably that growth is dependent on many nutrients, and just replacing vitamin A in a child's diet may do no more than allow more vitamin A storage until such time as the correct balance of nutrients in the diet is restored.

Haemopoiesis Vitamin A deficiency in humans and in experimental animals has been consistently associated with anaemia, and studies have shown that both vitamin A and iron are required to promote a full haematological response. The role of vitamin A in haemopoiesis is not fully understood. Vitamin A deficiency may interfere with the absorption, transport or storage of iron indirectly through infection and inflammation. Iron absorption and mobilization is depressed by infection and inflammation, therefore the haematological response following treatment with vitamin A may be due to improvements in health (Hess *et al.*, 2005).

11.4 Absorption, distribution and transport (Fig. 11.4)

11.4.1 Digestion

Vitamin A and its precursors are ingested in the food matrix. Proteolysis in the stomach may release some of the vitamin A and carotenoids from foods. However, to release pro-vitamin A carotenoids from vegetables, they should be thoroughly cooked and masticated, otherwise the carotenoids will remain within the cellulose structures and unavailable for absorption. Released vitamin A and carotenoids aggregate with lipids into globules and pass into the upper part of the small intestine. Here pancreatic lipase and other esterases hydrolyse lipids (triglycerides, etc.), retinyl esters and any esters of carotenoids. Bile salts assist in emulsifying the contents of the gut lumen and lipid micelles are formed.

11.4.2 Absorption

Lipid micelles are taken up by the cells lining the intestine and as much as 90% of retinol in foods is absorbed and utilized. The high efficiency of this process may be due to the existence of a specific cellular binding protein (CRBPII) in the mucosal cell that carries the retinol to the enzyme lecithin–retinol acyltransferase (LRAT) and this is the main intestinal enzyme that esterifies retinol and delivers it to the chylomicrons. Very little retinyl ester is absorbed but hydrolysis of the vitamin A esters in the gut is fairly efficient, so more than 50% of the vitamin A in large (pharmaceutical doses) is also absorbed. Carotenoids are also fairly efficiently absorbed at low doses (< 5 mg) but the amount absorbed falls off steeply as the dose rises. Carotene is also lost through enterocyte turnover. There is evidence that absorbed β-carotene is retained in the enterocyte, but if it is not taken up by the chylomicrons or converted to vitamin A, it can be subsequently lost in the faeces as epithelial cells are replaced. Light or moderate parasite infestations, such as with *Ascaris*, probably do not affect the absorption of vitamin A, but heavy infections are reported to do so.

Within the enterocyte, absorbed retinol is re-esterified to retinol palmitate and, together with triglycerides and other fat-soluble nutrients, is packaged into chylomicrons for transport to the liver. There are three potential fates for the carotenes absorbed. Some is metabolized by β-carotene-15,15′-dioxygenase to form first retinal, then retinol, and finally retinol palmitate. Some carotene is taken up by the chylomicrons unchanged while the epithelial

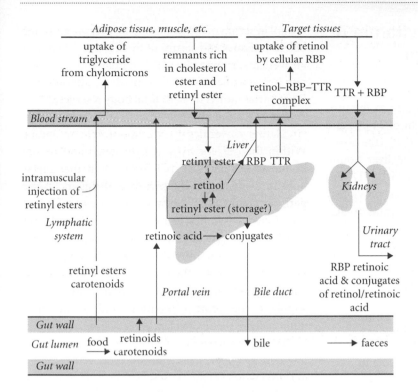

Fig. 11.4 Schematic representation of vitamin A metabolism; RBP, retinol-binding protein; TTR, transthyretin.

cell as described above retains the remainder. The amount of carotene converted to retinol is determined by a number of factors. Protein deficiency depresses the dioxygenase activity while vitamin A deficiency increases it. Zinc deficiency may also depress enzyme activity, as a zinc-dependent enzyme is needed to convert retinal to retinol. Failure to remove retinal would lead to substrate inhibition of dioxygenase activity. There is also evidence that other carotenoids in the diet, like lutein, may inhibit conversion of β-carotene to retinol if the molar ratio of lutein to β-carotene is greater than 3:1 and that β-carotene is preferentially metabolized in comparison with α-carotene or β-cryptoxanthin.

11.4.3 Transport from the gut to the liver

Retinol esters and carotenoids are transported from the gut in association with triglyceride in the core of chylomicrons via lymphatic vessels that drain into the jugular vein. The chylomicrons circulate around the body on their way to the liver. Most triglycerides are transferred to extra-hepatic tissues and there is also evidence to suggest that extra-hepatic cells using the same lipoprotein-receptor mechanisms take up some retinol palmitate, but most vitamin A is removed from the circulation by the liver's parenchymal cells when the chylomicron remnants (cholesterol esters, retinol palmitate, carotenoids and other fat-soluble vitamins) reach the liver.

The retinyl esters are hydrolysed in the parenchymal cells and then much of the retinol is transferred to the stellate cells in a process involving retinol-binding protein (RBP). Stellate cells are modified macrophages that comprise 7% of liver cells numbers but only 2% of the volume. Within the stellate cells, the retinol is mainly stored as retinol palmitate (> 90%). More than 80% of the total body vitamin A is stored in the liver and some in the kidney. Generally the amount of vitamin A in the liver increases with age. On average, a 70 kg man with a liver weighing 1.8 kg would have 150–300 mg of stored vitamin A—enough to last for a year or more of no intake.

11.4.4 Mobilization of vitamin A from the liver and serum transport

Retinol is released from the liver bound to the protein RBP. RBP has a molecular weight of 21 000 and one binding site for retinol. Holo-RBP (the RBP–retinol complex) is released from the liver bound to another protein—transthyretin (TTR). TTR has a molecular weight of 55 000 and was previously known as thyroxine-binding pre-albumin; it also has one binding site so the whole complex is a 1:1:1 structure. In plasma, 95% of the retinol is bound in the retinol–RBP–TTR complex, about 5% is present as retinol–RBP and less than 1% is present as free retinol.

The binding of retinol to RBP confers a number of physiological advantages:

- RBP (and all the vitamin A-binding proteins within the cell) facilitate the transport of a lipid-soluble compound through the aqueous environment of the plasma.

- Protection of retinol from oxidative damage during transport.

- Regulation of retinol mobilization.

- Delivery of retinol to specific sites on the surface of target cells.

- The complex is a large molecule that is not easily lost from the plasma during vasodilatation.

Holo-RBP is taken up by specific cell-surface receptors. Once the retinol is transferred within the cell, the apo-RBP (the free protein) is released from the receptor and can be recycled. Some of the apo-RBP is excreted by the kidney. Retinol inside the cell is bound to cellular RBP. Following an injection of ^{14}C-retinol in autologous plasma into three men, kinetic analysis indicates an average transit time of retinol in serum of 5.4 hours and an average recycling between tissues and serum of three times. There was an average turnover rate of 6.5 mg/day and a disposal rate (irreversible loss) of 1.71 mg/day—although the latter varies indirectly with total body reserves.

Some cells can also take up retinol palmitate from circulating chylomicrons via lipoprotein receptors. Within the cell, the ester is hydrolysed and retinol bound to cellular RBP (CRBP1) for further metabolism. Evidence for the presence of this metabolic pathway comes from the fact that persons who lack the ability to synthesize RBP can live normal lives in almost all respects, provided that their dietary requirements for vitamin A are regularly maintained. Night blindness was the only clinical sign of deficiency, suggesting that the eye does not have an adequate supply of lipoprotein receptors and is the most vulnerable tissue to deficiency as a result.

Plasma carotenes are transported mainly in the low-density lipoproteins while the more water-soluble xanthophylls are most concentrated in the high-density lipoproteins. Depletion studies suggest that half-lives of β- and α-carotene and β-cryptoxanthin are more than 2 weeks, lycopene is 2–4 weeks and lutein and zeaxanthin are 4–8 weeks. The shorter half-lives of the pro-vitamin A carotenoids may be evidence of their conversion to vitamin A in the tissues but the majority of retinol synthesis from carotenes (> 80%) takes place in the gut during absorption.

11.4.5 Vitamin A excretion

In a healthy person, no vitamin A is excreted *per se*. Oxidized metabolites can be found in the urine, and any conjugated vitamin A products that might be formed by vitamin A excess would be secreted into the bile and then lost in the faeces. During illness, particularly in persons with fever, retinol is lost in the urine together with RBP and the amounts can be as high as 500 µg retinol/day.

11.5 Vitamin A deficiency

11.5.1 Experimental deficiencies in animals

The most useful models for studying retinol metabolism are rats and mice. Rats convert almost all dietary carotene to retinol so they are not useful for studying carotene metabolism. Yellow-fat animals such as the rhesus monkey, mouse, domestic fowl and some ruminants absorb some carotene intact, but other animals are like the rat. Ferrets and fresh-water fish have been used by some investigators to study carotene metabolism. Fresh-water fish have also been used in the past to study vitamin A_2 formation. Apart from rodents, the chicken is probably the next most useful species to study vitamin A metabolism. It is also a useful species to study xanthophyll absorption and metabolism. In the laying hen, most of the absorbed xanthophyll is deposited in the egg. Viral diseases in the hen also provide a useful model to study the influence of infection on both retinol and carotenoid metabolism.

11.5.2 Experimental human deficiencies

The first important deficiency study in man was the Sheffield study (Hume and Krebs, 1949). Twenty men and three women, conscientious objectors to military service, volunteered to receive a diet containing no vitamin A_1 and < 7 µg RE of carotene. By 18 months only three of the volunteers actually showed early signs of vitamin A deficiency. However, intervention with carefully chosen amounts of retinol or β-carotene in arachis oil provided the information that established vitamin A requirements in the human adult to reverse signs of vitamin A deficiency to be 750 µg vitamin A_1 or 1800 µg β-carotene, and the bioequivalence of β-carotene to retinol (6 µg β-carotene ≡ 1 µg retinol). Subsequent depletion/repletion studies by Sauberlich *et al.* (1974) provided very similar conclusions—namely, that 1200 µg vitamin A_1 or 2400 µg β-carotene was required to maintain satisfactory serum retinol concentrations, and confirmed the bioequivalence of β-carotene and retinol.

11.5.3 Natural human deficiencies

For many years, the prevalence of vitamin A deficiency was defined by the number of persons showing signs of xerophthalmia (dry eyes). Using such criteria, Sommer and West (1996) estimated that over 40 million children under the age of 6 years have mild to moderate xerophthalmia, that 1% of them become blind each year, and that 50–75% of these will die within the year.

Early work with vitamin A showed that children at risk of xerophthalmia also have a high risk of infection. Hence the term 'anti-infective vitamin' was attached to vitamin A. As techniques to measure plasma retinol concentrations improved, this has been used as the preferred biomarker of vitamin A status and current estimates of vitamin A deficiency in the world are of the order of 500 million. Vitamin A deficiency is a particular problem in groups with the highest vitamin A requirements—infants, pre-school children, and pregnant and lactating women. Vitamin A status is commonly assessed in these groups using plasma retinol concentrations. Infection is particularly common in infants and children, and plasma retinol concentrations are depressed by inflammation. Since this has rarely been taken into account in assessing vitamin A status, current estimates of the risk of vitamin A deficiency in the world are probably overestimates. Nevertheless, vitamin A deficiency is a major risk to human health in many parts of Asia, south-east Asia, Africa, the Middle East, South America and central America. In addition to improving diets in these countries, major efforts are needed to improve sanitation, reduce infections and infestation, and improve literacy. Unless improvements are made in all these areas, the high risk of vitamin A deficiency is likely to continue.

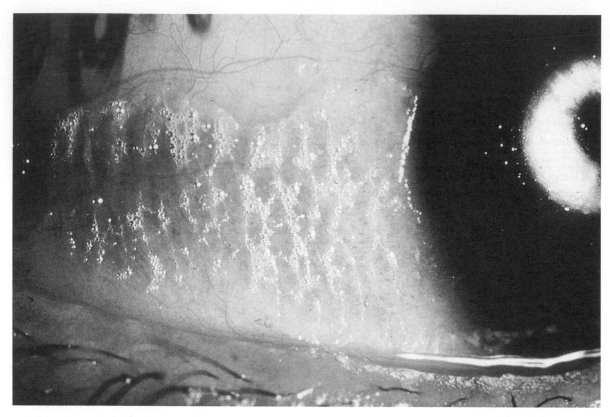

Fig. 11.5 Photograph of a Bitôt's spot.

11.5.4 Features of deficiency disease in man

Changes in the eye People with marginal vitamin A deficiency become less able to see in dim light. This is 'night blindness' and in communities where vitamin A deficiency exists, there is usually a specific word to describe the condition. The word frequently compares the person's behaviour to that of a chicken. Chickens have no rod cells in their retina and cannot see in the dark. If disturbed after night-fall, they bump into things when moving around. Night blindness correlates with low plasma levels of vitamin A, but note that retinol concentrations depressed by inflammation will not necessarily correlate with night blindness. Night blindness can occur in children and adults.

Another clinical indicator of early or marginal vitamin A deficiency is Bitôt's spots. These are foamy deposits found on the surface of the conjunctiva (Fig. 11.5). They are found more frequently in preschool and school-age children than in adults. The spot may indicate the inability of the eye to properly clean itself, and is associated with early xerosis. Both night blindness and Bitôt's spots disappear on treatment with vitamin A, with no lasting damage. In prolonged or more severe vitamin A deficiency, a series of changes can take place in the cornea, some of which are irreversible. The different stages of this xerophthalmia are graded X1, X2, X3 and XS, as summarized in Box 11.2.

Changes to other epithelial tissues The influence of vitamin A on cellular differentiation is reflected in the widespread effects of vitamin A deficiency on other epithelial tissues. Follicular hyperkeratosis seen in vitamin A-deficient adults is due to skin keratinization

---

BOX 11.2 Stages of xerophthalmia

- Conjunctival xerosis (X1A) consists of one or more patches of dry, non-wettable conjunctiva that has been described as 'emerging like sand banks at a receding tide at the sea-shore' when a child ceases to cry. The condition is due to changes in the epithelium of the conjunctiva and the lack of tear production.

- Bitôt's spots (X1B) are found in association with X1A and are a product of the same condition.

- Corneal xerosis (X2) is an extension of conjunctival xerosis to the cornea. The corneal surface also begins to lose its transparent appearance. A light shone at an angle on the surface of the eye will often reveal the ripple-like surface and irregular reflection of the source of illumination.

- Corneal ulceration (X3A) usually begins first at the edge of the cornea and is characterized by small holes, 1–3 mm in diameter, with steep sides. If treatment with vitamin A is initiated at this stage it may be possible to reverse the lesion and retain some sight.

- More extensive corneal ulceration (X3B) is characterized by larger defects that result in blindness. In Africa, it is reported that children with measles can develop X3B quickly without the appearance of the intermediate stages.

- Corneal scars (XS) result from the healing of the irreversible changes described above and may appear as white scar-like tissue in the cornea. On the other hand, if the cornea ruptures and the eye contents escape, a shrunken eyeball results.

Source: WHO (1982).

---

blocking sebaceous glands with horny plugs, though this may not be a specific vitamin A effect. Vitamin A deficiency also affects the epithelial cell lining of the respiratory, gastrointestinal and genitourinary tracts, as well as immune cell maturation. The different epithelia lose their characteristic structure and hence specialized function. The tracheal lining, for example, loses its cilia (which sweep foreign material up and out) and in severe cases the columnar epithelium is replaced by squamous epithelium in the intestine, and villi are flattened and mucus glands reduced.

Morbidity and mortality In 1928, Green and Mellanby showed that when animals were placed on vitamin A-deficient diets, practically all died with infective lesions. Likewise, the more recent work of Sommer and West in Indonesia (1996) showed that the death rate of children with mild xerophthalmia (night-blindness and Bitôt's spots) was on average four times higher than those with no xerophthalmia. Furthermore, meta-analysis of the results of intervention studies in countries where the risk of vitamin A

deficiency was high showed reduced overall mortality by a highly significant 23%. However, the effect of intervention with vitamin A on morbidity is much more difficult to demonstrate, possibly because the measures of morbidity are subjective.

Vitamin A and measles One particular infectious disease, measles, is much more severe, with a fatality rate of about 12%, in communities where xerophthalmia is seen. Even in countries where xerophthalmia does not occur, the benefit of vitamin A treatment in cases of measles is striking. WHO and UNICEF recommend that in developing countries all children with measles should be given a massive dose of vitamin A. This is also the advice for severe cases in developed countries.

Nutritional anaemia Human intervention studies with vitamin A have shown a specific effect of vitamin A on haemoglobin in the absence of additional dietary iron. Possible explanations for these effects are discussed above (in section 11.3.3) (Hess *et al.*, 2005).

11.6 Influence of disease/trauma on plasma retinol concentrations and mobilization of vitamin A from the liver

Infection or inflammation decreases plasma retinol concentrations and reduces mobilization of retinol from liver stores. The effects are part of the acute-phase response (APR) to stress. RBP is a negative acute-phase protein. Stimulation of the APR by infection, surgery or other stresses induces production of cytokines like interleukin-6 (IL-6) by macrophages that induce a wide variety of responses in the liver and elsewhere in the body. One effect is to reduce transcription of the messenger RNA for RBP synthesis. There is also increased vascular permeability, and some plasma retinol moves into extracellular fluid compartments. As much as 500 μg/day of retinol and RBP are lost in the urine. Fig. 11.6 shows plasma retinol concentrations following surgery.

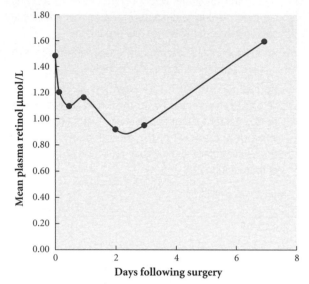

Fig. 11.6 Influence of surgery on plasma retinol concentrations in South African women.
Source: Data modified from Louw *et al.* (1992).

11.7 Biochemical tests for vitamin A deficiency

Biochemical tests for vitamin A status are summarized in Table 11.1. Plasma retinol is probably the most widely used method of assessing vitamin A status but it is influenced strongly by age (Fig. 11.7), female sex hormones and inflammation. Infection or inflammation decrease plasma retinol concentrations and reduce mobilization of retinol from liver stores. These effects can have a major impact on several methods of measurement, such as plasma retinol concentrations, plasma RBP concentrations and dose–response tests.

Recently a method of correcting plasma retinol has been suggested, which utilizes the plasma concentration of two acute-phase proteins, C-reactive protein (CRP) and α1-acid glycoprotein (AGP). CRP is a marker of the early phase of inflammation and is associated with large depressions in plasma retinol concentrations. In contrast, AGP is associated with chronic inflammation or late convalescence when plasma retinol concentrations are less depressed. The use of these two biomarkers enables plasma retinol concentrations to be corrected for the influence of inflammation (Thurnham *et al.*, 2003).

Probably the best (research) method of measuring total body vitamin A reserves are radioisotope dilution assays. These tests may be more or less unaffected by inflammation, as 3 weeks are allowed for equilibration of the labelled tracer with body stores of vitamin A. This period should allow sufficient time for any inflammation at the time of treatment to

Table 11.1 Biochemical tests for vitamin A deficiency

Test	Description	Advantages	Disadvantages	Thresholds of inadequacy
Blood retinol concentration	Measurement in fasting plasma or serum. Samples should be stored at < −20°C on collection. HPLC is the best method of analysis Concentrations <0.7 µmol/L indicate low liver stores of VA Adequacy should always be assessed by comparison with healthy controls of the same age (Fig. 11.7)	Samples easy to obtain and easily quantified	Concentration of retinol depressed by inflammation Concentration of CRP* and AGP** should be monitored Concentrations increased 20–50% by female sex hormones	< 0.35 µmol/L – severe deficiency (= 10 µg/dL) < 0.7 µmol/L – high risk of deficiency (= 20 µg/dL) < 1.05 µmol/L – in adults, possible risk of deficiency
Blood spot retinol concentration	Fasting blood spots can be collected on filter paper. After drying, store with desiccant. When volume of spot is unknown, various methods of correction must be applied	If volume of blood on spot is known, better to elute whole spot	As above. Uncertainties re validity still remain as of 2006	Similar thresholds as for blood retinol concentrations
Blood retinol-binding protein (RBP) concentrations	Same criteria as for blood retinol concentrations	RBP is more stable than plasma retinol	As for blood retinol concentrations	Similar thresholds as for blood retinol concentrations
RBP:trans-thyretin (TTR) ratio	Both RBP and TTR concentrations are depressed by inflammation but only RBP is depressed by both inflammation and dietary VAD Therefore a low ratio should only indicate a dietary VAD	Not influenced by inflammation	Currently no acceptable ratio yet established with which to assess VAD	None yet established
Relative dose response (RDR)	Relies on fact that plasma retinol concentration of VA adequate person is not influenced by a loading dose of VA. In deficiency, liver RBP binds rapidly to any	Indirect method of assessing low liver stores of VA	Influenced by inflammation that depresses RBP synthesis, so mobilization of loading dose does not occur	$RDR = (A5 − A0) \times 100/A5$ VAD when RDR is > 20% (A5 and A0 are concentrations of retinol at 5 and 0 hours, respectively)

Table 11.1 (*cont'd*)

Test	Description	Advantages	Disadvantages	Thresholds of inadequacy
	dietary VA, and retinol appears in plasma within 5 hours. Blood samples are taken at baseline and 5 hours, and the increase in retinol expressed as percentage			
Modified RDR (MRDR)	As above except that the loading dose of VA given is 3,4-didehydroretinol acetate (vitamin A_2)	As above and also only one blood sample required	As above and in addition vitamin A_2 is costly	MRDR = vitamin A_2/vitamin A_1 VAD when MRDR is > 0.06
Serum 30-day response	The test is similar to the RDR test except that the second blood sample is taken 30–45 days after the first.	Much less depression by inflammation due to elapsed time since treatment	Because of time loading, dose needs to be large and method is more applicable at the population level	Baseline and 30-day figures should be evaluated against reference VA for ages (Fig. 11.7)
Radioisotope dilution techniques	Dose of deuterium-labelled retinol given and concentrations in plasma assessed after 21 days. Dilution of the label in total retinol used to assess total body stores	Provides a measure of total body stores	Costly and time-consuming, requiring expensive equipment. Probably not influenced by inflammation	
Milk retinol concentration	Milk retinol palmitate concentration is fairly constant in healthy women of different ethnicities (1.75–2.45 µmol/L). When plasma VA concentration is low, milk VA concentration declines as well. Milk should also be determined using the creamatocrit#	Milk easily obtained during lactation	Concentration in milk declines through lactation and varies during the day	Risk of VAD when concentrations < 1.05 µmol/L or < 27.9 nmol/g fat

Legend:
*CRP is C-reactive protein, elevated in the early part of infection—associated with marked depression of plasma retinol or RBP concentrations.
**AGP is α1-acid glycoprotein, elevated in the latter part of infection and convalescence—associated with less depression of RBP than CRP.
#Creamatocrit—method of measuring the volume of fat in a milk sample by centrifugation to estimate the g fat/100 ml milk.
VA, Vitamin A; VAD, Vitamin A deficiency.

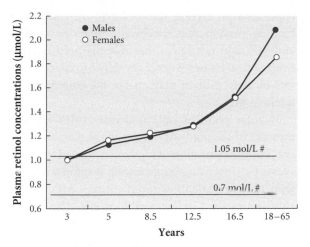

Fig. 11.7 Influence of age on plasma retinol concentrations from three national surveys in Great Britain.
Thresholds of biochemical deficiency; see blood retinol concentrations in Table 11.1.
Source: Thurnham *et al.*, 2005.

subside, and although there will be new infections during this period, most of the subjects should have a period of non-inflammation when equilibration of the tracer can take place.

The carotenoids are rarely used to measure vitamin A status, but when β-carotene is present in plasma, it can sometimes help interpretation of plasma retinol concentration when no acute-phase biomarkers are available. If a low plasma retinol concentration is accompanied by a satisfactory plasma β-carotene concentration, the low retinol is more likely to indicate inflammation than vitamin A deficiency. However, studies in both people and chickens have shown that the acute-phase response is also accompanied by depressed plasma carotenoid concentrations. Some of the depression in plasma carotenoid concentrations may be due to a loss of appetite during infection, but the rapid decline associated with an acute infection has not yet been satisfactorily explained.

11.8 Functions of carotenoids

11.8.1 Bioavailability and conversion of β-carotene to retinol

Carotenoids are fat soluble, so adequate fat in the diet at the time of consumption is necessary for optimal absorption of carotenoids. In plant leaves, carotenoids are present within pigment–protein complexes in the cell chloroplasts, and an important prerequisite for the satisfactory utilization of plant carotenoids is that the cellulose structure of cell walls is ruptured to release carotenoids into the luminal fluids of the gut. Cooking and chewing assist rupture of the cell walls of leaves during ingestion of food. However, in fruit, the cell wall structure is usually much weaker than in leaves, and carotenes are found in the lipid droplets in chromoplasts. Hence carotenoids from fruit are more easily bioavailable than those in leaves.

On the basis of data available to early committees, it was decided that on average only one-third of dietary plant carotene was absorbed. Furthermore, conversion of dietary β-carotene to retinol was also poorly efficient. Even when small amounts of pure β-

carotene dissolved in oil (< 2 mg) were fed to vitamin A-deficient volunteers, only 50% of the β-carotene was converted to retinol. Hence for many years the assumption was made that 6 μg β-carotene from plant sources was bioequivalent to 1 μg retinol. More recently, work in Indonesia and elsewhere has found that the bioequivalency of β-carotene, especially in plant material, was not as high as has been assumed and that far less was available for absorption. Hence the US Institute of Medicine (2000) decided that the bioequivalence in plant food was 12 μg β-carotene to 1 μg retinol (for β-cryptoxanthin and α-carotene, with only one β-ionone ring per molecule, the retinol activity equivalent in plant foods is 24:1).

11.8.2 Macular pigments, lutein, zeaxanthin and meso-zeaxanthin

(Fig. 11.8)

The retinal epithelium is unique in the human body in that it contains almost exclusively only the

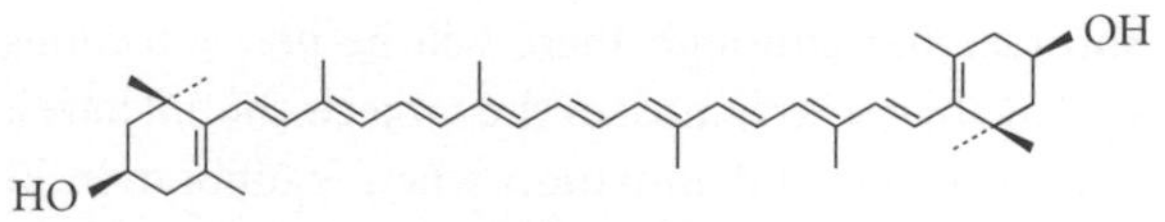

Zeaxanthin

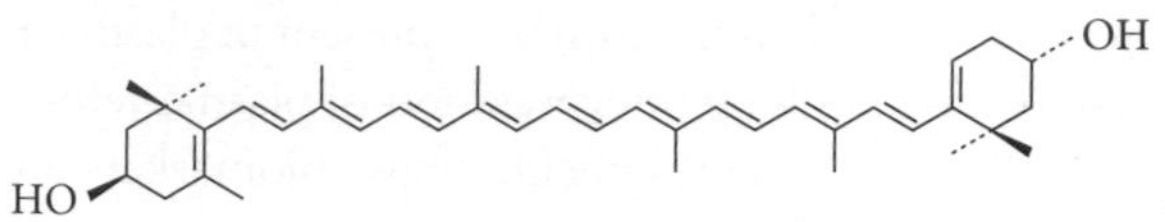

Meso-zeaxanthin

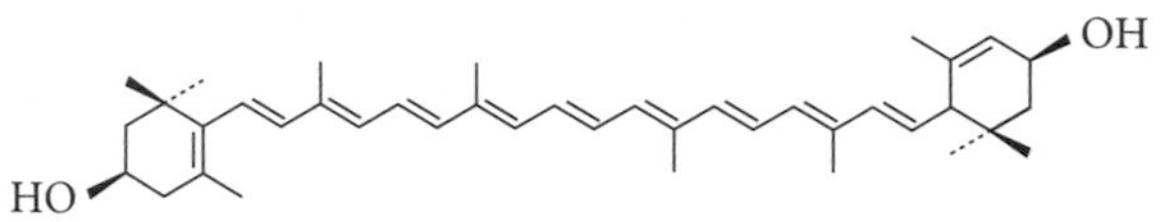

Lutein

Fig. 11.8 Main macular pigments showing zeaxanthin, meso-zeaxanthin and lutein.

three xanthophyll carotenoids—zeaxanthin, meso-zeaxanthin (MZ) and lutein. They are concentrated in the macula lutea in the centre of the retina and provide its yellow colour. Humans consume 1–3 mg lutein per day, and the ratio of lutein to zeaxanthin in the diet is about 5:1. Lutein and zeaxanthin occur in the blood in roughly the same proportions, but no MZ is found. The xanthophyll pigments occur widely in vegetables and fruits but MZ is found in only a few foods like shrimp, some fish and turtle meat. In spite of the amounts of the different xanthophylls in the diet, zeaxanthin and MZ occur in approximately equal amounts in the macula, and their combined concentration exceeds that of lutein. In addition, a binding protein that specifically binds zeaxanthin and MZ, and not lutein, has recently been isolated from optical tissues. There is evidence to suggest that this binding protein may enable the conversion of lutein to MZ.

Macular pigment optical density (MPOD) is a measure of the pigment density in the macula of the eye. The concentration of pigment extracted from the eyes of patients with macula disease at autopsy is lower than that of patients without disease. MPOD can also be measured in living subjects using physiological methods, and can be shown to increase following supplementation with pure lutein supplements and with vegetables like spinach. Once increased, MPOD remains elevated for several weeks or months after withdrawal of the supplement. Dark-green leafy vegetables are the richest source of dietary lutein, but egg yolks also contain lutein and zeaxanthin, which may be more bioavailable. MZ has been a component of a xanthophyll supplement added to chicken feed in Mexico for several years, but it is not yet in the food chain of other countries, either as a supplement or a nutraceutical.

Lycopene is the red pigment of tomatoes. It is often the most abundant of the carotenoids in human plasma. Having no β-ionine rings (Fig. 11.2), it is not a pro-vitamin A. It is, however, an antioxidant (as is β-carotene). Early reports of a negative association of tomato sauce consumption and prostate cancer await further substantiation.

11.9 Food sources of vitamin A and carotenoids

In most industrialized countries, the predominant dietary source of vitamin A activity is pre-formed vitamin A_1, mainly in the form of retinol palmitate in foods of animal origin. Liver is the richest source of vitamin A, but it is also found in milk, butter, cheese, egg yolk and some fatty fish. Margarine is enriched with vitamin A to levels similar to those in butter. Pro-vitamin A carotenes are also obtained from plant foods, the main ones being dark-green leafy vegetables and some yellow- or orange-coloured fruits.

In developing countries, plant sources of vitamin A are predominant in the diet. Certain foods like red palm oil, papayas, mangos and carrots are particularly rich in β-carotene and sometime also α-carotene and or β-cryptoxanthin. Plant sources of vitamin A are often seasonal, and seasonal fluctuations in vitamin A status are common in some tropical countries (for example, vitamin A status in West African countries improves with the mango season).

11.10 Recommended intakes

Vitamin A requirements vary with age and the requirement for growth is a major determinant. Thus requirements in infancy and childhood are higher per kg of body weight than in adults. Infants are born with almost no stores of vitamin A so it is critical that newborn infants obtain sufficient vitamin A to meet the needs of growth and a developing immune system, as well as to accumulate body stores. Hence the mother's colostrum and early milk is high in vitamin A; it progressively declines during lactation. The needs of the infant also increase the vitamin A requirements of lactating mothers. The British (1991) RDIs followed those of the FAO/WHO (1988) Consultation. Some of their recommended dietary intakes (RDIs) are lower than the more recent North American and Australia/New Zealand recommendations. They are summarized in Table 11.2.

Table 11.2 Summary of RDIs

	µg retinol equivalents/day
Infants	350–500
1–6 years	400
7–12 years	500
Adolescents	600
Men	600–900
Women	600–900
Pregnant	700–800
Lactating	850, 1100, 1300

11.11 Toxic effects of vitamin A

The most serious toxic effects of vitamin A are teratogenic as a result of overdose during the first trimester of pregnancy. Such effects include spontaneous abortions or fetal abnormalities including those of the cranium (microcephaly), face (hair lip), heart, kidney, thymus and central nervous system (deafness and lowered learning ability). Since embryogenesis is under the control of retinoic acid isomers, short-term increases in these compounds are probably responsible. In one experiment, large doses of vitamin A (> 300 000 IU, > 100 mg) given to ten women caused 10–100-fold increases in plasma retinoic acid concentrations at 4 hours. The half-life of retinoic acid is about 8 hours and normal concentrations of plasma retinoic acid are 1–2 nmol/L. Interestingly, the same amount of vitamin A given as liver only increased plasma retinoic acid concentrations 10-fold at 4 hours. Thus, women who are pregnant or who could become pregnant should not be exposed to retinoid therapy either for skin conditions or as supplements. Daily intakes should not exceed 10 000 IU (3 mg RE).

Acute and chronic toxic effects of vitamin A overdose can also occur in all individuals. Very high single doses can cause transient symptoms that may include a bulging fontanelle in infants, a headache in older children and adults, and vomiting, diarrhoea and loss of appetite in all age groups. It is rare for toxicity to occur from ingestion of food sources of vitamin A. When it does occur, it is usually due to the consumption of liver as, for example, in Arctic and Antarctic explorers who consumed polar bear, seal or dog liver. In these extreme circumstances, additional symptoms included blurred or double vision, vertigo, uncoordinated movements, elevated cerebrospinal pressure and skin exfoliation. Deaths have also occurred.

Single large doses of vitamin A in infancy and childhood have been reported to cause transient toxic effects, but these are usually avoided if the not more than 50 000 IU for infants younger than 6 months, or 100 000 IU for those aged 6–12 months, or 200 000 IU for children over 1 year. Doses are not usually given more frequently than once every 3 months but three doses of 50 000 IU given to infants at 2, 3 and 4 months of age was shown to be without any adverse effects in a recent study in The Gambia (Darbsoe *et al.* 2006).

Chronic toxicity is induced by consuming for a month or more at least ten times the recommended daily allowance (e.g. 10 mg RE/day or 33 300 IU). A wide range of symptoms have been reported including headache, bone and muscle pain, ataxia, visual impairment, skin disorders, alopecia, liver toxicity and hyperlipidaemia. It is usual to find high concentrations of retinol palmitate in the blood

(3–8 μmol/L). Normally, retinol palmitate is only found in the blood for 3–4 hours after a meal, in the chylomicron fraction.

High intakes of carotenoids, for example, from tomato or carrot juice or red palm oil, can lead to hypercarotenaemia and yellow coloration of the skin, especially the palms of the hands or the soles of the feet and the nasolabial folds (not the eyes); but they are not associated with toxic effects. High doses of β-carotene (180 mg/day) are used in the treatment of erythropoietic protoporphyria and have never been found to cause harm. The only worrying effects associated with carotenoids are the long-term use of β-carotene in smokers. Doses of 25–30 mg/day were found to increase the incidence of lung cancer in two large intervention studies.

11.12 Measures to prevent vitamin A deficiency

11.12.1 Using available foods

All nutritional deficiencies are due to a lack of food, and if sufficient food is available then most deficiencies will disappear. This of course means that deficiencies rarely occur alone, and that the clinical features of deficiencies in a community are those of the most serious deficiencies. In developing countries, vitamin A deficiency is a particular problem because dietary sources of pre-formed vitamin A (animal food products) are expensive and people are reliant on vegetable sources. As explained above, the bioavailability of carotene in plant food is poor. Fruit carotene is more bioavailable than that in vegetables but is often seasonal. In many places, there are a greater variety of plant foods to overcome seasonal shortages but thorough cooking of vegetables and fat (which improves carotene absorption) are necessary to optimize bioavailability. Cooking methods are part of the culture of a community and are not changed easily, and fat is very often an animal product and in short supply. Where vitamin A deficiencies exist, people need to be made aware of the diversity of foods that can provide vitamin A. Growing of mangos, papaya (yellow and orange varieties), red sweet potato and

plantain needs to be encouraged, as well as the introduction of chickens for their eggs, and fish where appropriate. As poverty is often the root cause of the lack of food, such schemes will need assistance and will take time to be effective. High-dose supplementation of vulnerable groups, food fortification and introduction of nutrient-enriched foods are short-term measures to rectify specific nutrient deficiencies and some may become part of the long-term solution to vitamin A deficiency.

Prevention—ideally eradication—of vitamin A deficiency is a priority for WHO and UNICEF. The deficiency is widespread; it causes death or blindness in many thousands of young children; measures of prevention are known, are safe and are practical, and need to be more generally applied by national governments and non-governmental agencies.

11.12.2 Massive dosing and supplementation

Massive dosing of communities with vitamin A to overcome vitamin A deficiency was first tried in the 1960s in India. Doses of 200 000–300 000 IU

(60–90 mg RE) were given to pre-school children, and any children showing side effects were noted. Specific problems included headaches, nausea, vomiting and a bulging fontanelle, but none of the side effects caused permanent damage, and the prevalence of signs like night blindness, Bitôt's spots and xerosis was reduced. Night blindness is cured first. Oral and intramuscular administration of vitamin A dissolved in oil were tested, and oral administration, by capsule or spoon, was found to be highly effective. Use of the method has extended to many countries and clear benefits in reduced mortality have been demonstrated (see section 11.5.4). Currently recommended treatments are shown in Box 11.3.

The high dose for a child provides sufficient vitamin A for a period of 4–6 months, so where vitamin A deficiency is a constant problem, treatment should be provided every 6 months. Women of child-bearing age should not be given high doses except immediately post-partum. The highest dose for a non-pregnant women is 10 000 IU (3 mg RE) or 1 mg RE daily. Children admitted to hospital with measles, xerophthalmia or malnutrition are given 200 000 IU of vitamin A therapeutically.

11.12.3 Fortification and enrichment

Fortification is the addition of vitamin A to a widely used food that would not normally contain the vitamin. Enrichment is the addition of vitamin A to a food to replace the vitamin lost during processing. Because vitamin A is lost during storage, the amount of vitamin added should usually be greater than the nominal amount required by legislation or shown on the package. Both processes are introduced where it is decided the community requires extra vitamin A. Margarine has been enriched with vitamin A at a level of the best summer butter (200 IU (60 µg RE) per 100 g) in many European and developing countries. Sugar fortification (1.5 mg RE/100 g sugar) has been successful in several Central American countries and is now being tried in Africa. Oil is also a useful vehicle for fortification, but with all methods the main problem is maintaining quality control of the product. If many manufacturers are involved, the costs of monitoring quality may be prohibitive.

11.12.4 Public health and other indirect methods

Poverty and disease are the main factors accompanying vitamin A deficiency in communities throughout Africa, Asia and South America. Immunization against infections and social improvements to address the issues of poverty, land reform, lack of education and improvements in agricultural diversity will all help to address the problem of vitamin A deficiency.

11.13 Influence of micronutrient deficiences and drugs on vitamin A status

11.13.1 Influence of other nutrients on vitamin A status

A balanced and adequate diet is necessary for optimal vitamin A status. Specific deficiencies of protein and zinc, and possibly vitamin E, may adversely affect status. Experimental protein deficiency reduces the activity of β-carotene-15,15′-dioxygenase activity, so may impair the conversion of β-carotene to retinal. Absorption of retinol is impaired in kwashiorkor, and serum retinol is low. It improves with re-feeding before vitamin A is given. Zinc-dependent enzymes convert retinol to retinal, and in one study night blindness in a group of alcoholics was explained by poor conversion of 11-*cis* retinol to 11-*cis* retinal in the eye, which is also dependent on zinc. Zinc is also involved in the synthesis of RBP, and RBP is particularly rich in zinc. Plasma retinol concentrations frequently correlate with plasma α-tocopherol concentrations. The precise reason is not known, but vitamin E may protect retinol from oxidation.

11.13.2 Interactions with drugs

Several drugs are known to affect the absorption of vitamin A, such as cholestyramine (an antihyperli-paemic), colchicine (for gout), mineral oil (a laxative), neomycin (an antibiotic that inactivates bile salts), olestra (antiobesity agent), phytostanols and phytosterols (for lowering obesity). However, unless their use is prolonged over many months, the large liver stores of vitamin A in adults will maintain vitamin A status.

Ethyl alcohol and the female sex hormones can potentially affect vitamin A status. Alcohol abuse results in a striking depletion of hepatic vitamin A. Increased ethanol-oxidizing capacity, as a result of alcohol abuse, may increase the oxidation and loss of retinol from the liver and cause the poor vitamin A status of many alcoholics. In contrast, oestrogen-containing drugs (oral contraceptives, hormone replacement therapy) can have a stimulatory effect on the concentration of plasma retinol.

11.14 Pharmaceutical uses of vitamin A

Several synthetic retinoids influence proliferation and differentiation of the skin epidermis, inhibit keratinization, reduce production of sebum and influence immune responses (especially cell-mediated immunity). These properties have been used in medicine particularly to treat such skin disorders as acne, seborrhoea (overproduction of sebum), some keratinizing dermatoses and psoriasis (areas covered by profuse silvery scales, especially on the elbows, knees and trunk of the body). One of the more effective drugs is 13-*cis* retinoic acid (isotretinoin, Roaccutane) but, even for topical applications, its use is restricted in women of child-bearing age because of the risk of teratogenesis. Topical use of all-*trans* retinoic acid can also reduce the wrinkling and hyperpigmentation caused by photo-ageing. All-*trans* retinoic acid and 13-*cis* retinoic acid have been used to treat certain acute myeloid leukaemias (AMLs) where the retinoids stop proliferation of the cells and induce terminal differentiation to the granulocyte. Unfortunately there are a number of different AMLs and only a limited number of patients respond.

Note: The International Vitamin A Consultative Group (IVACG) founded in 1976 provides a forum and network for scientists whose work aims at reducing vitamin A deficiency in the world. It holds annual meetings and publishes reports and newsletters. See http:ivacg.ilsi.org/.

FURTHER READING

1. Darboe, M.K. Thurnham, D.I. Morgan G., *et al.* (2006) Effectiveness of the new IVACG early high-dose vitamin A supplementation scheme compared to the standard WHO protocol: A randomised controlled trial in Gambian mothers and infants. *Lancet*, (submitted).

2. de Pee, S., West, C.E., Permaesih, D., Martuti, S., Muhilal, and Hautvast, G.A.J. (1998) Orange fruit is more effective than dark-green leafy vegetables in increasing serum concentrations of retinol and B$_6$ in schoolchildren in Indonesia. *Am J Clin Nutr*, **68**, 1058–67.

3. FAO/WHO Expert Consultation (1988) *Requirements of vitamin A, iron, folate and vitamin B-12*. FAO Food & Nutrition Series 23, Rome.

4. Hess, S.Y., Thurnham, D.I., and Hurrell, R.F. (2005) *Influence of provitamin A carotenoids on iron, zinc and vitamin A status*. Washington, International Food Policy Research Institute.

5. Hume, E.M., and Krebs, H.A. (1949) *Vitamin A requirements of human adults*. Report of the vitamin A sub-committee of the accessory food factors committee, No. 264. London, HMSO.

6. **Landrum, J.T., and Bone, R.A.** (2001) Minireview. Lutein, zeanthanthin and the macular pigment. *Arch Biochem Biophys*, **385**, 28–40.

7. **Louw, J.A., Werbeck, A., Louw, M.E.J., Kotze, T.J.W., Cooper, R., and Labadarios, D.** (1992) Blood vitamin concentrations during the acute-phase response. *Crit Care Med*, **20**, 934–41.

8. **McLaren, D.S., and Frigg, M.** (2001) *Sight and Life manual on vitamin A deficiency disorders*, 2nd edition. Basel, Sight and Life.

9. **Moore, T.** (1957) *Vitamin A* Amsterdam, Elsevier.

10. **Sauberlich, H.E., Hodges, R.E., Wallace, D.L., Kolder, H., Canham, J.E., Hood, J., Raica, N.Jr, Lowry, L.K.** (1974) Vitamin A metabolism and requirements in the human studied with the use of labelled retinol. *Vitam Horm*, **32**, 251–75.

11. **Sommer, A., and West, K.P.** (1996) *Vitamin A deficiency: Health, survival and vision*. New York, Oxford University Press.

12. **Thurnham, D.I., Mburu, A.S.W., Mwaniki, D.L., and de Wagt, A.** (2005) Micronutrients in childhood and the influence of subclinical inflammation. *Proc Nutr Soc*, **64**, 502–9.

13. **Thurnham, D.I., McCabe, G.P., Northrop-Clewes, C.A., and Nestel, P.** (2003) Effect of subclinical infection on plasma retinol concentrations and assessment of prevalence of vitamin A deficiency: meta-analysis. *Lancet*, **362**, 2052–8.

14. **US Institute of Medicine** (2000) *Dietary reference intakes for vitamin A, vitamin K, arsenic, boron, chromium, copper, iodine, iron, manganese, molybdenum, nickel, silicon, vanadium and zinc*. US Institute of Medicine, Food and Nutrition Board, Standing Committee on the Scientific Evaluation of Dietary Intakes. Washington, National Academic Press.

15. **WHO** (1982) *Control of vitamin A deficiency and xerophthalmia*. Report of a Joint WHO/USAID/Helen Keller International/IVACG Meeting. WHO Technical Report Series, No. 672. Geneva, World Health Organization.

To see topical and scientifically robust updates on nutrition associated with this textbook, and active web links to many of the journal articles in the Reference areas, please see the dedicated Online Resource Centre at www.oxfordtextbooks.co.uk/orc/mann3e/.

12 The B vitamins

Stewart Truswell

All the B vitamins are water soluble. The water-soluble B vitamin that McCollum differentiated from the fat-soluble A vitamin in 1915 was later shown to consist of several distinct essential nutrients, though often found in the same foods, like liver and yeast. As they were separately isolated, were named vitamin B_1, B_2, B_3 and so on at first, but some of these were the same as those that someone else had found in another laboratory and they fell by the wayside. There are now eight well-established vitamins from the original B complex. Most of them are now given their chemical names but B_1 is sometimes still used, and B_6 and B_{12} persist in common use.

12.1 Thiamin (vitamin B_1)

Eijkmann, a Dutch medical officer stationed in Java, discovered around 1897 that a polyneuritis resembling beri-beri (which was very common in South-east Asia at that time) could be produced in chickens fed on polished rice. Subsequently he and his successor, Grijns, showed that this polyneuritis could be cured with rice bran or polishings. This contained B_1, the first of the vitamins to be identified, but it was not until 1936 that R.R. Williams finally elucidated the unusual structure and synthesized thiamin.*

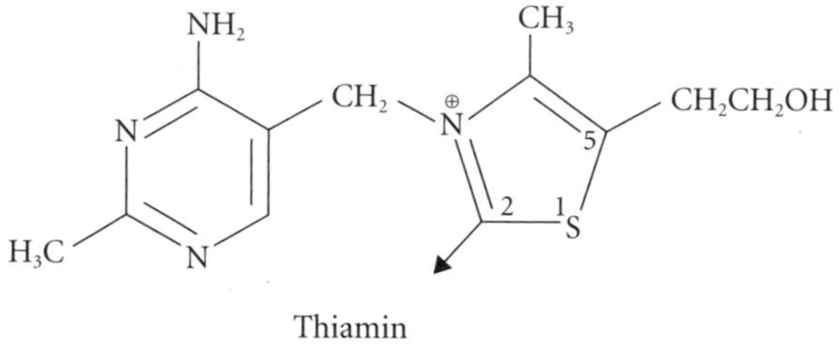

Thiamin

Fig. 12.1 Structure of thiamin.

12.1.1 Functions

Thiamin (Fig. 12.1) as the diphosphate (or 'pyrophosphate'), thiamin pyrophosphate (TTP) is a coenzyme

*We follow the spelling of the International Union of Nutritional Sciences for thiamin (no final 'e'). The pharmaceutical sciences still spell it 'thiamine'

for the following major decarboxylation steps in carbohydrate metabolism:

1. Pyruvate $\rightarrow$ acetyl CoA (pyruvate dehydrogenase complex) at the entry to the citric acid cycle. Hence, in thiamin deficiency, pyruvate and lactate accumulate.

2. α-Ketoglutarate → succinyl CoA (α-ketoglutarate dehydrogenase), half-way round the citric acid cycle.

3. Transketolase reactions in the hexose monophosphate shunt, an alternative pathway for oxidation of glucose. Hence, in thiamin deficiency, oxidation of glucose is impaired with no alternative route.

4. The second step in catabolism of the branched-chain amino acids, leucine, isoleucine and valine.

12.1.2 Absorption and metabolism

Thiamin is readily absorbed by active transport at low concentrations in the small intestine and by passive diffusion at high concentrations. Total body content is only 25–30 mg, mostly in the form of TPP in the tissues. There is another coenzyme form, thiamin triphosphate, in the brain. Thiamin is excreted both unchanged and as metabolites in the urine. It has a relatively high turnover rate in the body; there is really no store anywhere in the body. On a diet lacking in thiamin, signs of deficiency can occur after only 25–30 days.

12.1.3 Deficiency in animals

Pigeons and chickens are more susceptible than mammals. The characteristic effect is head retraction, called opisthotonus, from neurological dysfunction. In mammals with experimental deficiency, there is incoordination of muscle movements, progressing to paralysis, convulsions and death. The brain is dependent on glucose oxidation for its energy but the decrease in its pyruvate dehydrogenase and α-ketoglutarate dehydrogenase activities does not seem sufficient to explain the severe neurological dysfunction. Reduced formation of the neurotransmitter acetylcholine (because acetyl CoA is not being formed), and a role of thiamin triphosphate in nerve transmission are other possible mechanisms.

Loss of appetite, cardiac enlargement, oedema and increased pyruvate and lactate are also seen.

12.1.4 Deficiency in humans

There are two distinct major deficiency diseases, beri-beri and Wernicke–Korsakoff syndrome. They do not usually occur together.

Beri-beri is now rare in the countries where it was originally described—Japan, Indonesia and Malaysia (the name comes from the Singhalese language of Sri Lanka). In Western countries, occasional cases are seen in alcoholics. In *acute* beri-beri, there is a high-output cardiac failure, with warm extremities, bounding pulse, oedema and cardiac enlargement. These features appear to be the result of intense vasodilatation from accumulation of pyruvate and lactate in blood and tissues. There are few electrocardiographic abnormalities. Response to thiamin treatment is prompt, with diuresis, and usually a full recovery. In *chronic* beri-beri, the peripheral nerves are affected, rather than the cardiovascular system. There is inability to lift the foot up (foot drop), loss of sensation in the feet and absent ankle jerk reflexes.

Wernicke's encephalopathy is usually seen in people who have been drinking alcohol heavily for some weeks and eaten very little. Alcohol requires thiamin for its metabolism and alcoholic beverages do not contain it. Alcohol may also interfere with thiamin absorption. Occasional cases are seen in people on a prolonged fast (such as hunger strikers) or with persistent vomiting (as in Wernicke's first described case). Cases occurred in malnourished soldiers in Japanese prisoner-of-war camps in World War II. Clinically, there is a state of quiet confusion, a lowered level of consciousness and incoordination (fairly non-specific signs in an alcoholic). The characteristic feature is paralysis of one or more of the external movements of the eyes (ophthalmoplegia). This and the lowered consciousness respond to injection of thiamin within 2 days, but if treatment is delayed the memory may never recover. The memory disorder that is a sequel of Wernicke's encephalopathy is called Korsakoff's psychosis after the Russian psychologist who first described it. There is an inability to retain new memories and sometimes confabulation.

In people who die of Wernicke–Korsakoff syndrome, lesions are found in the mamillary bodies, mid-brain and cerebellum. It is not clear why one deficient person develops beri-beri and another develops Wernicke–Korsakoff syndrome, or why the two diseases seldom coincide. Possibly the cardiac disease occurs in people who use their muscles for heavy work and so accumulate large amounts of pyruvate, producing vasodilatation and increasing cardiac work, while encephalopathy is the first manifestation in inactive people.

12.1.5 Biochemical tests

Red cell transketolase activity, with and without TPP added *in vitro*, is a good test. However, heparinized whole blood must be used, it must be analysed fresh (or specially preserved) and the test will be normal if thiamin treatment has been already started. If the transketolase activity is increased more than 30% in the test tube with added TPP, this indicates at least some degree of biochemical thiamin deficiency. In Wernicke's encephalopathy, this 'TPP effect' can be higher than this, around 70% or even 100%. (Note: in this test, reported as 'TPP effect', high values are abnormal.)

12.1.6 Interactions with nutrients

The requirement for thiamin is proportional to the intake of carbohydrates + alcohol + protein. In homogeneous societies, where proportions of fat and carbohydrate do not greatly differ, the thiamin requirement is proportional to the total energy intake.

There are no real stores of thiamin and the body runs out of it after about 3 weeks of starvation. When a malnourished person is given food that uses thiamin, there is a danger of precipitating Wernicke's encephalopathy, for example, with an intravenous glucose/water infusion. Thiamin should always be given with re-feeding (cf. Chapter 40).

12.1.7 Food sources

There are no rich food sources of thiamin. The best sources in descending order are wheatgerm, whole wheat and its products, yeast and yeast extracts, pulses, nuts, pork, duck, oatmeal, fortified breakfast cereals, cod's roe and other meats. In many industrial countries (UK, North America, etc.), bread flour is enriched with thiamin and so are most breakfast cereals. Australia introduced mandatory fortification of bread flour with thiamin in 1991 and it has reduced that country's previously high rate of Wernicke–Korsakoff syndrome. Thiamin is readily destroyed by heat and by sulphite and by thiaminase (present in raw fish).

The recommended dietary intake of thiamin is 0.4 mg per 1000 kcal (0.1 mg/kJ) (i.e. about 1.0 mg/day in adults). The toxicity of thiamin is very low.

12.2 Riboflavin

Vitamin B was originally considered to have two components, heat-labile B_1 (= thiamin) and heat-stable B_2. In the 1930s, it was discovered that a yellow growth factor (riboflavin) in this latter fraction is distinct from the pellagra-preventing substance (niacin).

12.2.1 Structure

Riboflavin or 7,8-dimethyl-10-(1′-D-ribityl) isoalloxazine, comprises an alloxazine ring connected to a ribose alcohol—the ribityl side chain is required for full vitamin activity. It is a yellow-green fluorescent compound.

12.2.2 Functions

Riboflavin (Fig. 12.2) is part of two important coenzymes, flavin mononucleotide (FMN) and flavin adenine dinucleotide (FAD), which are oxidizing agents. They participate in flavoproteins in the oxidation chain in mitochondria. They are also cofactors for several enzymes, for example, NADH dehydrogenase,

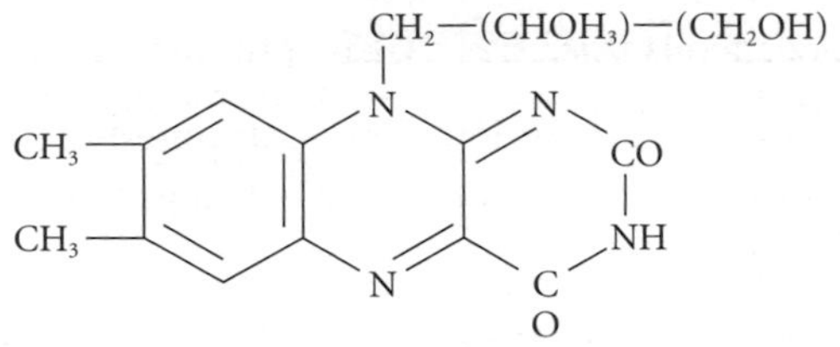

Riboflavin

Fig. 12.2 Structure of riboflavin. Ribitol is the alcohol form of the 5-carbon sugar, ribose. In FMN, two phosphates are attached to the end of the ribitol. In FAD, this is extended further with adenylate (ribose-adenine).

xanthine oxidase, L-amino acid oxidase, glutathione reductase, L-gulonolactone oxidase and methylene tetrahydrofolate reductase (MTHFR).

12.2.3 Absorption and metabolism

Absorption is by a specialized carrier system in the proximal small intestine, which is saturated at levels above 25 mg. The vitamin is transported as free riboflavin and FMN or bound to plasma albumin. The body contains only about 1 g of riboflavin, mostly found in the muscle as FAD. Riboflavin is excreted primarily in urine; urinary excretion tends to reflect dietary intake.

12.2.4 Deficiency in animals

The most common effects in animals are cessation of growth, dermatitis, hyperkeratosis, alopecia and vascularization of the cornea. Abortion or skeletal malformations of the fetus may occur. In some species, anaemia, fatty liver and neurological changes have also been reported.

12.2.5 Deficiency in humans

The clinical symptoms of deficiency: angular stomatitis, cheilosis, atrophy of the tongue papillae, nasolabial dyssebacea and anaemia, are surprisingly minor, presumably due to the body's ability to con-

serve riboflavin, and the high affinity of the coenzymes for their respective enzymes. Riboflavin deficiency (ariboflavinosis) is most commonly seen alongside other nutrient deficiencies (e.g. pellagra).

12.2.6 Biochemical tests

1. Erythrocyte glutathione reductase activity (EGRA) coefficient: FAD is a cofactor for this enzyme and its activity correlates with riboflavin status.

$$\text{The activity coefficient (or FAD effect)} = \frac{\text{EGRA with added FAD } in\ vitro}{\text{EGRA without FAD } in\ vitro}$$

Values of < 1.2 are considered to be acceptable, but values of 1.3–1.7 indicate inadequate riboflavin status. However, some doubts have been raised about the validity of the FAD effect, as it is elevated during exercise and pregnancy.

2. Measurement of urinary excretion of riboflavin: Non-vitamin flavins (from foods) can be excreted so an HPLC-fluorometric method should be used to separate the riboflavin. Levels below 100 µg riboflavin/day are low.

12.2.7 Interactions: drugs

Phenothiazine derivatives (e.g. chlorpromazine) and tricyclic antidepressants have similar structures and can interfere with riboflavin metabolism. Reduced riboflavin status is observed in alcoholics, but is due more to decreased dietary intake and absorption than to a direct effect of alcohol.

12.2.8 Food sources

Riboflavin is present in most foods although the best sources are milk and milk products, eggs, liver, kidney, yeast extracts and fortified breakfast cereals. Dairy products contribute significantly to riboflavin intake in Western diets. However, riboflavin is unstable in ultraviolet (UV) light, and after milk has been exposed to sunlight for 4 hours, up to 70% of riboflavin is lost.

The recommended dietary intake for adults is about 1.3 mg/day. The requirement is less in people with small energy intakes and more in those with large energy intakes.

12.3 Niacin

Niacin (Fig. 12.3) is a generic term for the related compounds that have activity as pellagra-preventing vitamins; the two that occur in foods are nicotinic acid (pyridine 3-carboxylic acid) and its amide, nicotinamide. They have apparently equal vitamin activity. Nicotinic acid is a fairly simple chemical (molecular weight 123) that was known long before its nutritional role was established. It was first isolated as an oxidation product of the natural alkaloid, nicotine, from which its name is derived. However, nicotinic acid and amide have very different physiological properties from nicotine (which is α-N-methyl-d-β-pyridyl pyrrolidine).

12.3.1 Functions

Nicotinamide is part of the coenzymes nicotinamide adenine dinucleotide (NAD) and nicotinamide adenine dinucleotide phosphate (NADP), the pyridine nucleotides. NAD has the structure: adenine-ribose-PO_4-PO_4-ribose-nicotinamide. It plays a central role in metabolism: it functions as the first hydrogen receptor in the electron chain during oxidative phosphorylation in the mitochondria. The pyridine ring

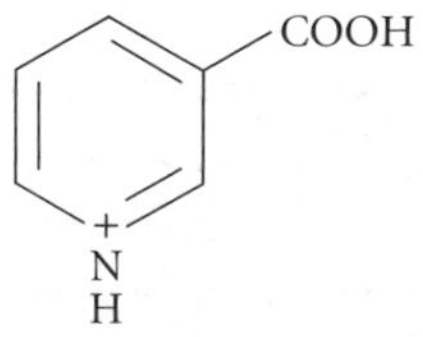

Fig. 12.3 Structure of nicotinic acid (niacin). Nicotinamide is the corresponding amide, with $CONH_2$ in the side chain.

12.2.9 Toxic effects

The toxicity is very low. The gastrointestinal tract cannot absorb more than about 20–25 mg of riboflavin in a single dose.

of the nicotinamide is the part of the molecule that takes up a hydrogen (NAD $\leftrightarrow$ NADH).

NADP has an extra PO_4 (phosphate) attached to the ribose adjacent to adenine. It has a more specialized function as hydrogen donor in fatty acid synthesis.

12.3.2 Absorption and metabolism

Nicotinic acid or its amide are water soluble and well absorbed from the stomach and small intestine and transported in solution in the plasma. Stores of niacin and its coenzymes are only small, and early features of pellagra can occur in human subjects after some 45 days of depletion.

12.3.3 Synthesis from tryptophan

A special feature of niacin is that in most conditions only about half of what is in the body is absorbed as pre-formed nicotinic acid or amide from the diet. About the same amount is synthesized in the liver from tryptophan, the indole amino acid, in a sequence of seven enzyme steps down the kynurenine pathway.

Most tryptophan in the body is used for protein synthesis—it is the least abundant in foods of all the essential amino acids—some also goes to serotonin. Normally, about one-sixth to one-tenth of the dietary tryptophan intake is converted in the liver to niacin (i.e. 60 mg tryptophan $\equiv$ 1 mg niacin). The first enzyme in the kynurenine pathway, hepatic tryptophan oxygenase, is under hormonal control and the amount of niacin formed appears to be increased in pregnancy. It is downregulated when the protein intake is inadequate (see Fig. 12.4).

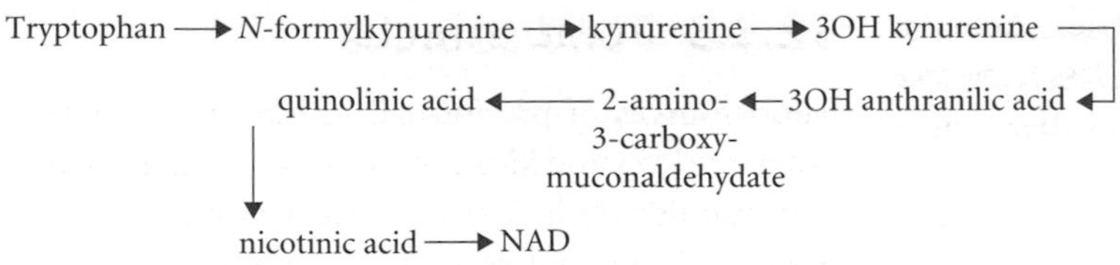

Tryptophan ⟶ *N*-formylkynurenine ⟶ kynurenine ⟶ 3OH kynurenine

quinolinic acid ◀——— 2-amino- ◀— 3OH anthranilic acid ◀
3-carboxy-
muconaldehyde

nicotinic acid ⟶ NAD

Fig. 12.4 Tryptophan → NAD (nicotinamide adenine dinucleotide).

12.3.4 Deficiency in animals

The classic animal model for pellagra is 'black tongue' in dogs. Puppies lose their appetite and have inflamed gums, dark tongue and diarrhoea with blood. Elvehjem's group at Wisconsin tested different fractions of liver for their ability to cure black tongue and in 1937 found that the 'pellagra-preventing factor' was nicotinamide.

12.3.5 Deficiency in humans

There is one deficiency disease, *pellagra* (the name means 'sour skin' in Italian). The skin is inflamed where it is exposed to sunlight, resembling severe sunburn, but the affected skin is sharply demarcated. The skin lesions progress to pigmentation, cracking and peeling. Often the skin of the neck is involved (Casal's collar) (see Fig. 12.5). Students are taught that pellagra is the disease of three Ds: dermatitis, diarrhoea and delirium or dementia. As well as diarrhoea, there is likely to be an inflamed tongue (glossitis). In mild chronic cases, mental symptoms (the third 'D') are not prominent. It is hard to explain the clinical manifestations by the known biochemical functions of niacin. Because some niacin is formed from tryptophan, pellagra can be cured by giving either niacin or a generous intake of easily assimilated protein.

Pellagra appeared in Europe after maize was introduced as a cereal crop from the New World after 1500, but the Mayans, Aztecs and indigenous North Americans do not seem to have suffered from pellagra.

There was a major epidemic of pellagra in poor people (share croppers) in the southern states of the USA from around 1905. It was generally thought to be an infectious disease but Joseph Goldberger, investigating for the Federal government between 1914 and 1929, demonstrated by epidemiology and crucial human experiments that it was due to a diet of maize grits and little else. He identified an animal model, black tongue in dogs (rats are not susceptible), cured by yeast in which the pellagra-preventing factor eventually turned out to be nicotinamide, already known in tissue culture biochemistry.

The niacin in cereals is in a complex, 'niacytin', which humans cannot absorb, so that although it appears in food tables (because the complex is split during extraction), it is not biologically available. If subsistence farmers eat a diet predominantly of maize, with few other foods, their niacin has to come from tryptophan in the protein of the cereal. However, the protein of maize is deficient in tryptophan, unlike

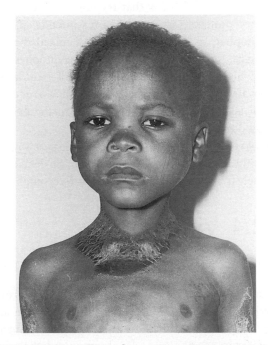

Fig. 12.5 A boy suffering from pellagra. Note the Casal's collar.

other cereals, so little or no niacin can be made in the body via the kynurenine pathway. All cereals are low in lysine but maize has less tryptophan than wheat and rice. In pre-Columban America, the ground maize was steeped in warm lime water (calcium hydroxide), which liberates the niacin (making it biologically available), and then made into tortillas, flat cakes—as it still is today in Mexico and Guatemala.

Pellagra is rare in developed countries. It occurs in parts of Africa.

12.3.6 Biochemical tests

1. Urinary N'-methylnicotinamide (and/or its 2-pyridone) is the best-known test but tests that require a 24-hour urine are inconvenient.

2. Red cell NAD concentration.

3. Fasting plasma tryptophan.

12.3.7 Interactions with nutrients

The most important is that tryptophan and hence dietary proteins (except in maize) provide niacin. Tryptophan makes up about 1% of mixed dietary proteins, so 6 g protein ($\rightarrow$ 60 mg tryptophan) $\equiv$ 1 mg niacin; hence a protein intake of 70 g/day is equivalent to about 12 mg niacin. The niacin requirement is thought to be proportional to the energy expenditure or energy intake.

Two of the enzymes in the kynurenine pathway are vitamin B_6-dependent so that vitamin B_6 deficiency is likely to reduce niacin synthesis from tryptophan.

12.4 Vitamin B_6

12.4.1 Structure

Vitamin B_6 (Fig. 12.6) occurs in nature in three forms: pyridoxine, pyridoxal and pyridoxamine, which are interconvertible within the body. Each form (vitamer) also occurs as a phosphorylated compound: the principal one in the body and in food is pyridoxal 5'-phosphate (PLP).

12.3.8 Food sources

Good sources of pre-formed niacin, in descending order, are liver and kidney (the richest sources), other meat, poultry, fish, brewer's yeast and yeast extracts, peanuts, bran, pulses and wholemeal wheat, and (surprisingly) there is some niacin in coffee, including instant coffee. Other foods that are rich in protein provide tryptophan. If food tables give values for milligram niacin equivalents (NE), this is pre-formed niacin (mg) + (tryptophan ÷ 60). The British food tables (McCance and Widdowson) have separate columns for 'nicotinic acid' and for 'potential nicotinic acid from tryptophan, mg tryptophan ÷ 60'. From this, one can see, for example, that 100 g fresh whole cow's milk provides 0.08 mg pre-formed niacin but 0.80 mg potential niacin from tryptophan.

The recommended dietary intake for niacin in adults, expressed as NE is 6.6 mg NE per 1000 kcal (1.6 mg NE/1000 kJ); in absolute numbers this is about 14 mg in women and 16 mg in men.

12.3.9 Pharmacological doses

Well above the nutrient dose, nicotinic acid (but not the amide) produces cutaneous flushing from histamine release, at doses of 100 mg/day or more; it has been used for chilblains. At doses of 3 g/day or more (200 × the RDI), it inhibits lipolysis in adipose tissue and lowers plasma triglyceride and cholesterol. It is in the pharmacopoeia as a second-line drug for combined hyperlipidaemia (i.e. high plasma cholesterol plus raised triglycerides). Side effects, as well as flushing, include gastric irritation, impaired glucose tolerance and disturbed liver function tests.

12.4.2 Functions

The major coenzyme form in the body is PLP. It functions in practically all the reactions involved in amino acid metabolism, including:

1. Transaminations, and synthesis of non-essential amino acids.

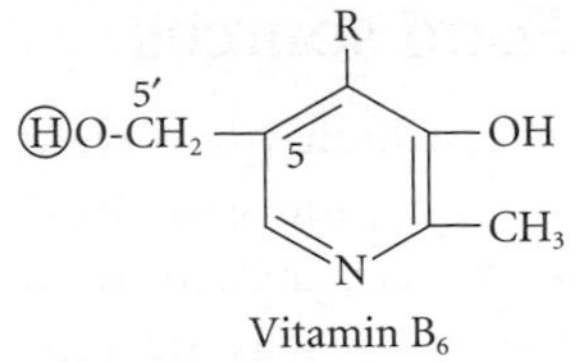

Fig. 12.6 Structure of vitamin B₆.

In pyridoxine, R = CH₂OH; in pyridoxal, R = CHO; in pyridoxamine, R = CH₂NH₂. In coenzyme forms, phosphate replaces the ringed H.

2. Deamination of serine and threonine.

3. Metabolism of sulphur-containing amino acids including homocysteine.

4. Decarboxylations:
    (a) formation of neurotransmitters adrenalin, noradrenalin, serotonin and γ-amino butyric acid (GABA)
    (b) formation of δ-aminolaevulinic acid, which is the first step in porphyrin synthesis, making haemoglobin
    (c) synthesis of sphingomyelin and phosphatidyl choline (lecithin)
    (d) synthesis of taurine, a conjugator of bile acids and important in eye and brain function.

5. Kynureninase: for the conversion of tryptophan to niacin. When this reaction is impaired, xanthurenic acid (major metabolite of 3(OH) kynurenine) accumulates in the urine, which is used as a biochemical marker for B₆ status.

However, the role of vitamin B₆ is not restricted to protein metabolism. Over half of total body B₆ is associated with glycogen phosphorylase enzyme in the muscles, which releases glucose as glucose 1-phosphate from glycogen stores. PLP may also have a role in modulating steroid hormone receptors.

12.4.3 Absorption and metabolism

In the small intestine, vitamin B₆ is absorbed by passive diffusion, mainly in the unphosphorylated form. Even large doses are well absorbed. The different forms of the vitamin are rapidly converted to pyridoxal in the intestinal cell, by the FMN-requiring enzyme, pyridoxal phosphate oxidase. Pyridoxal is transported in the circulation largely bound to albumin and haemoglobin, and after diffusion into cells, pyridoxal is rephosphorylated by pyridoxal kinase, which maintains it within the cells.

The total body content of vitamin B₆ is estimated to be between 50 and 150 mg in adults. Most of this (90%) is tightly bound in tissues. Vitamin B₆ in the liver, brain, kidney, spleen and muscle is bound to protein, which protects it from hydrolysis. The major metabolite of vitamin B₆ is 4-pyridoxic acid, which is inactive as a vitamin and excreted in the urine.

12.4.4 Deficiency in animals: animal studies

Dermatological and neurological changes are commonly observed in animals when vitamin B₆ is deficient. In rats, impaired growth, muscular weakness, irritability, dermatitis, anaemia, fatty liver, impaired immune function, hypertension and insulin insufficiency have all been observed. Neurological changes include convulsions.

12.4.5 Deficiency in humans

The symptoms of deficiency in humans are general weakness, sleeplessness, peripheral neuropathy, personality changes, dermatitis, cheilosis and glossitis (as in riboflavin deficiency), anaemia and impaired immunity. Deficiency on its own is rare; it is most often seen with deficiencies of other vitamins, or with protein deficiency. In 1953, a minor epidemic of convulsions in infants in the USA was traced to a milk formula that contained no vitamin B₆ because of a manufacturing error. Convulsions in pyridoxine deficiency are probably due to impaired synthesis of GABA, the major inhibitory neurotransmitter in the brain.

12.4.6 Secondary deficiency

A number of inborn errors of amino acid metabolism may respond to supranutritional doses of pyridoxine. Hyperhomocysteinaemia, a condition that may increase the risk of cardiovascular disease, responds to supplements of folate, vitamin B_{12} and sometimes B_6.

Low vitamin B_6 status is common in chronic alcoholics, who may have impaired absorption. Acetaldehyde (oxidation product of ethanol) can inhibit the conversion of pyridoxine to PLP.

Pregnant women have a decrease in plasma PLP levels. It is unclear whether this indicates a deficiency or is a normal physiological change.

12.4.7 Biochemical tests

1. Measurement of plasma PLP. Normal levels are above about 30 nmol/L.

2. Increased urinary xanthurenic acid after a load of the amino acid tryptophan.

3. Activity of erythrocyte alanine aminotransferase, with and without *in vitro* PLP.

4. Urinary 4-pyridoxic acid.

12.4.8 Interactions with other nutrients

High protein intakes increase metabolic demand for vitamin B_6.

12.4.9 Interactions with drugs

Isoniazid (used to treat tuberculosis) increases urinary excretion of vitamin B_6. Several drugs including cycloserine, gentamicin, penicillamine, L-dopa and phenelzine are vitamin B_6 antagonists. Some biochemical indices of vitamin B_6 state may be abnormal in a proportion of women taking oral contraceptives, but these are indirect indices (e.g. alanine aminotransferase).

12.4.10 Food sources

The vitamin is distributed in a wide range of unprocessed (or lightly processed) foods. Major food sources in the Western diet are meats, wholegrain products, vegetables, bananas and nuts. Refined cereal products such as white bread and white rice are not significant sources of vitamin B_6 due to milling losses.

The recommended dietary intake is 0.02 mg vitamin B_6 per gram of protein intake, which works out at about 1.5 mg/day in an average adult.

12.4.11 Pharmacological doses

Pharmaceutical preparations, tablets of pyridoxine HCl are indicated for several rare inborn errors of metabolism. They are used for radiation sickness and for premenstrual syndrome. The few controlled trials for the latter condition are unimpressive. Vitamin B_6 can contribute to lowering raised plasma homocysteine (though folic acid usually has more effect). Whether this has value in reducing the risk of cardiovascular disease is not clear at present.

12.4.12 Toxic effects

Vitamin B_6 toxicity was first reported in women taking supplements of very large doses of pyridoxine (2000–6000 mg/day). These supplements were taken for premenstrual syndrome or carpal tunnel syndrome and the women developed peripheral neuropathy and lost sensation in their feet. Intakes of supplements down to 200 mg/day ($133 \times$ RDA) have been associated with neuropathy. The upper intake level (UIL) set by the US Institute of Medicine is 100 mg/day. This can only be obtained from supplements. The amount of vitamin B_6 obtainable from foods is far below this.

12.5 Biotin

12.5.1 Functions

Biotin is a coenzyme for several carboxylase enzymes: pyruvate carboxylase (formation of oxaloacetate for the tricarboxylic acid cycle), acetyl CoA (coenzyme A), carboxylase (fatty acid synthesis), propionyl CoA carboxylase (catabolism of odd-chain fatty acids and some amino acids) and 3-methylcrotonyl CoA carboxylase (catabolism of the ketogenic amino acid leucine).

12.5.2 Deficiency in animals and humans

Biotin deficiency is very rare as biotin is found in a wide range of foods, and bacterial production in the large intestine appears to supplement dietary intake. Deficiency can, however, be produced when animals or humans eat large amounts of uncooked egg white, which contains avidin. This tightly binds biotin in the gut, preventing absorption. Avidin is destroyed by heating. 'Egg white injury' (e.g. biotin deficiency) impairs lipid and energy metabolism in animals. It produces seborrhoeic dermatitis, alopecia and paralysis of the hind limbs in rats and mice.

In humans, cases of biotin deficiency have been associated with a red scaly skin rash (altered fatty acid metabolism may contribute to this skin condition), glossitis, loss of hair, anorexia, depression and hyper-cholesterolaemia. Some cases of seborrhoeic dermatitis in young breast-fed infants have responded to administration of biotin to the mother. Human milk contains much less biotin than cows' milk. Biotin deficiency has been reported in patients on total parenteral nutrition whose infusions did not contain biotin. The human requirement is estimated to be about 30 µg/day. In experimental human biotin deficiency (feeding egg whites), the biochemical indicators have been reduced urinary biotin and increased 3-hydroxyisovaleric acid (which should normally be metabolized by 3-methylcrotonyl CoA carboxylase).

12.6 Pantothenic acid

Coenzymes often contain unusual structures—unusual in the sense that higher animals have lost the ability to form them and they must be supplied in the diet. For CoA, it is pantothenic acid.

12.6.1 Functions

Pantothenic acid is part of CoA and of acyl carrier protein (ACP). CoA and ACP are both carriers of acyl groups. Acetyl-CoA participates in the tricarboxylic acid cycle in the disposal of carbohydrates and ketogenic amino acids. CoA is also involved in the synthesis of lipids: fatty acids, glycerides, cholesterol, ketone bodies, sphingosine and in acylation of proteins. ACP is involved in chain elongation during fatty acid synthesis.

Pantothenic acid is transported primarily in the CoA form by red cells in the blood, and is taken up into cells by a specific carrier protein. The highest concentrations of the vitamin are found in the liver, adrenals, kidney, brain, heart and testes. Most is in the CoA form.

All tissues are able to synthesize CoA from pantothenic acid. ACP is synthesized from a 4- phosphopantetheine residue transferred from CoA. These metabolically active forms can be degraded to free pantothenic acid, which is the major form of excretion in the urine. Urinary pantothenic acid reflects dietary intake, ranging from 2 mg to 7 mg/day in adults.

12.6.2 Deficiency in animals

In most species, pantothenic acid deficiency is associated with dermatitis, changes to hair or feathers, anaemia, infertility, irritability, ataxia, paralysis, convulsions and even death. In rats, a condition called 'bloody whiskers' is caused by release of protoporphyrin via the nose and tear ducts.

12.6.3 Deficiency in humans

Spontaneous human deficiency has never been described. As pantothenic acid is so widely distributed in foods, any dietary deficiency in humans is usually associated with other nutrient deficiencies. The word *pantothen* means 'from everywhere' (Greek), but highly refined foods do not contain pantothenic acid.

Subjects given the antagonist ω-methylpantothenic acid developed a deficiency with symptoms of depression, fatigue, insomnia, vomiting, muscle weakness and a burning sensation in the feet. Changes in glucose tolerance, an increase in insulin sensitivity, postural hypotension and decreased antibody production were also noted.

During World War II, malnourished prisoners of war in the Far East developed 'burning feet syndrome', which appeared to respond to large doses of calcium-pantothenate, but not to other B-complex vitamins.

There is insufficient evidence to derive a requirement figure for pantothenate. The US/Canadian adequate intake (AI) is 5 mg/day, based on estimated usual intakes and urinary pantothenate excretion. It must be provided in total parenteral nutrition.

12.7 Folate

Folate is used as the generic name for compounds chemically related to pteroyl glutamic acid, folic acid. Deficiency of folate is quite common in hospital patients, secondary to diseases, especially intestinal, neoplastic and haematological. Requirements are notably increased in pregnancy. The word *folic* is from the Latin 'folia' (leaf), coined in 1941 for an early preparation of this vitamin from spinach leaves.

12.7.1 Structure (Fig. 12.7)

Folic acid (pteroyl glutamic acid) is the primary vitamin from the chemical point of view, and it is the pharmaceutical form (and used for food fortification) because of its stability. However, it is rare (naturally occurring) in foods and in the body. Most folates are in the reduced form, tetrahydrofolate (THF); they also have 1-carbon components (methyl or formyl) attached to nitrogen atom 5 or 10, or bridging between them (5,10-methylene THF). In addition, they have up to seven glutamic acid residues in a row (at the right in Fig. 12.7).

12.7.2 Functions

Tetrahydrofolate plays an essential role in 1-carbon transfers in the body. It receives 1-carbon radicals from, for example, serine, glycine, histidine and tryptophan, and donates them at two steps in purine synthesis and one important step in pyrimidine synthesis: insertion of the methyl group in deoxyuridylic acid to form thymidylic acid, the characteristic nucleotide of DNA. (The folate derivative involved here is 5,10-methylene THF.)

5-Methyl THF cooperates with vitamin B_{12} in the action of methionine synthase, which adds a methyl group to homocysteine and forms methionine and THF (from which 5,10-methylene THF can be formed). When vitamin B_{12} is deficient, folate is trapped as the 5-methyl compound and 5,10-methylene THF is not

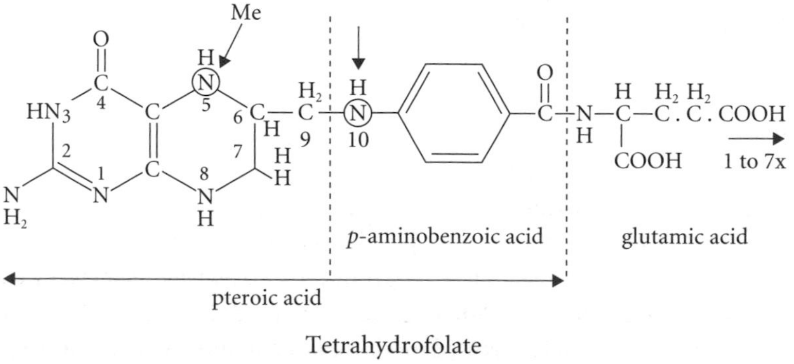

Fig. 12.7 Tetrahydrofolate (pteroyl glutamic acid) monoglutamate. This is folic acid with extra hydrogens at positions 5, 6, 7 and 8.

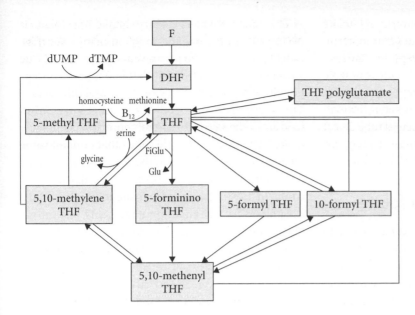

Fig. 12.8 Folate metabolism. Note that 5-methyl THF can only return to the pool for other functions if there is enough vitamin B_{12} for the homocysteine → methionine reaction, which takes up the methyl group. In the reaction of dUMP → dTMP, dTMP is thymidylate, one of the four essential bases of DNA. If there is insufficient 5,10-methylene THF (the specific cofactor), DNA synthesis is reduced or stops. F, folate; DHF, dihydrofolate; THF, tetrahydrofolate.

available to form thymidylate for DNA synthesis (Fig. 12.8).

12.7.3 Absorption and metabolism

It was formerly thought that the polyglutamyl forms ('conjugated' folate) are not as well absorbed as folic acid with only one to three glutamates ('free' folate) but folate with seven glutamates is nearly as well absorbed as pteroyl monoglutamate because there are conjugases in gastric and pancreatic juice and in the small intestinal epithelial cells. These split off the extra glutamates. More than half of folates in foods are in polyglutamyl form; after absorption, most folates in the plasma are in the monoglutamyl form. In the blood, red cells contain 30–50 times more folate than plasma. There is a small store of folate in the liver, mostly in polyglutamate form. Total body folate has been estimated at about 6–10 mg.

12.7.4 Deficiency in animals

Chicks show reduced growth, anaemia and impaired feather growth. In guinea-pigs, there is a low white blood cell count and growth failure.

12.7.5 Deficiency in humans

Folate is the final antimegaloblastic substance. In deficiency, the basic abnormality is reduced ability of cells to double their nuclear DNA, in order to divide, because of impaired synthesis of thymidylate.

There is megaloblastic anaemia (cells are enlarged, their nuclei large but with reduced density of chromatin) and similar changes in leucocytes, platelets and epithelial cells; there is also infertility and may be diarrhoea.

Pure dietary deficiency is seen occasionally. In a previously healthy physician, Victor Herbert, experimental depletion resulted in anaemia after 125 days, with biochemical and histological changes before this. However, when there is increased cell proliferation or interference with folate metabolism, features of deficiency appear earlier. Secondary deficiency is common in late pregnancy and in alcoholics and in haemolytic anaemias, uraemia, intensive hospital therapy and people with malabsorption.

12.7.6 Interactions

Vitamin B_{12} (see below). Vitamin C in foods reduces loss of folate in cooking. Several drugs interfere with folate metabolism, most of them by antagonizing dihydrofolate reductase (which converts 2H folate to 4H folate, i.e. THF): methotrexate, aminopterin, amethopterin (used for chemotherapy for cancer), pyrimethamine (antimalarial) and cotrimoxazole (anti-bacterial). Most of the antiepileptic drugs (carbamazepine, phenytoin, valproate) if taken through early pregnancy increase the risk of neural tube defect in the fetus. Folic acid, at the higher dose of 5 mg/day, should be taken periconceptionally.

12.7.7 Benefits of extra folate

Folate is important at both ends of pregnancy. In late pregnancy, some degree of megaloblastic anaemia is common and women are often given tablets of folic acid plus iron to prevent or treat this. This anaemia can sometimes first be noticed in the early weeks after childbirth.

Folic acid supplements have more recently been found to reduce the risk of a serious fetal malformation, neural tube defect, if taken around the time of conception. The neural tube closes at days 24–28 after conception and the extra folate must be taken before this (i.e. before the woman may be sure she is pregnant). In the Medical Research Council (UK) trial (1991), women who had previously had a baby affected by neural tube defect agreed to take one of four different nutritional supplements periconceptionally. It was found that those taking supplements containing folic acid had 70% fewer deformed babies. Other trials and cohort studies have been supportive. From studies of serum folate of women who were subsequently found to have an abnormal baby, it appears that neural tube defect is not caused by a deficiency but by a need for extra folate in some women at this time of embryonic development.

Observational evidence is accumulating that raised plasma homocysteine is a risk factor for cardiovascular diseases (Chapter 20). Folic acid in larger doses than the 200 μg/day to correct classical deficiency (in the range 0.5–5.0 mg/day) lowers plasma homocysteine. Extra vitamin B_6 and vitamin B_{12} may augment the effect. Plasma folate and dietary folate have been inversely associated with coronary heart disease in prospective cohort studies.

The recommended dietary intake for folate is 200 μg (0.2 g) per day for adults in many countries. In late pregnancy, 400 μg prevents the megaloblastic anaemia and it is estimated that 400 μg periconceptionally will prevent most cases of neural tube defect. This is approximately double the usual intake from food and is the reason for several countries encouraging folate enrichment of staple foods that contain some folate naturally. In the USA, the Institute of Medicine revised the RDA for folate up to 400 μg/day for most adults in 1998. This is more folate than most adults eat, unless they take vitamin supplements, but a growing number of foods are being fortified with folic acid.

As of 1 January 1998, the USA and Canada made it mandatory to fortify all cereal grains (bread, flour, pasta, breakfast cereal and rice) with folic acid at 140 μg per 100 g of grain food. Since then, people's intakes of folate and serum folates have increased considerably, prevalence of folate deficiency is much lower, plasma homocysteines are lower and so is the incidence of neural tube defects in the USA and Canada. There has been no evidence of more people with low vitamin B_{12} concentration without anaemia.

12.7.8 Genetics

A fairly common single nucleotide polymorphism in the gene for 5,10-methylene THF reductase (MTHFR), the 667C → T mutation, affects the activity of this enzyme. Overall around 10% of people are homozygous for the TT allele (with a range in different communities of 1 to 20%). They have reduced activity of MTHFR so that availability of methyl THF, and hence THF, is lower (see Fig. 12.8). They have been found to have lower blood folates (hence higher requirement) and also increased risk of neural tube defects and higher plasma homocysteines, but not more cardiovascular disease.

12.7.9 Biochemical tests

Serum folate reflects recent intake. The normal level is above 7 nmol/L (3 ng/mL). Red cell folate gives a better idea of cellular status. It is normally above 225 nmol/L (100 ng/mL).

12.7.10 Food sources

Although the name comes from the Latin 'folia' (leaf), and it does occur in leafy vegetables (spinach, broccoli, cabbage, lettuce), folate also occurs in other foods: liver, kidney, beans, beetroot, bran, peanuts, yeast extract, avocadoes, bananas, wholemeal bread, eggs and some fish. There is even a little folate in beer and tea. In the USA and Canada, all cereal products have to be fortified with folate. In other countries, voluntary fortification is permitted so that food tables may be out of date in their folate content of foods. Many breakfast cereals and some breads are now fortified with extra folic acid.

Pure folic acid as a supplement is about twice as bioavailable as most food folates. Also, the folic acid added in fortified food is more available than the intrinsic folate in most foods. The US Institute of Medicine has introduced the use of dietary folate equivalents (DFEs) for RDAs/RDIs.

$1\,\mu g$ of DFE $= 1\,\mu g$ of food folate $= 0.5\,\mu g$ of (pure) folic acid taken on an empty stomach $= 0.6\,\mu g$ of folic acid with meals. DFEs were adopted in the 2006 Australia New Zealand Nutrient Reference Values report.

Analysis of folate in foods is difficult because of the multiple compounds. Early analyses used microbiological assay but human cells may not respond to different folate compounds in the same way as bacteria. Some recent methods are based on the major peaks on HPLC. Folate is destroyed in foods by prolonged boiling.

12.7.11 Toxicity

The main concern is that if someone with vitamin B$_{12}$ deficiency (pernicious anaemia) is treated with a fairly high (supranutritional) dose of folic acid (5 mg/day) then the anaemia may improve, but the biochemical basis for the neurological symptoms of vitamin B$_{12}$ deficiency is not corrected, so correct biochemical diagnosis with serum B$_{12}$ *and* folate is essential before anyone is treated for anaemia with folic acid. Otherwise, the toxicity of folic acid is low.

12.8 Vitamin B$_{12}$

In the late 1920s, it was postulated that human gastric juice contained an 'intrinsic factor' that combined with an 'extrinsic factor' in animal protein foods (notably raw liver) and the combination would cure a type of anaemia that was until then untreatable —pernicious anaemia. In 1948, the extrinsic factor, vitamin B$_{12}$, was identified and human intrinsic factor was isolated in the 1960s.

12.8.1 Structure

Vitamin B$_{12}$ or cobalamin is a red compound containing a corrinoid ring (four pyrrole rings) with an atom of cobalt in its centre. It is only synthesized by bacteria. Vitamin B$_{12}$ has the largest molecule of the vitamins, with a molecular weight of 1355. The structure is large and three-dimensional—to view it, refer to a good textbook of biochemistry. Dorothy Hodgkin was awarded the Nobel Prize (for Chemistry in 1964) for elucidating the structure of vitamin B$_{12}$ by X-ray crystallography.

12.8.2 Functions

The coenzyme forms of vitamin B$_{12}$ are methylcobalamin and deoxyadenosylcobalamin. Only two B$_{12}$-dependent enzymes have been identified in humans: methylmalonyl-CoA mutase (which requires deoxyadenosylcobalamin) and methionine synthase (which requires methylcobalamin).

Methylmalonyl-CoA mutase is involved in the conversion of methylmalonyl-CoA to succinyl-CoA in the catabolism of propionate, in the mitochondria.

Methionine synthase, found in the cytosol, transfers a methyl group from the donor 5-methyl THF to homocysteine to produce methionine (see Fig. 12.8). Increased plasma homocysteine, a condition that may increase the risk for vascular disease, responds to supplements of vitamins B_{12}, B_6 and folate.

12.8.3 Absorption and metabolism

Absorption of vitamin B_{12} is by a highly specific mechanism. It first has to be released from its binding to animal proteins in food. This requires pepsin and acid in the stomach. When gastric acid is secreted after a meal, the parietal cells at the same time release the specific glycoprotein, intrinsic factor (IF). This does not attach to vitamin B_{12} until they are both in the duodenum. (While in the stomach, B_{12} is attached to R-binder (haptocorrin) from the saliva, which is removed by digestion in the duodenum.) The B_{12}–IF complex passes down the small intestine, and in the terminal ileum there are specific receptors for IF. The B_{12}–IF complex is absorbed and after 2–3 hours vitamin B_{12} appears in the blood stream carried on transcobalamin II (TCII), the main B_{12} transport protein.

Vitamin B_{12} is concentrated and stored in the liver. It is excreted in the bile into the duodenum where much of it combines with IF (secreted after a meal) and also gets absorbed in the terminal ileum. This enterohepatic cycle helps to conserve the vitamin.

Some anaerobic bacteria in the large intestine can synthesize vitamin B_{12}, but this is formed below the ileal receptor site so is not likely to be absorbed.

The total body store is estimated to range from only 3 to 5 mg but is enough for several years! Only about 0.2% of total body stores (2–5 µg) are excreted daily. The requirement is only 2 µg/day.

12.8.4 Deficiency in animals

The most common signs of deficiency in animals are lack of growth and reduced food intake. Alterations in lipid metabolism occur—fatty liver, increase in triglycerides and free fatty acids. In pigs, a mild anaemia is observed. Neurological changes have been observed in monkeys after 3–5 years on a vitamin B_{12}-deficient diet, and in fruit bats, after 7 months.

12.8.5 Deficiency in humans

Vegans Very strict vegetarian (vegan) diets that have no fish, poultry, eggs or dairy products, and are without vitamin supplements, contain practically no vitamin B_{12}. Vegans have low circulating levels of vitamin B_{12} but clinical symptoms are surprisingly uncommon. Normal body stores of the vitamin are sufficient to last for 2–5 years. Bacteria in the intestine produce some vitamin B_{12}, which might perhaps be absorbed from the caecum, but the bioavailability of such B_{12} is uncertain. However, infants breast-fed by strict vegan mothers are at serious risk of impaired neurological development, anaemia and even severe encephalopathy. Vegans are advised to take vitamin B_{12} tablets or foods fortified with B_{12} (produced micro-biologically, i.e. not from an animal source). However, for breast-fed vegan infants, vitamin B_{12} supplements are essential.

Pernicious anaemia and vitamin B_{12} neuropathy Inadequate dietary intake is not the usual cause of clinical vitamin B_{12} deficiency. Most common is malabsorption due to an autoimmune atrophy of the gastric mucosa so there is failure to produce IF. Other less common causes include total gastrectomy and disease of the terminal ileum. Severe vitamin B_{12} deficiency from gastric atrophy is called 'pernicious anaemia' because it used to be untreatable. There are two effects of vitamin B_{12} deficiency: megaloblastic anaemia and/or neurological dysfunction. Anaemia usually precedes neurological symptoms, but not always. Anaemia is megaloblastic, so called because the blood cells are characteristically large with reduced nuclear density, and white cells, platelets and epithelial cells are also affected the same way. Vitamin B_{12} deficiency interrupts normal nuclear division by 'trapping' folate, leading to a reduction in the synthesis of DNA (see section 12.7). The anaemia is morphologically the same in folate and vitamin B_{12} deficiency. Biochemical tests have to be used to distinguish between them. An injection of 100 µg/month will successfully treat pernicious anaemia but high oral doses (working by passive absorption) are also used.

The characteristic neuropathy of vitamin B$_{12}$ deficiency is subacute combined degeneration of the spinal cord. There is spastic weakness and loss of position sense in the lower limbs due to demyelination of the posterior and lateral (pyramidal) tracts (upper motor neurone). Sometimes the nervous system can be affected in other ways, e.g. with neuropsychiatric disorders. There is not always an accompanying anaemia. Serum vitamin B$_{12}$ is subnormal and symptoms should respond to vitamin B$_{12}$ treatment, though more slowly than the anaemia.

Spinal cord disease is not seen in folate deficiency. The biochemical basis of the pernicious anaemia involves an interaction with folate. The neurological disease does not. The most likely explanation of the neuropathy is impaired methylation of myelin basic protein from deficient methionine synthase.

Subclinical vitamin B$_{12}$ deficiency Pernicious anaemia—being a serious clinical disease—has been known since it was first described by Addison in 1894. However, in recent years, since serum vitamin B$_{12}$ assays have been generally available, it has been found that subnormal levels of serum B$_{12}$ occur in 10% or more of old people without anaemia in developed countries. Serum methylmalonate is raised, and absorption of crystalline vitamin B$_{12}$ is normal. In a proportion of cases, loss of gastric acid and failure to free B$_{12}$ from protein binding in food is the probable cause. Apart from raised homocysteine (a risk factor for cardiovascular disease), no consistent serious effect has been found. The Institute of Medicine recommends for older people that part of the intake of vitamin B$_{12}$ should be in crystalline form, e.g. fortified food or in multivitamins. Other recommended dietary intake committees (e.g. Australia and New Zealand) have not yet followed this advice.

12.8.6 Biochemical tests

Serum vitamin B$_{12}$ can be assessed by a radioligand binding assay or microbiological assay. Normal levels range from 200 to 900 pg/mL (pg = 10^{-12} g) or over 150 pmol/L. Deficiency is indicated by values below this.

Elevated serum or urinary excretion of methylmalonate and raised plasma homocysteine are the other biochemical tests indicating low B$_{12}$ status. Methylmalonate is more specific because homocysteine is also elevated with folate deficiency. The Schilling test is used to confirm the diagnosis of pernicious anaemia. It measures absorption of oral vitamin B$_{12}$ labelled with radioactive cobalt on two occasions, the first without and the second test with IF.

12.8.7 Interactions with nutrients

In vitamin B$_{12}$ deficiency, 5-methyl THF accumulates due to decreased activity of methionine synthase, thus holding folate in what is termed the 'methyl–folate trap'. The ultimate cause of megaloblastic anaemia is impaired conversion of deoxyuridylic acid to thymidylic acid and so DNA synthesis is impaired, because of lack of 5,10-methylene THF.

12.8.8 Food sources

As vitamin B$_{12}$ is synthesized by microorganisms, the vitamin is only found in bacterially fermented foods, or meat and offal from ruminant animals in which the vitamin is synthesized by ruminal microflora. The richest source of the vitamin is liver. Other sources include shellfish, fish, meat, eggs, milk, cheeses and yoghurt.

Not all corrinoids exhibit vitamin B$_{12}$ activity. In spirulina—a type of algae often promoted as a source of B$_{12}$ for vegetarians—80% of the corrinoids do not have vitamin B$_{12}$ activity. Up to 30% of the B$_{12}$ in supplement pills may be analogue(s) of B$_{12}$ with little or no activity.

The recommended dietary intake of vitamin B$_{12}$ is very small; in adults it is 2.5 µg/day.

12.8.9 Toxic effects

Oral intakes of several hundred times the nutritional requirement are safe, as intestinal absorption is specific and limited. Vitamin B$_{12}$ injections (a nice red colour) are used in medicine as a placebo.

FURTHER READING

Thiamin

1. **Carpenter, K.J.** (2000) *Beri beri, white rice, and vitamin B.* Berkeley, CA, University of California Press.

2. **Victor, M., Adams, R.D., and Collins, G.H.** (1989) *The Wernicke–Korsakoff syndrome and related neurologic disorders due to alcoholism and malnutrition*, 2nd edition. Philadelphia, PA: FA Davis.

Niacin

1. **Roe, D.A.** (1973) *A plague of corn. The social history of pellagra.* Ithaca and London, Cornell University Press.

Vitamin B$_6$

2. **Schaumberg, H., Kaplan, J., Windebank, A., *et al*.** (1983) Sensory neuropathy from pyridoxine abuse. *N Engl J Med*, **309**, 445–8.

Folate

1. **Bailey, L.B.** (1998) Dietary reference intakes for folate: the debut of dietary folate equivalents. *Nutr Rev*, **56**, 294–9.

2. **Department of Health** (2000) *Folic acid and the prevention of disease*. Report of the Committee on Medical Aspects of Food and Nutrition Policy. London, The Stationery Office.

3. **Ray, J.G.** (2004) Folic acid food fortification in Canada. *Nutr Rev*, **62**, 535–9.

Vitamin B$_{12}$

1. **Bates, C.J., Schneeds, J., Mishra, G., Prentice, A., and Mansoor, M.A.** (2003) Relationship between methylmalonic acid, homocysteine, vitamin B$_{12}$ intake and status and social-economic indices, in a subset of participants in the British National Diet and Nutrition Survey of people aged 65 years and over. *Eur J Clin Nutr*, **57**, 349–59.

2. **Von Shenck, U., Bender-Gotze, C., and Koletzo, B.** (1997) Persistence of neurological damage induced by dietary vitamin B$_{12}$ deficiency in infancy. *Arch Dis Childhood*, **77**, 137–9.

 To see topical and scientifically robust updates on nutrition associated with this textbook, and active web links to many of the journal articles in the Reference areas, please see the dedicated Online Resource Centre at www.oxfordtextbooks.co.uk/orc/mann3e/.

13 Vitamins C and E

Murray Skeaff

13.1 Vitamin C

13.1.1 History

> . . . For some lost all their strength, their legs became swollen, and inflamed, while the sinews contracted and turned as black as coal. In other cases the legs were found blotched with purple-coloured blood. Then the disease would mount to the hips, thighs, shoulders, arms, and neck. And all had their mouths so tainted, that the gums rotted away down to the roots of the teeth, which nearly all fell out. The disease spread among the three ships to such an extent, that in the middle of February, of the 110 men forming our company, there were not 10 in good health so that no one could aid the other, which was a grievous sight considering the place where we were.

The above passage describes the condition of Jacques Cartier's expedition in Quebec during the winter of 1535–6. It is one of the earliest descriptions of the vitamin C deficiency disease, scurvy, and the first report of a cure. On the advice of the local Indians, Cartier's party made a brew from the bark and leaves of a local tree—probably the white cedar (*Thuja occidentalis*):

> As soon as they had drunk it they felt better which must clearly be ascribed to miraculous causes; for after drinking it two or three times, they recovered health and strength and were cured of all the diseases they had ever had.

In modern times, the needles of the white cedar, like other leaves, have been shown to contain vitamin C. Despite this remarkable cure and Cartier's written record of it, the primitive nature of communication in early medicine meant that French and English voyagers to the same region would suffer the ravages of scurvy for at least another century.

Two centuries later, James Lind, a surgeon in the Royal Navy, after making several voyages during which serious outbreaks of scurvy occurred, undertook to discover the definitive cure for the disease in 1747. In what is now recognized as one of the first controlled dietary trials, Lind not only established 'that oranges and lemons were the most effectual remedies for this distemper at sea' but also (and of equal importance) he proved that other curative potions of the time were, with the exception of apple cider, without effect. It was another half century before the British Navy took heed of Lind's research and instituted lemon juice rations for all crews.

The discovery of vitamin C moved a step closer in 1907 when Hoist and Frölich, in Oslo, were able to produce scurvy in guinea-pigs. Until that time, experimental scurvy had not been produced in laboratory animals because most of them (e.g. rats, mice, rabbits) are not susceptible to the disease. This breakthrough opened the way for bioassays to be developed to test the relative potencies of antiscorbutic foods and extracts. Unrelated to the search for the antiscorbutic factor—now named vitamin C—Szent-Györgyi in 1928 isolated a crystalline substance he called 'hexuronic acid' from orange juice, cabbage juice and adrenal glands. Four years later, Szent-Györgyi shared some of these crystals with Svirbely, working in Hungary, who quickly showed it to cure scurvy in guinea-pigs; vitamin C had been discovered.

13.1.2 Terminology and biosynthesis

Vitamin C, formal chemical name L-ascorbic acid, is an odourless, stable, white solid, soluble in water, slightly soluble in ethanol, and insoluble in organic solvents. Ascorbic acid can be synthesized from glucose or galactose in a wide variety of plants and in most animal species (Fig. 13.1). The exceptions to this rule are humans and other primates, guinea-pigs, fruit-eating bats and many fish because they lack the final enzyme, L-gulonolactone oxidase, required to convert L-gulonolactone to L-ascorbic acid. Ascorbic acid is readily oxidized in the body to dehydroascorbic acid, which in turn can be reduced back to ascorbic acid. This ability to participate in oxidation-reduction reactions is the basis for most of the known functions of the vitamin.

13.1.3 Functions

Table 13.1 outlines some of the functions of vitamin C, which are discussed in detail below.

1. The best-defined function of vitamin C is its role in the synthesis of collagen, the principal connective tissue protein found in tendons, arteries, bone, skin and muscle. The protein is first synthesized with an abundance of proline and lysine residues, many of which are then converted by prolyl hydroxylase and lysyl hydroxylase to hydroxy proline and hydroxylysine, respectively. These hydroxy-amino acids provide the anchor for crosslinking of collagen molecules,

Table 13.1 Metabolic pathways requiring vitamin C

- Hydroxylation of proline and lysine for collagen synthesis
- Synthesis of noradrenaline from dopamine
- Synthesis of carnitine from lysine
- Activation of neuropeptides
- Catabolism of tyrosine
- General antioxidant function

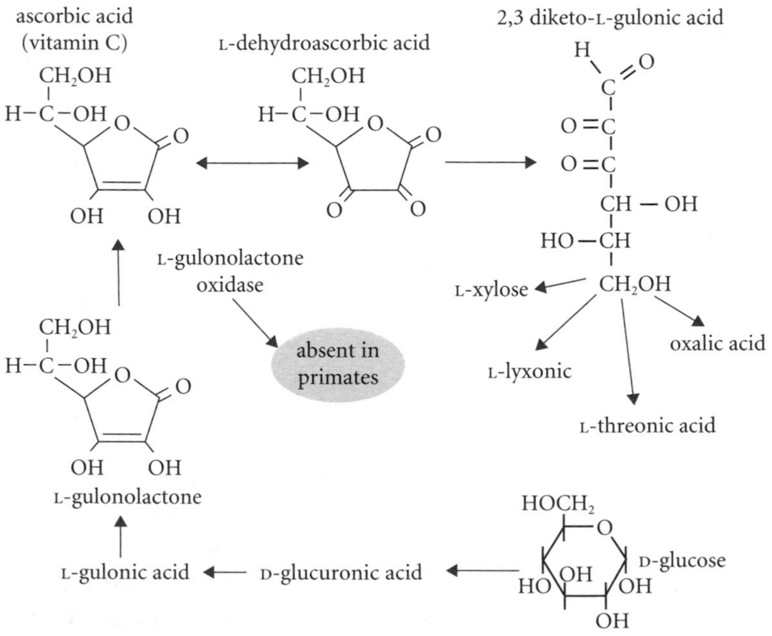

Fig. 13.1 Synthesis and metabolism of vitamin C.

which increases the strength and elasticity of connective tissue. The enzymes prolyl and lysyl hydroxylase require, along with amino acid substrates, vitamin C, ferrous ions (Fe^{2+}), molecular oxygen (O_2) and α-ketoglutarate to accomplish the hydroxylation reactions. Vitamin C does not participate directly in the hydroxylation reaction; rather, it is required to convert iron on the enzyme from the ferric state (Fe^{3+}) back to the ferrous state (Fe^{2+}). Reduced activity of these two hydroxylase enzymes during chronic deficiency of vitamin C leads to the connective tissue defects seen in scurvy. In scurvy, new connective tissue cannot be formed in sufficient amounts to replace ageing or injured connective tissue. Even minor injuries that might normally go unnoticed lead to tissue disruption and extensive bleeding.

2. A second hydroxylation reaction that requires vitamin C is the conversion of dopamine to norepinephrine (noradrenaline) by dopamine β-mono-oxygenase. Norepinephrine is an important neurotransmitter produced in neural tissues.

3. Vitamin C is required for conversion of lysine to carnitine (it participates at two steps). Carnitine plays an essential role in the transfer of long-chain fatty acids into the inner mitochondria where they can be converted to energy by way of β-oxidation. In tissues where fat is a significant source of energy, such as in heart and skeletal muscle, low levels of carnitine can impair muscle function. This may explain the fatigue and muscle weakness associated with severe chronic vitamin C deficiency.

4. Activation of various peptide hormones and hormone-releasing factors occurs through α-amidation of the hormone by the enzyme peptidylglycine α-amidating mono-oxygenase. This enzyme requires vitamin C and is involved in the synthesis of calcitonin, melanocyte-stimulating hormone and releasing factors for corticotropin, thyrotropin and growth hormone.

5. Vitamin C is required for one of the enzymes (4-hydroxyphenylpyruvate hydroxylase) involved in the catabolism of tyrosine to carbon and water.

6. Vitamin C deficiency in animals leads to a reduction in the activity of liver enzymes (i.e. mixed function oxidases) involved in the metabolism of hormones, cholesterol, drugs and carcinogens.

7. The rate-limiting step of bile acid synthesis in the liver involves the conversion of cholesterol to 7α-hydroxycholesterol by the enzyme 7α-hydroxylase. The activity of this pathway is reduced in vitamin C-deficient animals and is associated with elevated plasma cholesterol concentrations.

8. Considerable attention has recently been focused on the antioxidant function of vitamin C. The water-soluble nature of vitamin C permits it to act as an efficient antioxidant against a wide range of intra- and extracellular free radicals. Its role in the regeneration of vitamin E is discussed in section 13.2.4.

13.1.4 Food sources

Fruits and vegetables are the major sources of vitamin C in the diet, contributing together up to 90% of the vitamin intake in countries like New Zealand and the UK (Table 13.2). Fruit juices and drinks fortified with vitamin C are the most significant source in some groups, such as adolescents.

13.1.5 Digestion, absorption, transport and excretion

Vitamin C is readily absorbed in the small intestine by an energy-dependent mechanism, with 70–90% of average daily vitamin C intake (30–200 mg) being absorbed. The absorption decreases to 20% when a single 5 g dose of the vitamin is ingested and to 16% with a 12 g dose. The bioavailability of vitamin C from foods is similar to that from supplements.

In plasma, vitamin C is transported unbound to protein (i.e. free). Virtually all the extracellular vitamin is present as ascorbic acid (> 99.5%) with only trace (< 0.5%) amounts as dehydroascorbic acid. An energy-driven uptake mechanism serves to maintain a high concentration of vitamin C in intracellular, as compared with extracellular, fluid. The highest concentration of vitamin C in the body is found in pituitary and adrenal glands, eye lens, leukocytes, lymph glands, brain and other internal organs. The lowest levels are found in plasma and saliva.

Studies using isotopically labelled ascorbic acid have shown that the amount of vitamin C in the body

Table 13.2 Vitamin C content of common foods

Food	Vitamin C (mg/100 g)
Blackcurrants	200
Kiwifruit	122
Cauliflower	60
Broccoli	58
Potato crisps	51
Honeydew melon	50
Oranges	50
Strawberries	46
Grapefruit	40
Spinach	34
Pineapple	25
Tomatoes	24
Beef liver	22
Cabbage	21
Beef kidney	13
Potatoes	10
Peaches	10
Apples	9
Pears	3
Chicken liver	3
Milk	1
Wholemeal bread	0

Vitamin C is not stored for long in the body. When a vitamin C-free diet is consumed, approximately 3% of the total body pool is lost per day, although this proportion decreases considerably with duration of the diet. In the range of usual intake, almost half of the urinary metabolites of vitamin C appear as oxalic acid, while ascorbic acid, dehydroascorbic acid, 2,3-diketogulonate and ascorbate 2-sulphate make up the remainder. When vitamin C intake greatly exceeds physiological requirement, there is some increase in oxalate excretion but most of the vitamin is excreted as unmetabolized vitamin C. Despite the theoretical possibility of increased risk of calcium oxalate stones in the urinary tract of people who take vitamin C supplements, this has not found in practice.

13.1.6 Factors affecting metabolism

Cigarette smokers have lower concentrations of ascorbic acid in plasma and leukocytes. These lower levels are partly, but not entirely, the result of reduced consumption of vitamin C. Isotopic studies have shown that the metabolic turnover of vitamin C in smokers is twice that in non-smokers. Consequently, smokers require significantly more dietary vitamin C to maintain a body pool of vitamin C equivalent to that of non-smokers. Acute and chronic infections can reduce levels of vitamin C in plasma and leukocytes. However, in chronic disease, the poor vitamin C status is often due to poor diet. There is some evidence that excretion of vitamin C increases under acute infections and stressful conditions.

13.1.7 Deficiency

Scurvy is uncommon in populations unless there is a prolonged shortage of fruits and vegetables together with an overall reduced food supply, as in the Irish potato famine of the nineteenth century. More recent evidence of outbreaks comes from refugee camps in the Horn of Africa. During the famines of 1985–87, the incidence of scurvy in six refugee camps in Somalia and Sudan ranged from 14% to 44% of the camp

(i.e. body pool) plateaus at roughly 20 mg/kg body weight or 1500 mg for an average person. This body pool can be maintained with a daily vitamin C intake of 60–100 mg by all but a few in the population. Normal plasma vitamin C concentrations range from 23–87 µmol/L (4–15 mg/L) and it is difficult to raise the upper level, even when consuming very large doses. Beyond a daily intake of 200 mg, virtually all the excess vitamin C will be excreted in the urine within 24 hours.

populations. Those who participated in supplementary food programmes did not have a reduced incidence of scurvy. The supplementary foods, cereals, legumes and oil, were almost completely deficient in vitamin C. Accordingly, the World Health Organization (WHO) now advises that in this area of Africa vitamin C supplements be added to relief food at an early stage of a crisis.

In societies where food supply is plentiful and diverse, scurvy usually occurs only in those consuming extremely poor diets that have a complete lack of fruits and vegetables, for example, in young or elderly men living alone, alcoholics or illicit drug users. Scurvy can affect infants whose only source of food is cow's milk. There is no known genetic disorder of vitamin C metabolism.

There are several detailed reports of dedicated scientists, prisoners and paid volunteers in whom scurvy has been produced after adherence to a diet devoid of vitamin C. Symptoms such as weakness, fatigue, inflamed and bleeding gums, impaired wound healing, other skin haemorrhages and depression have been observed after 3–6 months on the scorbutic diets. The symptoms usually occur when the plasma concentration of vitamin C falls below 11 µmol/L (2 mg/L) or when the total body pool of the vitamin is less than 300 mg. Full recovery from the clinical manifestations of scurvy requires as little as 10 mg of vitamin C per day.

13.1.8 Nutrient interactions

Vitamin C enhances the absorption of non-haem iron when vitamin C and foods containing non-haem iron are consumed in the same meal (see section 9.4). Vitamin C achieves this effect in the small intestine by helping to convert dietary iron from the ferric state (Fe^{3+}) to the ferrous state (Fe^{2+}), and by binding to ferric iron (Fe^{3+}) to form soluble complexes. A high enhancing effect can be attained with a vitamin C intake of roughly 100 mg per meal. When body iron stores are low, the enhancing effect of vitamin C on non-haem iron absorption is markedly higher than when iron stores are high. Accordingly, it is common to recommend to vegetarians, many of whom have

lower than average iron stores, that foods containing vitamin C be consumed with meals.

In the stomach, vitamin C can inhibit the conversion of nitrates, commonly found in cured and pickled foods, to carcinogenic compounds known as nitrosamines. The incidence of nitrosamine-induced stomach cancer in animals can be reduced by vitamin C. In humans, an epidemiological association has been noted between low intakes of vitamin C, mainly from fruits and vegetables, and high rates of stomach cancer.

13.1.9 Higher-dose effects

One of the most commonly ascribed benefits of ingesting large doses of vitamin C (1–10 g/day), in the form of supplements, relates to prevention of the common cold. The most consistent finding from a review of controlled therapeutic supplementation trials is that vitamin C does not reduce the incidence of the common cold; however, some trials have demonstrated a slight decrease in the duration and severity of symptoms.

13.1.10 Toxicity

Toxicity of vitamin C is low, given the widespread chronic and acute use of supplements and the lack of reported harmful effects. There is some concern that vitamin C can increase oxidant stress in those susceptible to iron overload (e.g. with haemochromatosis) by reducing ferritin-bound iron from ferric iron (Fe^{3+}) to ferrous iron (Fe^{2+}), thereby promoting its release into the circulation. Discontinuation of high doses of vitamin C does cause a temporary drop in leukocyte ascorbic acid concentrations, below normal dose levels, but there is no evidence in humans that this is harmful or that 'rebound scurvy' occurs.

13.1.11 Biochemical assessment

Measurement of vitamin C in serum and leukocytes is the most common means of assessing vitamin C status (Table 13.3). Both correlate well with dietary intake in populations; in studies where participants

Table 13.3 Assessment of vitamin C status*

Test	Normal	Marginal	Deficient
Biochemical test			
Serum (μmol/l)	> 17	11–17	< 11
Leukocytes (nmol/10^8 cells)	> 85	45–85	< 45
Urine (24 h)			
Saliva			
Body pool size			< 300 mg
Functional test			
Capillary fragility test			

*Cut-off values and ranges have only been clearly established for some tests.

follow depletion and repletion diets, serum and leukocyte vitamin C are equally sensitive to changes in dietary vitamin C intake. For practical purposes, measurement of vitamin C in serum is preferred over leukocyte measurement.

Urinary excretion of vitamin C falls to undetectable levels during extended deficiency but is otherwise of limited use as a measure of vitamin status because it tends to reflect recent dietary intake. Measurement of urinary vitamin C in patients suspected of scurvy can provide supportive diagnostic information.

There are no reliable functional tests of vitamin C.

13.1.12 Recommended nutrient intakes

Recommended nutrient intakes vary considerably between countries and depend on the relative importance given to the various criteria for physiological requirement. At one extreme is the amount to prevent scurvy in adults (approximately 10 mg/day) while the other is the amount of vitamin C above which practically all ingested is excreted (approximately 200 mg/day). Most advisory bodies have chosen a level of intake sufficient to maintain a body pool of vitamin C that will provide a reasonable buffer against the onset of scorbutic symptoms when faced with a vitamin C-deficient diet.

The recommended nutrient intake for healthy adults is 40 mg/day in the UK, 45 mg in Australasia and 90 (M) and 75 (F) mg/day in the USA. With orange juice, potatoes and the wide availability of green vegetables and fruit, most people in affluent countries consume a good deal more than this.

13.2 Vitamin E

13.2.1 History

While investigating the relationship between fertility and nutrition, Evans and Bishop discovered in 1922 that female rats fed a diet containing rancid fat and deficient in a lipid-soluble factor were unable to support full-term development of a fetus. The death and ensuing resorption of the fetus could be prevented by adding small amounts of fresh lettuce, wheat germ or dried alfalfa leaves to the mother's diet. Over the next 10 years, vitamin E-deficient diets were found to produce sterility in male rats and chickens, nutritional muscular dystrophy in rabbits and guinea-pigs, and encephalomalacia (crazy chick disease) in chickens. The unidentified lipid-soluble factor that prevented fetal resorption in rats was named 'vitamin E' and subsequently also became known as tocopherol (from the Greek *tokos* for childbirth, *phereiu* meaning to bring forth and *ol* to represent the alcohol in its structure). The vitamin was isolated by Evans in 1936 and the chemical structure identified and synthesized in 1938. The necessity of the vitamin for humans was not clearly established until the 1960s.

13.2.2 Structure and terminology

Vitamin E is unique amongst vitamins because there are eight naturally occurring forms of it found in plants (Fig. 13.2): four tocopherols (alpha, α-; beta, β-; gamma, γ-; and delta, δ-) and four tocotrienols

Tocopherol

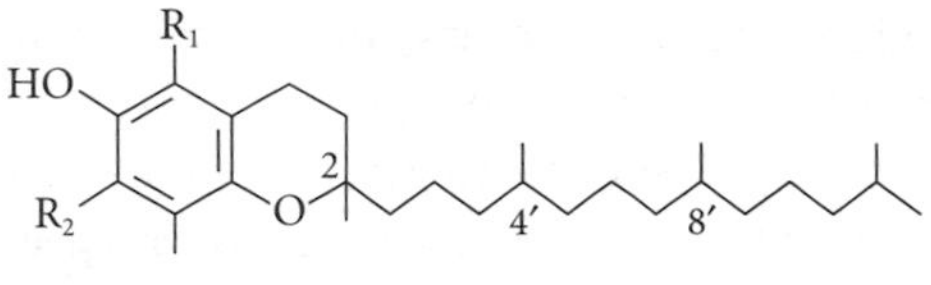

	R$_1$	R$_2$	
	CH$_3$	CH$_3$	α-tocopherol
	CH$_3$	H	β-tocopherol
	H	CH$_3$	γ-tocopherol
	H	H	δ-tocopherol

Tocotrienol

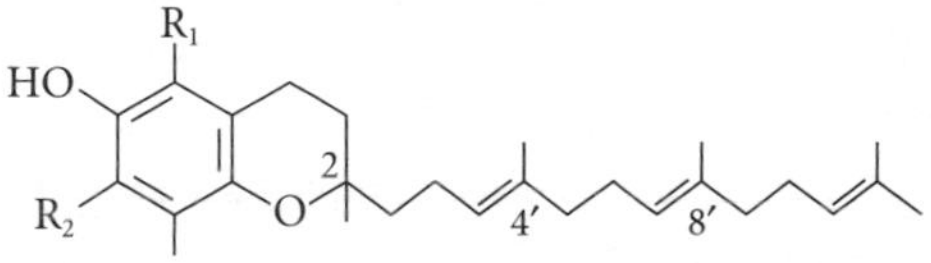

	R$_1$	R$_2$	
	CH$_3$	CH$_3$	α-tocotrienol
	CH$_3$	H	β-tocotrienol
	H	CH$_3$	γ-tocotrienol
	H	H	δ-tocotrienol

Fig. 13.2 Structure of tocopherols and tocotrienols.

(α-, β-, γ- and δ-). The structure common to all forms of vitamin E consists of a chromanol ring to which a hydrophobic 16-carbon isoprenoid tail is attached. The α-, β-, γ- and δ- forms of tocopherol differ in the position and number of methyl groups on the chromanol ring. The only structural difference between the four types of tocotrienols and their respective tocopherols is the presence of three double bonds in the isoprenoid or phytyl tail.

There are three asymmetric centres on the tocopherol or tocotrienol molecule that give rise to stereoisomers; namely, C2 on the chromanol ring, and C4′ and C8′ on the tail. There are, therefore, eight theoretical stereoisomers for each of the eight vitamin E compounds. The naturally occurring and most potent form of vitamin E is 2R, 4′R, 8′R-α-tocopherol (formerly termed *d*-α-tocopherol). Chemical synthesis of α-tocopherol results in the production of a mixture of equal amounts of eight stereoisomers known as all-*rac*-α-tocopherol (formerly termed *dl*-α-tocopherol).

13.2.3 Bioavailability

The abundance and biological activity of each form of naturally occurring vitamin E varies considerably (Table 13.4). The biological activities of the tocopherols and tocotrienols are usually determined by comparing the relative potencies of each form of the vitamin in animal model bioassays (e.g. prevention of rat fetal resorption). Using this method, the synthetic all-*rac*-α-tocopheryl acetate (tocopherol with an acetate molecule attached to the hydroxyl group) has an activity of 1.00 international units (IU) per mg, while the naturally occurring RRR-α-tocopherol has the highest activity of 1.49 IU/mg; of the tocotrienols only the alpha form shows any significant biological activity (0.45 IU/mg). Although there is a significant

Table 13.4 Biological activity of vitamin E

Form of vitamin E	Biological activity (IU/mg)	α-Tocopherol equivalents (α-TE/mg)
RRR-α-tocopherol	1.49	1.00
RRR-α-tocopheryl acetate	1.36	0.91
All-*rac*-α-tocopherol	1.10	0.74
All-*rac*-α-tocopheryl acetate	1.00	0.67
All-*rac*-β-tocopheryl acetate	0.45−0.60	0.30−0.40
All-*rac*-γ-tocopheryl acetate	0.11	0.10
All-*rac*-δ-tocopheryl acetate	0.015	0.01
RRR-α-tocotrienol	0.45	0.30

amount of γ-tocopherol in the diet, it makes only a minor contribution to overall vitamin E activity because of its low biological activity (0.11 IU/mg). Vitamin E content of the diet is often expressed as α-tocopherol equivalents (α-TE) where 1 α-TE is the activity of 1 mg of RRR-α-tocopherol.

13.2.4 Functions

Vitamin E is a powerful antioxidant that plays an essential role in protecting cell membranes and plasma lipoproteins from free-radical damage. Free radicals contain an unpaired electron and react readily with polyunsaturated fatty acids, proteins, carbohydrates and DNA. Vitamin E is able to 'neutralize' free radicals because the hydroxyl group on the chromanol ring readily gives up an electron or hydride group to the free radical. Through this oxidative reaction, the unpaired electron in the free radical becomes paired (less reactive); however, the hydroxyl group on the vitamin E now has an unpaired electron. This resultant vitamin E radical (Vit E•) can react with another free radical and be permanently inactivated to the stable vitamin E quinone (VIT E=O) or it can be regenerated to active vitamin E (Vit E—OH) by reacting with vitamin C or glutathione.

Fatty acids with two or more double bonds (i.e. polyunsaturated) are abundant in all cell membranes and have an important influence on membrane fluidity and function. However, their double bonds make them susceptible to oxidation by free radicals (Fig. 13.3). Fortunately, most vitamin E in the body is found in cell membranes where it functions to protect polyunsaturated fatty acids from free-radical attack. In the event that a fatty acid radical is produced, vitamin E stabilizes the free radical and prevents it from reacting with adjacent polyunsaturated fatty acids and propagating the reaction along the membrane with disastrous consequences.

There is an elaborate interrelationship between vitamin E and other antioxidant nutrient systems in the body. The most direct interaction is with vitamin C, which serves to regenerate vitamin E from its radical state. Glutathione can also regenerate vitamin E, thus explaining the interaction with sulphur amino acids. Antioxidant systems such as superoxide dis-

mutase, catalase, glutathione peroxidase and vitamin C help to eliminate free radicals, thereby reducing oxidant stress on membranes and preserving vitamin E. However, if membrane vitamin E is deficient, high levels of other antioxidants cannot prevent the peroxidation of membrane polyunsaturated fatty acids, although they may delay the damage.

Plasma lipoproteins, like cell membranes, contain an abundance of lipid including proportions of polyunsaturated fatty acids. They also contain fat-soluble vitamin E, which plays an essential role in protecting the lipoproteins from oxidative damage. This is particularly important in low-density lipoproteins (LDLs) because lipid peroxides can oxidize apolipoprotein B resulting in the formation of oxidatively modified LDL. This oxidized LDL accumulates in the walls of arteries at a greater rate than normal LDL (i.e. non-oxidized), thus accelerating the development of atherosclerotic plaques. (The role of oxidized LDL in the aetiology of cardiovascular disease is discussed in Chapter 20.)

13.2.5 Digestion, absorption, transport, and distribution

Vitamin E is absorbed in a manner similar to most other dietary lipids and requires fat digestion to be functioning normally. The presence of fat in the small intestine enhances vitamin E absorption because the products of triglyceride breakdown in the gut promote the formation of mixed micelles, the vehicle from which vitamin E is absorbed into the mucosal cells lining the small intestine. Absorption is normally quite efficient, from 50% to 70% of usual vitamin E intake, but it decreases substantially at high doses. Lack of bile acids or fat digestive enzymes, damage to the gastrointestinal lining, or an inability to synthesize chylomicrons will decrease vitamin E absorption. Diseases in which vitamin E absorption is reduced include: pancreatic diseases (e.g. cystic fibrosis), biliary obstruction, coeliac disease and a rare genetic inability to make chylomicrons (abetalipoproteinaemia).

Vitamin E is incorporated into chylomicrons and enters the circulation via the lymphatic system

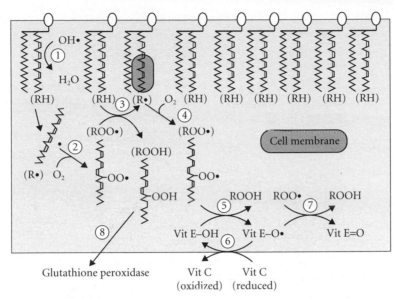

Fig. 13.3 Antioxidant function of vitamin E. (1) A free radical (e.g. hydroxyl free radical) abstracts hydrogen from a membrane polyunsaturated fatty acid (RH), converting it into a fatty acid free radical (R•). (2) A shift in the position of the double bond adjacent to the free radical followed by the uptake of oxygen results in the formation of a peroxy-fatty acid radical (ROO•). (3) The peroxy-fatty acid can be stabilized to a hydroperoxy-fatty acid (ROOH) by abstracting a hydrogen from another membrane polyunsaturated fatty acid (RH). The consequence of this is the propagation of the initial free radical damage along the membrane. (4) Isomerization and oxygen uptake occurs. (5) Vitamin E arrests the propagation of the free radical damage by converting the peroxy-fatty acid free radical (ROO•) to a hydroperoxy-fatty acid (ROOH). (6) The resulting vitamin E radical (Vit E•) can be regenerated to vitamin E (Vit E—OH) by oxidation of vitamin C. (7) Alternatively, the vitamin E radical can stabilize another peroxy-fatty acid radical to form the quinone form of vitamin E (Vit E=O). This form of vitamin E cannot be regenerated. (8) Hydroperoxy-fatty acids can be eliminated by glutathione peroxidase.

(Fig. 13.4). The profile of vitamin E forms incorporated into chylomicrons reflects that of the diet because there is little discrimination between the different forms of tocopherols and tocotrienols in gut absorption or in incorporation into chylomicrons. During catabolism of chylomicrons to chylomicron remnants by lipoprotein lipase, some vitamin E is transferred to muscle and adipose tissue. There is considerable exchange of vitamin E between chylomicrons and high-density lipoproteins (HDLs). Vitamin E acquired by HDL can be subsequently transferred to very-low-density lipoproteins (VLDLs) and LDL.

Vitamin E is distributed throughout the body mainly associated with cell membranes, plasma lipoproteins and adipose (i.e. triglyceride) deposits. Higher concentrations of the vitamin tend to be found in organs with a high fatty acid content (e.g. liver, brain and adipose tissue). The amount of vitamin E in the body reflects dietary intake, with excess to requirements deposited in adipose tissue. Adipose tissue vitamin E is not a freely available reserve against deficient intake since only small amounts of the vitamin are mobilized when plasma vitamin E is low. Movement of the excess vitamin E from adipose tissue to plasma can occur, but is the consequence of the breakdown of adipose triglycerides, as would occur during energy restriction, rather than a response to low plasma levels of the vitamin.

13.2.6 Metabolism and excretion

Vitamin E delivered to the liver by chylomicron remnants is incorporated into VLDL. However,

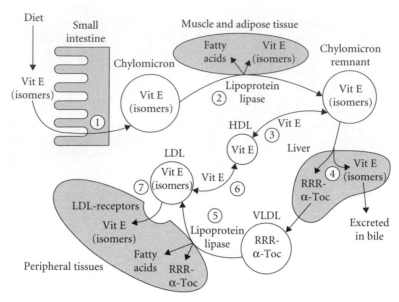

Fig. 13.4 Digestion, absorption, transport and distribution of vitamin E. (1) Vitamin E isomers of dietary origin are absorbed into the mucosal cell where they are incorporated into chylomicrons, which enter the circulation by way of the lymphatic vessels. (2) Vitamin E is transferred from chylomicrons to tissues during the catabolism of triacylglycerols by lipoprotein lipase. (3) Exchange of vitamin E isomers between chylomicron remnants and high-density lipoproteins (HDLs) can occur. (Individuals with familial isolated vitamin E (FIVE) deficiency must rely on this exchange mechanism for dietary α-tocopheral to be distributed to other lipoproteins.) (4) The remaining vitamin E isomers of dietary origin are removed from the circulation when chylomicron remnants are taken up by the liver. α-Tocopherol (Toc) transfer protein preferentially incorporates RRR-α-tocopherol into very-low-density lipoproteins (VLDLs), which are secreted from the liver. (5) Metabolism of triacylglycerol in VLDL by lipoprotein lipase leads to the transfer of α tocopherol to peripheral tissues. (6) Exchange of vitamin E isomers between HDL and low-density lipoprotein (LDL) occurs. (7) Vitamin E is also delivered to the peripheral tissues by way of the receptor-mediated uptake of LDL.

not all forms of vitamin E (α-, β-, γ- and δ-) are incorporated equally into VLDL. In the liver, α-tocopherol transfer protein preferentially incorporates RRR-α-tocopherol into VLDL as compared with RRR-γ-tocopherol or the other stereoisomers of α-tocopherol (see Fig. 13.4). Consequently, VLDL secreted from the liver is rich in RRR-α-tocopherol while most of the γ-tocopherol and stereoisomers of α-tocopherol are excreted in the bile. This shunting of RRR-α-tocopherol to VLDL helps to explain the fact that RRR-α-tocopherol is the predominant form of vitamin E delivered to the tissues, hence its higher biological activity (i.e. bioavailability).

Metabolism of VLDL to LDL results in the transfer of vitamin E to tissues and HDL in a manner analogous to chylomicron metabolism. Delivery of vitamin E in LDL to the tissues is accomplished by receptor-mediated uptake of the whole LDL particle.

On the basis of the preferential incorporation of α-tocopherol into VLDL, the Institute of Medicine in the USA, when setting the recommended nutrient intake for vitamin E, decided—somewhat controversially—that only dietary α-tocopherol could be considered to meet vitamin E requirements, despite evidence that other forms of vitamin E in the body, such as γ-tocopherol, are affected by dietary intake and have biological effects.

13.2.7 Deficiency

Symptomatic vitamin E deficiency disease has not been produced experimentally in humans; however, a genetically inherited disease called familial isolated vitamin E (FIVE) deficiency provides proof of the essentiality of vitamin E for humans. Individuals with this disease have normal lipid absorption and gastrointestinal function as well as normal incorporation of vitamin E into chylomicrons and subsequent delivery to the liver. Nevertheless, they have low or undetectable levels of plasma vitamin E. They develop reduced tendon reflexes by 3–4 years of age and more disabling cerebrospinal symptoms such as unsteadiness of gait, loss of touch and pain sense, limb ataxia (lack of coordination), ptosis, dysarthria and impaired eye movements by early adolescence. The genetic defect involves a mutation in the gene for the α-tocopherol transfer protein, thus blocking the liver's ability to incorporate α-tocopherol into VLDL. The clinical symptoms can be prevented by 1000 mg/day of oral all-*rac*-α-tocopherol. The therapy increases chylomicron vitamin E sufficiently to force enough vitamin E to be redistributed by direct transfer to other circulating lipoproteins from where it can be delivered to the tissues.

In diseases such as cholestatic liver disease, cystic fibrosis and abetalipoproteinaemia, where severe chronic fat malabsorption is present, neurological symptoms of vitamin E deficiency can develop. Children often develop the clinical symptoms of ataxia, areflexia or hyporeflexia (absent or low/slow reflexes) and loss of proprioception (position sense) within 2–3 years of the onset of fat malabsorption, whereas symptoms in adults may take up to 20 years to manifest. In some cases, there is a pigmentary retinopathy (retinitis pigmentosa). Typical treatment involves oral doses ranging from 5 to 25 IU/kg/day, although intramuscular injection has been used. Once started, the treatment normalizes plasma vitamin E levels rapidly and arrests further deterioration of clinical symptoms; however, full normalization of neurological function can take several years. Individuals with persistent steatorrhea (i.e. fatty stools) should have their plasma vitamin E levels monitored.

13.2.8 Toxicity

Reports of vitamin E toxicity are rare. Results from several randomized controlled trials of high-dose vitamin E supplements, taken for up to 5 years, have shown no consistent adverse effects on health. Intakes of 100–300 mg/day appear to be well tolerated.

13.2.9 Food sources

Plant foods high in fat, particularly polyunsaturated fat, are the best sources of vitamin E (Table 13.5). Wheat germ oil is the richest source. Tocopherols comprise the bulk of vitamin E in plant foods with the exception of oil, which contains more tocotrienols. Most vitamin E in animal foods is α-tocopherol (> 90%) with small amounts of γ-tocopherol (< 10%) and little tocotrienol. The relative amounts of α-, β-, γ- and δ-tocopherol varies considerably between plant foods, but in a diet, α- and γ-tocopherol tend to predominate.

13.2.10 Assessment of vitamin E status

Measurement of plasma vitamin E is the easiest and most common method of assessing vitamin E status (Table 13.6). Normal concentrations range from 12 to 30 μmol/L (5–13 mg/L), with more than 90% usually as α-tocopherol. A plasma concentration of vitamin E above 12 μmol/L (5 mg/L) is considered adequate.

When the concentration of plasma lipoproteins is elevated, plasma vitamin E is correspondingly high. To allow for this correlation, plasma vitamin E is frequently expressed per unit of plasma cholesterol. A plasma vitamin E to cholesterol ratio of greater than 2–2.5 μmol/mmol is judged to be normal.

Vitamin E can be measured in platelets, erythrocytes and adipose tissue, although these methods are more time-consuming and reference data are limited.

There are several functional tests of vitamin E status involving the measurement of oxidant stress. These tests are difficult to standardize and are not entirely specific for vitamin E status because other antioxidant systems can influence the results. The most common test is the erythrocyte fragility test in which erythrocytes are exposed to a standard concentration of hydrogen peroxide (2%) for 3 hours and the amount of haemolysis is measured. Poor vitamin E status is indicated when more than 5%

Table 13.5 Vitamin E content of common foods

Food	Vitamin E (mg/100 g)	Food	Vitamin E (mg/100 g)
Fats and oils		**Meat, poultry, fish**	
Wheat germ oil	137.0	Chicken	0.8
Palm oil	33.1	Cod	0.5
Soybean oil	16.3	Beef	0.3
Margarine	14.9	Lamb	0.2
Nuts		**Breads and cereals**	
Almonds (raw)	24.0	Wheat germ	22.6
Peanuts	10.1	Wholemeal flour	2.0
Fruits and vegetables		Bran cereal	1.9
Sweet potato	4.6	Rolled oats	1.6
Spinach	1.7	White flour	0.4
Peaches	1.3	Brown rice	0.3
Carrots	0.8	Wholemeal bread	0.2
Tomatoes	0.8	**Dairy products**	
Lettuce	0.8	Cheddar cheese	0.9
Apples	0.4	Cottage cheese	0.1
Honeydew melon	0.1	**Legumes**	
Broccoli	0.1	Mung beans	0.9
		Lentils	0.4
		Kidney beans	0.2

Source: New Zealand food composition database: (OCNZ97). Palmerston North: Crop and Food Research Institute, 1993.

of the erythrocytes haemolyse. The remaining tests involve measurement of metabolites produced during the *in vivo* peroxidation of polyunsaturated fatty acids; these include breath pentane and ethane, urinary malondialdehyde, and lipoprotein diene-conjugated fatty acids.

13.2.11 Recommended nutrient intakes

Recommended nutrient intakes for vitamin E are based on the usual intake in apparently healthy populations because clinical deficiency symptoms are rare, and there is no sensitive and specific biochemical measure of vitamin E status. Animal experiments confirm the theoretical prediction that vitamin E requirements (to prevent deficiency effects) are increased if the intake of polyunsaturated fatty acids is high. A ratio of 0.4 mg α-tocopherol per gram of poly-unsaturated fat intake is considered sufficient vitamin E to avoid any deficiency. Fortunately, increased intake of vitamin E is not difficult to achieve because of the natural association between vitamin E and polyunsaturated fatty acids in foods. A typical recommended nutrient intake is 10 mg α-tocopherol equivalents per day for healthy men and somewhat less for women.

There is considerable interest in using new criteria to establish nutrient recommendations for vitamin E. Minimizing free-radical damage is considered by many the future criterion for establishing recommended vitamin E intakes. The fact that free radicals have both beneficial and pathological effects in the body will make it challenging for nutritionists to decide, within the context of overall oxidant stress and antioxidant status, the level of vitamin E intake that achieves the optimal balance between these opposing effects.

Table 13.6 Assessment of vitamin E status*

Test	Normal	Marginal-deficient
Biochemical tests		
Plasma (μmol/L)	12–30	< 12
Erythrocytes		
Platelets		
Adipose tissue		
Vitamin E/lipid ratio		
Functional tests		
Erythrocyte haemolysis		
Breath pentane and ethane		
Erythrocyte malondialdehyde		
LDL oxidation		

*Cut-off values and ranges have only been clearly established for some tests.

Intakes of 50–200 mg/day appear in prospective epidemiological studies to be associated with a reduced risk of coronary heart disease. However, intakes as high as this cannot be achieved by ordinary diets; they require vitamin E supplements. The association between taking vitamin E supplements and reduced risk of coronary heart disease may be due to other confounding factors (i.e. the lifestyle of people who take vitamin supplements is likely to differ in other ways from people who do not take supplements). The results of several large clinical intervention trials have indicated that vitamin E supplements do not prevent ischaemic heart disease (see Chapter 20).

FURTHER READING

Vitamin C

1. **Carpenter, K.J.** (1986) *The history of scurvy and vitamin C*. Cambridge, Cambridge University Press.

2. **Carr, A.C., and Frei, B.** (1999) Toward a new recommended dietary allowance for vitamin C based on antioxidant and health effects in humans. *Am J Clin Nutr*, **69**, 1086–107.

3. **Daves, M.B., Austin, A., and Partridge, D.A.** (1991) *Vitamin C: its chemistry and biochemistry*. Cambridge, The Royal Society of Chemistry.

4. **Douglas, R.M., Hemila, H., Chalker, E., D'Souza, R.R.D., and Treacy, B.** (2006) Vitamin C for preventing and treating the common cold. *Cochrane Database Syst Rev*, **1**.

5. **Englard, S., and Seifter, S.** (1986) The biochemical functions of ascorbic acid. *Ann Rev Nutr*, **6**, 365–406.

6. **Hodges, R.E., Baker, E.M., Hood, J., Suberlich, H.E., and March, S.C.** (1969) Experimental scurvy in man. *Am J Clin Nutr*, **22**, 535–48.

7. **Sauberlich, H.E.** (1994) Pharmacology of vitamin C. *Ann Rev Nutr*, **14**, 371–91.

Vitamin E

1. **Brigelius-Flohe, R., Kelly, F.J., Salonen, J.T., Neuzil, J., Zingg, J-M., and Azzi, A.** (2002) The European perspective on vitamin E: current knowledge and future research. *Am J Clin Nutr*, **76**, 703–16.

2. **Horwitt, M.K.** (1960) Vitamin E and lipid metabolism in man. *Am J Clin Nutr*, **8**, 451–61.

3. **Kayden, H.T., and Traber, M.G.** (1993) Absorption, lipoprotein transport, and regulation of plasma concentrations of vitamin E in humans. *J Lipid Res*, **34**, 345–58.

4. **Leth, T., and Sondergaard, H.** (1977) Biological activity of vitamin E compounds and natural materials by the resorption-gestation test, and chemical determination of the vitamin E activity in foods and feeds. *J Nutr*, **107**, 2236–43.

5. **Meydani, M.** (1995) Vitamin E. *Lancet*, **345**, 170–5.

6. **Traber, M.G., and Arai, H.** (1999) Molecular mechanisms of vitamin E transport. *Ann Rev Nutr*, **19**, 343–55.

 To see topical and scientifically robust updates on nutrition associated with this textbook, and active web links to many of the journal articles in the Reference areas, please see the dedicated Online Resource Centre at www.oxfordtextbooks.co.uk/orc/mann3e/.

14 Vitamins D and K

Stewart Truswell

14.1 Vitamin D

14.1.1 History

In the first step towards identifying individual vitamins, E.V. McCollum, at the University of Wisconsin postulated (1915) two essential dietary factors as well as macronutrients and minerals—'fat-soluble A' and 'water-soluble B'. Fat-soluble A prevented growth failure and the eye disease xerophthalmia, in animals fed purified diets. In 1919, Edward Mellanby in London found that some fats would cure experimental dietary rickets in puppies kept indoors but others would not. Cod liver oil was very active against the bone disease rickets and against xerophthalmia (Chapter 11) but when heated, with oxygen bubbled through, its antixerophthalmia activity was lost, not its antirachitic (antirickets) activity, and McCollum realized in 1922 that there were two nutritional factors in cod liver oil. He designated the antirachitic factor vitamin D because 'water-soluble C' had been proposed for the antiscorbutic (antiscurvy) factor in 1919. Meanwhile, Harriette Chick, a British scientist, proved that rickets in children in Vienna after World War I could be cured either by cod liver oil or by exposure to an ultraviolet (UV) light lamp. Pure vitamin D_2 was first obtained by irradiating ergosterol with UV light in 1927. Its chemical structure was established by A. Windaus in Germany and F. Askew in England in 1932. In 1936, Windaus published the structure of vitamin D_3, the natural form of the vitamin made by UV light in the skin and present in cod liver oil.

14.1.2 Chemistry and metabolism

Vitamin D_3, cholecalciferol, is derived by the effect of UVB irradiation (wavelength 290–315 nm) on 7-dehydrocholesterol (cholesterol with a double bond at carbon 7), a minor companion of cholesterol, in the skin. There is a rearrangement of the molecule, with opening of the B ring of the steroid nucleus (Fig. 14.1). Cholecalciferol is the naturally occurring form of the vitamin in man and animals, for example, in cod liver oil, fatty fish, butter and animal liver.

Vitamin D_2 is derived from ergosterol (a fungal sterol) by irradiating it with UV light via the same sequence of chemical changes and is called ergocalciferol. It is used as a pharmaceutical (also called calciferol) and in some of the foods fortified with vitamin D (e.g. milk in North America, margarine). Ergosterol is a phytosterol (plant sterol). It and ergocalciferol differ from 7-dehydrocholesterol and cholecalciferol only in having an extra double bond at carbon 22 and a methyl group at carbon 24 in the side chain (Fig. 14.1). The original vitamin D_1

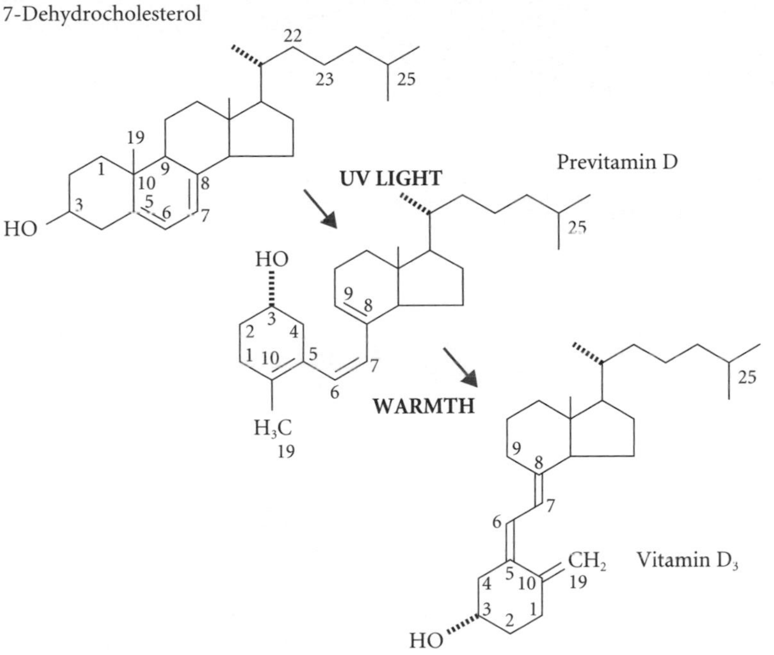

7-Dehydrocholesterol

Fig. 14.1 Formation of vitamin D_3 in the skin. 7-Dehydrocholesterol is present in the skin as a minor companion of cholesterol. Under the influence of short-wavelength UV light (290–315 nm) from sunlight, the B ring of the sterol opens to form a secosterol, previtamin D_3. The first step takes place rapidly. The second stage is a rearrangement of the secosterol to make vitamin D_3 (cholecalciferol). It takes place more slowly, under the influence of warmth.

turned out to be an impure mixture of sterols. Using the older quantitative unit for vitamin D, one international unit (IU) = 0.025 µg of cholecalciferol (so 1 µg = 40 IU).

In the tropical and subtropical regions of the world, enough vitamin D is made in the skin to meet the body's needs (unless people are housebound or completely covered). Since cholecalciferol is formed in one organ of the body (the skin) and transported by the blood to act on other organs (the bones, gut, kidneys), it can be called a hormone. However, when people live in high latitudes, are covered with clothes, spend nearly all their time indoors and the sky is polluted with smoke, there is insufficient UV exposure in the winter to make enough vitamin D in the skin. Dietary intake is required, so that the cholecalciferol present in a few foods and the ergocalciferol in fortified foods assume the role of a vitamin.

Inside the body, vitamin D itself is not active until it has been chemically modified (hydroxylated) twice. The first clue to this was the observation of a lag period of 8 hours before one could see an effect of administered vitamin D in experimental animals. Vitamin D, whether of cutaneous origin or absorbed

(D_3 or D_2), is carried in the plasma on a specific α_2-globulin, vitamin D-binding protein. In liver microsomes, the end of the side chain is hydroxylated to form 25-hydroxy-vitamin D (25(OH)D). This compound has a more stable concentration in the blood than that of vitamin D, which rises temporarily as some is absorbed or synthesized in the skin.

25(OH)D is still not the active metabolite. It has to have a third hydroxyl (OH) group put on at carbon 1. This is done by an enzyme, 1α-hydroxylase, in the kidneys (in the mitochondria of the proximal convoluted tubule) to make 1,25-dihydroxy vitamin D (1,25(OH)$_2$D) (Fig. 14.2). The plasma concentration of 1,25(OH)$_2$D is about one thousand times smaller than that of 25(OH)D. The activity of renal 1α-hydroxylase is tightly controlled so the rate of production of 1,25(OH)$_2$D is increased by any fall in plasma calcium or rise in parathyroid hormone level.

1,25(OH)$_2$D is one of the three hormones that normally act together to maintain the extracellular calcium concentration constant; the other two are parathormone and calcitonin (see Chapter 8). There are about 30 other known metabolites of vitamin D, probably all inactive.

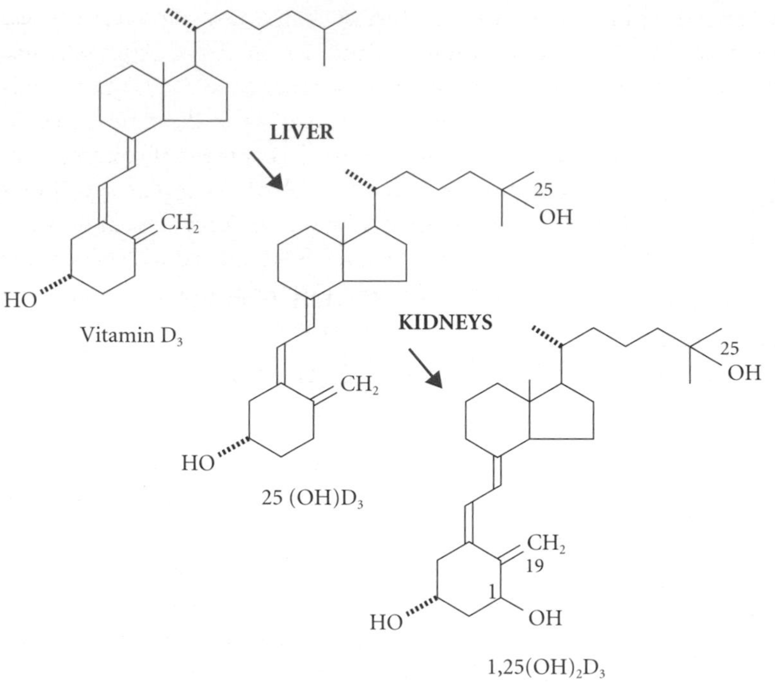

Fig. 14.2 Activation of vitamin D. In the liver parenchymal cells, vitamin D_3 (or D_2) is hydroxylated to 25-hydroxy-vitamin D (25(OH)D), which circulates in the blood. A small proportion of the available 25(OH)D is further hydroxylated by a specific 25(OH)D-1α-hydroxylase in the kidneys to the active form, 1,25(OH)$_2$ vitamin D. During pregnancy, some 1α-hydroxylation also takes place in the placenta.

1,25(OH)$_2$D acts in a similar manner to steroid hormones. There is a specific vitamin D receptor (VDR) protein in the cell nucleus, which has great affinity for 1,25(OH)$_2$D. It also has a DNA-binding domain. This receptor, when activated, switches on the gene that induces synthesis of a calcium transport protein (calbindin) in the epithelium of the small intestine. VDR has actually been found in a range of tissues but normally has its main effect in the small intestinal epithelium and the cells in bone, osteoblasts (that form new bone) and osteoclasts (that break bone down).

Less vitamin D is made in the skin of dark-skinned people than white-skinned people because the melanin in stin absorbs UV light. Old people also make less vitamin D after exposure to short-wave UV light; their skin contains less of the starting material, 7-dehydrocholesterol. Vitamin D taken by mouth is digested and absorbed, then transported from the upper small intestine on chylomicrons, like other lipids. Like other lipids, its absorption can be impaired in chronic biliary or intestinal disease with malabsorption. Excretion of vitamin D is in the bile, principally as more-polar metabolites.

14.1.3 Deficiency diseases

In *rickets*, there is reduced calcification of the growing ends (epiphyses) of bones. Thick seams of uncalcified osteoid cartilage are seen histologically. Rickets only occurs in young people, whose bones are still growing. *Osteomalacia* is the corresponding decalcifying bone disease in adults, whose epiphyses have fused so that the bones are no longer growing. Bone density is reduced. This is because the bones contain less calcium: the ratio of calcium to organic bone is reduced. Rickets can occur in premature infants and in children in northern Britain (especially of Asian origin). Surprisingly, rickets and osteomalacia can also occur in the tropics in dark-skinned children and women usually staying indoors and fully covered when outdoors. In affluent countries, osteomalacia is possible in elderly people confined indoors. Malabsorption increases the risk. Muscular weakness and susceptibility to infections in rickets or osteomalacia may reflect roles for VDR in the muscles and the immune system. In chronic kidney failure, 1α-hydroxylation is impaired. Renal osteomalacia does not respond to vitamin D (or sunlight), only to administration of 1,25(OH)$_2$D (pharmaceutical name 'calcitriol') or to 1α(OH)D (pharmaceutical name 'alphacalcidol'). This shows the critical importance of 1α-hydroxylation to normal vitamin D function.

14.1.4 Biochemical tests of vitamin D status

Plasma calcium and phosphate levels fall in severe vitamin D-deficient states. Plasma alkaline phosphatase (the isoenzyme originating in bone) is increased in mild as well as in severe rickets and osteomalacia. It can be elevated in some other bone diseases and does not directly indicate vitamin D status. This is best assessed by assaying plasma 25(OH)D levels and it can be seen how the concentration goes down in population samples at the end of the winter in those temperate countries that have little vitamin D fortification. Levels below 25 nmol/L indicate deficiency; 25–50 nmol/L is low or borderline; over 50 nmol/L is normal. In the alternative units (divide by 2.6), this normal level is 20 µg/mL. Plasma 1,25(OH)$_2$D can also be measured but is a specialized investigation.

14.1.5 Osteoporosis as well as osteomalacia

It used to be thought that vitamin D deficiency causes osteomalacia, not osteoporosis. (In osteoporosis, total bone is reduced—organic as well as calcium.) Now that vitamin D status can be quantified with serum 25(OH)D, it is becoming clear that as levels fall below 50 nmol/L there are compensatory secondary increases of parathyroid hormone and increased mobilization of bone. Some long-term prevention trials in older people using vitamin D (with or without calcium supplements) have shown delayed development of osteoporosis and fewer fractures.

14.1.6 Other possible roles for vitamin D

There is also accumulating evidence for non-calcaemic actions of vitamin D. Epidemiological clues are that some cancers (breast, colon and prostate) are less prevalent at sunny latitudes and so is multiple sclerosis. In tissue culture experiments 1,25(OH)$_2$D modulates function of activated T and B lymphocytes. In a 20-year trial in Finland, treatment of children with vitamin D reduced the risk of developing type 1 diabetes. Psoriasis has long been known to improve in the summer. It is now being treated with ointments containing 1,25(OH)$_2$D or derivatives.

14.1.7 Food sources

Fish liver oils (e.g. cod and halibut) and some fish and marine animal's livers are rich sources. Moderate sources are fatty fish (herring, sardine, salmon, etc.), margarines (which in most countries are fortified with vitamin D), infant milk formulas, eggs, red meat and liver. Milk is fortified with vitamin D in North America and Scandinavia. Human milk contains little vitamin D (moderate exposure to sunlight is good for babies).

14.1.8 Interactions

Inadequate calcium intake aggravates any insufficiency of vitamin D. Fraser (1995) suggests that low calcium intake increases formation of 1,25(OH)$_2$D and that this acts on the liver to increase destruction or reduce formation of 25(OH)D. Long-term use of anticonvulsants (e.g. for epilepsy), by inducing liver microsomes, may increase metabolic losses of vitamin D. Glucocorticoids (e.g. prednisone) inhibit vitamin D-dependent intestinal calcium absorption; patients on long-term steroids may benefit from additional vitamin D to maintain plasma 25(OH)D in the mid-normal range (above 50 nmol/L).

14.1.9 Recommended nutrient intake

The US Institute of Medicine estimates 'adequate intakes' (AI) of vitamin D for those with no sun-mediated synthesis in the skin. For ages 0–50 years (including pregnancy and lactation), the AI is 5 µg/day, for 51–70 years 10 µg/day and over 70 years of age

15 µg/day. Older people make less vitamin D in their skin and also tend to avoid sun exposure and use UV light-blocking sunscreen. If they are housebound and cannot get in the sun, they probably need vitamin D supplements because most diets provide under 5 µg vitamin D per day unless the milk is fortified. There is not enough UV light at the latitude of Boston (42°N) to make adequate vitamin D in the winter months. Vegans who avoid milk and fish are at risk of subclinical vitamin D deficiency if they live at high latitudes.

14.1.10 Toxicity

Exposure of the skin to sunlight, if excessive, causes sunburn and brings up the plasma 25(OH)D if it was low but does not lead to vitamin D toxicity because with excessive UV light, previtamin D_3 (7-dehydrocholesterol) is photoisomerized to biologically inert products (lumisterol and tachysterol). Vitamin D_3 is also photodegraded if it is not taken inside the body by vitamin D-binding protein. However, with oral intake, the margin between the upper limit of the nutritional dose and the lower limit of the toxic dose is quite narrow. Overdosage causes raised plasma calcium (hypercalcaemia), with thirst, anorexia, raised plasma levels of 25(OH)D, and risk of calcification of soft tissues and of urinary calcium stones. Infants are most at risk of hypervitaminosis D; a few children have developed hypercalcaemia on intakes of only 50 µg/day. The upper level of 50 µg (2 000 IU) per day for adults set by the US Institute of Medicine in 1997 has been shown to be unnecessarily cautious (Weaver and Fleet, 2004). In some conditions, people are unusually sensitive to vitamin D (e.g. in sarcoidosis and a rare condition in infants with elfin facial appearance, William syndrome).

14.2 Vitamin K

14.2.1 History

The name 'vitamin K' was proposed by Henrik Dam of Denmark in 1935. K was the next letter of the alphabet not already used for a vitamin at that time. It is also the first letter of the German word *koagulation*, which refers to its best-known function. While investigating the essentiality of cholesterol in the diet of chickens (their eggs, of course, are rich in cholesterol), Dam fed them rations from which the lipid had been extracted with organic solvents. They developed haemorrhages and their blood was slow to clot. This bleeding tendency could be corrected with alfalfa or with decayed fishmeal. The alfalfa was soon shown to provide vitamin K_1; bacteria in the fishmeal were responsible for producing vitamin K_2.

14.2.2 Chemistry

H.J. Almquist solved the chemical search in 1939, reporting that a lipid from the sheath of tubercle bacilli, phthiocol, had vitamin K activity (Fig. 14.3A). Vitamin K_1 and the K_2 series are all based on this 2-methyl-3-hydroxy-1,4-naphthoquinone. They have side chains in place of the 3-hydroxyl group. In vitamin K_1 (phylloquinone), the side chain is a 20 carbon terpenoid alcohol (four-fifths of the phytol side chain of chlorophyll) (Fig. 14.3B). It is found in green leaves.

Vitamin K_2 comprises a family of compounds, called menaquinones, whose side chain consists of repeated (5-carbon) isoprene units, from 1 to 14 of them (Fig. 14.3C). Depending on the number of isoprene units, they are referred to as MK1 to MK14. The menaquinones are synthesized by several bacterial species (*Bacteriodes*, *Enterobacteria*, etc.), some of which occur naturally in the large intestine of animals, including humans.

14.2.3 Functions

In the liver, vitamin K promotes the synthesis of a special amino acid with three carboxylic acid groups, γ-carboxyglutamic acid (Gla) (Fig. 14.4). The enzyme responsible for putting another carboxylic acid on to glutamic acid requires vitamin K as a cofactor.

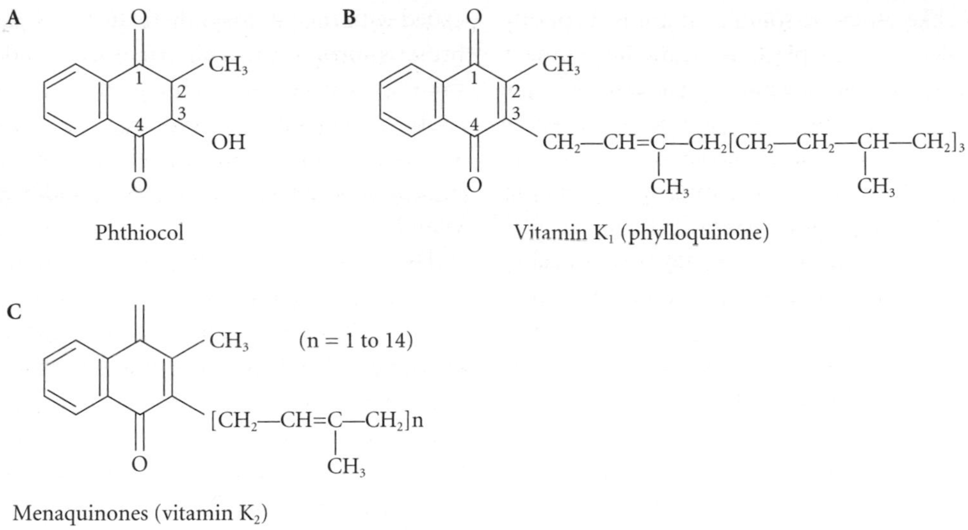

A

Phthiocol

B

Vitamin K$_1$ (phylloquinone)

C

Menaquinones (vitamin K$_2$)

Fig. 14.3 Structures of (A) phthiocol, (B) phylloquinone (vitamin K$_1$) and (C) menaquinones (vitamin K$_2$).

γ-Carboxyglutamic acid
(Gla)

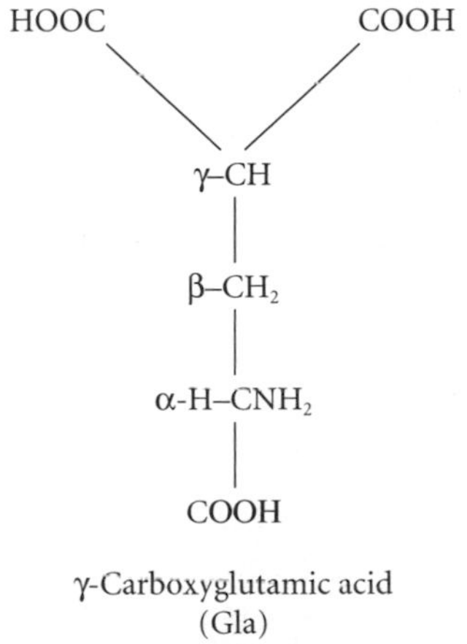

Fig. 14.4 γ-Carboxyglutamic acid (Gla).

Gla is an essential part of four of the coagulation factors, all proteins: prothrombin (factor II) and factors VII, IX and X. Factors II and VII contain 10 Gla residues per molecule; factors IX and X each contain 12. The Gla residues confer on these coagulation proteins the capacity to bind to phospholipid surfaces in the presence of calcium ions.

A few other proteins not involved in coagulation also contain Gla and require the presence of vitamin K for their synthesis. The best known is osteocalcin, a major protein of bone, made by the osteoblasts.

It also binds calcium and its plasma concentration indicates osteoblast activity.

Vitamin K, being fat-soluble, requires bile for its absorption. It is transported in the plasma on triglyceride-rich lipoproteins. Analysis of vitamin K in tissues has been difficult because the several compounds are present in very tiny (nanomolar) amounts. In adult liver, there is not only vitamin K$_1$ derived from green leaves in the diet, but also significant amounts of the K$_2$ vitamins MK7–MK13. As there is little K$_2$ in wholesome food, these must be synthesized by resident bacteria in the large intestine and absorbed, presumably from the caecum. In plasma, the major form of vitamin K appears to be K$_1$.

14.2.4 Deficiency disease

In vitamin K deficiency, there is a bleeding disorder, characterized by low plasma prothrombin activity (hypoprothrombinaemia). Vitamin K deficiency can occur in obstetric or paediatric practice, in surgical patients and in medical patients.

For most people in developed countries, the first injection of their life is vitamin K$_1$ given intramuscularly straight after birth to prevent haemorrhagic disease of the newborn. There is a small risk of haemorrhage in the first days after birth because vitamin K, like other fat-soluble vitamins, is poorly transported across the placenta from the mother's blood; the gut of the newborn is sterile (there are no resident bacteria so no vitamin K_2); it is some days before bacteria colonize the large intestine, and human milk has a low concentration of vitamin K (K_1).

In surgical practice, vitamin K status is critical in obstructive jaundice, whereby bile cannot flow into the small intestine so that vitamin K_1 is not absorbed. It is of course very dangerous to operate on someone with a coagulation defect, so before surgery on the bile duct, the prothrombin activity must be checked and vitamin K_1 given as a precaution. Vitamin K deficiency also occurs in patients with malabsorption, and sometimes following prolonged use of broad-spectrum antibiotics by mouth (which can destroy the colonic bacteria). In serious liver disease, the coagulation factors may not be adequately synthesized, but this is because of poor liver function, rather than vitamin K deficiency.

In internal medicine, the most common cause of vitamin K deficiency is the use of anticoagulant drugs, given to prevent clotting in veins: warfarin and dicoumarol, which owe their therapeutic action to blocking some of the enzymes that recycle vitamin K in the liver.

There are reports of low circulating vitamin K in elderly patients with femoral neck fractures or spinal crush fractures, suggesting that suboptimal vitamin K status may play a role in osteoporosis, presumably because osteocalcin is not made adequately.

It is not possible to measure vitamin K in plasma except as a difficult research procedure because its concentrations are so minute. Plasma prothrombin activity and its response, if it was low, to vitamin K_1 is the usual way of making the diagnosis of deficiency. A more specific method is to measure undercarboxylated prothrombin, that is des-γ-carboxyprothrombin (or PIVKA, protein induced by vitamin K absence).

14.2.5 Dietary sources

Vitamin K_1 is present in dark-green leaves eaten as foods. Some contain more than others. It is asso-

ciated with the photosynthetic tissues. Kale, spinach, brussels sprouts, broccoli, parsley, coriander, endive, mint, mustard greens, cabbage and lettuce are good sources (in descending order). Other good sources are some vegetable oils. Small amounts are present in beef liver, apples and green tea, and there is some vitamin K_2 in cheese.

There are no experimentally derived reference values yet for vitamin K but it is agreed that 1 µg/kg body weight is a safe and adequate intake (i.e. around 80 µg/day in men and 65 µg/day in women). Bone Gla protein may be more sensitive to low intakes than the Gla haemostatic proteins. Usual adult intakes are variously estimated at 60–200 µg/day.

No application has been devised for supernutritional doses of vitamin K_1 but even milligram doses by mouth have not been found toxic. However, the synthetic water-soluble pharmaceutical with vitamin K activity, menadione, can cause haemolytic anaemia and jaundice in newborn babies. It is now obsolete, superseded by vitamin K_1 since this became available in pharmaceutical form.

FURTHER READING

Vitamin D

1. Bischoff-Ferrari, H.A., Willett, W.C., Wong, J.B., Giovannucci, E., Dietrich, T., and Dawson-Hughes, T. (2005) Fracture prevention with vitamin D supplementation. A meta-analysis of randomized controlled trials. *J Am Med Assoc*, **293**, 2257–64.

2. Diamond, T.H., Eisman, J.A., Mason, R.S., *et al*. (2005) Vitamin D and adult bone health in Australia and New Zealand: a position statement. *Med J Aust*, **183**, 281–3.

3. Food and Nutrition Board, Institute of Medicine (1997) *Dietary reference intakes for calcium, phosphorus, magnesium, vitamin D and fluoride*. Washington, DC: National Academy Press.

4. Fraser, D.R. (1995) Vitamin D. *Lancet*, **345**, 104–7.

5. Holick, M.F. (2004) Sunlight and vitamin D for bone health and prevention of autoimmune diseases, cancers and cardiovascular disease. *Am J Clin Nutr*, **80**, 1678S–1688S.

6. **MacLaughlin, J., and Holick, M.F.** (1985) Ageing decreases the capacity of human skin to produce vitamin D$_3$. *J Clin Invest*, **76**, 1536–8.

7. **van Amerongen, B.M., Dijstra, C.D., Lips, P., and Polman, C.H.** (2004) Multiple sclerosis and vitamin D: an update. *Eur J Clin Nutr*, **58**, 1095–1109.

8. **Weaver, C.M., and Fleet, J.C.** (2004) Vitamin D requirements: current and future. *Am J Clin Nutr*, **80**, 1735S–1739S.

9. **Webb, A.R., Kline, L., and Holick, M.F.** (1988) Influence of season and latitude on the cutaneous synthesis of vitamin D$_3$: exposure to winter sunlight in Boston and Edmonton will not produce vitamin D$_3$ synthesis in human skin. *J Clin Endocrinol Metab*, **67**, 373–8.

Vitamin K

1. **Booth, S.L., Sadowski, J.A., Weikrauch, J.L., and Ferland, G.** (1998) Vitamin K (phylloquinone) content of foods: a provisional table. *J Food Comp Anal*, **6**, 109–20.

2. **Duggan, P., Cashman, K.D., Flynn, A., Bolton-Smith, C., and Kiely, M.** (2004) Phylloquinone (vitamin K$_1$) intakes and food sources in 18–64-year old Irish adults. *Br J Nutr*, **92**, 151–8.

3. **Feskanich, D., Weber, P., Willett, W.C., Rockett, H., Booth, S.L., and Colditz, G.A.** (1999) Vitamin K intake and hip fractures in women: a prospective study. *Am J Clin Nutr*, **69**, 74–9.

4. **Shearer, M.J.** (1995) Vitamin K. *Lancet*, **345**, 229–34.

 To see topical and scientifically robust updates on nutrition associated with this textbook, and active web links to many of the journal articles in the Reference areas, please see the dedicated Online Resource Centre at www.oxfordtextbooks.co.uk/orc/mann3e/.

15 Other biologically active substances in plant foods: phytochemicals

Claus Leitzmann and Bernhard Watzl

15.1 Introduction

Plants contain a wide range of secondary metabolites of low molecular weight that, in the broadest sense, are biologically active molecules that have evolved in the interaction between the plant and its environment, including ultraviolet light. When plant foods are consumed, a diverse range of secondary plant metabolites is ingested. In the past, emphasis was placed on secondary metabolites as natural toxicants that are present in plant foods (i.e. glycoalkaloids in potatoes and tomatoes, cyanogenic glycosides in cassava) and their potentially hazardous effects on humans. However, for the past two decades there has been increasing recognition of the health benefits of consuming diets rich in vegetables and fruits. Therefore, a resurgence of interest in secondary plant metabolites has evolved due to the overwhelming epidemiological evidence that has demonstrated a protective effect of vegetable and fruit intake against chronic illnesses such as cardiovascular disease and cancer.

Primary plant metabolites are substances that mainly contribute to energy metabolism and to the structure of the plant cell (i.e. carbohydrates including dietary fibre, proteins and fats). *Secondary* plant metabolites are non-nutritive dietary components (excluding vitamins) that have been referred to as *phytochemicals*. Secondary plant metabolites have various functions in the plant such as serving as a defence against destructive weeds, insects and micro-organisms, as growth regulators and as pigments. They are essential for the plant's interactions with its environment. Chemically, these secondary plant metabolites are quite diverse compounds and are found only in minute amounts, in contrast to the primary plant metabolites. Secondary plant metabolites have potentially pharmacological effects on humans, a thought that was already being discussed in the 1950s. More recently, nutrition scientists have systematically begun to investigate the health-promoting effects of these plant substances.

The total number of naturally occurring phytochemicals is not known. To date, the assumptions vary from 60 000 to 100 000 substances. With a mixed diet, around 1.5 g of secondary plant metabolites are ingested daily. On a vegetarian diet regimen, the intake of secondary plant metabolites can be distinctly higher.

Phytochemicals can have beneficial as well as detrimental health effects. Until a few years ago, they were merely seen under the aspect of toxicity and some were described as 'anti-nutritive' or even as 'toxic' metabolites because they restrict the availability of nutrients and increase the permeability of the intestinal wall. Our knowledge of adverse effects of phytochemicals is based on observations with farm animals usually fed exclusively one single fodder plant over a period of several months—a situation not comparable to human nutrition in industrialized countries. Under the usual conditions of food consumption, nearly all natural components—with a few exceptions such as solanine—are harmless when referring to natural toxic components of plant foods. Many phytochemicals that were previously regarded to have adverse effects on health may have a variety of health-promoting effects. This is exemplified by

protease inhibitors and glucosinolates of various *Cruciferae* species.

In the following sections, the health-promoting potential of phytochemicals is illustrated on the basis of experimental findings of their biological activity. The evidence found in epidemiological studies helps to estimate the importance that phytochemicals may have for human health.

15.2 Classification of phytochemicals

Phytochemicals are classified according to their chemical structure and their functional characteristics. The main groups of phytochemicals and their physiological effects show their great diversity (see Table 15.1).

15.2.1 Carotenoids

Carotenoids are widespread phytochemicals in fruits and vegetables and one of their main functions in

plants is to provide the red and yellow pigments essential for photosynthesis. They can be divided into oxygen-free and oxygen-containing (xanthophyll) carotenoids. Of the about 700 natural carotenoids, only around 40–50 are of significance in human nutrition. Depending on the carotenoid structure, several carotenoids possess provitamin A activity (Chapter 11). Human serum mainly contains the oxygen-free carotenoids, α- and β-carotene, lycopene,

Table 15.1   Classification of phytochemicals and their main effects

Phytochemical	Evidence for the following effects:								
	A	B	C	D	E	F	G	H	I
Carotenoids	X		X		X			X	
Phytosterols	X							X	
Saponins	X	X			X			X	
Glucosinolates	X	X						X	
Polyphenols	X	X	X	X	X	X	X		X
Protease inhibitors	X		X						X
Monoterpenes	X	X						X	
Phyto-oestrogens	X		X		X				
Sulphides	X	X	X	X	X	X	X	X	

A = anticarcinogenic
B = antimicrobial
C = antioxidative
D = antithrombotic
E = immunomodulatory properties
F = anti-inflammatory
G = influence on blood pressure
H = cholesterol-lowering effect
I = modulate blood glucose levels
Source: mod. from Watzl and Leitzmann, 2005.

Table 15.2 Absorption of phytochemicals in humans

Absorption		
High (> 15%)	**Medium (3–15%)**	**Low (< 3%)**
Carotenoids*	Phytosterols	Carotenoids**
Glucosinolates	Phenolic acids	Saponins
Flavonoids***	Protease inhibitors	Anthocyanins
Phyto-oestrogens		Flavones
Monoterpenes		
Sulphides		

*from heat-treated food, ** from raw food, ***flavonoids excluding anthocyanins and flavones.

as well as the xanthophylls lutein, zeaxanthin and β-cryptoxanthin, in varying proportions depending on the individual diet. Presently, the carotenoid lycopene is of special research interest because of its widespread physiological activities. At least 85% of the ingested lycopene derives from tomatoes and tomato products. β-Carotene accounts for 15–30% of the total serum carotenoids. Oxygen-free and oxygen-containing carotenoids differ mainly in their thermal stability. Whereas β-carotene in carrots and lycopene in tomatoes, for example, are heat-stable, xanthophylls (mainly in green vegetables) are sensitive to thermal processing. The total daily intake of carotenoids on a Western diet is about 6 mg. The absorption of carotenoids differs between raw and heat-treated vegetables and fruits (see Table 15.2).

15.2.2 Phytosterols

Phytosterols such as β-sitosterol, stigmasterol and campesterol are mainly found in plant seeds, nuts and oils. Chemically, phytosterols differ from cholesterol by an additional side chain only. The daily phytosterol intake amounts to 100–500 mg. In humans, absorption of phytosterols is low (0–10%) compared with > 40% for cholesterol. Absorbed phytosterols in the enterocytes are actively transported back to the intestinal lumen contributing to the low bioavailability of phytosterols. The cholesterol-lowering effect

of phytosterols has been known since the 1950s and is, in part, due to its property of inhibiting cholesterol absorption. This activity of phytosterols resulted in the generation of one of the first functional foods, a margarine enriched with phytosterol or phytostanol.

15.2.3 Saponins

Saponins are bitter-tasting, surface-active compounds that form complexes with proteins and lipids, such as cholesterol. Saponins are particularly abundant in legumes. The daily intake of saponins may be higher than 200 mg, depending on the dietary habits, but usually averages around 15 mg/day. Saponins have a low absorption rate (see Table 15.2) and therefore are primarily active in the intestinal tract. Due to their haemolytic properties, saponins were solely considered to be detrimental to health. In studies conducted with humans, however, this could not be confirmed. Some saponins have found approval as food additives within the European Union and in countries such as the USA and Canada as a foam stabilizer in beer and for soft drinks (E 999, *Quillaia saponaria* extract).

15.2.4 Glucosinolates

Glucosinolates are found in all plants belonging to the family of *Cruciferae*. Their degradation products contribute to the typical flavour of mustard, horse-radish and broccoli. Glucosinolates are sterically separated from the enzyme myrosinase, which degrades glucosinolates to the active metabolites isothiocyan-ates, thiocyanates and indoles. Mechanical damage of the plant tissue (cutting and chewing) eliminates the sterical separation between the enzyme and its sub-strates. Heating of cabbage reduces its glucosinolate content by 30–60% and inactivates its myrosinase activity. However, microbial myrosinase activity in the large intestine contributes to glucosinolate degra-dation. The total daily intake of glucosinolates is in the range of 10–50 mg. With vegetarian diets, the total daily intake can be as high as 100 mg. The glucosinolate metabolites, such as isothiocyanates, are completely absorbed in the small intestine (see Table 15.2). An isothiocyanate that has been intensely studied is sulphoraphane, which has an anticarcino-genic effect and induces antioxidant responses (see Table 15.1).

15.2.5 Polyphenols

The term polyphenol is used for all substances that are made up of phenol derivatives. Polyphenols mainly include phenolic acids (including hydroxycinnamic acids) and flavonoids (including flavonols, flavones, flavanols, flavanones and anthocyanins; see Fig. 15.1). Polyphenols normally occur bound to sugars and are rarely found as aglycones in plant foods. Besides monomeric flavonoids, oligomeric flavonoids (with two or more linked molecules) such as the flavanols (procyanidins) occur in red wine, tea, dark chocolate and apples. Fresh vegetables contain up to 0.1% poly-phenols, with the outer layer of fruits (e.g. apple skin) and vegetables (green leaves of lettuce) exhibiting relatively high amounts. The flavonoid content of green leafy vegetables is highest with increasing ripeness. Field-grown vegetables have a higher flavonoid con-tent than greenhouse produce. The most commonly found flavonoid is the flavonol quercetin, with a daily intake of about 25 mg. Recent findings suggest that some flavonoids, such as quercetin, can be absorbed by humans in health-relevant quantities, while other flavonoids such as the anthocyanins are hardly absorbed (see Table 15.2). Polyphenols exert a variety of physiological effects (see Table 15.1).

15.2.6 Protease inhibitors

Protease inhibitors are found especially in plant seeds (legumes and grains). Dependent on the mammalian species, protease inhibitors in the gut hamper the activity of endogenous proteases, such as trypsin. In response, the organism reacts with an increased synthesis of digestive enzymes. Humans synthesize a specific trypsin form, among others, that is resistant to protease inhibitors. Cooking significantly reduces the activity of protease inhibitors. Protease inhibitor intake averages about 300 mg daily. The protease in-hibitor intake of vegetarians with a diet high in grains and legumes can be considerably higher. Absorbed protease inhibitors can be detected in various tissues in biologically active form.

15.2.7 Monoterpenes

Active substances in herbs and spices such as menthol (peppermint), carvone (caraway seeds) and limonene (citrus oil) are examples of monoterpenes in food. The average daily intake of monoterpenes is up to 200 mg. Due to their fat solubility, monoterpenes display a high degree of bioavailability in humans (see Table 15.2). Limonene has been studied in animal models as an anticarcinogen and has been under-going preliminary trials in cancer patients.

15.2.8 Phyto-oestrogens

Phyto-oestrogens are plant components that bind to mammalian oestrogen receptors and have effects sim-ilar to those of endogenous oestrogens. Isoflavones and lignans, chemically both polyphenols, are the two major groups of the phyto-oestrogens in plant foods. Phyto-oestrogens have only about 0.1% of the efficacy that human oestrogens exhibit; however, their concentration in body fluids and tissues may be 100 to 10 000-fold higher. Therefore, phyto-oestrogens can act both as oestrogens and anti-oestrogens, depend-ing on the amount and concentration of endogenous

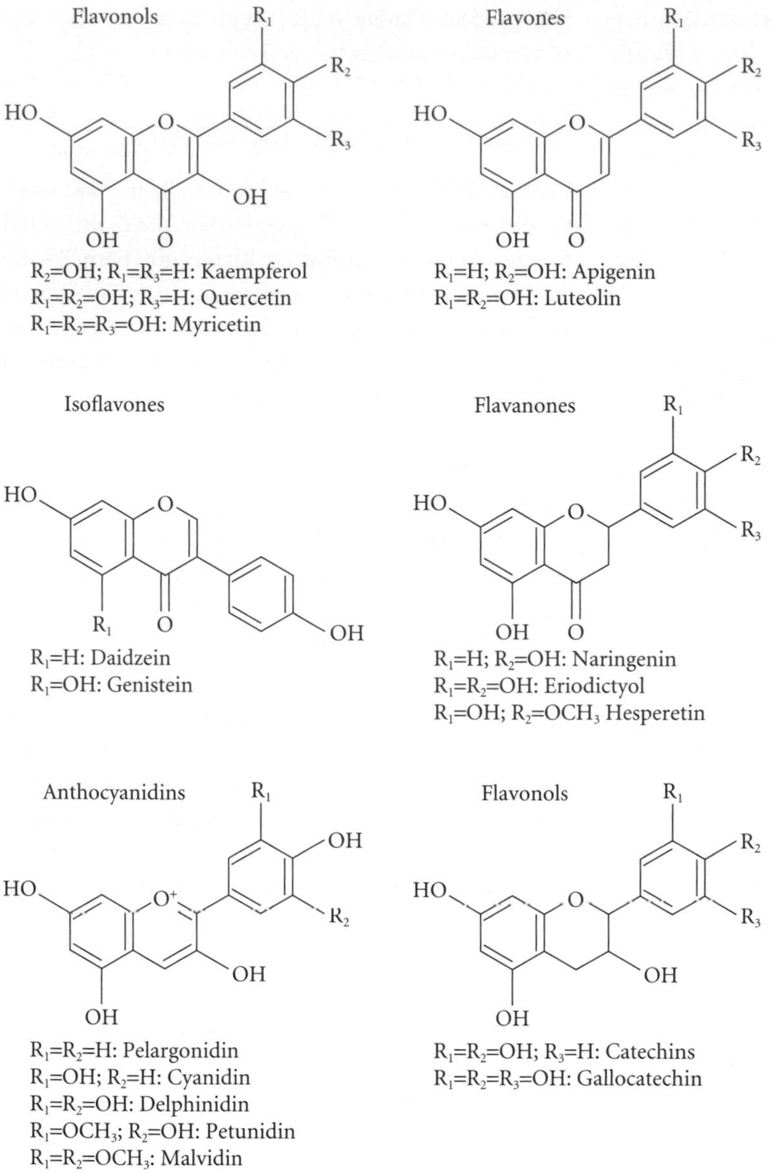

Flavonols

R$_2$=OH; R$_1$=R$_3$=H: Kaempferol
R$_1$=R$_2$=OH; R$_3$=H: Quercetin
R$_1$=R$_2$=R$_3$=OH: Myricetin

Flavones

R$_1$=H; R$_2$=OH: Apigenin
R$_1$=R$_2$=OH: Luteolin

Isoflavones

R$_1$=H: Daidzein
R$_1$=OH: Genistein

Flavanones

R$_1$=H; R$_2$=OH: Naringenin
R$_1$=R$_2$=OH: Eriodictyol
R$_1$=OH; R$_2$=OCH$_3$ Hesperetin

Anthocyanidins

R$_1$=R$_2$=H: Pelargonidin
R$_1$=OH; R$_2$=H: Cyanidin
R$_1$=R$_2$=OH: Delphinidin
R$_1$=OCH$_3$; R$_2$=OH: Petunidin
R$_1$=R$_2$=OCH$_3$: Malvidin

Flavonols

R$_1$=R$_2$=OH; R$_3$=H: Catechins
R$_1$=R$_2$=R$_3$=OH: Gallocatechin

Fig. 15.1 Chemical structures of flavonoids.

oestrogens. Isoflavones are almost exclusively found in soybeans and soybean products. Lignans are present in higher concentrations in flax seeds and wholegrain products. The major isoflavones in soy are the glycosides of genistein and daidzein. With traditional Asian diets and vegetarian diets, the phyto-oestrogen intake is high (15–40 mg/day), but Western diets provide little phyto-oestrogen (< 2 mg/day). Phyto-

oestrogens have a high absorption rate resulting in blood concentrations associated with various *in vitro* and *in vivo* effects (see Tables 15.1 and 15.2).

15.2.9 Sulphides

The sulphides among secondary plant metabolites include all organosulphur compounds of garlic and other bulbous plants. The main active substance of garlic is oxidized diallyl disulphide or allicin. Damage to the tissue in the garlic clove leads to the release of the enzyme alliinase, which produces allicin from the basic compound, alliin or *S*-allylcysteine sulphoxide.

15.2.10 Other phytochemicals

Apart from the secondary plant metabolites listed above, there are further phytochemicals that do not fit in the categories above. Lectins, for example, are present in legumes and grain products. They may have blood glucose-lowering effects. Other examples are glucarates, phthalides, chlorophyll and tocotrienols, as well as phytic acid.

15.3 Physiological effects of phytochemicals

The following is a short overview of the various effects of phytochemicals. For detailed information and references, see Watzl and Leitzmann (2005), Liu (2004) and Kris-Etherton *et al.* (2002).

15.3.1 Anticarcinogenic effects

Cancer is the second most frequent cause of death in industrialized countries. Nutrition is the major exogenous factor that modulates cancer risk and contributes to about one-third of all types of cancer. There are dietary factors that may promote carcinogenesis, but also others that may lower cancer risk. Evidence from epidemiological and animal experimental studies as well as information from biomarker and mechanistic studies indicates that a higher intake of vegetables and fruits is associated with a lower risk of various types of cancer. For all classes of phytochemicals occurring in vegetables and fruits, anticancer effects have been described. Based on the potential cancer preventive activity of plant foods, it has been recommended to increase the consumption of vegetables and fruits to at least five servings per day.

Phytochemicals may interfere and inhibit carcinogenesis at almost any stage in the multistep process of tumour initiation, promotion and progression (see Fig. 15.2). Knowledge of the anticarcinogenic effects of vegetables and fruits, and of isolated phytochemicals, has been obtained from different experimental systems (*in vitro*, animal and human). Animal experiments yield direct information about the extent of suppression of spontaneous and chemically induced

tumours by ingestion of certain plant foods or isolated phytochemicals (dose–effect studies). However, human studies, especially epidemiological, intervention and biomarker-related studies, are of particular relevance.

Carcinogens (e.g. nitrosamines) are usually ingested in their inactive form. Their endogenous activation by phase I enzymes (e.g. cytochrome P450-dependent mono-oxygenases) is a prerequisite for the interaction with DNA and genotoxic activity. Phase II enzymes (e.g. glutathione *S*-transferase, GST) usually detoxify activated carcinogens. In general, phytochemicals (glucosinolates, polyphenols, monoterpenes, sulphides) can inhibit carcinogenesis by inhibiting phase I enzymes and inducing phase II enzymes in cell cultures and in animal experiments, thereby acting as blocking agents (see Fig. 15.2). In this manner, the risk of DNA damage and tumour initiation is reduced. As an example, the isothiocyanate sulphoraphane, that can be isolated from broccoli activates the phase II detoxifying enzyme quinone reductase in cell culture systems. In human studies, 300 g brussels sprouts per day led to increased levels of α-GST (a phase II enzyme) in male subjects, but not in female subjects.

Recent data on genetic polymorphisms in humans have contributed to a better understanding of the cancer-preventive activity of phytochemicals and of vegetables and fruits. According to new studies, the potential effects of phytochemicals such as carotenoids and isothiocyanates on cancer prevention, as an example, highly depend on GST genotypes. In subjects

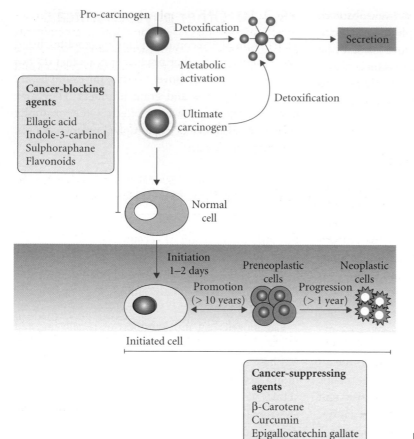

Fig. 15.2 Dietary phytochemicals that block or suppress multistage carcinogenesis.

Source: Surh, Y.-J. (2003) *Nat Rev Cancer*, **3**, 768–80.

with deletions of certain GST isotypes, a high intake of these phytochemicals is associated with a lower cancer risk.

An influence on hormone metabolism has been demonstrated by phyto-oestrogens. This is an example of cancer-suppressive activities of phytochemicals during tumour promotion and progression (see Fig. 15.2). Animal experiments have shown that phyto-oestrogens and the glucosinolate metabolite indole-3-carbinol influence oestrogen metabolism in such a manner that oestrogens known for their low-promoting tumour-growth properties are produced (i.e. catechol oestrogen). Furthermore, phyto-oestrogens induce the synthesis of the sex-hormone-binding globulin in the human liver, leading to an increase of oestrogens bound to this transport protein, thus making them less active. In prospective studies, however, phyto-oestrogens were not associated with lower cancer risk. Genistein, an isoflavone and phyto-oestrogen present in soybeans that can be detected in humans after soybean consumption inhibits the growth of blood vessels *in vitro*, possibly having an effect on the growth and metastasis of tumours.

A further point of attack for anticarcinogenic phytochemicals is the regulation of cell growth (proliferation) and programmed cell death (apoptosis).

Tumour cells distinguish themselves by a distorted regulation of cell proliferation and apoptosis. Phytochemicals such as isothiocyanates and carotenoids could intervene in such a twisted regulation by modulating the endogenous formation of cell growth-promoting substances and the process of intracellular signal transduction.

15.3.2 Antioxidative effects

The pathogenesis of cancer and cardiovascular diseases has been associated with the presence of reactive oxygen molecules and free radicals. The human body is equipped with several protective mechanisms against these reactive substances, including enzyme systems, superoxide dismutase and glutathione peroxidase, as well as endogenous antioxidants (uric acid, glutathione, α-lipoic acid, coenzyme Q_{10}). Essential nutrients with antioxidant activity include vitamins E and C. Additionally, phytochemicals (carotenoids, polyphenols, phyto-oestrogens and sulphides) exhibit antioxidative effects.

Certain carotenoids, such as β-carotene, lycopene and canthaxanthin, provide effective protection against singlet oxygen or oxygen radicals *in vitro*. However, human studies have failed to demonstrate an antioxidative effect of carotenoid supplements in well-nourished individuals. Of all antioxidants in plant foods, polyphenols *in vitro* have the highest potential in terms of quantity and effect. While most human studies could not demonstrate an antioxidative effect of polyphenols *in vivo*, recent studies using dark chocolate or tea showed an effect on plasma antioxidant capacity of polyphenol-rich foods.

Certain vegetable species influence the level of naturally occurring oxidative DNA damage. A daily consumption of 300 g brussels sprouts over a 3-week period led to a significant decrease of oxidative DNA damage (shown by urinary excretion of 8-oxo-7,8-dihydro-2-deoxyguanosine) compared with subjects that consumed 300 g glucosinolate-free vegetables per day over the same time period. Essential nutrients with antioxidative potential are ingested in amounts of around 100 mg/day. In contrast, the daily ingested amount of phytochemicals with antioxidant potential may exceed 1 g. This emphasizes the potential physiological importance of phytochemicals as antioxidants and as agents for other mechanisms that reduce the risk of cancer by consumption of vegetables and fruits.

15.3.3 Immunomodulatory effects

The immune system, primarily responsible for the defence against pathogens and transformed cells, is also involved in pathophysiological processes that lead to cancer and cardiovascular disease. Adequate nutrition is the basis for an optimally functioning immune system. Of special importance in this respect are total energy intake, quantity and quality of fats, and certain micronutrients.

Immunomodulatory activities of phytochemicals are a further mechanism through which plant foods may reduce disease risk. The immunomodulatory effects of phytochemicals have so far only been investigated to a very small extent, except for carotenoids. The stimulating effects of various carotenoids and carotenoid-rich foods on the immune system have been demonstrated in numerous animal experiments and human intervention studies.

Flavonoids, in contrast to the carotenoids, have been almost exclusively studied *in vitro*. Most studies demonstrate immunosuppressive activity of the flavonoids. Saponins, sulphides, phyto-oestrogens and phytic acid show immunomodulatory effects. As human studies with pure phytochemicals are lacking, with the exception of certain carotenoids, the evaluation of their immunomodulatory effects in humans is not yet possible. For some phytochemicals, however, such an effect seems likely.

15.3.4 Antimicrobial effects

Vegetables, fruits and spices have been used to treat infections since antiquity. The discovery of sulphonamides and microbial antibiotics and their successful use in treating infections resulted in a decline of interest in antimicrobial constituents in food. Only recently has there been a renewed interest in plant foods with antimicrobial effects.

Earlier studies clearly verified the antimicrobial action of sulphides from bulbous plants. Recent studies also demonstrated an inhibitory effect of garlic sulphides against *Helicobacter pylori in vitro*. Eliminating allicin from garlic prevented this effect, suggesting that this sulphide is causally related to the effect. The glucosinolate metabolites isothiocyanate and thiocyanate have likewise been shown to have antimicrobial activity. They are present in bacteriostatic concentrations in the urinary tract after consumption of garden cress, nasturtium and horseradish roots. However, the consumption of these plants alone will not lead to successful therapy.

In naturopathy, some berries such as cranberries and blueberries are frequently used for the prevention and therapy of infectious diseases. Data from several human intervention studies indicate that the daily intake of 300 mL cranberry juice as well as of other berries significantly reduces the risk of urinary tract infections. Juice consumption increased the intake of polyphenols (procyanidins) that inhibit the adherence of infectious bacteria to the urinary tract epithelium.

15.3.5 Cholesterol-lowering effects

Phytosterols, saponins, sulphides and lycopene have been found to lower serum cholesterol levels in both animal experiments and in clinical studies. The extent to which cholesterol levels are reduced depends on the cholesterol and fat content of the diet. The minimal effective dose of phytosterol is 1 g/day, while 170–440 mg/day is consumed in a typical Western diet. Margarines enriched with the esters of phytosterol or phytostanol provide 1.5–3.0 g/day, resulting in a 10–15% reduction of LDL-cholesterol (also see Chapter 20).

Although the cholesterol-lowering effect has been known for over 50 years, the underlying mechanism is still not clear. Several mechanisms may be responsible for this. Saponins bind to primary bile acids in the gut and form micelles. These micelles are too large to pass through the intestinal wall, thus leading to reduced absorption of bile acid and, in turn, to their excretion. As a consequence, an increased synthesis of primary bile acids in the liver from the endogenous cholesterol pool is initiated, leading to a decrease of the serum cholesterol level. Phytosterols probably also retard cholesterol absorption by driving cholesterol out of the micelles that normally help to absorb cholesterol from the gut.

Phytochemicals can also inhibit key enzymes of cholesterol synthesis in the liver. Of these key enzymes, the most important is 3-hydroxy-3-methylglutaryl-CoA-reductase, which is inhibited by monoterpenes and sulphides in animals.

15.3.6 Phytochemicals affecting drug metabolism

Phytochemicals in grapefruit juice interact with the metabolism of a variety of drugs. Drinking a single glass of grapefruit juice before administration of these drugs can severely affect drug bioavailability and the pharmacokinetics of the drug. The mechanism for this effect is the post-transcriptional inhibition of the cytochrome P450 3A4 enzyme in the small intestine, without affecting the same enzyme system in the large intestine or in the liver. This results in a reduction of pre-systemic metabolism of the drug followed by enhanced drug effects. A further mechanism could be the inhibition of a transporter system (P-glycoprotein) that normally carries drugs from the enterocyte back to the small intestinal lumen. While human experimental data support the contribution of furanocoumarins to this effect, it is likely that no single component of grapefruit juice is mediating this effect.

Other health-promoting effects of phytochemicals include regulation of blood pressure, blood glucose levels, blood coagulation and inhibition of inflammatory processes (see Table 15.1). Furthermore, carotenoids may be involved in the prevention of macular degeneration in the retina as well as other diseases of the eye (see section 11.8.2).

15.4 Epidemiological evidence for the protective effects of vegetables and fruits and phytochemicals

A number of case–control studies analysed by the World Cancer Research Fund, the American Institute for Cancer Research, and the International Agency for Research on Cancer of the WHO suggest that a high intake of vegetables and fruits is inversely associated with cancer risk. While the outcome of recent prospective cohort studies was less supportive for a cancer-protective effect of vegetables and fruits, overall the totality of evidence still suggests that constituents in plant foods protect against cancer. In addition, data from prospective studies analysing associations at the level of phytochemical intakes and cancer risk suggest that phytochemicals are related to the reduction of cancer risk. As well as evidence about cancer, a number of prospective cohort studies have reported a reduction of risk of cardiovascular disease by 30% in subjects consuming high amounts of vegetables and fruits compared with subjects with a low intake. Similar trends were observed for the intake of specific phytochemicals.

At the present state of knowledge, it is hard to differentiate to what degree the various components in vegetables and fruits (essential nutrients, dietary fibre, phytochemicals) contribute to the observed reduction in disease risk. Human intervention studies are needed to investigate whether the health-promoting effects of vegetables and fruits observed in epidemiological studies are causally related to the intake of phytochemicals.

15.5 Conclusions

Present knowledge of the effects of phytochemicals allows us to conclude that these non-nutritive dietary compounds of plant foods can have health-promoting effects. Phytochemicals, along with vitamins, minerals, trace elements, fatty acids and dietary fibre, are responsible for the protective effects of vegetables and fruits, nuts, cereals and legumes against cancer and cardiovascular disease. Clearly, there is no evidence that a single phytochemical is especially effective in the prevention of cancer or cardiovascular disease. The most protective effect is observed when a large number of different phytochemicals is consumed with plant foods, which presumably exerts cumulative or synergistic effects. For many phytochemicals, detection methods in foods and body fluids have been established. Although the determination of phytochemicals in terms of content, bioavailability and biokinetics is now possible, only key phytochemicals of the individual classes have been carefully studied. Further epidemiological and experimental studies should elucidate the links between the inges-tion of certain phytochemicals and the incidence of specific diseases including mechanisms of protection. In short-term intervention studies, biomarkers need to be identified that yield indications for long-term preventive effects of phytochemicals in humans.

The toxic potential of phytochemicals is negligible, as long as consumption habits are restricted to whole food and avoid extracts or isolates from food. So far, no adverse effects of phytochemicals as part of wholesome foods have been reported, even in subjects on predominantely vegetarian diets.

Nutritional recommendations do not need to be modified in the light of the latest understanding of the health benefits of phytochemicals. Recommended dietary allowances for certain foods of plant origin for prevention or therapy of certain diseases cannot be given at this point in time. However, most nutritional recommendations include an increase in the consumption of plant-derived foods (five-a-day) based on epidemiological evidence that phytochemicals have beneficial effects on the health and wellbeing of humans.

FURTHER READING

1. **Adlercreutz, H., Heinonen, S.M., and Penalvo-Garcia, J.** (2004) Phytoestrogens, cancer and coronary heart disease. *Biofactors*, **22**, 229–36.

2. **Dahan, A., and Altman, H.** (2004) Food–drug interaction: grapefruit juice augments drug bioavailability—mechanism, extent and relevance. *Eur J Clin Nutr*, **58**, 1–9.

3. **Gu, L.** (2003) Concentrations of proanthocyanidins in common food and estimations of normal consumption. *J Nutr*, **134**, 613–7.

4. **Huang, H.C., Joshipura, K.J., Jiang, R.,** *et al.* (2004) Fruit and vegetable intake and risk of major chronic disease. *J Natl Cancer Inst*, **96**, 1577–84.

5. **International Agency for Research on Cancer** (2003) *IARC handbooks of cancer prevention, Vol. 8. Fruit and vegetables*. Lyon, IARC Press.

6. **Kris-Etherton, P.M., Hecker, K.D., Bonanome, A.,** *et al*. (2002) Bioactive compounds in foods: their role in the prevention of cardiovascular disease and cancer. *Am J Med*, **113** (9B), 71S–88S.

7. **Liu, R.H.** (2004) Potential synergy of phytochemicals in cancer prevention: mechanism of action. *J Nutr*, **134**, 3479S–3485S.

8. **Manach, C., Williamson, G. Morand, C.,** *et al.* (2005) Bioavailability and bioefficacy of polyphenols in humans. I. Review of 97 bioavailability studies. *Am J Clin Nutr*, **81** (Suppl. 1), 230S–242S.

9. **Mithen, R.F., Dekker, M., Verkerk, R., Rabot, S., and Johnson, I.T.** (2000) The nutritional significance, biosynthesis and bioavailability of glucosinolates in human foods. *J Sci Food Agric*, **80**, 967–84.

10. **Ostlund, R.E.** (2002) Phytosterols in human nutrition. *Ann Rev Nutr*, **22**, 533–49.

11. **Shi, J., Arunasalam, K., Yeung, D., Kakuda, Y., Mittal, G., and Jiang, Y.** (2004) Saponins from edible legumes: chemistry, processing, and health benefits. *J Med Food*, **7**, 67–78.

12. **Surh, Y.J.** (2003) Cancer chemoprevention with dietary phytochemicals. *Nat Rev Cancer*, **3**, 768–80.

13. **Watzl, B., and Leitzmann, C.** (2005) *Bioaktive Substanzen in Lebensmitteln*, 3rd edition. Stuttgart: Hippokrates.

14. **Webb, A.L., and McCullough, M.L.** (2005) Dietary lignans: potential role in cancer prevention. *Nutr Canc*, **51**, 117–31.

15. **Williamson, G., and Manach, C.** (2005) Bioavailability and bioefficiency of polyphenols in humans. II. Review of 93 intervention studies. *Am J Clin Nutr*, **81** (Suppl. 1), 243S–235S.

 To see topical and scientifically robust updates on nutrition associated with this textbook, and active web links to many of the journal articles in the Reference areas, please see the dedicated Online Resource Centre at www.oxfordtextbooks.co.uk/orc/mann3e/.

PART 3

Nutrition-related disorders

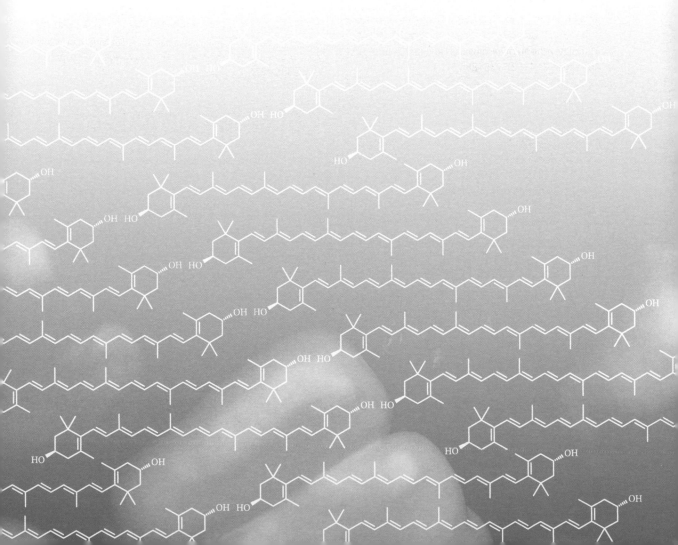

16 Overweight and obesity

Abdullah Omari and Ian D. Caterson

Overweight and obesity are very common conditions in developed societies, and they are becoming more common in developing countries and those in transition. Indeed, the increased prevalence of these disorders in many societies and countries has been accompanied by an increased risk of many associated diseases and health disorders as well as premature mortality. This chapter discusses the prevalence, aetiology, consequences, management and possibilities for prevention of excess adiposity.

16.1 Definition and measurement

Obesity is a condition in which the fat stores (adiposity) are excessive for an individual's height, weight, gender and race to an extent that produces adverse health outcomes. Several measures for assessing and defining obesity exist (Box 16.1). In clinical practice

---

BOX 16.1 Techniques for measuring adiposity

- Body mass index (BMI)
- Waist circumference
- Waist/hip ratio
- Skinfold thickness
- Hydrodensitometry (underwater weighing)
- Bioelectrical impedance
- Dual energy X-ray absorptiometry (DEXA)
- Computerized tomography (CT)
- Nuclear magnetic resonance spectroscopy
- Near-infrared spectroscopy

---

and epidemiological research, obesity is most often defined by the body mass index (BMI), a calculation that gives a reasonable approximation of adiposity. BMI is derived by dividing an individual's weight in kilograms by height in metres squared (kg per m^2). Adults with a BMI between 25 and 29.9 kg/m^2 are categorized as overweight, and those with a BMI greater than 30 kg/m^2 are categorized as obese (Table 16.1). However, in children, or the aged, or the very fit and muscular, the BMI definitions given above are not as useful as an obesity measure. In children, BMI-for-age charts may be used to assess overweight and obesity in this age group (see Chapter 32).

These BMI cut-offs were based on epidemiological studies that showed a steady increase in risk of the consequences of obesity (see section 16.8) as BMI increased above 25. However, these studies were undertaken in Western populations. In some other ethnic groups, the proportions of adipose tissue and lean body mass for a given BMI may differ from that which might be predicted from studies in those

Table 16.1 Recommended definition of obesity according to WHO (2000) for European populations and WHO (Western Pacific Region) /IOTF (2000) for Asian populations

Classification	BMI (kg/m²)		Risk of comorbidities
	Caucasian	Asian	
Underweight	< 18.5	< 18.5	Low (but risk of other clinical problems increased)
Normal range	18.5–24.9	18.5–22.9	Average
Overweight	≥ 25.0	≥ 23.0	
Pre-obese	25–29.9	23.0–24.9	Mildly increased
Obese	≥ 30.0	≥ 25.0	
Class I	30.0–34.9	25.0–29.9	Moderate
Class II	35.0–39.9	≥ 30.0	High
Class III	≥ 40.0		Very high

of European descent. Some Asian populations (notably those from the Indian subcontinent and China) tend to have a greater fat mass (which is more likely to be centrally distributed) and less lean body mass than Europeans for a given BMI. Therefore, the Western Pacific Region of the World Health Organization (WHO) and the International Obesity Taskforce (IOTF) have suggested different cut-off points for Asian adults. It has been suggested that those with a BMI between 23 and 24.9 kg/m² are categorized as overweight or 'at risk' and those with a BMI over 25 kg/m² are categorized as obese (Table 16.1). This range has been accepted by Japan, as an example, while other countries are still considering appropriate action points. Different ranges are being considered for other ethnic groups such as people of Polynesian descent who have more lean body mass than Europeans for a given BMI.

The site of the increased fat tissue is known to be important in identifying individuals at increased risk of obesity-related disease. In particular, excess abdominal (visceral) adipose tissue is associated with considerable risk of cardiovascular disease and metabolic disorders such as diabetes, dyslipidaemia and the metabolic syndrome (see section 16.7 and Chapter 22). Therefore, it is important to measure abdominal fat. Scanning techniques (e.g. DEXA, CT), are used for research purposes but in clinical practice and epidemiological research, measuring waist circumference provides a satisfactory surrogate measure of abdominal obesity. Measurements > 102 cm in men and > 88 cm in women indicate a greatly increased risk of metabolic disease. Measurements exceeding 94 cm in men and > 80 cm in women suggest an increased risk. Those of Asian extraction tend to have more abdominal fat and it has been suggested that waist circumferences > 90 cm in men and > 80 cm in women signify increased risk in Asians. The waist, or abdominal circumference, is measured by placing a non-stretchable measuring tape in a horizontal plane around the abdomen at the level midway between the iliac crest and the lowest rib margin in the mid-axillary lines. Clothing from around the waist should be removed to ensure correct positioning of the tape and the measurement is made at a normal minimal respiration. The waist (W) to hip (H) ratio (W/H ratio) can also be used as a measure of abdominal adiposity. (The hips are measured around the maximal protrusion of the buttocks). A W/H ratio of > 0.8 in women and > 0.9 in men suggests abdominal obesity.

Underwater weighing is now rarely used.

Skinfold thickness measured at several sites is associated with a high level of observer error unless the observers have been formally trained. The remaining methods (Box 16.1) are more costly and are used predominantly for research purposes, though several of the more elaborate techniques are becoming more widely available and are increasingly being used in a clinical setting.

16.2 Prevalence

Obesity and overweight are very common and affect most regions in the world, despite the many public health interventions that have been implemented over the past several decades. Obesity increases with age, and in the developed world, prevalence is greater amongst lower socioeconomic groups than amongst the more affluent. Obesity prevalence has been increasing steadily in most countries over the last few decades. Prevalence data for four countries are illustrated in Fig. 16.1. At all ages, and throughout the world, women are generally found to have a higher mean BMI and higher rates of obesity than men. Overall, the prevalence of obesity in men in developed or Western societies is approximately 20%, while in women it tends to be a few percentage points higher. In the USA prevalence of obesity is greater amongst African–American people than amongst those of European ethnicity. Obesity is very prevalent in eastern European countries. In the Middle East almost

25% of the population is obese. Alarming statistics have been reported from some African countries. For example, 44% of the black female population in the Cape Peninsula in South Africa were found to be obese using current criteria. This is in contrast to Ghana where only 0.8% of the population is obese. South American and Asian countries have not been spared from the obesity epidemic.

Overweight is far more common than obesity, though interestingly in some countries men have higher rates of overweight than women, despite the reverse applying to obesity rates. For example, in Australia, 62% of adult males and approximately 50% of adult females are overweight, whereas almost 20% of adults are obese. In China, 27% of men and 31% of women are overweight, using BMI cut-offs more appropriate for European populations. This is of particular concern since it suggests that the degree of adiposity and associated disorders has been underestimated.

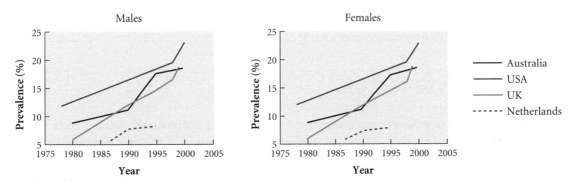

Fig. 16.1 Changing obesity prevalence rates in four countries.

16.3 Perceptions

Perceptions of body size differ from country to country and influence public health and clinical approaches to the management of obesity. In most Western countries, those who are obese are perceived poorly by the community and health professionals and the patients themselves often have low self-esteem. Women tend to see themselves as fatter than they are and seek to be thinner than is necessary or practically possible, predisposing any overweight or obese woman to failure in a treatment programme due to unrealistic expectations. In contrast, men often do not see overweight as a problem and tend not to present for weight control or treatment, unless persuaded to do so as a result of a comorbidity associated with obesity. In some cultures (e.g. Polynesian), overweight and obesity may be regarded as desirable attributes.

16.4 Genetics of obesity

There is strong evidence that genetic factors play an important role in determining weight gain and obesity. For example, Stunkard and colleagues (1986) have shown in an adoption study that the weight of adults adopted as children is related to the weight of their biological parents, rather than the weight of their adopting family. In addition, Bouchard's over-feeding study (Bouchard *et al.*, 1990) involving twins demonstrated a strong genetic component in the amount of weight gained with the same amount of over-feeding. Adoption, twin and family studies indicate that adiposity is highly heritable and the estimated genetic and shared environment contribution to BMI ranges between 60% and 84%.

Many genes are involved in contributing to overweight and obesity in most people (i.e. the inherited tendency is polygenic). However, a number of single gene mutations that cause obesity have been discovered. Some of the genes are listed in Box 16.2. These monogenic causes of obesity are uncommon and usually involve mechanisms associated with energy homeostasis (e.g. appetite regulation). Single gene mutations are typically associated with massive obesity. In addition, pleiotropic syndromes where obesity is a clinical feature have also been described, and they are often associated with mental retardation, organ abnormalities and dysmorphism. The molecular mechanisms by which these genes act to produce obesity are not clear, but the use of mouse models of obesity has greatly enhanced our understanding.

BOX 16.2 Examples of single genes, mutations of which may be associated with massive obesity

Melanocortin-4 receptor
Leptin
Leptin receptor
Pro-opiomelanocortin
Prohormone convertase 1

16.5 Adipocyte factors

Traditionally thought of as an inert mass acting as a reservoir for energy storage, adipose tissue is now known to be an active endocrine organ playing key roles in energy and metabolism homeostasis. This dynamic organ exerts its effects via endocrine, paracrine and autocrine functions, secreting hormones and cytokines (adipokines) that influence the body's energy, immune and autonomic systems.

The recent discoveries of novel adipocyte-related proteins, and the understanding that many proteins initially thought of as not having a role in energy homeostasis do exert effects on such pathways,

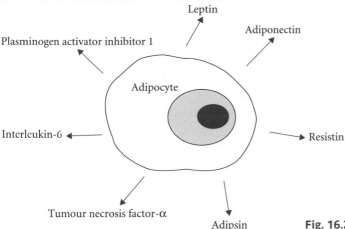

Fig. 16.2 Adipocyte hormones and cytokines.

have fuelled research interest into the adipocyte (fat cell). Two of the adipocyte hormones, leptin and adiponectin, are discussed briefly below. For a discussion of the many other hormones and proteins associated with the adipocyte (Fig. 16.2), the reader is referred to the review by Kershaw and Flier (2004).

16.5.1 Leptin

Leptin is a polypeptide protein produced by adipocytes and secreted in direct proportion to adipose tissue mass and the individual's nutritional status. Leptin levels are high in obese individuals and low in lean people, with females tending to have higher leptin levels than men. More leptin is secreted from subcutaneous than visceral adipose tissue; and when adults lose weight, leptin levels fall. Leptin's main actions are on energy balance (intake and expenditure) predominantly acting via central hypothalamic pathways, with some effects on peripheral tissues such as muscle. In humans, leptin may act as a signal of adequate fat stores for puberty and fertility, or as a signal of famine. Secretion of leptin is influenced by many factors such as glucose metabolism (insulin), inflammation (tumour necrosis factor-α (TNF-α)) and steroid pathways (glucocorticoids and oestrogens), indicating leptin's complex interactions with physiological systems. Deficiency of leptin results in hyperphagia,

decreased energy expenditure and severe obesity. In those rare cases where leptin deficiency exists, treatment with leptin results in a reduction in energy intake and weight loss.

16.5.2 Adiponectin

Adiponectin, a polypeptide secreted exclusively by adipocytes, circulates at high concentrations in the bloodstream. Unlike leptin, adiponectin is inversely associated with adipose tissue mass, and among the obese, levels of adiponectin are reduced. In addition, inflammatory and insulin-resistant states and coronary heart disease are associated with decreased adiponectin levels. Acting on the liver, muscle and blood vessels, adiponectin exerts a wide range of effects that include insulin sensitization, anti-inflammatory effects by antagonizing pro-inflammatory cytokines such as TNF-α, and anti-atherogenic properties by decreasing monocyte adhesion and smooth muscle proliferation in vessel walls. Weight loss and improvement in insulin sensitivity are associated with increasing levels of adiponectin. Also, treatment with thiazolidenediones (a class of antidiabetic drug) is associated with increased levels of adiponectin.

Thus, the adipocyte clearly has many roles other than as a storage organ. These will be further clarified as the complexities of the control of eating and nutrient storage continue to be unravelled.

16.6 Energy balance

Weight stability implies a balance between energy intake (calories consumed) and energy expenditure (calories expended). Despite energy balance oscillating from meal to meal and from day to day, under normal conditions there are no persistent changes in body stores. However, when such a balance is positive for considerable periods, then obesity is likely to occur. Feeding behaviour is influenced by many factors including energy deficiency, social influences, palatability of food and mood. This is balanced by energy expenditure, which includes basal metabolic rate, dietary thermogenesis (meal-induced heat production) and physical activity (Chapter 5).

Energy homeostasis involves complex mechanisms that exist centrally (brain) and peripherally (adipose tissue and gut). Appetite and consequently food intake may be initiated by both environmental factors and biochemical interactions. Environmental factors include cultural and psychological influences, and olefactory and visual stimuli. The biochemical interactions that control appetite occur principally in the arcuate nucleus of the hypothalamus in response to peripheral stimuli. The appetite-stimulating pathway is situated in the ventromedial part of this nucleus. Decreased leptin levels activate neurones that express two neuropeptides that increase appetite: neuropeptide Y (NPY) and agouti-related protein (AGRP). Ghrelin, secreted by the stomach during fasting, also stimulates the neurones that express NPY and AGRP. The central appetite-suppressing pathway is situated in the dorsolateral part of the arcuate nucleus. This pathway is stimulated by leptin and insulin via the expression of melanocortins and corticotrophins. Cholecystokinin (CCK) and peptide YY (PYY) are gut-derived factors that are released after eating and also stimulate the appetite suppression pathway. Thus, leptin, which circulates in proportion to adipose tissue mass, may be regarded as a long-term signal to appetite control, whereas insulin, CCK and PYY are more acute responses to meal ingestion. In theory, these complex biochemical interactions should ensure energy balance and weight stability. However, psychological factors, and the presentation and energy density of food (high fat, high sugar) may override the control mechanisms and lead to weight gain. It is important to appreciate that a very small daily excess of energy may lead to a large accumulation of fat over a prolonged period. For example, a 44 kJ (10.5 kcal) daily excess would lead to a 10 kg weight gain over 20 years.

16.7 Environmental and lifestyle factors

Despite the genetic factors underlying overweight and obesity, environmental and lifestyle factors are very important determinants of the current obesity epidemic. Obesity rates have increased over the last several decades (see Fig. 16.1), while the gene pool has been stable. The potential for environmental factors to overpower genetic effects is well illustrated by two groups of genetically similar Pima Indians. Those living on reservations in Arizona in the USA do little physical activity and consume much energy-dense food. They have exceptionally high rates of obesity and comorbidities. Those following their traditional subsistence lifestyles in mountainous areas of Mexico have low rates of obesity and associated diseases. Transition from traditional to more Western ways of life seems to explain the relatively rapid increase in rates. Attempts have been made to unravel the components of this obesogenic environment and determine the cause more precisely.

16.7.1 Food intake

It is difficult to quantify with any degree of certainty the extent to which total amount of food consumed contributes to obesity. Individuals who are overweight or obese tend to underestimate their total energy consumption, sometimes by as much as 50%. National statistics regarding energy consumption are also not particularly reliable, though in a number of countries it appears that total energy intake may have declined, despite the increase in BMI and obesity. This suggests that a decline in activity must play an important role in the increasing rates of obesity. However, it seems unlikely that the increased prevalence of obesity is entirely explained by a reduction in energy output and that an increase in intake must in some way contribute to the excess accumulation of body fat. The methods for measuring energy intake accurately cannot be used in epidemiological studies easily. Therefore, the nature of the food consumed has been the focus of more recent research. Foods, food groups and nutrients are more easily measured than total energy intake. The WHO/FAO Expert Consultation on Diet, Nutrition and the Prevention of Chronic Diseases (TRS 916) has identified a number of lifestyle-related factors that are considered to promote or protect against excessive weight gain (Table 16.2). A high intake of energy-dense foods (which are typically also micronutrient poor) is considered promotive and a high intake of non-starch polysaccharide is considered to be protective factors. Energy-dense foods are high in fat, free sugars and starches, and may be more easily over-consumed than other foods. Trials that have covertly manipulated fat content and energy density have established that the resultant passive overconsumption can lead to excessive intakes of total energy. High intakes of sugars, sweetened soft drinks and fruit juices are also regarded as probable causal factors contributing to overweight and obesity. The environment may provide a range of societal determinants that alter food intake and contribute to excessive intake. For example, a home and school environment that supports appropriate food choices will probably be associated with a decreased risk, whereas heavy marketing of energy-dense foods is likely to increase the risk. Also, foods high in fat and sugar tend to be cheap to produce and so may be more readily purchased by those in lower socio-economic situations.

Table 16.2 Summary of strength of evidence of factors that might promote or protect against weight gain and obesity

Evidence	Decreased risk	No relationship	Increased risk
Convincing	Regular physical activity High dietary intake of non-starch polysaccharide		Sedentary lifestyles High intake of energy-dense, micronutrient-poor foods
Probable	Home and school environments that support healthy food choices for children Breastfeeding		Heavy marketing of energy-dense foods and fast-food outlets High intake of sugar-sweetened soft drinks and fruit juices Adverse socioeconomic conditions*
Possible	Low glycaemic index foods	Protein content of the diet	Large portions High proportion of food prepared outside the home (developed countries) 'Rigid restraint/periodic disinhibition' eating patterns
Insufficient	Increased eating frequency		Alcohol

Adapted from WHO Technical Report Series 916. Diet, nutrition and the prevention of chronic diseases.
*Especially for women in developed countries.

16.7.2 Exercise

Low levels of voluntary and incidental activity are also important factors in weight gain. This may result from changes in lifestyle (giving up competitive sport, taking on more sedentary job responsibilities, having children), ageing or disease (such as arthritis, which restricts mobility, or respiratory or cardiovascular disease, which reduce exercise capacity). Also, urbanization, affluence and modernization of lifestyle have resulted in changes to exercise amount and pattern. The modern lifestyle relies more on technology and the incidental activities of daily living have been reduced. The prevalence of obesity in children has been related directly to hours of television viewed. Television watching may result in obesity because of reduced activity, reduced resting metabolic rate while viewing, excessive food intake during periods of inactivity, or because of inappropriate food intake resulting from television advertising.

16.7.3 Other factors

Other possible factors in aetiology include cessation of smoking (a 1–4 kg weight gain is usual), pregnancy or initiation of treatment with some medications, particularly some antidiabetics, some antiepileptics and antipsychotics (Box 16.3). Hormonal alterations are often blamed as the cause of obesity, but in reality such diseases rarely produce obesity. The weight gain associated with endocrine conditions (see Box 16.4) is usually of the order of 5–10 kg. Type 2 diabetes mellitus is often associated with obesity but it is not yet clear whether the two conditions have the same genetic predisposing factors, or whether type 2 diabetes is caused by the insulin resistance of obesity.

BOX 16.3 Medications associated with weight gain

- Diabetes management
  - Insulin
  - Sulphonylureas
  - Thiazolidinediones
- Steroids
- Antipsychotic medications (including newer anti-psychotics)
- Antidepressants
- Lithium
- Antiepileptics
  - Valproate
- Beta-blockers
- Antihistamines

BOX 16.4 Hormonal conditions associated with weight gain

- Hypothyroidism
- Acromegaly
- Cushing's syndrome
- Polycystic ovarian syndrome
- Hyperprolactinaemia
- Insulin resistance

16.8 Consequences of obesity

There is no doubt regarding the adverse health consequences of obesity, with some of these listed in Box 16.5. Being overweight is associated with a modest increase in risk of the conditions discussed below and the risks increase with the degree of obesity, so that for those with a BMI > 30 kg/m^2, total mortality rates are 2 (for women) to 2.5 (for men) times greater than for those with a BMI in the healthy range. These data are based on Caucasian populations, and the risks of metabolic disease may be much greater in Asians. In addition, the distribution of obesity is an important determinant of the health risks associated with

---

BOX 16.5 Consequences of obesity

- *Metabolic*:
  Insulin resistance, impaired glucose tolerance and type 2 diabetes
  Dyslipidaemia
  – Increased VLDL, triglyceride, increased LDL cholesterol
  – Reduced HDL cholesterol
  – Increased apo B lipoprotein (small dense molecules)
  Fatty liver/non-alcoholic steatohepatitis (NASH)
  Gallstones
  Polycystic ovarian syndrome / infertility in women
- *Cardiovascular*:
  Hypertension
  Coronary heart disease
  Varicose veins
  Peripheral oedema

- *Cancer*:
  Breast
  Endometrium
  Prostate
  Kidney
  Pancreas
  Colon
- *Mechanical*:
  Osteoarthritis
  Spinal complications
  Obstructive sleep apnoea
- *Social*:
  Low self-esteem
  Adverse judgement by society
- *Other*:
  Increased anaesthetic risk
  Increased risk of fractures in children

---

obesity. The metabolic complications of obesity, listed in the box, are associated with increased visceral fat, even if the BMI is within the desirable range.

While weight reduction is associated with a reduction in the various risks, the evidence that life can be prolonged by intentional weight loss is inconclusive and is being clarified in a number of clinical trials.

16.8.1 Metabolic consequences

Secondary dyslipidaemias (abnormalities in plasma lipids) are common in those who are obese, especially in those with increased waist circumference or high W/H ratio. These dyslipidaemias are characterized by raised levels of very-low-density lipoproteins (VLDLs), raised triglycerides, low levels of high-density lipoprotein (HDL) cholesterol and atypical low-density lipoprotein (LDL) particles, which tend to be smaller and denser than usual. LDL levels may also be raised. Abnormalities of carbohydrate metabolism, manifesting as insulin resistance, impaired glucose tolerance (IGT) and often type 2 diabetes, are associated with central adiposity, as are elevated liver transaminases. In the absence of excess alcohol consumption, the latter suggests the diagnosis of fatty liver, non-alcoholic steatohepatitis (NASH). This condition is associated with increasing rates of liver cirrhosis. This clustering of metabolic abnormalities along with hypertension that is associated with central obesity is often referred to as the metabolic syndrome, and while the precise mechanism is not understood, insulin resistance is believed to play an important role (see Chapter 22).

The prevalence of gallstones increases with increasing age and weight. Polycystic ovarian syndrome and associated decreased fertility are associated with obesity. Of note, many of those women undergoing *in vitro* fertilization programmes are overweight or obese and with weight loss the success of such programmes increases substantially.

16.8.2 Cardiovascular consequences

Obesity is an important risk factor for the development of cardiovascular disease. In part, this may be due to the constellation of metabolic and other abnormalities associated with the metabolic syndrome. Obesity particularly increases the risk of coronary heart disease in those younger than 50. Varicose veins and peripheral oedema occur more commonly in obese than normal-weight individuals and cardiac abnormalities such as cor pulmonale and lymphoedema may occur with gross obesity.

16.8.3 Obesity-associated cancer

Recent studies have emphasized that several cancers are increasing and that this increased cancer prevalence is strongly associated with obesity. The cancers implicated are the hormone-dependent cancers (breast, endometrial and prostatic) and cancer of the colon. Decreasing weight reduces the number of colonic polyps that may be the precursors to malignancy. Cancers of the kidney and pancreas occur less frequently but are also associated with obesity.

16.8.4 Mechanical consequences

Osteoarthritis of both the weight-bearing and non-weight-bearing joints (e.g. in the hands) is more common in obesity. Occasionally, chest pain may be caused by spinal complications in the lower cervical and upper thoracic region, resulting in referred pain.

Obstructive sleep apnoea is common among obese individuals, especially in men. They often report symptoms such as snoring, stopping breathing during sleep (apnoea), morning headache, daytime sleepiness and difficulty in concentration. These symptoms can be successfully treated with weight loss, and/or with continuous positive airways pressure administered by a nasal mask while the patient sleeps.

16.8.5 Social consequences

Obese people, particularly those who have made many unsuccessful attempts to lose weight, often have low self-esteem. Obesity or its medical consequences may prevent individuals from doing many activities that they enjoy, resulting in impairment of quality of life. Children see obesity as a disability, and often may be teased at school or feel socially isolated. In some societies, there is a poor perception of obesity by the community at large and obese individuals may experience discrimination in various forms, including reduced employment opportunities. This does not apply to all societies. In many Polynesian and some African countries, being overweight or obese is regarded as a desirable state, although there is evidence to suggest the younger generation may be adopting more Western views of body image.

16.9 Management

16.9.1 Whom to treat?

Given the high prevalence of overweight and obesity in many countries, individualized care for all would place an unsustainable burden on health care resources. Public health approaches (see section 16.10) to reduce the risks of becoming overweight or obese are a priority for those who are already overweight, and societal attempts to reduce the 'obesogenicity' of the environment will facilitate weight loss. For the healthy overweight and obese individuals and those with no family history of diabetes and heart disease, nutrition advice and encouragement to increase activity may suffice. However, it is important to provide

ongoing encouragement and follow-up to ensure that lifestyle changes are sustained.

For those with a BMI > 27 and abdominal adiposity, the metabolic syndrome, or other medical complications, and those with BMI > 30, both intensive dietary advice (preferably from a dietitian or nutritionist) and medical supervision (to decide if adjunctive treatment is required if there is no weight loss with diet and increased activity alone) are necessary (Table 16.3). In Asians, because of the greater risk and higher prevalence of metabolic diseases at lower BMIs, active intervention for overweight should be considered earlier.

Table 16.3 Outline of obesity management approach

BMI	INTERVENTION			
	General Advice	Lifestyle programme	Adjunctive therapy	Possibilities
18.5–24.9	Maintain weight			
25–29.9		Use		
High risk*		Use	Consider	Pharmacotherapy
30–34.9		Use	Consider/use	Pharmacotherapy or VLCDs
High risk*		Use	Use	Pharmacotherapy +/− VLCDs
35–39.9		Use	Use	Pharmacotherapy +/− VLCDs
High risk*		Use	Use	Pharmacotherapy + VLCDs or surgery
40+		Use	Use	Pharmacotherapy + VLCDs or surgery

*Individuals at high risk for a given BMI are those with high waist circumference and the presence of comorbidities (e.g. type 2 diabetes, impaired glucose intolerance, coronary heart disease, dyslipidaemia)
VLCDs, very-low-calorie diets.

16.9.2 Basic interventions

At the outset, it is important to for patients to appreciate that weight-loss therapy involves appreciable lifestyle changes that have to be maintained long term. There are two phases of therapy, active weight loss and weight maintenance. The basic interventions involve a change in eating and exercise habits and such changes invariably involve behaviour modification. It is important to set achievable goals for each individual and these should extend beyond the number of kilograms to be lost (see Table 16.4). Weight loss should be planned in stages. Goals should be recorded and discussed at subsequent visits, and the attaining of goals acknowledged. Patients should be aware that even a modest weight loss (of the order of 5–10% of original weight) may be expected to result in clinically important benefits (Box 16.6).

An 'eating plan' rather than a 'diet' is recommended. Most overweight and obese people will be aware of at least some of the many available diet books. The Atkins, Zone, South Beach, Low GI (glycaemic index) and CSIRO approaches and various low-fat diets (Box 16.7) have been best sellers. Regardless of which eating plan is to be implemented, patients need to understand and accept that weight loss only occurs when energy intake is less than energy output. Reducing energy intake is principally achieved by consuming smaller portions and reducing energy-dense foods. The latter are high in fat and sugars.

Table 16.4 Goals of obesity therapy

- Weight loss—set realistic losses, in stages
- Change in body shape and size (less abdominal fat)
- Control of associated disorders:
  impaired carbohydrate metabolism (diabetes, impaired glucose tolerance)
  dyslipidaemia
  hypertension
  sleep apnoea
  arthritis
- Mobility
- Reduction in medications
- Improved cardiovascular fitness
- Psychological and social factors
- Individual goals:
  fitting into clothes
  need for, or ability to have, operation
  reduction in pain

BOX 16.6 Major benefits of moderate weight loss (10%)

Mortality
  Decreased overall as well as diabetes and cancer-related mortality with intentional weight loss

Reduced blood pressure
  10 mm Hg decrease

Improved serum lipids
  Decreased LDL-cholesterol and triglycerides
  Increased HDL-cholesterol

Reduced rate of progression from impaired glucose tolerance to type 2 diabetes

Better diabetes control

BOX 16.7 Frequently recommended weight-loss diets

Low fat/high carbohydrate:	reduced total fat high in fibre-rich carbohydrates
Reduced carbohydrate:	Zone, relatively high in protein South Beach, relatively high in protein CSIRO, relatively high in protein Atkins, very low carbohydrate, high fat/high protein
Improved carbohydrate:	low-glycaemic index diet

This in turn may possibly be facilitated by increasing carbohydrates rich in non-starch polysaccharides (dietary fibre) and which have a low GI. Such foods are satiating, as is protein, and an increase of either in the diet may help weight loss. These principles constitute the conventional approach to weight loss. Several of the novel approaches to weight loss rely to some extent on the satiating effects of protein (Zone, South Beach, CSIRO, Atkins), though the novelty and prescriptive nature of some may also account for the reduced energy intakes. The ketosis associated with very high intakes of fat recommended in the Atkins approach may result in nausea, which in turn reduces appetite. Several of these approaches result in enhanced weight loss during the early phase of adoption but by 1 year there appears to be little difference between these 'new' and the 'conventional' approaches using low-fat, low-energy-dense foods and less total energy. While the newer high-fat and high-protein approaches do not appear to be associated in the short term with adverse effects on cardiovascular risk factors, no long-term follow-up studies of safety or efficacy have been undertaken.

These novel approaches may be suitable for some people but it is essential to have an individualized approach for each patient. For example, there is little point in recommending a high-fibre, high-carbohydrate diet to a farmer accustomed to large meat meals. Far more effective would be to reduce portion size and ensure lean meat intake, with some small changes to food choices. 'Calorie counting' may be useful for some patients who require highly prescriptive advice to achieve weight loss. However, for many people, ensuring appropriate food choices, with quantitative advice regarding particularly energy-dense foods or with regard to fat and free sugars, is usually sufficient. It is obviously essential to ensure that energy-reduced diets are nutritionally adequate in all respects. Encouraging a variety of foods from the different food groups will usually ensure this.

Not all obese and overweight people have an excessive caloric intake all the time. They may be binge eaters, overeating periodically. Such binges tend to be produced by emotional problems or stress and be the cause of regaining weight after satisfactory loss. Patients can be helped to recognize stress cues and learn alternative ways of dealing with them. Alcohol may be an important source of extra energy intake in some overweight and obese men, and this needs to be considered in their eating programme. The use of low-alcohol beers is often a good starting point.

Exercise is a most important part of any programme. In itself it may not produce major weight loss, but it helps to alter body composition favourably, reducing fat mass and increasing muscle. It also increases mobility and induces a feeling of wellbeing and improves the metabolic and clinical comorbidities of obesity. For the obese and overweight, low-intensity but prolonged exercise produces these changes, even if cardiovascular fitness is not achieved. Increasing the 'volume' of activity (volume = time × occurrences × intensity) should be emphasized. One way of doing this is by increasing 'incidental activity' (or taking the active choice) wherever possible; it may involve using the stairs, walking to the shops, and even such small changes as not using the television remote control. Increasing exercise to a sufficient extent to achieve cardiovascular fitness confers additional benefit since, regardless of BMI, these levels of activity appear to confer benefit. An individual with a high degree of cardiovascular fitness will be at lower risk than someone with the same BMI who does not have this greater level of fitness, and it is important to note that weight loss (reduced BMI) reduces the cardiovascular risk even more.

Behaviour modification is an integral and important part of therapy and it is essential to prevent regain of weight by aiming to change habits in the long term. The techniques used include the keeping of food and exercise logs, cognitive restructuring (removing the guilt from eating), awareness and changing of habits, and improving self-esteem. Such therapy may be given to individuals or in groups.

16.9.3 Adjunctive therapies

If lifestyle interventions alone do not achieve the set goals, it is necessary to consider whether any additional adjunctive therapies are required. Drug therapy may be of value and should be considered in those who are markedly obese or when the comorbidities of obesity have developed, when there has been no weight loss, or inadequate loss, after 12 weeks on a lifestyle programme.

Despite both perceived and real problems with the earlier drugs to treat obesity, the newer drugs, studied in clinical trials for up to 4 years, are effective and appear to be relatively free of major side effects (Box 16.8).

Orlistat is an intestinal lipase inhibitor. By this action, it reduces fat absorption (30% of fat eaten is malabsorbed). This can cause gastrointestinal prob-

---

BOX 16.8 Drugs used to treat obesity

Centrally acting
- Sibutramine (+ some thermogenesis)
- (Rimonabant)

Peripheral action in gastrointestinal tract
- Orlistat

Less commonly used

Centrally acting
- Phentermine
- Fluoxetine
- Topiramate

Peripheral action
- Metformin

---

lems so that people using the drug must be given a low-fat diet. Treatment with Orlistat produces an extra 70% weight loss over that with an intensive life-style programme alone. It is associated with reductions in cholesterol over that to be expected with weight loss, falls in blood pressure and serum triglycerides, and improvement of insulin sensitivity. Diabetes control is improved in those who have already developed the condition. The major side effects of this drug are gastrointestinal and are controlled by adherence to a low-fat diet. In theory, absorption of fat-soluble vitamins might be compromised with long-term usage, but levels of these vitamins remain in the normal range after 4 years of treatment. However, a wise precaution is to supplement these vitamins (at night) if a course of treatment of more than 1 year is contemplated.

Sibutramine is a central appetite suppressant and also has a mild thermogenic action. It is a derivative of fluoxetine, and is a selective serotonin reuptake inhibitor (SSRI) as well as a selective norepinephrine reuptake inhibitor (SNRI). Sibutramine produces a 50–100% additional weight loss above that associated with a lifestyle intervention. Comorbidities of obesity are reduced in proportion to the weight lost. However, there does appear to be a specific effect of sibutramine on raising HDL-cholesterol quite markedly.

In those who are depressed, the SSRI antidepressant drugs (e.g. fluoxetine) may assist weight reduction. Metformin is used in insulin-resistant patients. The antiepileptic drug topiramate is very effective but its use is limited by side effects.

Rimonabant is one potentially interesting new agent. It is a blocker of the endocannabinoid system and thus has an entirely different action from other drugs. It produces the same amount of additional weight loss as the other drugs, reduces triglycerides and, like sibutramine, appears to have a specific effect in increasing HDL cholesterol levels. Part of its effect on metabolism may be because it increases adiponectin levels. It is likely to be available for routine clinical use in the near future.

Very-low-calorie diets (VLCDs), which contain between 400 and 800 calories per day, are largely protein-based with essential fatty acids, vitamins and minerals and very little carbohydrate. They are effective at producing rapid and early weight loss in the very obese but the weight loss at longer-term follow-up may not be greater than that achieved by following a standard programme. However, they have been shown to produce weight loss that can be sustained for 4–5 years when used for 2–3 months to replace two meals a day and then replacing one or two meals daily. They are of particular use when rapid weight reduction is needed for medical reasons (e.g. pre-operatively). When consumed as replacements for all meals, VLCDs should only be used under medical (or nutritionist) supervision because there are potential dangers, including cardiac arrhythmias, electrolyte abnormalities and gout. Particular care should be taken when VLCDs are used by those on multiple medications, especially insulin or sulphonylureas, when there is a greater risk of hypoglycaemic reactions. Reducing the dosage of these agents when the VLCDs are commenced and monitoring blood sugar levels thereafter is necessary. VLCDs are generally administered as outpatient care as part of a programme that includes exercise and behaviour modification, regular follow-ups and preparation for the reintroduction of normal eating. Their use should follow a period of intensive education regarding the lifestyle changes necessary to lose weight and maintain such weight loss.

Surgery for the management of obesity is the most effective form of therapy. This specialized surgery is called 'bariatric surgery'. With this surgery, and in conjunction with a lifestyle programme and regular follow-up, substantial weight loss (20–30 kg) has been maintained for up to 10 years. This weight loss is associated with resolution of many of the associated disorders, particularly type 2 diabetes. However, it is relevant that hypertension has been found to return after 8 years despite continued weight loss (i.e. weight loss has delayed some other gene/effect, which causes hypertension by 8 years). The operations used today tend to be variations on gastric bypass or the far less invasive gastric banding (an inflatable band is inserted laparoscopically). The side effects of surgery are due to the restriction the surgery places on eating, and large meals or some particular foods may cause vomiting. There are also potential problems with band slippage, or ulceration at the site of the bypass operation, but these are rare in the hands of an experienced surgeon. Those who have had bariatric surgery need to have regular nutritional follow-up consultations (especially years after the surgery) to ensure their intake is nutritionally adequate.

Bariatric surgery is effective and should be considered in those with grade 2 obesity (BMI > 35) who have associated diseases or in those with BMI > 40.

16.9.4 Maintenance therapy

The planned maintenance phase is critical to all weight-reduction programmes. This may consist of regular reinforcement visits and regular weigh-ins, as well as the continued application of behaviour modification principles and techniques. Even when weight loss is achieved, the predisposing factors remain and so does the propensity for weight regain. Weight regain should be identified early so that appropriate treatment may be reintroduced. It is possible that the newer drugs mentioned above may be used to help weight maintenance. Repeated short courses of

VLCDs (for 1 month every 6 months or so) may be considered.

Weight-reduction programmes are undertaken by commercial organizations, but general practitioners working in conjunction with dietitians, physiotherapists and exercise physiologists, and other specialists, have a particularly important role to play because they know their patients well and are trusted. Programmes run by dietitians (and/or other health professionals) in the context of general practice can be particularly effective.

16.10 Prevention of obesity

The rapidly increasing prevalence of overweight and obesity in many countries and the difficulties involved in achieving and maintaining satisfactory weight loss in those who are already obese mean that preventive approaches offer the only meaningful long-term solution to reversing the worldwide epidemic of obesity. Many approaches have been tried to date, but thus far no country has been able to reverse the escalating rates in the population as a whole. However, the fact that there is now less overweight in those of higher socioeconomic status in Western societies shows that despite the role of genetic factors, obesity is partially preventable. Several clinical trials suggest that increased physical activity in children and reduced consumption of sugary drinks may slow the rate of excessive weight gain.

Targeted preventative programmes need to be developed and evaluated. For children, the most appropriate first step is to ensure that some planned physical activity is done each day at school and that there is a correct approach to nutrition and eating in the curriculum and school canteen. Lack of time and cost seem to be the justification for rejection of this approach by schools or education authorities. In order to make major inroads into the obesity epidemic, further environmental changes will also be necessary. These will require changes in attitudes and political will.

Facilities for physical activities are required in both urban and rural environments. Appropriate food choices must be available at reasonable cost. Advertising of energy-dense food and drinks to children should be restricted. The development of programmes that aim to prevent excessive weight gain in children and adults and that are appropriate for specific groups must be one of the most important challenges for preventive medicine in both affluent and developing countries. Reducing the obesogenic environment will not only help to stem the tide of the obesity epidemic and its consequences, but will facilitate weight reduction in those who are already overweight and obese.

FURTHER READING

1. **Astrup, A., Meinert Larsen, T., and Harper, A.** (2004) Atkins and other low-carbohydrate diets: hoax or an effective tool for weight loss? *Lancet*, **364**, 897–9.

2. **Astrup, A., Caterson, I., Zelissen, P.,** *et al.* (2004) Topiramate: long-term maintenance of weight loss induced by a low-calorie diet in obese subjects. *Obes Res*, **12**, 1658–69.

3. **Bouchard, C., Després, J.-P., and Mauriege, P.** (1993) Genetic and non-genetic determinants of regional fat distribution. *Endocrine Rev*, **14**, 72–93.

4. **Bouchard, C., Tremblay, A., Després, J.-P.,** *et al.* (1990) The response to long-term over-feeding in identical twins. *N Engl J Med*, **322**, 1477–82.

5. **Cole, T.J., Bellizzi, M.C., Flegal, K.M., and Dietz, W.C.** (2000) Establishing a standard definition for child overweight and obesity worldwide: international survey. *Br Med J*, **320**, 1240–3.

6. **Ebbeling, C.B., Leidig, M.M., Sinclair, K.B.,** *et al.* (2005) Effects of an ad libitum low-glycaemic load diet on cardiovascular disease risk factors in obese young adults. *Amer J Clin Nutr*, **81**, 976–82.

7. **Foster, G.D., Wyatt, H.R., Hill, J.O.,** *et al.* (2003) A randomized trial of a low-carbohydrate diet for obesity. *N Engl J Med*, **348**, 2082–90.

8. **Gill, T.P.** (2001) Cardiovascular risk in the Asia–Pacific region from a nutrition and metabolic point of view: abdominal obesity. *Asia Pacific J Clin Nutr*, **10**, 85–9.

9. **Gu, D., Reynolds, K., Wu, X., et al.** (2005) Prevalence of the metabolic syndrome and overweight among adults in China. *Lancet*, **365**, 1398–405.

10. **James, W.P., Astrup, A., Finer, N., et al.** (2000) Effect of sibutramine on weight maintenance after weight loss: a randomized trial. STORM Study Group. Sibutramine trial of obesity reduction and maintenance. *Lancet*, **356**, 2119–25.

11. **James, W.P.T., Jackson-Leach, R., and Mhurchu, C.** (2004) Overweight and obesity (high body mass index). In: Ezzati, M., Lopez, A.D., Rodgers, A., and Murray, C.J.L. (eds) *Comparative quantification of health risks: global and regional burden of disease attributable to selected major risk factors*. Geneva, World Health Organization, pp. 497–596.

12. **Kershaw, E.E., and Flier, J.S.** (2004) Adipose tissue as an endocrine organ. *J Clin Endocrinol Metab*, **89**, 2548–56.

13. **Kopelman, P., Caterson, I., and Dietz, W.** (2005) *Clinical obesity*, 2nd edition. Melbourne, Blackwell.

14. **Noakes, M., Keogh, J.B., Foster, P.R., et al.** (2005) Effect of an energy-restricted, high-protein, low-fat diet relative to a conventional high-carbohydrate, low-fat diet on weight loss, body composition, nutritional status, and markers of cardiovascular health in obese women. *Am J Clin Nutr*, **81**, 1298–306.

15. **Samaha, F.F., Iqbal, N., Seshadri, P., et al.** (2003) A low-carbohydrate as compared with a low-fat diet in severe obesity. *N Engl J Med*, **348**, 2074–81.

16. **Segal-Isaacson, C.J., Johnson, S., Tomuta, V., et al.** (2004) A randomized trial comparing low-fat and low-carbohydrate diets matched for energy and protein. *Obes Res*, **12** (Suppl. 2), 130S–140S.

17. **Sjostrom, L., Rissanen, A., Andersen, T., et al.** (1998) Randomized placebo-controlled trial of orlistat for weight loss and prevention of weight regain in obese patients. European Multicentre Orlistat Study Group. *Lancet*, **352**, 167–72 (see comment).

18. **Stern, L., Iqbal, N., Seshadri, P., et al.** (2004) The effects of low-carbohydrate versus conventional weight loss diets in severely obese adults: one-year follow-up of a randomized trial. *Ann Intern Med*, **140**, 778–85.

19. **Stunkard, A.J., Sorensen, T.I., Hanis, C., et al.** (1986) An adoption study of human obesity. *N Engl J Med*, **314**, 193–8.

20. **Toubro, S., and Astrup, A.** (1997) Randomized comparison of diets for maintaining obese subjects' weight after major weight loss: ad lib, low fat, high carbohydrate diet v fixed energy intake. *Br Med J*, **314**, 29–34.

21. **Van Gaal, L.F., Rissanen, A.M., Scheen, A.J., et al.** (2005) Effects of the cannabinoid-1 receptor blocker rimonabant on weight reduction and cardiovascular risk factors in overweight patients: 1-year experience from the RIO-Europe study. *Lancet*, **365**, 1389–97. (Erratum: *Lancet*, **9483**, 370.)

22. **WHO** (2000) *Obesity: preventing and managing the global epidemic*. Report of a WHO consultation. Technical Report Series 894. Geneva, World Health Organization.

23. **Wolf, A.M., and Colditz, G.A.** (1998) Current estimates of the economic cost of obesity in the USA. *Obes Res*, **6**, 97–106.

24. **Zimmet, P., and Inoue, S.** (2002) *The Asia–Pacific perspective: Redefining obesity and its treatment*. WHO, IOTF, IASO.

 To see topical and scientifically robust updates on nutrition associated with this textbook, and active web links to many of the journal articles in the Reference areas, please see the dedicated Online Resource Centre at www.oxfordtextbooks.co.uk/orc/mann3e/.

17 The challenge of the chronic diseases epidemic for science and society

Phil James and Neville Rigby

17.1 The impact of chronic diseases and their relationship to diet

The term 'chronic diseases' usually refers to the adult conditions of cardiovascular disease, cancers, diabetes and obesity. The non-communicable diseases include mental illnesses, respiratory diseases and many other conditions, which are not traditionally considered to relate to nutritional problems.

Cardiovascular diseases are the principal causes of premature death (< 75 years) and disability in the world and are predicted to remain so for the next 20 years. Fig. 17.1 shows the main causes of death in the developing world as assessed in 2001. Cardiovascular diseases and cancers have been the principal causes of death in the developed world for many years. There are, however, nearly twice as many deaths from cardiovascular disease in the developing world as there are in affluent societies, with rising rates in many countries and with a major impact on both the overwhelmed health services and the economy of many lower-income countries.

Nutritional factors make major contributions to the biggest risk factors inducing disease, disability and premature death in the world as shown in Fig. 17.2. Smoking is of great importance, but the major effects of nutrition and physical inactivity on many of the other risk factors make diet-induced or related diseases the biggest contributor to premature death in the world.

The detailed analysis of the relative importance of each nutritional factor in determining the develop-

ment of a particular risk factor is difficult to calculate, but Table 17.1 gives an estimate of the possible contributors to high blood pressure. When people reduce weight, this can have a substantial, beneficial effect in lowering blood pressure, but part of the fall reflects the direct impact of dietary changes such as reduced fat and increased fruit and vegetable intakes, which are used to induce the weight loss. The relative effects of different dietary factors are calculated from short-term studies in adults, but there seem to be other longer-term effects of diet on blood pressure, starting with inappropriate fetal nutrition, which may establish the life-long trends in blood pressure or the magnitude to which the child and adult's blood pressure responds to diet. Early exposure of infants to high-salt diets seems to programme a child to greater increases in their future blood pressure and perhaps a greater sensitivity to some nutritional factors. Thus the classic INTERSALT studies showed that in some very isolated societies, where salt intakes are very low, blood pressures do not rise with age and hypertension is almost unknown. The subjects tend, however, also to be thin, on low-fat diets and with ample vegetable and fruit intakes—three conditions that help to reduce blood pressure. Fig. 17.3 sets out a range of nutritional factors that contribute to the chronic diseases.

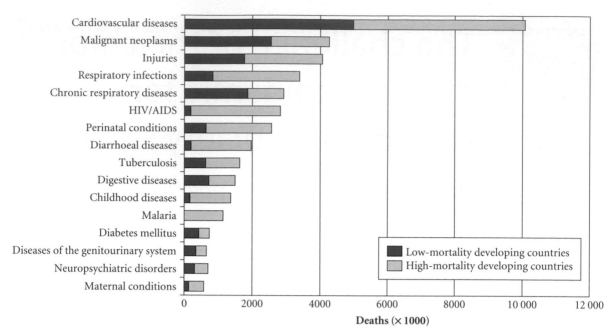

Fig. 17.1 The 16 leading causes of death in developing countries in 2001.

Source: WHO (2003) The World Health Report. Geneva, WHO.

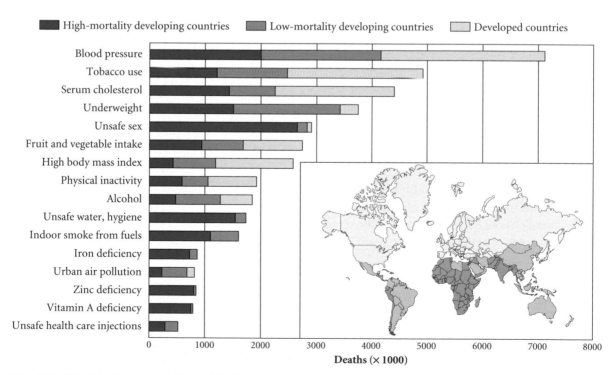

Fig. 17.2 Global deaths attributable to 16 leading risk factors in 2001.

Source: WHO (2003) The World Health Report. Geneva, WHO.

Table 17.1 The relative merits of dietary change and weight loss in determining blood pressure in normal and hypertensive adults

	Systolic BP change (mmHg)		Diastolic BP change (mmHg)	
	Normotensives	Hypertensives	Normotensives	Hypertensives
Increase fruit and vegetable by 200 g/day*	−0.8	−7.2	−0.3	−2.8
Reduce fat intake by 10% energy*	−2.7	−4.1	−1.8	−2.6
Reduce salt from 10 g/day to 4 g/day*	−1.6	−7.6	Average −3.5	
Total weight-independent dietary benefit*	−7.1	−11.5	Average −4.5	
Increased free sugars intake of 145 g/day	+6.9		+5.3	
Reduce weight by 10 kg or 10%	Average −6.1 for 10% loss		Average −3.7 for 10 kg loss	

*The basis for these analyses are set out by Haslam and James (2005).

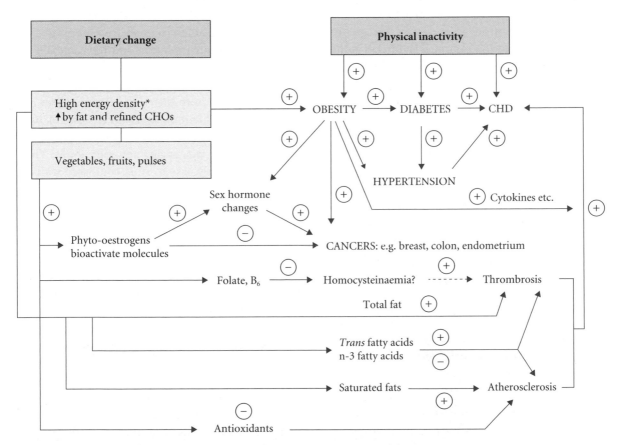

* Energy density reduced by water-holding, bulky foods, e.g. tubers, cereals, vegetables, fruits, pulses.

Fig. 17.3 A summary of some of the potential roles of different dietary factors and physical inactivity in the development of obesity and its principal comorbidities. CHD, coronary heart disease; CHO, carbohydrate.

17.2 Optimum intakes of nutrients

The original Seven Country studies on the relationship of coronary heart disease to environmental factors showed that smoking, high blood pressure and high total serum cholesterol levels were the three biggest risk factors. However, in Japan in the 1950s, men smoked heavily and had the highest blood pressures of all seven countries, but the lowest coronary heart disease. Their high blood pressure was explained by their extraordinarily high salt intakes amounting to 20–30 g/day compared with the goal of less than 5 g/day, but their low rate of coronary heart disease was explained by their very low saturated fat intakes in an average total fat intake of only 14% and therefore very low blood cholesterol levels. Similar findings in China in the 1980s showed that with total fat intakes varying from 4% to 24% (average 14%), the correspondingly low saturated fat intakes induced very low cholesterol levels in the blood, and coronary heart disease rates were also exceptionally low and in proportion to the cholesterol concentrations at levels down to 3 mmol/L. These low levels were never observed in Western studies where total fat intakes were > 40% energy, saturated fat intakes > 20% and blood cholesterol levels > 6 mmol/L! So again the low blood cholesterol levels were the main determinant of the low risk of coronary heart disease, despite the high blood pressures of the Chinese and the high smoking rates in men. Since then, it has become clear that smoking and high blood pressure amplify the atherosclerotic and thrombotic processes, but these are primarily caused by diet-induced alterations in blood lipids. The lipid changes are therefore the permissive factor that allows the other risk factors to become so important. The latest data from intervention trials to lower cholesterol levels with the use of statin drugs suggest that the lower the cholesterol levels the better, and the data are now beginning to reproduce the pre-existing data from Asia about optimum cholesterol levels and therefore the optimum saturated and total fat intake levels. Thus, the first classical 1982 World Health Organization (WHO) report on the prevention of coronary heart disease set the total fat intake goals at 20–30% energy and saturated fat intakes at < 10%, simply because with exceptionally high intakes of fat in US and European diets the experts could not bring themselves to really consider fat levels of 15% with negligible saturated fat intakes as the optimum—they therefore presented, in practice, intermediate targets.

Currently, the average blood pressures of populations in almost all countries of the world are high because salt has been such a sought-after condiment for millennia: huge trade routes were developed for the commodity, which had proven so useful for food preservation as well as for making food more attractive. The word 'salary' comes from the practice of paying Roman soldiers with salt! The salt receptors in the tongue explain the human drive for a rare commodity during our evolution and the same applies to the sugar-responsive sweet-taste receptor and the newly discovered essential fatty acid receptor. So as societies transfer from their rural environments and become more affluent, their serum cholesterol, body weights and blood pressures rise as they gain easier access to dietary fats, sugars and salty foods. These foods are relatively easy to store compared with the problem of transporting vegetables and fruit from the countryside. This 'nutritional transition' continues to affect hundreds of millions in countries such as China, India, Indonesia and many African and Latin American countries.

Although cardiovascular disease and cancers are now the major causes of death in most countries, there has also been a remarkable rise in both obesity and type 2 diabetes in the last 20 years. There are now more than a billion people who are overweight or obese globally, with more obese in the developing countries than in the developed world. Excess weight gain amplifies insulin resistance and precipitates the development of type 2 diabetes. Both these conditions increase the risks of cardiovascular disease, but in the West, the rates of stroke and coronary heart disease have been until recently going down, despite obesity and diabetes rates rapidly increasing. This is explained by the progressive fall in blood cholesterol levels in these societies over the last 30 years as dietary saturated and *trans* fatty acids were replaced by mainly n-6 polyunsaturated fats. These fats still, unfortunately, promote obesity and therefore type 2 diabetes, even if the dietary fat changes have advantageous effects on the atherosclerotic and thrombotic processes.

17.3 The global nutritional transition

The diet changes markedly as a population's wealth increases. Animal foods and sugar intakes rise with a fall in unprocessed cereal and vegetable intakes. In Asia, rheumatic heart disease is still a problem, but haemorrhagic strokes, precipitated by salt-induced high blood pressures, are the dominant causes of cardiovascular disease and premature death. Then, as oil imports (e.g. palm oil) increase, body weight and blood cholesterol levels also rise, with ischaemic stroke and coronary artery disease now emerging as major problems together with breast, colon and prostate cancers.

Western countries slowly began to respond to the nutritional transition in the 1960s with public health measures including changes in agriculture policies aimed at combating the epidemic of coronary heart disease, as shown in Norway in Fig. 17.4. To understand why lower income countries are now experiencing the same chronic diseases epidemic as seen in the Western world 50 years ago one needs to understand why diets have been changing so rapidly. The story goes back about 100 years.

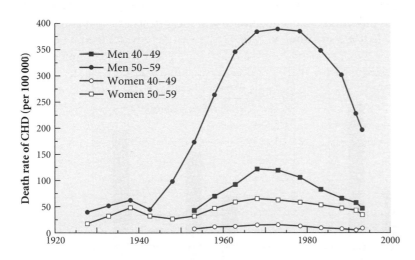

Fig. 17.4 The changing rates of coronary heart disease (CHD) in adults in Norway.

17.4 The cycle of global nutrition transitions: the discovery of vitamins and national survival

A hundred years ago, nutrition was exciting and at the centre of a huge public debate. The British were worried that their Empire might collapse because the fighting strength of their soldiers had deteriorated and they had suffered some alarming defeats in the Boer wars in South Africa. The army was no longer able to recruit tall, strong young soldiers from Scotland to serve in so many of the world-famous regiments. Instead of being 1.8 m tall as in the 1850s, they were now puny, pale 1.5 m tall adolescents who were unable to carry the required weight, sustain prolonged marches and then endure the usual severe combat conditions. The poor working classes in the new Scottish cities, which had expanded rapidly in the previous century as a result of the Scottish clearances, were also breeding too rapidly compared with the tall, strong aristocratic classes, so the issue was whether the country was deteriorating genetically because of the excessive breeding of the lower classes!

Then Gowland Hopkins described strange accessory food factors as crucial to growth, needing to be added to the list of what were thought to be the vital amines already discovered and needed for the avoidance of such diseases as pellagra. These scientific discoveries of the 'vitamins' were important because they proved to be essential dietary factors in special feeding experiments on both animals and children. Thus, when groups of stunted children were given milk, they grew taller, and thin children became heavier when given extra butter or sugar (see Fig. 17.5). Boyd Orr also showed in the Carnegie Survey that it was the poor who had appallingly limited diets, and

were thin, small, anaemic and clinically undernourished, so suddenly the threatened collapse of the British army was seen as being potentially avoidable!

The Carnegie data were crucial in persuading Winston Churchill, as British Prime Minister in the early part of World War II when the German submarines were destroying the majority of ships carrying food from the colonies, that food rationing had to be based on the new scientific principles if Germany was not to win the war by starving the British into defeat. Churchill also insisted that pregnant and lactating women, as well as children, had extra milk, orange juice and cod liver oil; he also decreed that all children should have a good meal at school to ensure their wellbeing and limit the work of their mothers, now recruited into the war effort. Thus, the recent groundbreaking animal experiments, the controlled feeding trials in children, and the detailed national epidemiological surveys of the nutritional state of poor families all contributed to major government policies affecting health and social policies—and also now to

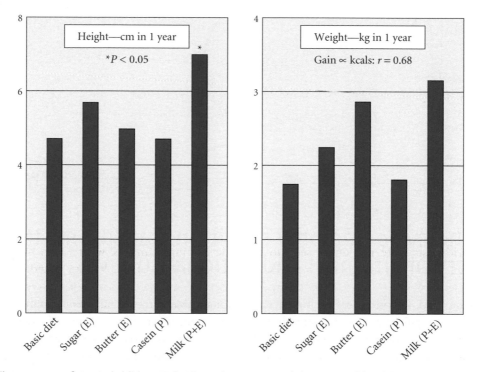

Fig. 17.5 The response of stunted children to food supplements containing energy (E) either with or without additional protein (P).

national security and even survival policies during the war!

The British survived, and the national experiment was hailed as a great success. Hopkins and Orr received their Nobel prizes for science and peace, and the world became convinced that milk, meat, butter and sugar were dietary guarantees of a good protein and energy supply, as well as containing a multitude of special vitamins and minerals. Thus, the world put a priority on their production as a fundamental issue of national security. Vast subsidies, guaranteed prices and a variety of schemes including the European Common Agricultural Policy (CAP) were started to nurture the farming community with the aim of producing far more cheaply the luxury foods of meat, milk and butter and plentiful, purified sugar, previously only readily available for the rich. A cheap food policy, approved by all concerned nutritionists, would allow even the disadvantaged and poor to eat and grow well.

Figure 17.4 above shows what happened in Norway as a result. Nutritionists continued to emphasize the importance of a balanced diet with a variety of foods and the message that 'a little bit of what you fancy does you good'—particularly after a war when food had been scarce and great efforts were needed to make food taste interesting and varied. Now, however, there was no need to be deprived of luxury foods, so the birthday parties children experienced, with the wonders of different cakes, biscuits, sweets, trifles, chocolates and fizzy pop drinks, became the weekly and then the daily aspiration of everybody. The reintroduction of treats such as ice cream became an instant hit.

Chapter 20 describes the underlying basis for the epidemic of heart disease that became the principal cause of death in the Western world during the 1950s with the resurgence of ever-more-intensive agriculture and the development of a much stronger food industry. Animal fat intakes rose as meat, cream, butter and milk consumption were promoted by government, the farming community and many in the nutritional community. Nutritionists joined forces with the food industry to advise them on the new opportunities to develop suitable energy-packed products, with snacks being seen as another way of ensuring adequate intakes in children and those workers who were physically very active. Most nutritionists were then perplexed when Keys and his colleagues in the Seven Country Study showed that the higher the saturated fat intake, the greater the incidence and death rates from coronary heart disease in a community. Since Keys, Hegsted and others had already demonstrated in tightly controlled month-long feeding studies that the response in serum cholesterol, although varying individually, could be predicted from the nature of the dietary fatty acids, it became clear that the nutritional messages needed to change with a new emphasis on the crude assessment of the polyunsaturated/saturated (P/S) ratio in the dietary fat.

17.5 The emergence of a powerful farming and food industry: local food becomes global food

Post-war nutritionists were no longer seen to be involved in particularly exciting research because the principal problems must have been solved! Now the real challenge was how best to cope with the huge numbers of children suffering from kwashiorkor and other forms of malnutrition in the developing world. Protein deficiency seemed to fit with previous concepts of essential food ingredients so a controversy started about the so-called 'protein gap' in so many 'developing countries' where, with the exception of centres in India, the Lebanon, Uganda, South Africa, Mexico, Chile and Jamaica, there were few nutritionists undertaking fundamental research with modern techniques. The top nutritionists linked their work to the earlier pre-war concepts and recognized that these undernourished children would do better if the poor countries followed the West's example and fed children more milk, meat, butter and other forms of energy and that agriculture should be developed on Western lines.

Animal nutritionists came to dominate the nutritional world because cheap meat, butter and milk were national priorities. It was then shown that feeding ruminants such as cows and sheep with cereals rather than grass allowed them to grow far faster, producing more milk and meat cheaply. Thus, cereal growing for animals rather than for humans became the top agricultural priority. Vegetable oil production was also favoured because this would prove a marvellous source of energy for both human and animal feeding. Thus, new agriculture policies were set across the world with huge agriculture budgets for subsidizing the farmers; those in the new European Community (EC) accounted for nearly the total EC budget! Networks of special national agricultural institutes and extra international institutes funded through the UN system and referred to as the CGIAR institutes dominated government (and particularly agricultural ministry) thinking across the world. In 2001, the total farming subsidies still amounted in the OECD countries to US$230.7 billion annually, amounting to almost a third of the total farmers' income. Some countries now provide negligible support, e.g. New Zealand, whereas Korean, Norwegian and Swiss governments subsidise 64–69% of farm incomes.

The food industry also blossomed because the wartime experience had shown that housewives could manage to bring up their children as well as being in the workforce if they were able to buy more convenience and readily cooked meals that used processed ingredients. The national economy benefited enormously from mobilizing the female workforce so the food industry was a crucial contributor to governments' economic policies.

The power of the food industry then grew remarkably; it is now the biggest manufacturer in the European Union accounting for 13% of total manufacturing capacity. As intense competition developed, it was possible with good air and ship transport systems and standard cultivation, harvesting and storage systems to provide quality guaranteed products throughout the year for wealthy societies. African and Latin American governments as well as other developing countries were then manoeuvred by powerful food companies into producing foods for export and consumption within days of collecting. So there is now no such thing as a seasonal cycle in food availability because the crops can be grown in different parts of the world throughout the year and shipped or air freighted into the rich countries.

17.6 Profitability in the food industry: manipulating the price, availability and marketing of products as the determinants of societal intakes

The food industry then had to develop under the same commercial pressures as any other business— they have to make more money and bigger profits each year to be distributed to the owners or shareholders. Thus, there are constant food wars as companies compete for market share. Table 17.2 lists some recent strategies for persuading consumers to buy their products. The price of the food is a critical issue. Indeed, food prices are a crucial part of governments' inflation analyses and social policies. They are also critical for the poorer consumers since they use 80–

100% of their income on food in the poorest developing world, whereas in the developed world this proportion has been steadily dropping for years. In the UK, it is 11% for the richest tenth of the population compared with 15% for the poorest. However, the poorest have much less to spend and still focus on price when buying food; economists for years have calculated the 'price elasticity' of different foods, which shows how intakes fall when prices rise. Thus, in the annual review of the European CAP pricing policies for milk, butter, meat and sugar, they used to

Table 17.2 Fifteen strategies to improve profitability in the food industry, often to the disadvantage of health

1. Design foods to appeal to the palate by reducing bulk and ensuring fat, sugar and salt sufficient for maximum impact on primary taste buds.

2. Engage new flavour specialists to identify the thousands of flavours in a food or drink, which contribute to activating specific olfactory receptors, through molecular techniques. Identify which flavours lock into cerebral pleasure responses using novel brain imaging techniques, taking account of genetic diversity of the population's receptors, sex differences in responses and the combination effects of other ingredients, e.g. alcohol if the desired target is increased alcohol consumption in young women.

3. Reduce prices paid to farmers.

4. Offer larger portion sizes for 'value' where ingredient costs are small and fixed costs of production and distribution the same: the consumer purchases a larger portion but the manufacture gets a much bigger profit.

5. Provide ready-to-eat meals, e.g. hamburgers, fried chicken and pizzas: sell for immediate consumption with maximum convenience.

6. Provide food in ready-to-eat or -drink cartons for 'take away'. (Develop the market concept of eating and drinking on the move because distracted purchasers will eat and buy more.)

7. Increase the availability of outlets for purchase, e.g. in vending machines, specialist shops (e.g. coffee, hamburger) and other specialist outlets where populations congregate, e.g. in town centres.

8. Build 'brand value' by intensive marketing using famous popular figures, e.g. football stars.

9. Target children, preferably below the age of five when particularly amenable to image building and acceptance of all messages. Employ child psychologists to gear messages to bypass parents and increase the 'pester power' of children to overcome parental resistance.

10. Extend the variety of marketing approaches: TV advertising is progressively less important: place foods and drinks as routine scenes in soap operas, boost internet marketing, and use 'viral marketing' where key children are paid to receive and pass on text messages on mobile phones.

11. Prompt children to go to food outlets by geo-satellite monitoring of mobile positions in relation to desired food outlets.

12. Take over school food and drink supplies and give schools a minor profit share to encourage removal of alterative water and food sources at school.

13. Fundamental new drive on the developing world with huge investments dominating economic and social policy thinking of the recipient countries: get in early and establish market dominance, especially in major societies, e.g. China, India, Indonesia, Brazil, Mexico.

14. Employ media-friendly nutritional experts to sanction ideas based on values of pleasure and quality of food for maximum individual choice in a 'balanced diet'; use economic influence to access ministers and prime ministers; consider inducements.

15. Target opponents' scientific or personal credentials if they criticize new developments.

juggle the subsidies and price guarantees to farmers in order to change the price of the foods in the market place. This then allowed an increase or decrease in the mountains of frozen foods, which had originally been kept for national emergencies. Changes in the consumption of these foods by the population could be very accurately predicted if the price was changed.

The food industry has got around the problem of raising prices by reducing their costs through a number of mechanisms including merging and acquiring new businesses, closing factories, mechanizing for mass production, and using as few employees as possible, focusing on a relatively small number of branded goods and buying up small competitors to remove them from the market place.

Apart from the price of foods and convenience preprepared meals, the other factors profoundly affecting food purchases are the ready availability of a variety of foods so that consumers can gain easy access to them at any time. Then there is the marketing of foods. The food industry manipulates portion size to make foods appear cheaper and they also pay supermarkets to have their products placed at particular points and shelf heights in the supermarkets to promote sales. Local councils, schools and work sites are also offered special deals to ensure that their products are immediately available. Thus, one hamburger chain suggests 4 minutes as the appropriate maximum time for anybody to have to drive to get to their outlet within any reasonably sized town in the USA, and soft-drink companies ensure there is an outlet and advertising of their products in every reasonably sized village throughout the world! Marketing is also directed to the most susceptible and responsive groups are the young children. Commercial interests therefore now target young children before they are able to discriminate marketing from general information and try to manipulate the educative processes by providing schools with teaching materials that have the companies' products as suitable examples.

To keep the rising expectations of company profits (when, biologically, children and adults in the affluent world cannot eat any more food), the Western food companies now have to take over the food system of the developing world—as one of their highest priorities. They promise prime ministers and policy makers huge investments to establish soft-drink and fast-food factories, and often provide financial and other inducements to ensure the deals are agreed. Some indication of the power of the food industry is shown in Table 17.3. While the food companies have become powerful, so too have the supermarkets—now, individually, they also often have a greater turnover than many countries. Thus, the biggest, Wal-Mart, a US-based company operating in ten countries, had

Table 17.3 Analysis of the power of the industry

1. The global food advertising budget is over $40 billion—more than the total income of 70% of the world's countries.

2. The food industry spends 500 times more on promoting high-energy-density Western diets than the total governmental prevention budget on promoting good nutrition.

3. Food advertising accounts for half of all adverts on children's TV; 75% are for high-energy, low-nutrient foods.

4. Transitional economies (e.g. Eastern Europe) find 60% of foreign investment is for sugar, confectionary and soft drinks—10 times the investment in vegetable and fruit production.

annual retail sales of US$250 billion in 2003; in most affluent countries > 70% of food sales are through a small number of huge supermarkets. This then gives major food companies a major negotiating power for influencing consumers and governments throughout the world. They also control what farming communities earn and produce. The most rapidly expanding Western supermarkets are now in most middle income countries where their sales are already growing far faster than in the West. This then explains the huge and overwhelming epidemic of chronic diseases in developing countries.

17.6.1 Implications for prevention

The massive global epidemic of obesity, type 2 diabetes and other chronic diseases is guaranteed to continue unless the nutritional world focuses on the prime drivers affecting the food system, and recognizes that individuals have to be very well educated, affluent and motivated to create their own 'micro-environment' when they live in what is now termed 'a toxic obesogenic environment'. Traditionally, nutritionists are trained to expect that patients or individuals given advice will act upon it, and therefore they can be made responsible for their own nutritional wellbeing. It is, however, exceptionally difficult for even discerning consumers to understand current food labels because they are set out for the benefit of regulators and analysts who can readily understand the sodium or fat content/100 g of a product. Consumers, however, cannot work out how to limit their fat or saturated fat intake given the usual advice, for example, about limiting total fat to < 30% and saturated fat to < 10% energy, when almost nobody knows what their own energy needs are. Many surveys show that a traffic-light signalling system is much preferred by the public, but such systems have been opposed by some sectors of the food industry who reiterate the old mantra that there are no 'good' or 'bad' foods, only wrongly balanced diets. Unfortunately, many nutritionists also pedantically endorse the concept that there are no 'good' or 'bad' foods, while the food companies now promote their own version of good healthy foods or 'functional foods' at premium prices! When the more responsible nutritionists insist on a food having an appropriate nutritional profile (e.g. with the food being low in total fat, saturated fat, sugars and salt) before any health claim is made, this is resisted intensively by the food industrial consortia using tactics analogous to those used by the tobacco industry—confusing policy makers with spurious claims, targeting personally the nutritional critics of their marketing strategies, and rewarding some industry-friendly nutritionists who dispute the nutritional evidence. Thus, even some of the prominent nutritionists of the world are targeted to ensure they do not create trouble for the marketing of major food brands.

Nutritional education has now been shown to be a hopelessly inadequate approach for dealing with the population's public health problems. This means that nutritionists are going to have to learn completely different approaches involving policy making and a changed role for themselves in society if they are really going to help people. The huge environmental pressures to eat the wrong foods and remain physically inactive are overwhelming most people's desire to remain healthy, so a new outlook by nutritionists is now needed. Clearly, economic and other policy methods analogous to those involved in the control of tobacco and alcohol will be required to limit the intense promotion of nutrient-poor, energy-dense foods.

FURTHER READING

1. **Corry Mann, H.C.** (1926) *Diets for boys during the school years*. MRC Special Report Series 105. London, HMSO.

2. **Ezzati, M., Lopez, A.D., Rodgers, A., Vander Hoorn, S., and Murray, C.J.** (2002) Comparative Risk Assessment Collaborating Group. Selected major risk factors and global and regional burden of disease. *Lancet*, **360**, 1347–60.

3. **Haslam, D.W., James, W.P.** (2005) Obesity *Lancet*. **366**, 1197–209. (Review.)

4. **James, W.P.T., Norum, K., Smitasiri, S., et al.** (2000) Ending malnutrition by 2020: an agenda for change in the millennium. Final Report to the ACC/SCN by the Commission on the Nutrition Challenges of the 21st Century. *Food Nutr Bull*, **21** (Suppl. 3), 1–88.

5. **James, W.P.T., and Rigby, N.J.** (2005) Nutrition policy: national strategies for dietary change. In: Marmot, M. and Elliott, P. (eds) *Coronary heart disease epidemiology: From etiology to public health*, 2nd edition. Oxford, Oxford University Press, pp. 805–18.

6. **Johansson, L., Drevon, C.A., and Bjorneboe, G.-E.** (1996) The Norwegian diet during the last hundred years in relation to coronary heart disease. *Eur J Clin Nutr*, **50**, 277–83.

7. **Lang, T., and Heasman, M.** (2004) *Food wars: the global battle for mouths, minds and markets*. London, Earthscan.

8. **Popkin, B.M.** (2004) The nutrition transition: an overview of world patterns of change. *Nutr Rev*, **62**, S140–S143. (Review.)

9. **Schlosser, E.** (2001) *Fast food nation. The dark side of the all-American meal*. London, Allen Lane/Penguin Press.

10. **WHO** (2003) *Diet, nutrition and the prevention of chronic diseases*. Report of a Joint WHO/FAO Expert Consultation. WHO Technical Report Series No. 916. Geneva: World Health Organization.

18 Protein-energy malnutrition

Stewart Truswell

People, young or old, who eat less food than they usually eat, and need, lose body weight; the deficit of energy (or calories) in the diet is made up by drawing on the body's energy reserves: first fat, later muscle. The weight loss is carbon dioxide (breathed out) and water (excreted) from oxidation of fat.

$$2(C_{55}H_{106}O_6) + 157O_2 \rightarrow 110CO_2 + 106H_2O + heat$$

(This representative fat molecule is a triglyceride with oleic (18:1), linoleic (18:2) and palmitic (16:1) acids). This is undernutrition.

Undernutrition can be mild or severe, beneficial (in someone who was obese) or dangerous. The loss of weight is a manifestation of energy depletion. Essential nutrients, protein and micronutrients are likely to be depleted at the same time but some micronutrients have large stores in the body, and requirements of some others are lower when energy intake is reduced. In children, who have higher protein requirements than adults, important depletion of protein is likely to accompany serious undernutrition.

Protein depletion can affect the body in two different ways:

1. *In somatic protein depletion*, the loss of tissue shows as general wasting of muscles, which together contain the largest amount of the body's protein.

2. *In visceral protein depletion*, the brunt of the protein loss is borne by the liver, pancreas and gut. This is the less common type of protein malnutrition and nutritional scientists still do not fully agree why it occurs.

Protein-energy malnutrition (PEM) occurs in three situations:

1. In young children in poor communities, usually in developing countries.

2. In adults, even in affluent countries, due to severe illness (hospital malnutrition).

3. In people of all ages in a famine.

BOX 18.1 Definitions of malnutrition

- Undernutrition is depletion of energy (calories)
- Malnutrition is serious depletion of any of the essential nutrients (other than energy)
- Fasting is voluntary abstention from food
- Starvation is involuntary lack of food
- Famine is severe food shortage of a whole community
- Wasting is loss of substance, especially muscle (from insufficient food, disuse or disease).

18.1 Protein-energy malnutrition in young children

There are two forms of severe PEM: marasmus and kwashiorkor.

18.1.1 Nutritional marasmus

Nutritional marasmus is the common form; it is starvation in an infant or young child. (The word is from the Greek *marasmus* meaning 'wasting'). The child is very thin. Weight is less than 60% of the median reference weight-for-age and there is marked wasting (Fig. 18.1). There is no oedema.

There is loss of almost all the adipose tissue and (to a smaller extent) wasting of the voluntary muscles. Growth has stopped and it has taken weeks

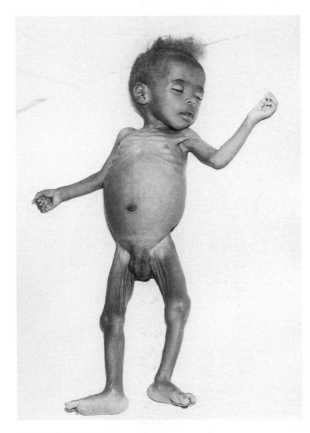

Fig. 18.1 Marasmus.

of inadequate feeding for a child to become very wasted like this. The cause is a diet very low in total energy, that is, not enough food, for example, early weaning from the breast on to dilute food, because of poverty or ignorance. Poor food hygiene leads to gastroenteritis, diarrhoea and vomiting. This leads to poor appetite so more dilute feeds are given. Further depletion in turn leads to intestinal atrophy and more susceptibility to diarrhoea.

'Not enough food' implies 'not enough protein', because most foods contain some protein. It is most unlikely that child not getting enough food would still be eating protein-rich food since such foods are expensive. With negative energy balance, the major fuel to maintain life is free fatty acids, drawn from the adipose tissue. Blood glucose needed for tissues that can only metabolize glucose (brain, red blood cells) is maintained by gluconeogenesis of glucogenic amino acids (e.g. alanine) drawn from the body's proteins, usually the muscles, sometimes the viscera. Although energy depletion predominates in marasmus, there is inevitably insufficient protein intake and loss of protein inside the body.

Inside the body, the heart, brain, liver and kidneys are least wasted, but in advanced cases, the heart becomes atrophied (wasted) and brain weight is reduced. There is increased mobilization of free fatty acids from adipose tissue, with ketosis (increased concentration of 3-hydroxybutyrate and acetoacetate). The blood glucose may be subnormal. The basal metabolic rate goes down; an increased proportion of triiodothyronine is in the inactive rT3 form. Plasma insulin is low and leptin is low.

Infections that are only a temporary nuisance in well-nourished children become life-threatening in children with severe PEM. Their bodies are not capable of producing the usual responses to common bacterial infections of pyrexia and increased white blood cells (leukocytosis). Cell-mediated immunity, the main defence against viruses and tuberculosis, is impaired. Pathogenic bacteria in the intestines can more easily gain access to the blood circulation.

Table 18.1 Classification of PEM in young children

Condition	Body weight as percentage of international standard*	Oedema	Deficit in weight-for-length
Kwashiorkor	80–60	+	+
Marasmic kwashiorkor	< 60	+	++
Marasmus	< 60	0	++
Nutritional stunting	< 60	0	Minimal
Underweight child	80–60	0	+

*The 50th percentile line, weight forage, of the World Health Organization reference values.

18.1.2 Kwashiorkor

Marasmus has been known for centuries, but the other type of severe PEM (Table 18.1), i.e. kwashiorkor, was not generally recognized until the 1950s. The classic description was by Cecily Williams in the *Lancet* in 1935. She wrote from Accra in Ghana, giving the syndrome the name that the mothers used there, in the Ga language.

Typically, a child with kwashiorkor (Fig. 18.2) develops oedema, which is generalized. The child is miserable, withdrawn, obviously ill and will not eat. Changes can be seen in the skin; there are areas of pigmentation, which are symmetrical in distribution, most commonly in the nappy area. The skin later shows cracks and the superficial layer peels off. The hair is thinned and discoloured, blonde or red or grey, instead of black. There is diarrhoea. Inside the body, the liver is enlarged and its parenchymal cells contain numerous fat droplets. The protein in the liver is reduced and two of the main features of kwashiorkor can be explained by failure of the liver to make two important (export) plasma proteins. Failure to synthesize albumin and the consequent very low plasma albumin may, because of low plasma osmotic pressure, at least partly explain the oedema. Failure to synthesize very-low-density lipoproteins and an inability to transport fat out of the liver to the periphery explain the accumulation of fat in the liver. There is an abnormal and characteristic pattern of amino acids in plasma (Table 18.2).

Kwashiorkor develops more quickly than marasmus. One day the oedema appears and the mother seeks medical help—though changes in skin and hair must have been developing over a longer period. The child with kwashiorkor is not necessarily underweight.

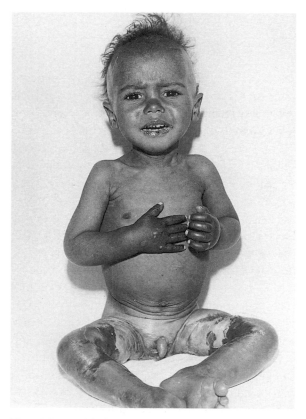

Fig. 18.2 Kwashiorkor.

Table 18.2 Biochemical findings in kwashiorkor compared with marasmus (on admission to hospital)

	Kwashiorkor	Marasmus
Plasma albumin	Very low	Usually normal
Plasma amino acids	Reduced branch chain and tryosine	More normal
Serum amylase	Very low	Normal/low normal
Plasma (total) cholesterol	Very low	Normal/low normal
Plasma free fatty acids	Increased	Increased
Plasma growth hormone	Raised	Not as high
Red cell glutathione	Low	Normal
Fasting blood glucose	Low to normal	Low
T lymphocytes	Low	Low
Plasma retinol	Low	Low
Somatomedin-C (IGF-1)	Low	Not as low
Plasma transferrin	Very low	Low to normal
Plasma urea	Low	Not as low
Plasma urate	Low	Raised
Plasma zinc	Low	Not as low

The original meaning of kwashiorkor is 'the deposed child' or 'first second'. Mothers in Accra thought that this illness might affect a child when a second baby follows and displaces them from the breast.

There are two schools of thought on the cause of kwashiorkor. The question is, why is there an acute depletion of protein from the liver and other viscera rather than from the muscles in these cases of PEM?

The original theory is that a child who develops kwashiorkor has been fed on a diet moderately adequate in carbohydrate but very low in protein so that there is a relative deficiency of protein to energy (i.e. protein malnutrition), whereas the diet that leads to marasmus is low in both energy and protein. Researchers who disagree with this classical theory argue that in their experience dietary histories are indistinguishable between children with kwashiorkor and children with marasmus. Something else must explain the visceral protein depletion—'dysadaptation', mycotoxins or free-radical damage have been suggested. A practical trial of antioxidants in over

2000 pre-school children in Malawi failed to prevent kwashiorkor (Ciliberto *et al.*, 2005).

Individual dietary histories are not likely to be scientifically reliable from the carer(s) of a child who has become severely malnourished. Kwashiorkor children are not necessarily underweight (= energy-deficient). Their very low blood and urinary urea levels indicate low protein intakes. Cure of kwashiorkor has been initiated with a diet consisting only of 18 pure amino acids plus only 30% energy from glucose. Kwashiorkor occurs in countries where the staple diets for weaned children have very low protein/energy ratios (e.g. cassava, plantains, sweet potato or refined maize). R.G. Whitehead (1977) made observations comparing children in The Gambia, where the usual form of severe PEM is marasmus, with children in Uganda, where kwashiorkor occurs. Ugandan children grew more in weight and height and had more subcutaneous fat but lower plasma albumin concentrations. They had higher plasma insulin levels and lower plasma cortisols. Protein/energy ratios of their food were lower. Whitehead suggested that with a very low protein diet, but with adequate carbohydrate, the carbohydrate stimulates insulin, and this is known to favour deposition of amino acids in muscles. On a very low protein diet, amino acids are in short supply, so muscle proteins can only be maintained at the expense of the liver (and other viscera). The liver is stimulated by infection to put much of its protein-synthetic effort into making 'acute-phase' plasma proteins that should help to fight the infection. Syndromes resembling kwashiorkor can be produced in monkeys on a diet of cassava with added sugar, and in young rats on a 5% protein ration.

18.1.3 The spectrum of severe protein-energy malnutrition

Kwashiorkor and marasmus are distinct diseases, but in communities where both occur, cases of severe PEM often have some features of both (e.g. these children are very underweight and also have skin or hair changes). This is marasmic kwashiorkor.

PEM does not only affect protein and energy. The Spanish name *syndrome policarencial infantile* means the 'polynutritional syndrome of infants'. Deficiencies of some micronutrients commonly occur in severe PEM, notably vitamin A deficiency: xerophthalmia (Chapter 11) and potassium depletion from diarrhoea, which contributes to oedema (Chapter 7). There may also be evidence of zinc (Chapter 10), folate and/or niacin (Chapter 12) and/or calcium deficiency.

Children with severe PEM have diarrhoea. An infection may have brought on the severe illness. These children stand infections poorly; measles is especially lethal.

18.1.4 Treatment of severe protein-energy malnutrition

Treatment of severe PEM is in three stages and is similar for marasmus and kwashiorkor:

1. *Treatment of acute complications*: correction of dehydration and/or electrolyte disturbance and/or very low blood glucose and/or low body temperature (hypothermia) and start of treatment for infections. Clinical signs of infections are difficult to elicit (e.g.

no pyrexia or leukocytosis). Many paediatricians give broad-spectrum antibiotics on the presumption of some infection. The fluid given to rehydrate malnourished children should contain less sodium and more potassium than the standard UNICEF oral rehydration solution. ReSoMal contains, per litre of water, only 45 mmol sodium, but 40 mmol potassium, more glucose and some magnesium and zinc.

2. *Initiation of cure*: refeeding, gradually working up the energy and protein intake and giving multivitamin drops and potassium and magnesium supplements. Children with kwashiorkor have poor appetites. They have to be hand fed, with frequent feeds, preferably in the lap of their mother or a nurse they know. To start refeeding, the standard 'formula' is F75 recommended by the World Health Organization (WHO), which provides 75 kcal and 1 g protein/ 100 mL. This is given for the first few days, in small amounts that add up to around 100 mL/kg/day. Although the child is malnourished, energy and protein must be limited at the start to avoid metabolic stress. When the child is starting to recover, F100 is introduced, which contains 100 kcal and 29 g protein/ 100 mL. This can be given to satiety. F75 and F100 are available as powders that can be reconstituted with water. They contain dried skimmed milk, sugar, vegetable oil electrolyte/mineral solution. Equivalent formulas can be made up from appropriate local foods. Different examples are in the literature (e.g. Torún, 2005).

3. *Nutritional rehabilitation*: after about 3 weeks, the child should be obviously better, with oedema cleared, and mentally bright with good appetite, yet still below the standard (reference) weight-for-height. At this stage, catch-up growth should occur if the child is well looked after and given nutritious combinations of local, familiar foods. If the child has been in hospital, they have to go back to their family, unless a nutrition rehabilitation unit is available.

Prognosis: Even in well-equipped hospitals, the death rate of children with severe PEM is around 20%. In those who survive, are there lasting effects? Follow-up biopsies after kwashiorkor have shown that the liver returns to normal; the fatty change does not progress to cirrhosis (unlike in alcoholics). In marasmic children who have become severely wasted in the first 2 years of life, growth of the head (circumference easily measured) is retarded, so the brain must be smaller than normal, and such children may subsequently have impaired intelligence unless they are fortunate thereafter and brought up in an excellent environment.

18.2 Mild to moderate protein-energy malnutrition

For every florid case of marasmus or kwashiorkor, there must be 7–10 children in the community with mild to moderate PEM. Like an iceberg, there is more malnutrition below the surface and it is not easily recognized. Mothers often do not realize that their child is malnourished because he or she is similar in size and vitality to many of the same age in an impoverished neighbourhood. Most children with mild to moderate PEM can be detected, however, by their weight-for-age, which is less than 80% of the international standard (Table 18.1). Such children are either wasted with subnormal weight-for-height/length or *stunted* (nutritional dwarfism), with subnormal height-for-age (but not wasted)—or both. Wasted children have used up body fat, and some muscle, to maintain their fuel supply. Stunted children have adapted in a different way, by stopping or slowing their growth. Reference tables (or graphs) are available from WHO for weight-for-age, height/length-for-age and weight-for-height for prepubertal children (see Chapter 32).

In many developing countries, around 2% of preschool children have severe PEM, and 20% (in some places more) have mild to moderate PEM. The importance of this mild to moderate PEM is that affected children are growing up smaller than their genetic potential and have increased susceptibility to severe gastroenteritis and respiratory infections. Mild to moderate PEM is probably a major underlying reason why the 1–4-year mortality in developing countries is 30–60 times higher than in Europe or North America (in some places higher).

18.3 Prevention of protein-energy malnutrition

Kwashiorkor most often occurs in the second year of life; marasmus mostly in the first year. Kwashiorkor is more amenable to the medical model of education, for example, education of mothers about the need for protein foods for weaned children and encouraging their provision at the political level. Marasmus is a more intractable problem, bound up with poverty, the status and education of women, lack of contraceptive resources and poor sanitation. UNICEF has achieved reductions in rates of PEM with four simple measures, represented by the acronym GOBI (see Box 18.2).

BOX 18.2 UNICEFs inexpensive measures to prevent PEM

G *for growth monitoring*. The mother keeps the simple weight-for-age chart in a cellophane envelope and brings the child to a maternal and child health clinic regularly for weighing and advice.

O *for oral rehydration*. The UNICEF ORS formula (NaCl 3.5 g, $NaHCO_3$ 2.5 g, KCl 1.5 g, glucose 20 g in clean water to 1 litre) is saving many lives from gastroenteritis.

B *for breast-feeding*. This has overwhelming advantages for a baby in a poor community with no facilities for hygiene. It should be continued as long as possible while solid foods are added. Additional foods, which should be prepared from locally available foods, are not usually needed before 6 months of age.

I *for immunization*. For a few dollars, a child can be protected against measles, diptheria, pertussis, tetanus, tuberculosis, poliomyelitis, etc., infections that predispose to and aggravate malnutrition.

18.4 Famine

The worst famines in recent times have been in areas torn by civil war. The hostilities greatly hamper communication of early warning and confirmation of the severity of the food shortage and transport of relief food into the area.

When there is not enough food for an entire community, the children stop growing and the children and adults lose weight. Starving people feel cold and weak and crave food. Subcutaneous fat disappears and muscles waste. The pulse is slow and blood pressure is low. The abdomen is distended. Diarrhoea is common. Infections are to be expected, especially gastrointestinal infections, pneumonia, tuberculosis and typhus.

The problem in a famine is not so much loss of food as loss of ability to obtain it. People have to sell all their assets in the attempt to buy food. The community's social and economic structures break down.

Aid professionals in relief operations should expect to have a mainly administrative and organizational role. It is impossible to give most time to treatment of a few very sick individuals. Therapeutic feeding is not an effective use of resources. Field workers have three options for distribution of food where supplies are insufficient to provide the minimum requirements of 1900 kcal/day (7.9 mJ/day): (i) where community and family structure are still intact and community representatives can be identified, let the community decide how the limited food is to be distributed; (ii) where community structures have been disrupted, distribute food selectively to those assessed to be at the highest risk of mortality; or (iii) ensure equitable distribution of the same basic ration to all members of the affected population with selection of particularly vulnerable members. The standard food-aid rations usually consist of cereals, legumes and some oil. If the cereal is wholegrain, milling equipment is necessary. Milk powder is used for malnourished children. Provision of clean water is a priority. Care must be taken that the population gets the critical micronutrients, which are not the same in different areas and situations (e.g. vitamin C, potassium).

To assess the degree of undernutrition in individuals, two measures are commonly used: mid-upper arm circumference (MUAC) and weight-for-height in children or body mass index (BMI, kg/m²) in adults. MUAC is obviously quicker and tape measures can be given to several workers. Weight and height are slower to measure. In children, low MUAC tends to select younger children as malnourished, and misses older children with low weight-for-height (or BMI). In adults, MUAC and BMI appear to correlate fairly well. A MUAC of 220 mm in men or 210 mm in women corresponds approximately to a critical BMI of 16 kg/m². As a general rule, moderate starvation = weight-for-height 80–71% of reference (in children), BMI of 18–16 kg/m² (in adults); severe starvation = weight-for-height ≥ 70% of reference (in children) or BMI ≥ 15.7 (in adults).

The clinical photographs in this chapter were kindly provided by Professor J.D.L. Hansen of Cape Town.

FURTHER READING

Five major books have been written (in English) on PEM of children, the first in 1954. The three most recent are those by Alleyne *et al.* (1977), Suskin and Lewinter-Susking (1990), and Waterlow (1992).

1. **Alleyne, G.A.O., Hay, R.W., Picou, D.I., Stanfield, J.P., and Whitehead, R.G.** (1977) *Protein-energy malnutrition*. London, Edward Arnold.

2. **Bhan, M.K., Bhandari, N., and Bahl, R.** (2003) Management of the severely malnourished child: perspective from developing countries. *Br Med J*, **326**, 146–51.

3. **Ciliberto, J.H., Ciliberto, M., Briend, A., Ashorn, P., Bier, D., and Manary, M.** (2005) Antioxidant supplementation for the prevention of kwashiorkor in Malawian children: randomized, doubled blind, placebo controlled trial. *Br Med J*, **330**, 1109–11.

4. **Suskind, R.M., and Lewinter-Suskind, L.** (1990) *The malnourished child*. New York, Raven Press.

5. **Torún, B.** (2005) Protein-energy malnutrition. In: Shils, M.E., Shike, M., Ross, A.C., Caballero, B., and Cousins, R.J. (eds) *Modern nutrition in health and disease*, 10th

edition. Philadelphia, Lippincott, Williams, and Wilkins, pp. 881–908.

6. **Waterlow, J.C.** (1992) *Protein-energy malnutrition*, London, Edward Arnold.

7. **Whitehead, R.G., Coward, W.A., Lunn, P.G.,** *et al.* (1977) A comparison of the pathogenesis of protein energy malnutrition in Uganda and the Gambia. *Trans R Soc Trop Med Hyg*, **71**, 189–95.

8. **WHO** (1991) *Management of severe malnutrition: a manual for physicians and other senior health workers*. Geneva, World Health Organization.

9. **WHO** (2004) *United Nations Standing Committee on Nutrition. Fifth Report on the World Nutrition Situation*. Geneva, World Health Organization.

To see topical and scientifically robust updates on nutrition associated with this textbook, and active web links to many of the journal articles in the Reference areas, please see the dedicated Online Resource Centre at www.oxfordtextbooks.co.uk/orc/mann3e/.

19 Nutritional crises

Alain Mourey and Jennifer McMahon

Nutritional crises occur when individuals or populations are unable to sustain the feeding process. This occurs when they cannot obtain adequate supplies of food, or are unable to consume or utilize food. A nutritional crisis involves two phases: a *preliminary phase* during which progression of the crisis may be averted by adaptation, utilization of reserves or other defence mechanisms[a] and an *acute phase* where the protective mechanisms fail, systems disintegrate and the feeding process breaks down to the extent that hunger and ultimately nutritional inadequacy and starvation associated with famine occur. Identification of the preliminary phase represents a major challenge to local and national governments and

humanitarian organizations since there may be opportunities to facilitate interventions that have the potential to halt progression to the acute phase. The crisis process is initiated when an event (generally referred to as a phenomenon) strikes a vulnerable target group or population (see Fig. 19.1). A single event such as an isolated drought episode in an arid setting is unlikely to pose a serious threat because the population is accustomed to responding with adaptive mechanisms to recurrent, and therefore familiar, phenomena. However, several drought episodes in rapid succession are likely to deplete adaptive mechanisms and enhance the vulnerability of the population.

19.1 Causes of nutritional crises

Phenomena causing crises stem from either the human community (war, economic, social and cultural crises) or the natural environment. Environmental phenomena may be geophysical (earthquakes, volcanic eruption, tidal waves), or natural climatic variation (drought, floods, hurricanes, erosion), or non-human predators. However, human activities such as over-farming and inappropriate farming practices may

also contribute to adverse environmental phenomena, including erosion, desertification, drought, global warming and pollution.

19.1.1 Human phenomena

Political War is a major trigger of nutritional crises. Looting, destruction, danger, restrictions on access and movement, population displacements, confinement, occupation, terror and harassment, seizure of goods, embargoes and conscription all undermine household economy and food security. Displacement

[a]Governments sometimes suppress information relating to an impending crisis and prevent such news from reaching the international community.

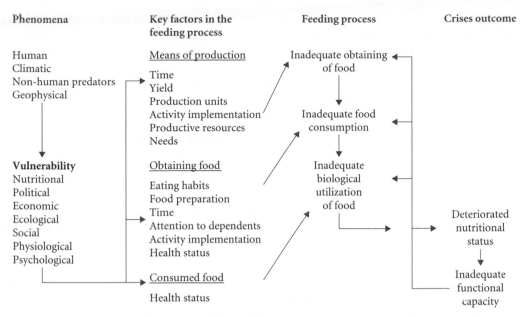

Fig. 19.1 Progression of events leading to a nutritional crisis.

of populations may result in epidemics of infectious disease with direct consequences to consumption and utilization of food, further reducing production potential.

Economic Economic phenomena induce poverty and restrict choice. Speculation by market traders and power struggles and shortages cause a rise in prices of essential commodities. Farmers may be forced to sell produce to those who trade outside their region, or even abroad, leading to reduced local availability or excessive prices, especially if harvest yields are poor. Devaluation of currency can have devastating effects on pensioners and others living on fixed incomes. Following currency devaluation and price inflation in Abkhazia (the western region of Georgia), pensioners were in a desperate position when the price of bread increased approximately 10 000-fold.

Economic subjugation and its consequences result when small domestic economies become dependent on altered agricultural practices and costly imports. Compared with traditional crops, hybrid or genetically modified seeds require annual purchases, appreciably greater use of fertilizers and pesticides, and

often controlled irrigation. A community in Angola would almost certainly have experienced a nutritional crisis without humanitarian aid in 1999 as it became isolated due to war and was dependent on such seeds and related inputs, which were no longer obtainable.

Misguided economic development policies may result in environmental deterioration—erosion, desertification, soil salinity, deforestation, resource depletion and pollution—from excessive exploitation. This is turn contributes to a rural exodus towards urban centres, resulting in the impoverishment of both migrants and residents who remain in the areas.

Social Population growth is considered to be an important phenomenon that has been countered in affluent societies by industrial and agricultural development, often accompanied by adverse environmental consequences in the countries themselves, and indirectly in developing countries through the importation of food. In the developing world, population growth results in competition for scarce resources, risk of conflict, misguided development policies, deterioration of the environment and disintegration of the social fabric, which can profoundly increase the risk of nutritional crises.

Cultural Social phenomena can occur in any society, but cultural phenomena are specific to communities. For example, the belligerent nature of Somali clans led to suppression and looting of those without strong family affiliations and perceived wealth. This individualistic behaviour led to one of the last century's most devastating famines. Such behaviour is acquired, and is thus eminently cultural. Some weaning and infant-feeding practices also have serious consequences for the consumption and biological utilization of food. For instance, the Baganda children of Uganda are weaned from maternal milk by a sudden shift to mostly starchy food, which is low in protein and other nutrients, and poor in energy. In addition, they lose the immune protection of breastfeeding while the weaning food exposes them to new forms of bacterial contamination. Thus, their appetite is satiated without their nutritional requirements being met. Infective illness compounds the problem, and severe malnutrition frequently results (see section 18.1.2).

Accidents and illnesses Accidents can cause massive pollution, such as the mercury poisoning in Minamata, Japan, the toxic gas and chemical leak in Bhopal, India, and the nuclear explosion in Chernobyl, Ukraine. They can contaminate entire regions, making them uninhabitable for large population groups. Workplace and traffic accidents and illness affect individuals and households to an extent that may predispose to nutritional crises, especially in societies with limited support systems.

19.1.2 Climatic environmental phenomena

Drought Especially when combined with war, drought may have devastating consequences. This has been seen in recent times in Ethiopia, Angola, Mozambique, Somalia and Sudan. An isolated drought episode in a country prone to yearly variation in rainfall rarely results in a nutritional crisis because the population may be able to implement tried and tested adaptive mechanisms. However, pendulum variations, in which relatively humid years and dry spells may last for around 5 years (as occurs in southern Africa) or as long as 10–18 years (as in the Sahel), and permanent climatic changes are of far greater concern. Climatic changes have occurred as natural phenomena over time and it is unclear whether the apparent increase in drought in many countries in recent years is as a result of such an occurrence or whether environmental overexploitation (particularly by deforestation) and global warming are responsible. However, regardless of the cause, there is no doubt that persistent drought is resulting in devastating consequences in many parts of Africa. In the totally arid areas of northern Mali, for example, pools lined with shell residues provided a supply of permanent water until 1972. Since then, because of the severity of drought, they have dried up completely. Angola and Mozambique were countries that seldom experienced drought, but since the late 1980s and early 1990s, consecutive drought years have been relatively commonplace. In Angola, endemic malaria is occurring at higher altitudes than previously, indicating rising temperatures.

Floods Flooding principally leads to a crisis situation when it occurs during the main planting season, when it follows a drought, when repeated flooding occurs, and when the geographic and political environment preclude efficient action. Like droughts, floods may be natural climatic phenomena or may be a consequence of human activity, especially deforestation.

Hurricanes, earthquakes, volcanic eruptions and tidal waves These climatic phenomena are invariably of short duration but may predispose to nutritional crises by destroying crops, devastating arable land and displacing communities from their homes and properties to areas where they must depend on international agencies or on others who are barely in a position to feed themselves.

19.1.3 Non-human predators

Plagues of locusts, caterpillars, other insects and birds can devastate crops. Insects and rodents can attack stored harvests. Parasites and infectious diseases can affect livestock and endanger pastoral economies.

19.1.4 Impact of infectious disease on the feeding process

Epidemics of infectious disease have the potential to precipitate nutritional crises by reducing the capacity of sick individuals to produce or secure food. Severe infections may not only undermine the household economy, but if infections reach epidemic proportions then the economy of a country or region may be slowed. At an individual level, severe infections may influence consumption and utilization of food. Infants and young children are particularly vulnerable.

19.2 Vulnerability

The phenomena described in section 19.1 are most likely to result in nutritional crises when imposed on groups that are vulnerable to them. Vulnerability is determined by a range of factors, several of which are closely associated with the phenomena considered to be causes of nutritional crises.

19.2.1 Nutritional vulnerability

Young children, pregnant and lactating women, elderly people and ill people are universally regarded as vulnerable. When exposed to a range of adverse circumstances, these groups are likely to be first to meet the consequences of a breakdown of the feeding process. Nutritional vulnerability results from difficultly in obtaining food (see Box 19.1), failure to consume adequate and appropriate food (see Box 19.2), or inability to utilize food (see Box 19.3).

BOX 19.1 Difficulties in obtaining food may result from:

- Poor health, affecting functional capacity.
- Low food availability within the society resulting in price rises of essential commodities.
- Insufficient economic production at household level (indicating an inadequate economic performance).
- Losses before and after harvest.
- Loss of reserves through excessive sale, consumption or looting.
- Impoverishment from the use of reserves to cover essential needs.
- Any increase in time to find or produce food.
- Climate change influencing harvests, hunting, collecting and fishing activities.
- Disturbances in market forces from shortages, infrastructural damage and/or transport disruptions.
- Government favouring certain communities and regions, and neglecting others.

BOX 19.2 Failure to consume adequate and appropriate food results from:

- Inability to obtain sufficient food.
- Disturbed eating habits from changes in availability of food products, the time available for preparation and sharing of food, and weaning practices.
- Lack of means and knowledge for caring for dependents when circumstances change and imposed measures are unfamiliar or impossible to apply.
- Lack of adequate health care and exposure to infectious diseases when living conditions change.
- Health problems affecting food consumption (most often anorexia).

BOX 19.3 Inability to utilize food results from:

- Reduced and inadequate food consumption.
- Gastrointestinal pathology associated with reduced digestion and absorption of nutrients.
- Infectious disease having an impact on metabolism and nutrient requirements.

19.2.2 Political vulnerability

Political instability is often associated with the risk of conflict, repression and discrimination, and it also results in an inability to arrest the crisis process. Transport services are usually inadequate. Disregard of human rights may lead to particular groups being disadvantaged, sometimes affecting all but a privileged few.

19.2.3 Economic vulnerability

Economic vulnerability occurs when human and natural phenomena undermine production activities and their yield, thus affecting the ability of communities and entire populations to secure food.

19.3 Pathology of nutritional crises

Famine represents the acute phase of a nutritional crisis. The immediate causes of famine are summarized in Box 19.4. The severity of a famine depends on the level of food insufficiency, its duration, and the persistence of the predisposing phenomena, which then function as aggravating factors.

It is noteworthy that famine is a relatively rare event when one considers how often the famine process is initiated. Famine only develops when household/

BOX 19.4 Immediate causes of famine (one or more may apply)

- Household food production is insufficient or non-existent.
- Harvesting, hunting or fishing activities are insufficient or non-existent.
- Household means to buy food in the market are insufficient because of inadequate supply or high price.
- No food in market place following infrastructure destruction, problems of security or isolation.
- Local mutual aid and social aid systems are exhausted or non-existent.
- National support systems against famine are insufficient, neglected, non-functioning or non-existent.
- International support has not been given to humanitarian agencies to help feed the population.
- Humanitarian agencies unable to access.

---

population vulnerabilities are progressively exploited by repetitive phenomena and reserves to cover nutritional needs are depleted.

Each famine situation is different, but the effect on household economy is the same. Four stages can be identified, although there tends to be overlap between the stages:

1. *Adaptation* This stage overlaps the preliminary phase of the nutritional crisis. Households modify their activities to maximize economic output and productive activities. Reserves may be used to preserve normal life.

2. *Impoverishment* There is an increase in activities usually found loathsome or demeaning; the sale or exchange of non-productive items, termination of reserves, spending limited to the absolute minimum, strict control of food consumption, and increase in access and use of social support networks. Seeds and means of production are preserved in order to maximize chances of recuperation. Food restriction may result in early signs of nutritional inadequacy.

3. *Decapitalization* Households exploit all possible means of income generation, by sale or exchange of their remaining non-productive items. Further food restrictions are initiated, resulting in more advanced nutritional inadequacies and reduced functional capacity. Social services can no longer cope, and social norms disintegrate alongside economic degradation. Individuals struggle to remain alive, at whatever cost.

4. *Hunger and exhaustion* This stage represents the full-blown picture of famine. All reserves are

exhausted, and mortality from malnutrition and infectious diseases reaches epidemic proportions. The international community usually intervenes at this stage.

The extent to which households and communities recover from famine depends upon the stage at which the famine is alleviated by outside intervention or reversal of causal phenomena or aggravating factors.

19.4 Diagnosing a crisis: the need for surveys

Frequently when a nutritional crisis occurs, there is a call from local and international media, local authorities and the world at large for instant humanitarian assistance. While the situation is often dire, it is imperative to undertake a full evaluation and develop a logical plan of action before implementing an appropriate programme. Ideally surveys should be undertaken prior to the development of the acute phase of the crisis since it may be possible for the full consequence of the causal phenomena to be averted.

The purpose of the initial survey is to define the extent of the problem and to determine the immediate and future needs of the affected groups as well as the phenomena responsible for the existing or impending crisis. While standard information is required, the precise strategies for obtaining the necessary information will need to be adapted to individual circumstances.

An experienced multidisciplinary team is required to gather appropriate information. Expertise in nutrition, public health, water and shelter and from the appropriate economic sector is needed. For a subsistence agricultural population, advice from an agronomist is required. In a situation such as existed after the break-up of Yugoslavia, input is required from an economist specialized in urban and war-affected economies.

19.4.1 Identification of existing or potential problems

The steps to be followed may appear obvious, but if they are not followed, there will be an inappropriate response. Once the affected regions and populations have been identified, a range of quantitative and qualitative information is required, especially as it relates to the most vulnerable sections of the affected

population (see Box 19.5). The nutritional status of the population must be defined, and the extent to which this can be formally assessed depends upon circumstances.

In order to determine the extent of support that will be required to maintain the feeding process, it is necessary to make quantitative assessments of the remaining food stocks and expected agricultural production. To this is added a qualitative assessment of what might be available from forage activities, exchange and purchase, taking into account the changed circumstances. For example, in normal circumstances, forage activities may produce nuts and fish of high nutritive value, but in a crisis may only produce green leaves and wild grains of limited nutritive value. Home-brewed beer and gathered firewood may in good times generate income or provide items for exchange, but during a crisis others may be attempting similar activities and their value is thus reduced. For those who rely habitually, or during a crisis, on food purchase for family needs, the extent to which available income can meet food costs must be established. In general, when as much as 80% of available income is required for food purchase, a critical phase has been reached. Although the gap between means and needs is difficult to assess, such information is essential.

In addition to assessing the absolute severity of the crisis, it is important to discover how the situation differs from 'normal'. Access to food (quality as well as quantity), food preparation, distribution within the family, and means of distributing the food need to be compared. It is also important to establish how the population or high-risk groups have coped with comparable problems in the past. Box 19.6 gives an example of the initial assessment of a crisis in Irian Jaya.

BOX 19.5 Summary of initial survey (*with methods to obtain the required information*)

1. Geographic localization of the affected area (*maps and views in cross-section*).
2. Identification of the population groups affected by the crisis.

For each population, undertake and determine:

3. Subdivision of each group to economic classes (poor, average, rich), an economic profile for each class (number and types of economic activity), both in usual times and at the time of the survey (*functional classification; proportional piling*).
4. Assess the relative importance and proportion of activity for each economic class in the economy: when the situation is normal; when the situation is the worst they remember; when the situation is the best they remember; and the situation at the time of the survey; incorporating food consumption, both qualitatively and quantitatively, and the general system of social obligation in different situations (*proportional piling and study of food consumption*).

5. Minimum economic resources for economic self-sufficiency in usual times (*household economy models with budget equilibrium*).
6. Usual means of adaptation or modification to normal variations in the economy and climate (*proportional piling and seasonal calendars*).
7. Methods that might be employed to alleviate particular crises.
8. Stages of the famine process, including assessment of nutritional status (*model of household activities; anthropometry; evaluation of nutritional resources*).
9. Causes of the present situation (*diagrams of events; graphical representation of market prices; income/exchange rates*).
10. Events that could ameliorate or worsen the situation.
11. Problems faced by the population (*class in order of priority*).
12. Requirements for aid (*class in order of priority*).
13. Programme required to deliver aid (*identify all actions, Strengths, Weaknesses, Opportunities, Threats (SWOT) analysis, decision-making tree*).

BOX 19.6 Initial assessment of the 1997 crisis in Irian Jaya

In 1997, rumours circulated that El Nino would lead to an unprecedented drought in Irian Jaya, leading to a risk of famine. The signal led to a preliminary survey. The approach to the situation consisted of documenting the climate, mode of living of the inhabitants and factors that could influence progress of the survey. The nutritionist in the survey team learned that, despite the drought, it rained heavily in some places and field conditions were extremely difficult with village access almost impossible without helicopter. The population lived essentially on sweet potato and forage. There were almost no health posts, malaria was rampant and communication with the local people required translators. Initial preparation involved obtaining as much local information as possible, including information on the cultivation and nutritional value of sweet potatoes. Such preliminary data gathering helped to define the logistical constraints should an assistance

programme prove necessary. Once in the field, the rumours of the drought and the famine were confirmed, despite not being able to verify the effects directly on the affected population. The surveying nutritionist believed that despite the drought being well-established, it was necessary to verify the effects on the population as the people are well known for their resilience and abilities to forage, hunt and fish. In the first village visited, it was clear that the population already had signs of severe malnutrition. Thus, the approach was changed. Levels of malnutrition were measured and a state of famine due to drought declared. Visits to the agricultural areas confirmed the virtual absence of production due to drought. General poor health resulting from malaria, chest infections and diarrhoea, exacerbated by the reappearance of rain and cold, aggravated the situation. The situation could only be relieved by humanitarian aid.

Working through the list of phenomena with a potential to cause vulnerability and precipitate the acute phase of the crisis is an integral part of the initial survey, and it is an essential prerequisite to determining the solution. For example, if in a subsistence agricultural zone the cause of the famine is drought, one might expect the harvest after the next rainy season to relieve the problem, and this might require only temporary food assistance. However, if the famine is a result of armed conflict, prolonged support and intensive negotiation with military authorities may be necessary. Table 19.1 summarizes the phenomena

Table 19.1 Access to food (in order of importance), phenomena and difficulties encountered and the responses made in the course of the famine in a region in southern Sudan

Access to food	Phenomena and difficulties	Population responses
Milk from the herd (normal access)	– Attacks against the cattle herd in 1991–1992 – Seasonal migration	– Agriculture – Fishing – Forage for wild resources – Marriage – Salaried employment – Social obligations
Cattle sales for sorghum purchase (normal access)	– War between 1989 and 1994	– Agriculture – Salaried employment
Agriculture (seasonal activity, normally marginal)	– Drought in 1993 – Destruction by insects in 1993 and 1994 – Lack of tools and seeds – Seasonal factors – Forced displacement between 1988 and 1992	– Fishing – Forage for wild resources – Salaried employment – Social obligations
Fishing (seasonal activity, normally marginal)	– Drought in 1993 – Lack of equipment – Seasonal factors – Forced displacement between 1988 and 1992	– Forage for wild resources – Salaried employment – Social obligations – Reduction in food consumption
Forage for wild resources (seasonal activity, normally marginal)	– Drought in 1993 – Seasonal factors – Competition for natural resources	– Salaried employment – Social obligations – Reduction in food consumption
Salaried employment (activity undertaken only in cases of necessity)	– More workers than work available – Insecurity impedes access to work – Unable to fulfil employers' requirement	– Social obligations – Reduction in food consumption
Social obligations (reciprocal assistance)	– Poor overall economic situation for the community – Relationships breakdown	– Reduction in food consumption – Humanitarian aid in 1993
Humanitarian aid (occasional, irregular, rather rare)	– Political constraints in 1994 – Season access factors – Donor fatigue in 1994	– Reduction in food consumption
Reduction in food consumption (response to the crisis situation)	– Physiological reserves already made poor	– No more response possible – Significantly increased mortality

that influenced access to food, the difficulties encountered and the responses made during the course of the prolonged famine in southern Sudan. Despite the wide ranging and desperate responses made by the population to the phenomena, the stage was reached when outside aid offered the only means of survival.

19.4.2 In-depth survey, continuing surveillance and evaluation

An action plan is generally developed after the initial survey. However, there is often need for more in-depth information to ensure the most appropriate level and type of support. This includes consideration of any possible untoward effects of the intervention, obtaining a better understanding of relevant cultural issues (specifically those related to food) and identification of the vulnerable groups. Much useful information is often obtained from discussion with community leaders and affected individuals. Once the plan has been implemented, ongoing surveillance is essential, as is a final evaluation to ensure that lessons learned can inform future interventions and that resources have been appropriately utilized.

19.5 Planning the intervention

Box 19.7 lists the eight stages of the development of an intervention plan. In defining priorities, the two most important factors are ensuring the protection of individual rights and providing assistance for survival, if the population is no longer self-sufficient in productive activities. This may involve general food distributions, rehabilitational feeding programmes, selective feeding programmes and nutrition education. Economic support and rehabilitation must also be considered. Once priorities have been established, it is important that these are followed, regardless of the logistical or security constraints. Every effort must be made to overcome the difficulties because 'second-best' strategies are seldom successful. The protection

---

BOX 19.7 Planning an intervention programme

1. Define the priorities, ensuring protection of human rights and assistance necessary for survival.

2. Define the objectives
Statement of the problem including who and how many will benefit, and time required for stated outcome.

3. A plan of activities and resources
Qualitative and quantitative plan including human resources, material, logistics and financial requirements in order of priority.

4. Plan mobilizing resources
Includes finding required personnel, material, the approach to donors and time period in which resources can be obtained.

5. Plan of the tasks
Implementation includes the roles and responsibilities of the personnel, the logistic chain, a calendar of activities, administration for personnel (lodging, regulations and security), work plans and coordination with others involved.
Surveillance includes methods to identify key indicators, persons responsible for surveillance and reports methods and timing.

6. Plan to evaluate the intervention's impact
Includes measuring against identified key indicators, and who is responsible.

7. Awareness of the possibility of adjustment to intervention if necessary.

8. Plan for disengagement
This includes a calendar for withdrawal, use of remaining resources and follow-up after withdrawal.

of rights to access food are an integral component of Protocols of the Geneva Conventions and the Declaration of International Human Rights.

Once the priorities and objectives have been defined, the activities and resources and the means of mobilizing them need to be determined. The implementation plan includes the development of detailed work plans, coordination with others politically involved in providing relief including local authorities, the roles and responsibilities of personnel, security and such details as lodging for personnel. At the outset, it is necessary not only to establish the means for adjustment if surveillance and evaluation demonstrate that this is necessary, but the terms of disengagement (total or partial) are also defined at this stage. This will occur if objectives have been met, if the intervention is made obsolete by a change in the situation, if adverse effects result from the intervention or if insecurity, a deteriorating political situation or other logistical issues result in an untenable situation. The terms and methods of withdrawal also need to be considered.

19.6 Nutrition-related programmes in the management of a crisis

19.6.1 General food distribution

Ideally, a general food distribution to families or households should be implemented before a famine situation in order to avoid the crisis and preserve their way of life. However, usually it is a means to provide macronutrients and micronutrients to a population already in a famine situation in order to prevent deterioration, or in the early recuperative phase to facilitate recovery. Food rations appropriate to individual situations are distributed regularly to restore or protect functional capacity. A general food distribution is usually accompanied by programmes necessary to provide water, shelter (especially in the case of displaced populations), health services and opportunities for the restoration of the economy. General food assistance depends less upon the nutritional status of a population than the capacity to procure food, since food assistance may prolong a crisis, result in sale of distributed items and lead to what has been described as 'assistance syndrome'. Detailed planning will precede any such distribution (see section 19.5).

Distribution rations may be made to households or groups by a humanitarian organization (the preferred method) or by giving the food to a community for redistribution amongst its members. Rations may be given either as bulk food items to be taken home, survival rations or as prepared meals for immediate consumption. Survival rations are based on the average nutritional needs of a population with appropriate quantities provided for each household. A complete ration theoretically provides all necessary macronutrients and micronutrients. In reality, there is often a need to supplement this in some way from local sources (e.g. foraging). It is essential that rations provide food in acceptable forms. For predominantly agricultural populations, this is relatively easy because cereals and legumes can be distributed in dried form. The situation is far more complex for groups who traditionally consume tubers and bananas, or who are pastoralists, or who rely on fish. Diversity is essential in the foods provided in order to avoid deficiencies.

Food rations are based on energy requirements (see Table 19.2) and typically contain a principal energy source (usually a cereal), a concentrated energy source (e.g. oil enriched with vitamin A), a protein source (legumes, tinned fish or meat, dried fish), iodized salt, complementary food to provide micronutrients or micronutrient tablets, and spices, condiments, tea, coffee and sugar.

Rations that form part of a general food distribution may need to be augmented in certain situations. Where nutritional rehabilitation is required, an appreciable increase in both energy and protein is necessary. If grain, which needs to be milled, is provided (rather than cereal flour), the inevitable loss of energy

Table 19.2 Reference rations based on average weight by age group, gender and level of physical activity

WHO 1			WHO 2		
Age (years)	%[1]	Energy needs (kcal (kJ))	Age (years)	%[1]	Energy needs (kcal (kJ))
0–1	3	820 (3 290)	0–4	12.37	1290 (5 390)
2–3	9	1360 (5 680)	5–9	11.69	1860 (7 770)
4–6	8.7	1830 (7 650)	10–14	10.53	2210 (9 240)
7–9	8.5	2190 (9 150)	15–19	9.54	2420 (10 120)
10–14 M	6.3	2800 (11 700)	20–59	48.63	2230 (9 320)
10–14 F	6.2	2450 (10 240)	60+	7.24	1890 (7 900)
Adults M	29.2	3000 (12 540)	Pregnant (supplem.)	2.4	285 (1 190)
Adults F	26.2	2200 (9 200)	Lactating (supplem.)	2.6	500 (2 090)
Pregnant	1.5	2550 (10 660)			
Lactating	1.4	2750 (11 490)			
Average		2350 (9 820)			2080 (8 690)

[1]Approximate proportion of age group in the population.

WHO 1—Basic ration for a developing country. The population is considered to be moderately active with an average weight of 65 kg for men and 55 kg for women. This ration is used by the International Committee of the Red Cross rounded to 2400 kcal/person/day.

WHO 2—Reference ration for a developing country. The population is considered to be lightly active with average weights of 60 kg and 52 kg for men and women. This ration is used by the WHO, the World Food Programme and the High Commission for Refugees. In practice, the absolute minimum ration of 1900 kcal/person/day is usually distributed.

Energy requirements should be increased with reductions in the ambient temperature or with increased requirements for physical activity.

and nutrients needs to be taken into account, as does the cost of milling. However, grain is often preferred over flour because it travels and stores better and it is cheaper. Flour, on the other hand, can be consumed immediately and can be fortified, and is regarded as preferable in dire situations when an immediate source of energy and micronutrients is required. Theft can be a major problem that prevents food aid from reaching the target group, and humanitarian organizations are often faced with finding ways to ensure that armed groups, sometimes government agencies, do not redirect the aid for their own purposes.

Putting in place a general food distribution, in practice, involves creating a beneficiary population and establishing good relations with the population and their traditional authorities, starting from the moment of the initial survey. If the general food assistance is to be provided to households rather than the community or local government, there needs to be a population census and the provision of distribution cards that provide access to the assistance programme. Recipients need to understand the process by which the food distribution will take place. Explanation regarding place, frequency, quantity and control of distribution is essential to avoid frustration, cheating and misunderstanding. Firmness and reliability relating to procedures ensures respect of the population and authorities, and helps to guarantee security in conflict zones. It also facilitates the logistical chain and is important *vis-a-vis* donors, media and political authorities.

Complementary rations A complementary ration can be considered if a population is not self-sufficient in acquiring food and/or it is too dangerous to complete all activities to acquire sufficient food. The complementary ration furnishes the foodstuffs unable to be found (partially or totally), or is of replacement value to allow continued survival. While the concept of complementary rations is straightforward, the principles involved in planning and implementing a programme involve a process that is similar to that required for a general food distribution.

Targeting a population Targeting a beneficiary population for general food assistance reduces wastage by not assisting those who have no real need. Targeting can be geographical or can be of specific households within communities. Although it can be difficult to find objective criteria to differentiate between the extremely poor and the very poor, targeting too far may also be dangerous because those who do not qualify for inclusion in the programme may be resentful and may retaliate. It can also be important to target the host community, to ensure the displaced people under their care help will be well accepted and integrated. Protocols as described for a general food distribution are required.

Feeding kitchens Feeding kitchens may be required to meet the food needs of a population if a beneficiary population has no means of cooking their own meals, or security situations prevent carrying food items to homes. They may also be required in institutions. Community kitchens provide the same energy and protein requirements as would a general food ration and they require the census and control mechanisms described earlier.

19.6.2 Rehabilitational feeding

Rehabilitational feeding is necessary to treat severe malnutrition and specific deficiencies, which almost invariably occur in a famine situation. The purpose is to identify such individuals and restore them to a satisfactory nutritional status to permit survival in their natural environment, even if this involves dependence on other humanitarian programmes. If the target population is concentrated in an area, it is conceptually relatively easy to establish a rehabilitational centre, although invariably there are logistical difficulties to overcome to ensure security, an uninterrupted supply line of medications and provisions, and adequate supplies of water. If, on the other hand, the population is a nomadic one, it may be impossible to implement a rehabilitation programme.

Ideally, a rehabilitation programme involves four phases (cf. section 18.1.4). Early treatment includes rehydration, correction of electrolyte imbalance and treatment of infections; nutritional rehabilitation follows. Thereafter, the malnourished child or adult should return to a normal food supply. Surveillance should continue once the patient has returned 'home' so that corrective measures can be resumed in the event of a relapse.

Detailed methods to achieve rehabilitation can be found in handbooks published by the International Committee of the Red Cross, Médicins Sans Frontières and the WHO. An example from the Planalto of Angola describes the two main means for achieving nutritional rehabilitation and the required parallel programmes (see Box 19.8).

19.6.3 Supplementary feeding programmes

Supplementary feeding programmes involve distribution of a food supplement to individuals or groups considered vulnerable, in order to prevent deterioration in nutritional status. Conceptually it is a hybrid measure, somewhere in between a small general food assistance and the provision of a partial nutritional rehabilitation centre. Because what little food distributed is often further redistributed by the beneficiary, it is generally not a particularly appropriate or successful measure and is usually implemented when there are insufficient resources for general food assistance.

BOX 19.8 Nutritional programmes required to relieve a crisis in Angola

In late 1993, a nutritional evaluation on the Planalto of Angola revealed a drought situation exacerbated by inaccessibility to other areas as a result of on-going conflict, with no access to work or means of food procurement.

Increasing mortality associated with severe malnutrition required rapid intervention. The closure of road access by landmines left an airlift as the only means for logistical supply. A 3000 metric tonnes per month supply pipeline capacity required the setting of priorities. While bulk food items were assembled for distribution, a census of the population was undertaken, rehabilitational feeding centres established (a total of five for the young severely malnourished), with 18 community kitchens (to provide energy and essential nutrients ensuring rehabilitation for those able to eat sufficient bulk food to achieve adequate weight gain), water supplies protected, and provision of medicines to medical facilities and vaccination programmes initiated.

Once monthly general food assistance was meeting the food needs of the population, and nutritional rehab-

ilitation and health programmes functioning, non-food (blankets, soap and kitchen sets) and agricultural distributions (seeds and tools) were undertaken at appropriate seasonal interludes.

Disengagement of activities in this instance was precipitated by military activity. However, a resumption of nutrition programmes was unnecessary as nutrition rehabilitation had been achieved and a deterioration in status was not expected following a satisfactory harvest and the reopening of road transport routes to the coast facilitating trade. However, a programme of continued surveillance with random cluster surveys measuring nutritional status and following food access ensured adequate monitoring.

In this case, the full range of approaches was required to deliver an adequate food supply to 600 000 beneficiaries and the daily rehabilitation of 21 000 people to reduce mortality. Co-operation and collaboration between the implementing agencies enabled survival of the population.

RECOMMENDED READING

1. **Mourey, A.** (2004) *Manuel de nutrition pour l'intervention humanitaire*. Geneva, Comité International de la Croix-Rouge (CICR). (English version expected in 2007.)

FURTHER READING

1. **De Ville de Goyet, C.** (1978) *The management of nutritional emergencies in large populations*. Geneva, World Health Organization.

2. **FAO/WHO/UN** (1985) *Energy and protein requirements*. Report of a Joint FAO/WHO/UNU Expert Consultation. Technical Report Series 724. Geneva, World Health Organization.

3. **MSF** (1995) *Nutrition guidelines*. Paris: Médicins Sans Frontières.

4. **Pratt, B., and Boyden, J.** (1985) *The field director's handbook. An Oxfam manual for development workers*. London, Oxfam.

5. **Shoham, J.** (1995) *Emergency supplementary feeding programmes. Good practice review 2. Relief and rehabilitation network*. London, Overseas Development Institute.

6. **Sphere Project** (1998) *Humanitarian Charter and Minimum Standards in Disaster Response*. A programme of The Steering Committee for Humanitarian Response and InterAction with VOICE, ICRC, ICVA. Geneva, The Sphere Project.

7. **UNICEF** (1986) *Assisting in emergencies. A resource handbook for UNICEF field staff*. New York, United Nation Children's Fund.

8. **WFP/UNHCR** (1997) *Guidelines for estimating food and nutritional needs in emergencies*. World Food Programme and United Nations High Commissioner for Refugees.

9. **WHO** (1999) *Management of severe malnutrition: A manual for physicians and other senior health workers*. Geneva, World Health Organization.

10. **WHO** (2000) *The management of nutrition in major emergencies*. Geneva, World Health Organization.

Editor's note

At the time of going to print, *The Lancet* had once again drawn attention to the fact that starvation is the biggest killer in the world and contributes significantly to the 10.9 million deaths annually among children under 5 years. The current drought, reportedly more severe than those reported previously, in north-eastern Kenya has killed 40% of the country's cattle. Desperate pastoralists are sharing their meals with livestock in a bid to save the few remaining animals that have not yet died, thus exacerbating the human consequences of famine. Kenya has appealed for US$245 million to help an estimated 3.5 million people, including 500 000 children in need of urgent humanitarian assistance. The World Food Programme has highlighted the expanding geography of famine. The band of malnutrition between the tropics of Cancer and Capricorn is now extending north to the Commonwealth of Independent States and China. Over 800 million people worldwide are considered to be at risk. The consequences of lack of rain are exacerbated by chronic inadequate external investment in infrastructure. While short-term emergency food aid is essential, and will continue to be necessary in Kenya and other areas where nutritional crises exist, to avoid mass starvation, such aid should be seen to resemble the interest payment on an accumulating debt. Longer-term strategies are urgently required to address the local factors that tip the balance from drought to famine.

1. **Anon.** (2006) A global famine. *Lancet*, **367**, 876.

2. **Wakabi, W.** (2006) *'Worst drought in a decade' leaves Kenya crippled. Lancet*, **367**, 891–2.

 To see topical and scientifically robust updates on nutrition associated with this textbook, and active web links to many of the journal articles in the Reference areas, please see the dedicated Online Resource Centre at www.oxfordtextbooks.co.uk/orc/mann3e/.

20 Cardiovascular diseases

Jim Mann and Alexandra Chisholm

Cardiovascular disease includes coronary heart disease (CHD) (also referred to as coronary artery disease or ischaemic heart disease, cerebrovascular disease and peripheral arterial disease). A similar pathological process underlies each of these three groups of conditions which affect the heart, the brain and peripheral arteries. Inappropriate nutrition has most consistently been linked with CHD, and this chapter deals primarily with CHD and those risk factors for the disease which are influenced by diet.

Coronary heart disease

CHD is a common condition in most affluent and some developing societies. In most industrialized countries, it is the commonest single cause of death, often accounting for around one-third of all deaths. In addition, each year there are about as many non-fatal cases as there are deaths. A high proportion of the health care budget in these countries is spent treating CHD and its consequences. Genetic as well as nutritional factors contribute to the aetiology of the condition, but lifestyle modification is undoubtedly the most effective means of reducing CHD risk in high-risk populations and individuals. Dietary modification is also important in the treatment of people who have already developed CHD.

20.1 Pathological and clinical aspects

The basic pathological lesion underlying CHD is the atheromatous plaque, which bulges on the inside of one or more of the coronary arteries that supply blood to the heart muscle (myocardium). In addtion, a superimposed thrombus or clot may further occlude the artery (Fig. 20.1). A variety of cells and lipids are involved in the pathogenesis of the atherosclerotic plaque and the arterial thrombus, including lipoproteins, cholesterol, triglycerides, platelets, monocytes, endothelial cells, fibroblasts and smooth muscle cells.

Nutrition can influence the development of CHD by modifying either atherogenesis or thrombogenesis or both these processes. Two readily identifiable clinical conditions result from these pathological processes:

1. *Angina pectoris* is characterized by pain in the centre of the chest, which is brought on by exertion or stress, and which may radiate down the left arm or to the neck. It results from a reduction or temporary block to the blood flow through the coronary artery

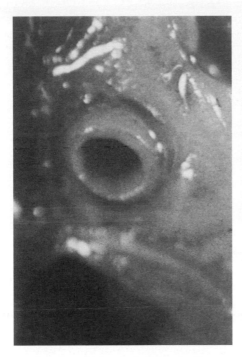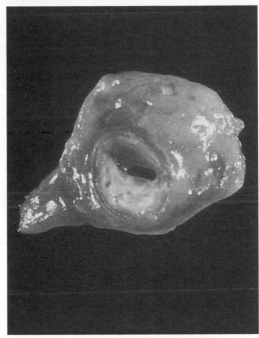

Fig. 20.1 A normal coronary artery is contrasted with an artery showing atheromatous deposits.

to the heart muscle. The pain usually passes with rest and seldom lasts for more than 15 minutes.

2. *Coronary thrombosis* or *myocardial infarction* results from total occlusion of the artery, which causes infarction or death of some of the heart muscle cells and is associated with prolonged, and usually excruciating, central chest pain. The terms coronary thrombosis and myocardial infarction are used to describe the same clinical condition, although they really describe its two distinct pathological processes.

20.2 Epidemiological aspects

There are marked international differences in rates of CHD (Fig. 20.2). Overall rates are higher in men than women, though as women age, CHD contributes a greater proportion of total mortality. Mortality rates are more than seven times higher in some Eastern European countries than they are in Japan and within Europe, and there is an almost threefold difference between France, Spain and Portugal on the one hand and some of the more northern countries such as Scotland, Northern Ireland and Finland. The experience of migrants and changing rates in various countries suggest that environmental and behavioural differences account for much of the variation between countries. People who have migrated from a low-risk country (e.g. Japan) to a relatively high-risk country (e.g. the USA) tend to have rates approaching the host country. There is also some evidence for the reverse: Finns living in Sweden have appreciably lower rates than those in their country of origin. In the UK, where CHD rates are higher in Scotland and Northern Ireland than in England, CHD risk depends upon country of residence at the time of death rather than country of birth.

Some examples of the rapidly changing rates (increases as well as decreases) are shown in Fig. 20.3. Some of the most striking changes have been the increase in many European countries, North America, Australia and New Zealand during the third quarter

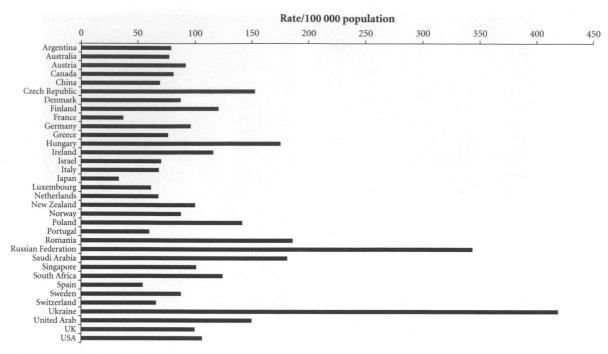

Fig. 20.2 International differences in estimated ischaemic heart disease death rates. League Label for 2002: mortality in men and women aged 40–69 years.

Source: WHO (2002) *Death and DALY estimates* (http://www.who.int/healthinfo/en/).

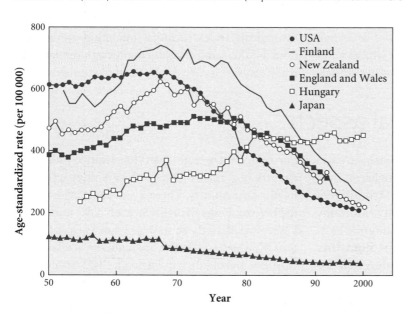

Fig. 20.3 Trends in age-standardized coronary heart disease mortality rates in men aged 40–69 years, in six countries from 1950 to 2000.

Source: Modified from Beaglehole, R. (1999) International trends in coronary heart disease mortality and incidence rates. *J Cardiovasc Risk*, **6**, 63–8.

of the twentieth century. Then, in the fourth quarter, rates declined appreciably in those countries but increased strikingly in most countries of Eastern Europe. In general, a decline has occurred in those

countries where the attempt to reduce cardiovascular risk factors has been most active. The situation is particularly complex in some countries where affluence and poverty coexist and which are said to be in a state of nutrition transition. In such countries, (e.g. India, South Africa), CHD rates are high amongst the relatively affluent and those rapidly accumulating wealth, whereas diseases of undernutrition remain prevalent amongst the poor and underprivileged. This situation is the reverse of what has been observed in more affluent societies where the socioeconomically disadvantaged have higher CHD rates than better-educated, more affluent groups in the community.

Projections suggest that CHD will become an increasingly important health issue in developing countries and that the majority of cases and deaths worldwide will be in developing rather than developed

countries. The changes that have occurred are compatible with lifestyle changes that have occurred in these countries, but given the complex interactions between various lifestyle attributes that may influence CHD rates, it is very difficult from such data to disentangle individual effects. This may be done using more sophisticated epidemiological and experimental approaches discussed later. The observation that changes in CHD rates have occurred over relatively short time periods encourages the belief that CHD is to some extent preventable. The hope is to reduce morbidity and mortality from CHD in those who are in the prime of life.

20.3 Foods and nutrients in the aetiology of coronary heart disease: the development of the diet–heart hypothesis

Early studies investigating the role of dietary factors in the causation of CHD involved correlating national dietary intakes (based on food balance data) with CHD death rates (mortality) in countries with varying rates or with changes in CHD mortality over time in individual countries. Positive associations between CHD death rate (age standardized) and saturated fat, sucrose, animal protein and coffee consumption and negative correlations with flour (and other foods rich in complex carbohydrates) and vegetables are some of the most clearly described. However, both food balance data and mortality statistics can be unreliable. Studies that measure food intake of individuals and relate this information about food and nutrients to accurately recorded information regarding CHD events and mortality are much more reliable.

It was the pioneering Seven Country Study that was started around a half-century ago, coordinated by Ancel Keys and colleagues, which gave credence to the diet–heart hypothesis. Food consumption of people in 16 defined cohorts in seven countries, selected because of their widely varying rates of CHD, was related to subsequent CHD incidence. The strongest correlation was observed between CHD and percentage of energy derived from saturated fat (Fig. 20.4).

Weak inverse associations (suggesting protective effects) were found with percentages of energy from mono- and polyunsaturated fat and CHD. Total fat did not correlate with CHD, and of the other well-known risk factors for CHD (see below) only plasma (total) cholesterol and blood pressure appeared to

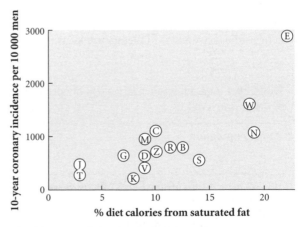

Fig. 20.4 Association between CHD and percentage energy derived from saturated fatty acids in the Seven Country Study. Letters on the graph indicate the location of the cohorts in the seven countries.

Source: Keys, A. (1980). *Seven countries: a multivarate analysis of death and coronary heart disease*. Massachusetts, Havard University Press.

explain part of the geographic variation in the frequency of this condition. These observations led to the suggestion that nutrition-related factors may be particularly important in determining whether countries are likely to have high CHD rates and that the diet–heart disease link was principally mediated via an effect of saturated fat on plasma cholesterol, which in turn increased the risk of CHD. The Seven Country Study also provided evidence that the degree of risk conferred by other lifestyle factors is strongly influenced by nutrition-related factors: the relationship between cigarette smoking and CHD is much more powerful in those countries where saturated fat intake and mean plasma cholesterol levels are high (e.g. in the USA and northern European countries) than in southern Europe and Japan, where saturated fat intake and cholesterol levels are lower.

A few well-conducted prospective studies have examined the relationship between foods and nutrients and the subsequent development of CHD within a single population. In addition to the problems associated with the long-term follow-up of tens of thousands of individuals, there are particular difficulties associated with establishing nutritional aetiology in this way: no methods for measuring dietary intake are fully reliable, and a single assessment does not necessarily provide a truly representative indication of lifelong, or even long-term dietary practices. Some more recent studies have assessed dietary intake using more sophisticated food frequency questionnaires administered several times during the follow-up period and have used biological markers as surrogate measures of dietary intake (e.g. plasma levels of antioxidants; fatty acid composition of red cells, platelets or adipose tissue as indicators of the nature of dietary fat).

Among the best known and most meticulous of the prospective studies have been those undertaken by the Harvard group, led by Willett, and based on follow-up of huge cohorts of female nurses and male health professionals. These studies are impressive because of their size and excellent retention rates, the detailed and validated food frequency questionnaires from which intakes of foods and nutrients are computed, and the sophisticated statistical analyses that have examined the effects of potential confounding by other factors related to CHD. The Harvard and other longitudinal studies have suggested several foods and nutrients that may be protective against CHD: fish, wholegrain cereals, fruits and vegetables, nuts, garlic, moderate intakes of red wine and some other alcoholic drinks, antioxidant nutrients (B_6, vitamins C and E, flavonoids), non-starch polysaccharides and folic acid and several long-chain unsaturated fatty acids—C18:2, ω-6; C18:3, ω-3; C20:5, ω-3—and three that might increase risk—dietary cholesterol, *trans* unsaturated fatty acids and coffee. Some examples of the studies in which these associations have been demonstrated are given in Table 20.1. It

Table 20.1 Age-adjusted relative risk of coronary heart disease according to quintile of intake of certain foods or nutrients

Study population	Relative risk according to quintile of intake					*P* for trend
	1	2	3	4	5	
43 757 male health professionals (40–75 years) (Rimm *et al.*, 1996)	Total dietary fibre					
	1.00	0.97	0.91	0.87	0.59	< 0.001
75 521 female nurses (38–63 years) (Liu *et al.*, 2000)	Wholegrain consumption					
	1.00	0.87	0.82	0.72	0.67	< 0.001
87 245 female nurses (34–59 years) (Stampfer and Rimm, 1995)	Total vitamin E intake					
	1.00	0.90	1.00	0.68	0.59	< 0.001
39 910 male health professionals (40–75 years) (Rimm *et al.*, 1996)	Carotene intake					
	1.00	0.93	0.93	0.86	0.71	0.02

should be noted that, even in longitudinal studies where dietary intake has been carefully measured and endpoints accurately assessed, it may be extremely difficult to determine whether any demonstrated association is causal. Further information on causality may be obtained from studies examining the effect of foods and nutrients on cardiovascular risk factors (section 20.4) and intervention trials (section 20.5).

20.4 Cardiovascular risk factors and their nutritional determinants

Attempts to explain the pathological process underlying CHD and to identify individuals at risk suggest that there is no single cause of the disease. An understanding of the characteristics that put individuals at particular risk of developing CHD provides a useful background against which to examine in more detail the role of diet in the aetiology. The term 'risk factor' is used to describe features of lifestyle and behaviour, as well as physical and biochemical attributes that predict an increased likelihood of developing CHD. Potential risk factors are often identified when comparisons are made between people who have developed CHD and healthy controls (case–control studies) and are confirmed by cohort (prospective) studies in which these factors are measured in a large group of apparently healthy people who are then followed to see if they develop the disease or not at some future date. The presence, absence or degree of each factor can then be related to the risk of developing CHD. Table 20.2 lists most of the important risk factors for CHD that have been identified in this way. The effect of risk factors is synergistic if they are

Table 20.2 Risk factors for coronary heart disease

Irreversible	• Masculine gender • Increasing age • Genetic traits, including monogenic and polygenic disorders of lipid metabolism • Body build
Potentially reversible	• Cigarette smoking • Dyslipidaemia: increased levels of cholesterol, triglyceride, low-density and very-low-density lipoprotein and apolipoprotein B; low levels of high-density lipoprotein; atypical lipoproteins • Oxidizability of low-density lipoprotein • Obesity, especially when associated with high waist circumference or waist/hip ratio • Hypertension • Physical inactivity • Diabetes, hyperglycaemia and insulin resistance • Increased thrombosis: increased haemostatic factors and enhanced platelet aggregation • High levels of homocysteine • High levels of inflammatory markers (e.g. CRP, IL-6, TNFα) • Impaired fetal nutrition
Psychosocial	• Stressful situations • Coronary-prone behaviour patterns: type A behaviour
Geographic	• Climate and season: cold weather • Soft drinking water

truly independent, that is, when more than one risk factor is present, the combined increase in risk is greater than might be expected from simply adding together the risk associated with each. The irreversible psychosocial and geographic factors, as well as cigarette smoking and physical activity, are reviewed in textbooks of medicine and epidemiology. This chapter concentrates on potentially reversible factors that have been shown to be influenced by diet.

20.4.1 Dyslipidaemia

Altered levels of blood lipids and lipoproteins (see Chapter 3) may place individuals at increased risk of CHD in three ways. First, a relatively small proportion of people have an exceptionally high risk because of a clearly inherited increase of plasma lipids and lipoproteins. Second, a large number of people

(perhaps as many as half the adult population in high-risk countries) have a slight to moderately increased risk because their blood lipids are higher than desirable as a result of an interaction between polygenic (many genes involved) and lifestyle-related factors. They are described as having 'polygenic' or 'common' hyperlipidaemia. Third, some people are also at increased CHD risk because of low levels of high-density lipoprotein (HDL).

Genetically determined disorders of lipid metabolism The clearly defined genetically determined disorders of lipid metabolism, which are usually characterized by an increase in one or more lipoprotein fractions, are described in Table 20.3. *Familial hypercholesterolaemia* is the best known. It is characterized by marked elevation of plasma total and low-density lipoprotein (LDL) cholesterol, with xanthomas

Table 20.3 'Genetic–metabolic' classification of hyperlipidaemia

	Atherosclerosis risk	Inheritance	Relative prevalence	Lipid abnormalities
Familial hypercholesterolaemia	+++	Autosomal dominant	++	Cholesterol and LDL ↑↑ Triglyceride N or slightly ↑
Familial combined hyperlipidaemia	++	Uncertain	+++	Cholesterol and LDL ↑ Triglyceride and VLDL ↑
Remnant hyperlipoproteinaemia	++	Apo EIII deficiency and other factors	+	Cholesterol ↑↑ Triglyceride ↑↑ Intermediate-density lipoprotein ↑
Familial hypertriglyceridaemia Excessive synthesis	Uncertain	Probably autosomal dominant	+	Triglyceride and VLDL ↑↑ Chylomicrons ↑
Lipoprotein lipase/apo CII deficiency	Uncertain	Probably recessive	Rare	Triglyceride ↑↑ Chylomicrons ↑↑ VLDL ↑
Polygenic hypercholesterolaemia	+	Polygenic	++++	Cholesterol and LDL ↑

↑ = raised; ↑↑ = markedly raised; N = normal; + = relatively low; ++++ = extremely high; LDL = low-density lipoproteins; VLDL = very-low-density lipoproteins.
Source: Lewis, (1987) B. Disorders of lipid transport. In: Weatherall D.J., Ledingham J.G.G., and Warrell D.A. (eds) *The Oxford Textbook of Medicine*, 2nd edition. Oxford, Oxford University Press.

(nodules) in tendons and a very high risk of premature CHD. Untreated, 85% of males with this condition will have had a myocardial infarction before the age of 60 years. The metabolic abnormality and clinical consequences result from impaired removal of LDL from the circulation because of a reduction in LDL receptors on the surface of cells. The other common inherited hyperlipidaemia, *familial combined hyperlipidaemia*, is characterized by increased LDL and increased very-low-density lipoprotein (VLDL), which result from increased production of these lipoproteins. The mode of inheritance is not so clearly understood, but the condition is associated with an equally high risk of cardiovascular disease. *Remnant hyperlipidaemia* and the *familial hypertriglyceridaemic* states are relatively rare. In addition to the diagnostic categories shown in Table 20.3, some individuals will be at risk because they have increased levels of atypical lipoproteins. Concentrations of lipoprotein (a), which is assembled from LDL and apolipoprotein (a), may vary from near zero to over 1000 mg/L. Case–control studies suggest a strong independent association with CHD, but no data are available from prospective studies. Finally, some individuals appear to have high levels of LDL, that are smaller and more dense than typical LDL particles. These small, dense LDL particles appear to be more atherogenic than typical LDL. Diet and other lifestyle factors are relatively unimportant in the aetiology of these conditions, but play a role in their management.

Polygenic hypercholesterolaemia Hypercholesterolaemia, with elevated LDL or VLDL, or both, is one of the most clearly described CHD risk factors. In over 40 longitudinal studies in different countries, total cholesterol has been shown to be related to the rate of CHD. The association is independent of other risk factors and characterized by a gradient of risk with increasing plasma cholesterol concentration (Fig. 20.5). Cholesterol is a major constituent of the atheromatous plaque. Average cholesterol levels are similar in adult men and women, but this similarity hides the different age trends observed in cross-sectional studies (Fig. 20.6). Hormonal factors may in part explain the gender differences but the fact that

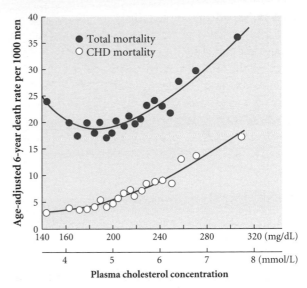

Fig. 20.5 Within-population relationship between plasma cholesterol and CHD and total mortality.

Source: Martin, M.J., Hulley, S.B., Browner, W.S., *et al.* (1968) Serum cholesterol, blood pressure, and mortality: implications from a cohort of 361,662 men. *Lancet*, **2**, 933–6.

populations and groups with low average cholesterol levels do not show such marked increases with age suggest that lifestyle-related factors may also be involved.

LDL which transports the bulk of cholesterol in the blood stream, is taken up by macrophages after being oxidized and may then become deposited in the atheromatous plaque. Dietary antioxidants (vitamins E and C and carotenoids, and possibly flavonoids and selenium) may protect LDL against oxidation (see Chapters 11 and 13) and help slow the progression of atherosclerosis and thus influence the degree of risk conferred by a particular level of plasma cholesterol. High intakes of antioxidants may explain the relatively low rates of CHD in France despite cholesterol and saturated fat intakes that do not differ appreciably from other countries with much higher CHD rates (the 'French paradox', see Box 6.4).

Levels of total and LDL-cholesterol are profoundly influenced by the dietary factors described in Chapter 3 (section 3.3.4). It seems very likely that the deleterious effect of saturated fat on CHD in epidemiological studies is largely explained by the ability

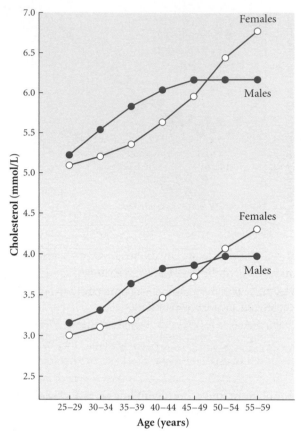

Fig. 20.6 Relationship between total and LDL cholesterol, gender and age. Upper lines: total cholesterol (mmol/L). Lower lines: LDL cholesterol (mmol/L).

Source: Mann, J.I., Lewis, B., Shepherd, J., *et al.* (1988) Blood lipid concentrations and other cardiovascular risk factors: distribution, prevalence, and detection in Britain. *Br Med J*, **296**, 1702–6.

of myristic, palmitic and perhaps also lauric acids to elevate LDL and total cholesterol and the protective effects of ω-6 polyunsaturated fatty acids (PUFA) by their cholesterol-lowering properties.

Hypertriglyceridaemia This is a less clearly defined risk factor. People who have had myocardial infarctions tend to have higher levels of triglycerides and VLDL than controls and this association is confirmed by prospective studies. However, it is not clear whether the association between triglycerides and VLDL and CHD is independent of other factors known to be associated with both raised levels of triglycerides and cardiovascular risk (e.g. obesity,

hyperglycaemia, hypercholesterolaemia and hypertension). It has been suggested that raised levels of triglycerides may only be important in the presence of reduced HDL cholesterol. Raised plasma triglycerides appear to be particularly important in determining cardiovascular risk in people with diabetes. Determinants of plasma triglyceride and VLDL levels are discussed in section 3.3.4.

Reduced high-density lipoprotein concentrations There has been considerable interest in plasma HDL as a protective factor. Women have higher levels of HDL and lower risk of CHD. An attempt to aggregate the findings of four large American studies suggests that an increase of 1 mg/100 mL (0.026 mmol/L) HDL cholesterol is associated with a 2–3% reduction in CHD. HDL levels do not differ markedly with age, are reduced in heavy cigarette smokers, and are increased by physical activity and alcohol intake (Chapter 6). Nutritional determinants are considered in section 3.3.4.

Apolipoproteins Apoprotein B (apo B) and apoproteins A1 (apo A1) are the major apoproteins of LDL and HDL, respectively, and therefore, not surprisingly, the former is predictive of CHD and the latter protective against CHD. However, interestingly the effects appear to be independent of total cholesterol, LDL and HDL. The interaction between diet and the apolipoproteins is complex. Dietary factors that influence LDL and HDL also have an effect on apo B and apo A1, but genetic variation appears to explain some of the variation in LDL and HDL response among individuals to dietary change.

20.4.2 Thrombogenesis

Factors that increase the tendency to thrombosis (either as a result of increased platelet aggregation or a high level of coagulability of blood) have received less attention than those influencing lipids and lipoproteins. They are more difficult to study and much of the relevant research is based on *in vitro* tests, which may not correspond to what goes on inside the body. One clue to the potential for dietary factors to

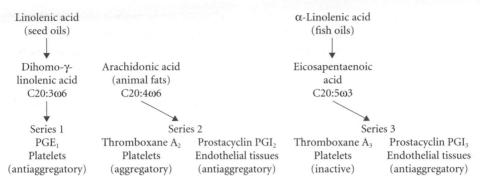

Fig. 20.7 Prostanoids formed from different fatty acids.

Source: Ulbricht, T.L.V., and Southgate, D.A.T. (1991) Coronary heart disease: seven dietary factors. *Lancet*, **330**, 985–92.

enhance or reduce the tendency for platelets to aggregate stems from observations made on the Eskimo people (Inuits) of Greenland. They have low rates of CHD and reduced platelet aggregation compared with Western nations, despite high intakes of total fat. However, this fat comes largely from marine foods rich in ω-3 fatty acids (eicosapentaenoate, C20:5, and docosahexaenoate, C22:6), which form the antiaggregatory prostanoid, PGI_3. Platelet aggregation is largely controlled by a balance between the proaggregatory compound thromboxane A_2 (synthesized from arachidonic acid released from the platelet membrane after injury to the blood vessel wall) and the antiaggregatory substance prostacyclin PGI_2 (also synthesized from arachidonic acid in the endothelial cells of the arterial wall). C20:5 and C22:6 inhibit conversion of arachidonic acid to thromboxane A_2 as well as facilitate the production of the additional antiaggregatory substance PGI_3 (Fig. 20.7). Polyunsaturated fatty acids of the ω-6 series may also reduce platelet aggregation by providing the series 1 prostanoid PGE_1, which is also antiaggregatory. Oleic acid may also act as a inhibitor of platelet aggregation, though the effect is less than for polyunsaturated fatty acids.

Although there have been studies of the antithrombogenic effect of polyunsaturated fatty acids in humans, the thrombogenic effect of saturated fatty acids has been more extensively studied in laboratory animals. The findings are consistent: the longer-chain saturated fatty acids (C14:0, C16:0 and C18:0) all appear to accelerate thrombosis. One mechanism may be via inhibition of antiaggregatory prostacyclin. Stearic acid (C18:0), which appears not to raise LDL, has thrombogenic properties.

Dietary factors may also influence thrombogenesis via an effect on the *coagulation system*. The physiological function of coagulation is to secure haemostasis after an injury. Thrombin is produced, which enables the conversion of soluble fibrinogen to insoluble fibrin. Several prospective studies suggest that factors involved in the coagulation system (notably factor VII and fibrinogen) are important predictors of CHD. Too high a level of coagulability might predispose to thrombosis. High levels of fibrinogen are associated with obesity and cigarette smoking. Factor VII is associated to a greater extent with dietary factors: increasing dietary fat can increase it within 24 hours. Levels of a range of clotting factors, including factor VII, are lower in populations and groups eating a low-fat, high-polyunsaturated/saturated-ratio, high-fibre diet, and individuals changing to such a diet show reduction in these factors. Levels of another prothrombotic agent, plasminogen activator inhibitor-1 (PAI-1) are reduced on low-glycaemic-index diets.

20.4.3 Diabetes, hyperglycaemia and insulin resistance

Many studies have shown that people with diabetes have an increased risk of CHD. Genetic factors play important roles in the aetiology of type 2 diabetes, but nutrition-related factors are also important. Obesity (body mass index > 30) is associated with a considerable increase in risk of diabetes and there is evidence that those who are overweight are also at increased risk. High intakes of saturated fat and low intakes of dietary fibre and low-glycaemic-index foods increase the risk of developing type 2 diabetes. This effect appears to be independent of the relationship between low fibre intakes and obesity. Impaired glucose tolerance, raised levels of fasting glucose and insulin resistance, pre-diabetic states that have a similar aetiology to type 2 diabetes, are also associated with increased cardiovascular risk.

20.4.4 Hypertension

Increasing levels of both systolic and diastolic blood pressure are associated with increased rates of CHD, strokes (cerebral vascular disease) and peripheral vascular disease. Fewer than half of the adults in the USA are considered to have optimal blood pressure and nearly a quarter have hypertension.

Sodium (salt) Over 30 years ago, Dahl drew attention to the correlation between salt intake and prevalence of hypertension in populations. This and other similar studies were flawed by methodological difficulties associated with measuring salt intake and blood pressure. Also, the association may not be causal because increased salt intake is associated with greater acculturation and many other lifestyle-related attributes of a 'Western' diet could explain the link with CHD. The best available method for assessing sodium intake is 24-hour urinary sodium excretion. This method and standardized blood pressure measurements were used in the Intersalt Study (Elliott *et al.*, 1996), which collected data on 10 000 people in 32 countries. The results suggested that a reduction in sodium intake of 100 mmol/day would be expected to result in differences of approximately 10 mmHg in systolic blood pressure and 6 mmHg in diastolic blood pressure over a 30-year period. Meta-analyses of published observational studies, as well as randomized controlled trials, of sodium restriction have demonstrated broadly comparable results.

Even a more modest reduction in dietary sodium (to 50 mmol/day or about 3 g/day of salt) might be expected to lower systolic blood pressure by about 6 mmHg, on average, with more marked reductions in those with higher blood pressures. It has been estimated that a reduction in blood pressure of this magnitude would reduce the incidence of stroke by 26% and CHD by 15%. Several mechanisms have been suggested to explain the association between salt intake and blood pressure, including reduced urinary sodium excretion and fluid retention by some individuals, increased sympathetic nervous system activity and impaired baroreflex function and alterations of ion transport in vascular smooth muscle. The heterogeneity in the response of individuals to sodium restriction suggests the possible existence of a group of hyper-responders, but there is as yet no simple test by which such individuals might be identified.

Potassium In the Intersalt Study, urinary potassium excretion—an assumed indicator of intake—was negatively related to blood pressure. A pooled analysis of a number of intervention trials suggests that potassium supplementation might reduce blood pressure in both normotensive and hypertensive people by an average of 5.9–3.4 mmHg. However, several limitations reduce the likely effectiveness of increasing potassium intake as an important means of treating hypertension. The effect of potassium appears to be relatively small when compared with a reduction in sodium intake. The amount of potassium required to reduce blood pressure is relatively high so that supplements rather than dietary modification would be necessary to achieve appreciable blood pressure lowering. No foods contain sufficient to provide the increase in intake achieved in the trials—between 50 and 140 mmol potassium per day.

Body weight Obese people have higher blood pressures than lean people and if they lose weight their blood pressure falls, even if usual salt intake is maintained on the calorie-restricted diet. Raised blood pressure is particularly associated with obesity that is centrally rather than peripherally distributed. The Intersalt Study showed a highly significant correlation between body mass index as an index of obesity and blood pressure. An Australian study showed, in a clinical trial setting, that dietary weight reduction (mean loss of 7.4 kg) compared favourably with a standard β-blocker drug, metoprolol, in the treatment of mild hypertension. Furthermore, diet was associated with an improvement in the lipid profile, which was not seen with the drug.

Calcium Intracellular calcium is an important determinant of arteriolar tone, and some claims have been made that increased calcium intake can reduce blood pressure. However, two meta-analyses summarizing the results of more than 20 trials showed that intakes of 1000 mg or more of calcium per day have only a trivial effect on blood pressure levels. Calcium supplements or a high-calcium diet might be useful in a very small number of hypertensive patients who have low serum calcium levels or increased plasma parathyroid levels.

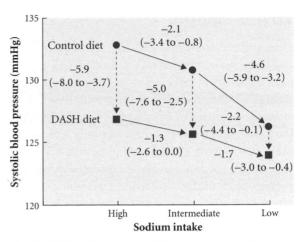

Fig. 20.8 The effect on systolic blood pressure with a control diet when sodium is reduced (●) and on the DASH diet with similar reductions in sodium (■). Differences between DASH and control diets are significant at each level of sodium intake but smallest when sodium intake is low (1.5 g/day).

Source: Sacks *et al.* (2001).

Combining dietary factors It is conceivable that combining the effects of the various nutrients that appear to influence blood pressure levels will have a far greater effect than altering a single nutrient. In the series of DASH (Dietary Approaches to Stop Hypertension) trials (Sacks *et al.*, 2001), the effects on blood pressure of specific diets were compared with control diets—these diets were rich in: fruit and vegetables; fruit, vegetables and low-fat dairy products; fruit, vegetables and low-fat dairy products and low in sodium. As shown in Fig. 20.8, the effect of increasing fruit, vegetable and low-fat dairy products is greatest when sodium intake is also reduced, the reduction in both systolic and diastolic blood pressure being greatest when blood pressures are raised. These effects are comparable with those resulting from some blood pressure-lowering medications.

Comparable data exist regarding the effects of a vegetarian diet on blood pressure. A series of carefully controlled studies from Perth, Western Australia, have shown that significant reductions in systolic and diastolic pressures occur when healthy subjects are changed from a typical Western diet to a vegetarian diet and salt intake is kept constant. Both the vegetarian diet and the combination diet of the DASH trial have many nutritional attributes that could be contributing to the blood pressure-lowering effect, and it is probably impossible as well as clinically unhelpful to attempt to disentangle which have the greatest effect.

Alcohol In epidemiological studies, blood pressure increases progressively when reported alcohol intake increases above three drinks per day. Several intervention studies have shown that reduction of alcohol intake can produce an appreciable reduction in blood pressure amongst hypertensive heavy drinkers. For example, one study showed that replacing standard beer (5% alcohol) with a reduced alcohol beer (0.9% alcohol) produced a reduction in alcohol intake from 450–64 mL/week and a significant fall in blood pressure.

Other factors Small and inconsistent inverse associations have been reported between blood pressure and polyunsaturated fatty acids, magnesium, protein and dietary fibre. A small positive association with caffeine has also been reported.

20.4.5 Obesity

Obesity is a major risk factor for CHD. While increasing body mass index shows a modest and graded association with myocardial infarction, increasing waist circumference and waist/hip ratio show a more striking relationship. The effect is not surprising given the association between excess adiposity and several other risk factors, notably dyslipidaemia, hypertension, insulin resistance and type 2 diabetes. Weight loss corrects most of the clinical and metabolic derangements seen in overweight and obese individuals (see Chapter 16).

20.4.6 Inflammatory markers

Inflammation is now acknowledged as a process that can appreciably increase cardiovascular risk to the extent that high-sensitivity C-reactive protein (CRP) is regarded as a useful risk indicator. Information regarding the extent to which nutritional factors can influence the inflammatory response is limited. However, diets very low in fat have been shown to reduce levels of high-sensitivity CRP. Moderately high intakes of ω-3 fatty acids may also reduce the inflammatory response.

20.4.7 Impaired fetal nutrition

Robinson and Barker (2002) in Southampton observed some time ago that low-birthweight babies, especially those who tended to gain weight rapidly in early life, were more prone than those of normal weight to a range of clinical and metabolic abnormalities (including obesity, hypertension, dyslipidaemia, insulin resistance) that predispose to the increased risk of CHD and diabetes in later life. The fetal-origins hypothesis (Barker) suggests that maternal malnutrition at critical stages of fetal development leads to intrauterine growth retardation, including decreased pancreatic islet β cells, decreased number of nephrons, insulin resistance, and a range of other abnormalities that are *not* associated with later chronic diseases if the child remains in a relatively deprived nutritional environment. However, problems are proposed to occur if the malnourished fetus is born into conditions of adequate nutrition or over-nutrition and rapid catch-up growth occurs. Much debate and research centres around the explanation for the observation, but the hypothesis has been offered as an explanation for the massive increase in cardiovascular disease and type 2 diabetes that has occurred with increasing affluence in some developing countries. The main message to be taken from this research at this stage is the importance of adequate and appropriate nutrition for women of childbearing age. There is insufficient evidence to recommend altering current advice regarding infant feeding practices (see Chapter 31).

20.4.8 Raised plasma homocysteine levels

Patients with inborn errors of homocysteine metabolism have very high levels of plasma homocysteine, homocysteinuria and a high risk of cardiovascular disease. It has also been found that in the general population there is a gradient of CHD risk associated with increasing levels of plasma homocysteine, i.e. homocysteine is an independent risk factor for CHD. Interest in this relatively newly identified risk factor centres around the fact that folic acid and vitamins B_6 and B_{12} can reduce raised homocysteine levels. There is as yet no definitive evidence that reducing homocysteine levels can reduce clinical CHD.

20.5 Clinical trials of dietary modification

Ideally, evidence from epidemiological and experimental studies should be confirmed in randomized controlled trials involving clinical endpoints in order to establish causal links between individual foods and nutrients and CHD. As with other chronic diseases there are major methodological difficulties in undertaking such trials (see Chapter 1). However, several trials have been undertaken and these demonstrate the potential of dietary modification to reduce cardiovascular risk. The early trials all attempted to lower cholesterol levels, usually by increasing the poly-unsaturated/saturated (P/S) ratio, i.e. they were single-factor intervention trials. More recent trials have involved multifactorial interventions, including dietary change intended to improve all nutritionrelated risk indicators, as well as attempts to modify other risk factors that are not diet related (e.g. cigarette smoking). Dietary intervention trials have been undertaken in people with and without evidence of CHD at the time the trial was started (i.e. secondary and primary prevention trials). This section describes briefly a few landmark trials (Table 20.4) and presents an overview of all of the important investigations of this kind.

Los Angeles Veterans Administration Study This was the first of the major intervention trials, in which 846 male volunteers (aged 55–89 years) were randomly allocated to 'experimental' and 'control' diets taken in different dining rooms. The control diet was intended to be typically North American (40% energy from fat, mostly saturated). The experimental diet contained half as much cholesterol, and predominantly polyunsaturated vegetable oils (ω-6 PUFA) replaced approximately two-thirds of the animal fat, achieving a P/S ratio of 2. With skilled food technology, the trial was conducted under double-blind conditions. During the 8 years of trial, plasma cholesterol in the experimental group was 13% lower, and coronary events, as well as deaths due to cardiovascular disease, were appreciably reduced

Table 20.4 Results of selected intervention trials. (Confidence intervals are given in parenthesis)

Trial	No of subjects	% reduction in cholesterol	Odds ratio (experimental vs control)	
			Total mortality	Fatal and non-fatal CHD
Veterans Administration (Dayton *et al.*, 1969)	846	13	0.98 (0.83–1.15)	0.77
Oslo (Hjermann *et al.*, 1981)	1232	13	0.64 (0.37–1.12)	0.56
DART Fat advice	2033	3.5	0.98 (0.77–1.26)	0.92
Fish advice	2033	Negligible	0.74 (0.57–0.93)	0.85
Lyons Heart (de Lorgeril *et al.*, 1994)	605	Negligible	0.30 (0.11–0.82)	0.24
CHAOS (Stephens *et al.*, 1996)	2002	NA	1.30	0.60
GISSI-Prevenzione n-3 fatty acids	2836	NA	0.80 (0.67–0.94)	0.80
Vitamin E	2830	NA	0.86 (0.72–1.02)	0.88
HOPE (2000)	1511	NA	1.00 (0.89–1.13)	1.05

NA, not available.

compared with the controls (Table 20.4). The beneficial effect of the cholesterol-lowering diet was most evident in those with high cholesterol levels at the start of the study. Deaths due to other and uncertain causes occurred more frequently in the experimental group, though no single other cause predominated. This increase in non-cardiovascular mortality in the experimental group raised for the first time the possibility that cholesterol lowering might be harmful in some respects, despite the reduction in CHD. This has not been substantiated in subsequent studies.

Oslo Trial Middle-aged men at high risk of CHD (smokers or those having a cholesterol in the range 7.5–9.8 mmol/L) were divided into two groups; half received intensive dietary education and advice to stop smoking, the other half served as a control group (Hjermann *et al.*, 1981). An impressive reduction in total coronary events was observed (Table 20.4) in association with a 13% fall in serum cholesterol and a 65% reduction in tobacco consumption. There was also an improvement in total mortality and no significant difference between the two groups with regard to non-cardiac causes of death. Statistical analysis suggested that approximately 60% of the CHD reduction could be attributed to serum cholesterol change and 25% to smoking reduction. The composition of the experimental diet was quite different from that used in the Veterans Administration trial: total and saturated fat were markedly reduced without any appreciable increase in ω-6 PUFA, and fibre-rich carbohydrate was increased. These differences, as well as the fact that the participants in the Oslo Trial were younger, could have accounted for the different results with regard to non-cardiovascular diseases.

Diet and Reinfarction Trial (DART) This was the first trial to examine the effects of diets high in ω-3 PUFA. Burr *et al.* (1989) randomized 2033 men who had survived myocardial infarction to receive or not receive advice on each of three dietary factors: a reduction of fat intake and an increase in the ratio of polyunsaturated to saturated fat, an increase in fatty fish intake, and an increase in cereal fibre. For those unable to eat fatty fish, a fish oil supplement was

recommended. Within the short (2-year) follow-up period, the subjects advised to eat fatty fish had a 26% reduction in all causes of mortality compared with those not so advised. The other two diets were not associated with significant differences in mortality, but in view of the fact that fat modification only achieved a 3–4% reduction in serum cholesterol, compliance with the fat-modified and high-fibre diets may have been less than that on the fish diet. Furthermore, diets aimed to reduce atherogenicity (ω-6 PUFA) are likely to take longer to show a beneficial effect than those aimed at reducing thrombogenicity (ω-3 PUFA). These results are the first to find that very simple advice aimed at reducing thrombogenicity (at least two weekly portions, 200–400 g, of fatty fish) appears to reduce mortality appreciably. Results of follow-up long after the completion of the intervention phase were inconclusive.

Lyons Heart Study This study (de Logeril *et al.*, 1994) is the most recent in the series of multifactorial dietary intervention studies in the secondary prevention of cardiovascular disease, in which 605 individuals with clinical CHD received conventional dietary advice or advice to follow a type of Mediterranean diet. The experimental diet was lower in total and saturated fat (30% and 8% total energy) than the control diet (33% and 12% total energy) and contained more oleic (13% vs 10% total energy) and α-linolenic acid (0.80% vs 0.27%). Dietary linoleic acid was higher in the control group (5.3% vs 3.6%). The Mediterranean diet included more bread, legumes, vegetables and fruit, and less meat and dairy products. Those in the experimental group were also provided with a margarine rich in α-linolenate (C18:3, n-3). The marked reductions in risk ratios for cardiovascular events as well as total mortality associated with the experimental diet are difficult to interpret. The confidence intervals are wide and it is difficult to understand why cholesterol levels did not fall despite the reduced intake of saturated fatty acids. The latter observation has led to the suggestion that the beneficial effect must have resulted from an antithrombogenic effect of the diet or a reduction in the risk of dysrythmias. The study has been widely quoted as providing evidence for the health benefits associated with the Mediterranean diet, though it should be noted that the experimental diet cannot be regarded as a traditional Mediterranean diet given the important role of n-3-supplemented margarine in the intervention diet.

Cambridge Heart Antioxidant Study (CHAOS) Several early clinical trials involving supplementation with antioxidant nutrients (vitamins C and E and β-carotene) without concomitant dietary change suggested no benefit in terms of cardiovascular risk reduction despite strong evidence of a cardioprotective effect in epidemiological studies. This study from Cambridge (Stephens *et al.*, 1996) involved the randomization of over 2000 participants with pre-existing cardiovascular disease to receive either placebo or 400 IU or 800 IU α-tocopherol daily. After 1.4 years, non-fatal myocardial infarction was substantially reduced in the α-tocopherol group (14 out of 1035) as compared with the control group (41 out of 967). However, there were marginally more total deaths in the α-tocopherol than the control group (36 out of 1035 compared with 26 out of 967).

GISSI–Prevenzione Study This large study (GISSI, 1999) examined the effect of supplementation with very-long-chain ω-3 fatty acids (eicosapentaenoic acid, EPA, and docosahexaenoic acid, DHA) or vitamin E (300 mg), or both, in 2830 subjects who had had a myocardial infarction. The trial was not conducted in a double-blind manner but was nevertheless interesting in view of its size and otherwise appropriate conduct. Supplementation with ω-3 fatty acids was associated with a statistically significant 15–20% reduction in all of the important endpoints (non-fatal myocardial infarction, cardiovascular deaths and total mortality). A smaller reduction in event rate in association with vitamin E supplementation did not achieve statistical significance.

Heart Outcomes Prevention Evaluation (HOPE) Study Patients at high risk of cardiovascular events because they had cardiovascular disease or diabetes and one other risk factor were randomized to receive placebo, 400 IU vitamin E or drug treatment (an angiotensin-converting enzyme (ACE) inhibitor, ramipril) and were followed for 4.5 years. A primary outcome event (myocardial infarction, stroke or death from a cardiovascular cause) occurred in 16.2% (772 out of 4761) patients assigned to the vitamin E group and 15.5% (739 out of 4780) assigned the placebo. Furthermore, there were no differences between the two groups when considering total mortality or indeed any other cardiovascular endpoint.

Overall perspective of the trials

It is inappropriate to aggregate the results of the dietary intervention trials in a meta-analysis in view of the wide range of interventions that have been employed. Nevertheless, certain conclusions may be drawn from the results of the various studies. There is convincing evidence that cholesterol lowering by dietary means reduces coronary events in the context of both primary and secondary prevention. Indeed there is confirmation of the rule derived from observational epidemiology that a 2–3% reduction in coronary events results from each 1% of cholesterol lowering achieved. Such benefit is further confirmed in trials of pharmaceutical reduction of total cholesterol by statin drugs.

There would seem to be reasonably strong evidence that lowering of total cholesterol (reflecting principally a reduction in LDL cholesterol) should primarily be achieved by reducing total and saturated fatty acids. While increasing ω-6 polyunsaturated fatty acids (chiefly linoleic acid C18:2, ω-6) might further decrease LDL, the clinical trials do not suggest that replacement energy be derived entirely from this source. Rather, they suggest that when substitution is required, oleic acid (C18:1, ω9), carbohydrate from lightly processed cereals (whole grains), vegetables and fruit as well as linoleic acid might all contribute replacement energy.

Two trials provide some support for the suggestion that dietary modification has the potential to reduce cardiovascular risk by means other than cholesterol lowering. The DART and GISSI trials achieved appreciable reductions in cardiovascular mortality with minimal change in cholesterol, presumably because the increase in C20:5, ω-3 and C22:6, ω-3 in the fish or fish oil supplements resulted in reduced tendency to thrombosis or perhaps reduced the risk of dysrythmias. Similarly, the experimental diet in the Lyons Heart Study was not associated with appreciable lowering of cholesterol. It is impossible to identify which of the many nutritional changes might have been responsible for the beneficial effects observed in this study. There was undoubtedly an increase in a range of antioxidant nutrients, which may have reduced oxidizability of LDL, despite minimal change in cholesterol. Non-starch polysaccharide (dietary fibre) as well as starch increased because of the increase in cereals, vegetables and fruit. Total saturated fatty acids decreased while oleic and α-linolenic acids increased. The authors of the study regarded the last-mentioned change to be of particular importance. However, it would seem more plausible to suggest that a combination of all of these factors contributed to the overall risk reduction resulting from favourable modification of several of the risk factors listed in Table 20.2. Although widely quoted, it should be noted that the Lyons Heart Study

is relatively small and the estimate of risk reduction subject to wide confidence intervals.

The trials of nutrient supplements have generally been disappointing apart perhaps from the GISSI-Prevenzione study, which suggests potential benefit of supplementation with modest amounts of fish oils. Several trials published subsequent to the HOPE Study and a meta-analysis provide convincing evidence for the absence of a benefit of supplemental vitamin E for high-risk individuals. There is no clear explanation as to why the vitamin E and other antioxidant nutrient supplementation trials have been largely negative despite strong suggestions of benefit from epidemiological data. The most likely explanation would seem to be either that a longer time frame might be necessary in order to demonstrate benefit or that a blend of these nutrients in proportions similar to those found in foods might be required to produce benefit, rather than a pharmacological dose of a single antioxidant nutrient. Large trials are presently underway to determine whether supplementation with folic acid and other dietary determinants of homocysteine levels have the potential to reduce cardiovascular risk. Early underpowered trials have generated contradictory results.

20.6 Foods and nutrients as causes of coronary heart disease: strength of evidence

The epidemiological and experimental evidence discussed above has generated a large number of associations between foods and nutrients and CHD. A WHO/FAO Expert Consultation (2003) considered the strength of evidence for all of the putative lifestyle-related variables and categorized them as being convincingly, probably or possibly causal. For some, the evidence was regarded as insufficient (Table 20.5). Associations graded as convincing or probable were deemed to be sufficient to translate into recommendations. Most of these associations have been discussed in the preceding sections and in Chapter 3, but are reviewed briefly below to justify the evidence gradings and resultant recommendations.

20.6.1 Fatty acids and dietary cholesterol

Myristic and palmitic acids, derived from dairy products and meat, comprise a substantial proportion of total intake of saturated fatty acids in countries with high fat intakes and high CHD rates. They have a more marked LDL-raising effect than other saturated fatty acids and reducing their intake has been shown, in randomized controlled trials, to be associated with reduced rates of CHD regardless of replacement energy. *trans*-Unsaturated fatty acids, mostly found in deep-fried fast foods, baked goods and some fat spreads, are associated with an even more atherogenic

Table 20.5 Summary of strength of evidence on lifestyle factors and risk of developing cardiovascular diseases

Evidence	Decreased risk	No relationship	Increased risk
Convincing	Regular physical activity Linoleic acid Fish and fish oils (EPA and DHA) Vegetables and fruits (including berries) Potassium Low to moderate alcohol intake (for coronary heart disease)	Vitamin E supplements	Myristic and palmitic acids *trans* fatty acids High sodium intake Overweight High alcohol intake (for stroke)
Probable	α-Linolenic acid Oleic acid NSP Wholegrain cereals Nuts (unsalted) Plant sterols/stanols Folate	Stearic acid	Dietary cholesterol Unfiltered boiled coffee
Possible	Flavonoids Soy products		Fats rich in lauric acid Impaired fetal nutrition β-Carotene supplements
Insufficient	Calcium Magnesium Vitamin C		Carbohydrates Iron

EPA, eicosapentaenoic acid; DHA, docosahexaenoic acid; NSP, non-starch polysaccharides.
Source: WHO/FAO (2003)

plasma lipid profile (increased LDL and lipoprotein (a) and decreased HDL) than saturated fatty acids. Furthermore, several large cohort studies have reported a linear association between their intake and subsequent CHD risk. Polyunsaturated vegetable oils supplying linoleic acid, found especially in sunflower and soybean oils, lower LDL, and when used as a replacement energy for saturated fat in clinical trials have been shown to be associated with reduced disease rates. However, excessive intakes (PUFA > 10% total energy) may reduce HDL levels and might promote oxidation of LDL and should be avoided.

ω-3 Polyunsaturated oils (EPA and DHA from fish oils) have potentially powerful beneficial effects on several cardiovascular risk factors (notably they are antiplatelet and anti-inflammatory) and physiology (endothelial function, arterial compliance, vascular reactivity, cardiac electrophysiology) and randomized trials suggest clinical benefit. Although these fatty acids can lower triglycerides, the benefit is believed to be mediated principally through pathways other than lipoproteins. While the evidence relating to the protective effects of these polyunsaturated fatty acids is regarded as convincing, the potentially protective effects of oleic acid, derived from olive oil, canola and nuts and plant sources of ω-3 fatty acids (α-linolenic acid, high in flaxseed, canola and soybean oils) are considered to be probable. The beneficial effect of oleic acid on LDL is less marked, and while there is epidemiological evidence for a protective role, oleic acid has not been used as a sole replacement for saturated fat in any randomized controlled trial. α-Linolenic acid (see section 18.3) from plant foods has been found to be inversely related to CHD in prospective studies, but in the Lyons Heart trial, in which intake was increased, it was only one of the dietary variables that was modified. Stearic acid, another important saturated fatty acid, does not appear to adversely influence lipoproteins, and although there is a suggestion that it might be thrombogenic in animals, there are no comparable data in humans, hence the suggestion that there is probably no risk of CHD associated with its consumption. Lauric acid, on the other hand, does elevate LDL but is also associated with an almost equivalent increase in HDL, which may mitigate at least to some extent any lipoprotein-mediated adverse effects. There is also no corroborative epidemiological evidence of increased CHD risk, hence its classification as a possibly related factor.

Cholesterol in the blood is derived from endogenous synthesis and dietary intake, principally from dairy fat and meat, which are also important sources of saturated fatty acids, and eggs, which are not. Dietary cholesterol raises plasma LDL and plasma cholesterol, especially when consumed in substantial amounts and when intake of saturated fatty acids is also high. There is some, though not entirely consistent, evidence from observational studies that increasing intakes are associated with increasing CHD risk. However, no clinical trial has examined the effect of reducing dietary cholesterol without also substantially reducing saturated fatty acids. From a practical point of view, restriction of saturated fatty acids will be associated with a reduction in the dietary cholesterol except in individuals with an unusually high intake of egg yolk. Plant sterols and stanols, when incorporated into functional foods, notably margarines and spreads, are associated with appreciable reductions in LDL and cholesterol, by inhibiting cholesterol absorption. Products are widely available but long-term effects have not been examined.

20.6.2 Sodium and potassium

Sodium and potassium are considered to be, respectively, convincingly promotive and protective against cardiovascular disease because of their effects on blood pressure (reviewed in section 20.4.4). Although potassium supplements have been shown to be associated with reductions in blood pressure, fruit and vegetables, which are rich sources of potassium, rather than supplements, are recommended.

20.6.3 Dietary fibre (non-starch polysaccharides) and wholegrain cereals

Dietary fibre is a heterogeneous mixture of polysaccharides and lignins that are not degraded by the endogenous enzymes. Water-soluble fibres (notably pectins, gums, mucilages and some hemicelluloses) reduce total and LDL cholesterol, and several large cohort studies have reported that high intakes of dietary fibre, as well as diets high in wholegrain cereals, were associated with CHD. Thus, although the mechanisms are not clear, dietary fibres are regarded as probably protective factors against CHD.

20.6.4 Antioxidant nutrients and flavonoids

Experimental evidence has clearly demonstrated the potential for antioxidant nutrients (vitamin E, vitamin C, β-carotene) to reduce the oxidizability of LDL *in vitro*, and prospective studies have shown a decreasing risk of CHD with increasing intakes of these nutrients and flavonoids, which occur in a variety of foods of vegetable origin such as onions, berries, apples and tea. However, several large clinical trials in which vitamins E and C and β-carotene have been given as supplements have shown no consistent benefit. Indeed, vitamin E supplementation has been studied in a sufficient number of studies for meta-analyses to confirm absence of benefit in terms of reducing cardiovascular risk (Table 20.5). Failure of supplementation to confirm experimental and observational data may result from the need for prolonged exposure to produce benefit or the requirement for a blend of antioxidants and flavonoids such as may be found in foods rather than in supplements supplying pharmacological doses of a single nutrient.

20.6.5 B vitamins

Increasing homocysteine levels appear to increase CHD risk in case–control and cohort studies. Dietary folate and folic acid as a supplement or fortificant result in lowering of homocysteine by facilitating the methylation of homocysteine to methionine (see Chapter 12) and vitamins B_6 and B_{12} may further reduce homocysteine by enhancing its conversion to cysteine. Although the first trial of homocysteine lowering by supplemental B vitamins suggested clinical cardiovascular benefit, the results have been inconsistent in subsequent randomized controlled trials. The results of further larger trials are awaited.

20.6.6 Food items and food groups

Fruit and vegetables Consumption of fruit and vegetables has long been believed to promote good health, but it is only relatively recently that ecological and prospective studies have reported their potential to reduce both CHD and stroke. The series of DASH trials have shown convincing benefits in terms of reducing blood pressure levels, especially when consumed together with relatively high intakes of low-fat dairy products and a reduced intake of sodium. Additional benefit in terms of cardiovascular risk reduction may accrue as a result of the high intake of antioxidant nutrients and flavonoids in fruits, berries and vegetables, some of which may also be high in dietary fibre.

Fish Many prospective studies have shown a reduced risk of CHD in association with fish consumption, especially fatty fish, with one recent systematic review suggesting that high-risk populations might halve CHD deaths if fish intake was increased to 40–60 g/day. All-cause mortality may also be reduced by an increase in fish consumption. The DART and GISSI-Prevenzione trials support the clinical benefits of regular consumption of fish and fish oils (C20:5, C22:6), which may reduce cardiovascular risk via several different mechanisms.

Nuts Several large epidemiological studies have reported decreased CHD risk in association with frequent consumption of nuts. The studies have generally considered nuts as a group. Nuts are high in unsaturated fats and regular consumption results in a favourable alteration in the fatty acid profile of plasma lipids, as well as some reduction in atherogenic lipoproteins. It is clearly impossible to conduct a long-term clinical trial in which increased intake of nuts is the sole dietary modification. Nevertheless, the evidence is deemed to be sufficient to regard nuts as probably protective against CHD. Any recommendations to include nuts in the diet must be tempered with a reminder of their relatively high energy content to ensure that an increase in intake does not result in energy imbalance.

Soy Soy protein has a favourable effect on several cardiovascular risk factors. An overview of 38 clinical studies suggests that a consumption of 47 g of soy protein daily leads to a 9% decline in total cholesterol and a 13% fall in LDL-cholesterol. Soy isoflavones have been shown to lower blood pressure, and there is some evidence of beneficial effects on vascular and endothelial function, platelet aggregation, smooth muscle cell proliferation and LDL oxidation. Soy protein has been shown to inhibit atherosclerosis in animals, but human data are regarded as insufficient to classify the potential benefits as being greater than 'possible'.

Alcohol Ecological, case–control and cohort studies all suggest a protective effect of low to moderate alcohol consumption. The effect is apparent for all alcoholic drinks and has been attributed to the HDL-raising effect of alcohol, or perhaps to the antioxidant content of some alcoholic beverages. It is noteworthy that the benefits in absolute terms apply only to middle-aged and older individuals. Other cardiovascular and health risks associated with alcohol, especially when consumed in excess, argue strongly against a general recommendation for its use.

Coffee Boiled unfiltered coffee raises total and LDL-cholesterol because of the cafestol content of coffee beans. Such unfiltered coffee is still widely consumed in Greece, the Middle East and Turkey. A shift from coffee prepared in this way to filtered coffee is reported to have contributed appreciably to the decline in plasma cholesterol in Finland.

20.6.7 Dietary patterns

Early dietary advice aimed at reducing cardiovascular risk centred principally around a reduction in saturated and an increase in polyunsaturated fatty acids. More recently, there has been interest in certain dietary patterns that are regarded as protective against CHD. The traditional Mediterranean diets of Italy, Greece and Spain have been singled out as being of particular benefit, perhaps because populations consuming the traditional diets of countries surrounding the Mediterranean Sea had remarkably low rates of CHD, and probably also because of the widespread publicity surrounding the Lyons Heart Study. The fact that, from a culinary point of view, such dietary patterns are regarded as especially attractive may also have contributed.

Vegetarian diets have also been promoted for their apparent cardioprotective effect. Vegetarians are indeed at lower risk of CHD than meat eaters, but it has not been established which attributes of the vegetarian diet might be protective since there are many aspects other than the avoidance of meat that characterize these diets. One study suggests that the lower rates might be due to the relatively low intake of saturated fatty acids rather than meat avoidance.

The substantial body of epidemiological, experimental and clinical trial data reviewed above provide strong evidence that there are other equally cardioprotective dietary patterns. The attributes of cardioprotective diets listed in Table 20.6 are seen in many traditional diets (e.g. most Asian diets) and indeed the so-called typical Western diet can be modified to follow these dietary principles. It is important to note that adopting individual attributes of potentially appropriate cardioprotective diets may not confer benefit. For example, consuming substantial quantities of olive oil in the context of an otherwise inappropriate diet may confer little or no advantage. Failure to ensure appropriate energy balance may negate the benefits of adhering to many of the other attributes listed in Table 20.6 because obesity-mediated cardiovascular risk (see Chapter 16) may outweigh favourable trends in other risk factors. Unfortunately, some populations that previously consumed cardioprotective diets and had low rates of CHD have introduced foods not traditionally consumed. For instance, some modern Mediterranean or Asian diets may be high in saturated fatty acids and thus, at least to some extent, have lost their health benefits.

Table 20.6 Attributes of cardioprotective dietary patterns

- Low intakes of saturated fatty acids
- High intakes of raw or appropriately prepared fruits and vegetables
- Wholegrains and lightly processed cereal foods are preferred
- Fat intakes are predominantly derived from unmodified vegetable oils[a]
- Fish, nuts, seeds and vegetable protein sources are important dietary components
- Meat, when consumed, is lean and eaten in small quantities
- Energy balance reduces rates of obesity

[a]Coconut oil and palm oil are not encouraged because they tend to elevate cholesterol and LDL

20.7 Nutritional strategies for high-risk populations

It is essential in countries with high CHD rates to have in place a nutritional strategy that is aimed at the entire population. Individuals with extreme levels of risk factors or with several different risk factors are at the highest risk of CHD and will benefit most, as individuals, from dietary modification. However, the majority of cases of CHD will occur in people at moderate risk, i.e. those with one or two risk factors that may be modestly elevated. This is simply because there are far more such individuals in the population than people at very high risk. Thus, in order to reduce (or in those countries where rates are already coming down to further reduce) the epidemic proportions of CHD, population change is essential. The disadvantage of the 'population approach' is that many individuals are being asked to make changes that are likely to produce a relatively small reduction in their personal CHD risk (the 'prevention paradox') and those who are at high risk will still need to be individually identified because they are likely to require more radical and individually designed lifestyle changes and perhaps medication.

Most high-risk countries have in place nutrient and food targets aimed at reducing CHD rates and more global targets have been set by the WHO. Table 20.7 compares the UK targets with those suggested by WHO/FAO. While at first glance there appear to be some striking differences, these principally reflect local and international requirements. A total fat intake target of 35% may be a realistic goal in a country such as the UK where present average intake may be higher. For international purposes, the WHO-recommended range acknowledges that, on the one hand, many countries have a low total fat intake and there is no justification for an increase; on the other hand, for countries with a high fat consumption at present, reduction to an intake of around 30% may be a target achievable in the long term and one that might facilitate the reduction of obesity as well as more directly helping to reduce CHD risk by reducing saturated and *trans*-unsaturated fatty acids.

20.8 Dietary advice for high-risk individuals

High-risk individuals are those who have markedly elevated levels of a single risk factor (e.g. those with familial hyperlipidaemia), those with multiple risk factors (see Table 20.2), or those who have already developed clinical CHD. They may be identified because of a personal or family history of CHD or in screening programmes. It is clearly important in such individuals to attempt to achieve the lowest possible degree of risk with regard to all identifiable risk factors. From a dietary point of view, the principles are similar to those recommended for the general population, but further changes from the current Western diet are often required. Food lists such as those given in Table 20.8 are helpful, but individually tailored advice from a dietitian and regular monitoring of dietary intake and risk factor levels are usually necessary. Emphasis on dietary advice specific to particular risk factors is required. For those who are overweight or obese, weight loss should be a primary consideration (see Chapter 16). For most high-risk individuals, saturated fatty acids should be reduced to 8% or less of total energy in order to help achieve the lowest possible levels of LDL. Regular intakes of soluble-fibre-rich foods and the use of margarines and spreads to which plant sterols or stanols have been added also facilitate LDL reduction. For those with high triglyceride and low HDL levels, rapidly digested (high-GI) carbohydrate intake should be as low as possible and carbohydrate should principally be derived from intact fruits, vegetables and wholegrain cereals. It may be helpful for such individuals to have a lower than average intake of total carbohydrate provided that any relative increase in fat intake derives from mono- and polyunsaturated fatty acids

Table 20.7 Ranges of population nutrient intake goals as recommended by WHO and FAO[a] and in the UK[b] (unless otherwise stated, the goals are expressed as percentage of total energy)

	WHO/FAO	UK
Total fat	15–30%	35%
Saturated fatty acids (SFA)	< 10%	< 10%
cis Polyunsaturated fatty acids (PFA)	6–10%	++
n-6 PUFA	5–8%	< 10%
n-3 PUFA	1–2%	1.5 g/week[+]
cis Monounsaturated fatty acids	By difference[c]	++
trans Fatty acids (TFA)	< 1%	< 2%
Dietary cholesterol	< 300 mg/day	Approx. 245 mg/day
Total carbohydrate	55–75%	50%
Free sugars[d]	< 10%	Fruits and vegetables encouraged
Dietary fibre (NSP)	From foods	Complex carbohydrates encouraged
Protein	10–15%	++
Sodium chloride	< 5 g/day	6 g/day (100 mmol/day)
Potassium		3.5 g/day
Fruit and vegetables	> 400 g/day	Encouraged

[a] WHO/FAO (2003).
[b] Report of the Cardiovascular Review Group Committee on Medical Aspects of Food Policy. *Nutritional Aspects of Cardiovascular Disease*, Department of Health, Report on Health and Social Subjects 46, London 1994.
[c] Total fat – SFA + PFA + TFA.
[d] All monosaccharides and disaccharides added to foods by manufacturer, cook or consumer, plus sugars naturally present in honey, syrups and fruit juices.
[+] Mainly from oily fish.
++No specific recommendation.

with *cis* configuration and that energy balance is maintained. The presence of hypertension necessitates emphasis on salt restriction and increased intake of fruit, vegetables and low-fat dairy products. The absence of clinical trial data showing the benefits of dietary change in the elderly does not mean that they should not be given dietary advice. The absolute risk of cardiovascular disease increases steadily with age, although the relative risk associated with individual risk factors might decrease. No doubt there is an age beyond which there are minimal advantages to dietary change, but those who might be expected to

otherwise have a reasonable life expectancy should be given advice similar to that given to younger people. When giving lipid-lowering advice to older people, it is necessary to ensure an adequate intake of essential nutrients because they usually have a reduced intake of total energy.

The widespread use of several cardioprotective drugs shown in randomized controlled trials to be of benefit to people at high risk of cardiovascular disease in no way reduces the need to comply with dietary advice. Statins are principally prescribed to reduce total and LDL-cholesterol, β-blockers and

ACE inhibitors to lower blood pressure, and aspirin and other antiplatelet drugs to reduce the risk of thrombosis. While these drugs may have some benefits beyond favourably altering the risk factors for which they have been prescribed, a cardioprotective diet influences a wide range of risk determinants. In addition, dietary compliance may enhance the effect

of the drug. For example, appreciable reduction of saturated fatty acids will result in lipid lowering beyond that which can routinely be achieved by statins and strict salt restriction, and other dietary measures to lower blood pressure will enhance the blood pressure-lowering effect of hypotensive agents.

20.9 Gene–nutrient interactions

It has long been appreciated that not everyone exposed to a risk factor for CHD will develop the disease and that exposure to foods or nutrients known to influence risk factors will produce a range of responses within a group of individuals all consuming the same diet. For example, while increasing saturated fatty acids can elevate total and LDL-cholesterol to an extent that may, in a population or group of individuals, be predicted by a formula (see Box 20.1), some individuals may show little or no change, whereas others will have striking changes in their levels when the nature of dietary fat changes (see Fig. 20.9). In the clinical context, failure to respond to dietary modification has often been attributed to failure to

comply with dietary advice. While non-compliance is indeed associated with absence of response or reduced response, variation in response has been confirmed in carefully controlled dietary experiments in which all participants were fed identical diets. Genetic factors undoubtedly account for this variability, and several genetic polymorphisms that predict plasma lipid responses to change in dietary fat have now been identified. For example, individuals carrying the *APO E4* allele of the *APO E* gene will show a more marked reduction in total and LDL-cholesterol than those who do not carry it, when changed to a diet that is reduced in both fat and cholesterol. A common genetic polymorphism in the promoter region

---

BOX 20.1 Predictive equations for estimating changes in plasma cholesterol and lipoprotein concentrations in response to changes in dietary fatty acids and cholesterol. More sophisticated equations were developed when the effects of different saturated and unsaturated fatty acids were identified. TC and LDL-C given in mg/dL. For mmol/L, multiply by 0.02586

Authors	Equations
Keys *et al.* (1957)	$\Delta TC = 1.35\,(2\Delta S - \Delta P) + 1.52\Delta Z$
Mensink and Katan (1992)	$\Delta TC = 1.51\Delta S - 0.12\Delta M - 0.60\Delta P$ $\Delta LDL\text{-}C = 1.28\Delta S - 0.24\Delta M - 0.55\Delta P$
Yu *et al.* (1995)	$\Delta TC = 2.02\,(\Delta C12{:}0 + \Delta 14{:}0 + \Delta 16{:}0) - 0.03\,(\Delta 18{:}0) - 0.48\Delta MUFA - 0.96\Delta PUFA$ $\Delta LDL\text{-}C = 1.46\,(\Delta 12{:}0 + \Delta 14{:}0 + \Delta 16{:}0) + 0.07\,(\Delta 18{:}0) - 0.69\Delta MUFA - 0.96\Delta PUFA$

Abbreviations:
Δ = change, TC = total cholesterol, LDL-C = LDL cholesterol, S = percentage of saturated fatty acids, M/MUFA = percentage of monounsaturated fatty acids, P/PUFA = percentage of polyunsaturated fatty acids; all as percentage of total energy intake.
C12:0, C14:0, C16:0 = percentage saturated fatty acids with 12, 14 or 16 carbon atoms
Z = square root of daily dietary cholesterol
Source: Kris-Etherton, Y., Yu-Poth, S. Sabaté, J., *et al.* (1999) Nuts and their bioactive constituents: effects on serum lipids and other factors that affect disease risk. *Am J Clin Nutr*, **70**, 5045–115.

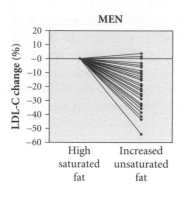
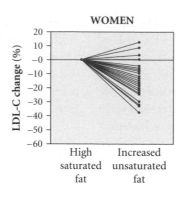

Fig. 20.9 Individual changes in LDL cholesterol when *cis*-unsaturated fatty acids replace some of the saturated fatty acids in the diet.

of the *APO AI* gene determines the extent to which HDL responds to substantial increases in polyunsaturated fatty acids.

Such observations have led to speculation that this study of 'nutrigenetics' will soon lead to the development of 'designer diets', which will enable individualized dietary advice to be based on genetic characteristics. However, while this type of nutrigenetic research will no doubt continue to flourish, such expectations are premature for several reasons: polygenic rather than monogenic factors are almost certainly responsible for most of the heterogeneity in risk factor response to diet; no studies carried out thus far have involved sufficient participants to study the interaction of many genes; most research to date has centred on the variability in plasma lipid and lipoprotein response to changes in nature of dietary fat, and

many other risk factors and nutrients are involved; and finally—and perhaps of greatest importance— there is convincing evidence that compliance with cardioprotective dietary patterns can profoundly reduce cardiovascular risk in high-risk populations and the majority of individuals who have raised risk-factor levels.

Nutrigenomic research explores how nutrients influence gene expression rather than the inter-individual differences in relation to the effects of nutrients. Of particular relevance to cardiovascular disease has been the research that has shown the profound effect of ω-3 fatty acids on the activation of nuclear receptors, which are associated with inflammation and lipid metabolism, thus helping to explain their cardioprotective effect.

Cerebrovascular disease

Cerebrovascular disease presents clinically as a stroke, which, like the clinical manifestations of CHD, also has a major impact on public health because of its high frequency in most affluent and developing countries. There are several different types of stroke.

One cause of stroke is a bleed from one of the cerebral arteries (haemorrhagic stroke); it may be associated with a congenital abnormality (aneurysm) and/or raised levels of blood pressure. Thus, nutritional determinants of hypertension are contributory causal factors. Ischaemic strokes are more common and result from thrombosis and atheroma, the process being similar to that which results in myocardial infarction.

The clinical features of stroke (typically loss or slurring of speech and weakness of one side of the body) result from the loss of blood supply to a section of the brain. Although the nutritional determinants have been far less studied than is the case for CHD, the risk factors for the two sets of conditions are similar, and therefore nutritional factors that predispose to CHD should also apply. However, in the relatively limited number of studies of stroke that have been carried out, some food groups emerge as being particularly relevant. Most striking is the protective effect of fruit and vegetables, as demonstrated in six of the seven large prospective studies that examined the relationship. Although it appears most categories of fruit and vegetables may be protective, the effect is particularly striking for cruciferous vegetables, green leafy vegetables and citrus fruits. Blood pressure is also a particularly important risk factor for ischaemic stroke, so that, once again, all the nutritional determinants of hypertension can be regarded as especially relevant. Of the remaining nutrients and food groups that have been identified as causal or protective in terms of CHD, ω-3 fatty acids, regular fish consumption and intake of whole grains have been shown to be protective against ischaemic stroke.

Thus, although there have been no intervention studies specifically to examine the effect on clinical outcome, implementing a cardioprotective dietary pattern (see Table 20.8) can be expected to reduce the risk of both haemorrhagic and ischaemic stroke.

Table 20.8 Guidelines for a lipid-lowering diet

Food	Advisable	Daily/weekly amounts, serving size, comments	May be eaten in moderation	Should be avoided or eaten rarely
Fats, and oils	All fats should be limited to no more than the daily amount unless otherwise directed. If following a weight-reducing diet, use reduced fat MUFA or PUFA spreads and the 'light' sterol or stanol spreads.	3–5 teaspoons/day Per serving/ 1–1$^1/_2$ teaspoon	Monounsaturated (MUFA) or polyunsaturated (PUFA) table spreads/margarine. Mono- or polyunsaturated oils, e.g. olive, canola, peanut, soybean, avocado; sunflower, corn, safflower, wheatgerm, grapeseed, sesame; nut oils, e.g. walnut, hazel nut, almond, avocado. If following a weight-reducing diet use reduced-fat mono- or polyunsaturated spreads.	Butter, dripping, suet, lard, palm oil, coconut oil. Margarines/table spreads not labelled poly- or monounsaturated. Cooking or vegetable oils of unknown origin. Hydrogenated fats and oils and partially hydrogenated fats and oils.
	20–25 g/day sterol or stanol spreads will help reduce blood cholesterol	Equivalent to 4–5 teaspoons/day	Avocado may be used as a spread instead of margarine or table spread.	
Meat— red meat and poultry	Mixed light and dark poultry meat (skinned), 3–5 times/week. Very lean red meat or game.	Serving: – (cooked weight) High risk 100–150 g women; 150–200 g men < 3 times/week Moderate 100–250 g 3–5 times/week	Mixed light and dark poultry meat (skinned). Lean beef, lamb, pork, steak mince, ham. Average serving liver or kidneys no more than once a fortnight.	Visible fat on meat (including crackling), belly pork, streaky bacon, salami, pate, scotch eggs, duck, goose, pork pies, poultry skin. Sausages and luncheon meat, fried meats, rolled roasts, pressed meats.

Table 20.8 (*Cont'd*)

Food	Advisable	Daily/weekly amounts, serving size, comments	May be eaten in moderation	Should be avoided or eaten rarely
Dairy products	Low-fat (less than 1% fat) milk, skimmed milk.	Dairy 2–3 servings daily 1 glass = 200 ml 50 ml	Semi-skimmed 1.5% and 2% fat milk. Low-fat whipped topping.	Full-cream milk, evaporated or condensed milk, double cream, whipping cream, imitation cream, reduced cream.
	Low-fat yoghurt, soya yoghurts, Greek yoghurt 3–4% fat. Virtually fat-free fromage frais.	1 serving = 1 individual container; size range 100–200 g/serving	Half-fat yoghurt, whole milk yoghurt. Half-fat, half-cream, crème fraîche. Light sourcream 3% fat or less.	Greek yoghurt, thick and creamy yoghurt, crème fraîche 40% fat, sourcream 20% fat. Full-fat yoghurt.
Cheese	Low-fat cheeses, i.e. cottage cheese, low-fat quark, curd cheese. Hard and semi-soft cheese can be included up to 3 times weekly in very small amounts.	⅓ cup cottage cheese ½ cup low-fat cottage cheese ⅓ cup quark or ricotto 2 tbsp Parmesan or 3 tbsp grated Cheddar cheese 2 cm cube Cheddar cheese 3 cm cube standard Brie, Edam, Camembert, Fetta, Mozzarella	Medium-fat cheeses, i.e. those with 24% total fat (45% fat content in dry matter) or less, e.g. standard Brie, Camembert, Edam, Mozarella, Parmesan, special processed and blue (12–13% fat) cheeses. Hard and semi-soft cheese can be included up to 4 times weekly in small amounts.	Full-fat cheeses, e.g. Stilton, Cheddar, Cheshire, full-fat blue cheeses, cream cheeses. High-fat soft cheeses, e.g. Brie, Camembert, Mascarpone.
Eggs	Egg whites free. Eggs—up to 3 egg yolks per week including those in cooking and baking.		3–6 egg yolks per week including those in cooking and baking.	Fried eggs, eggs cooked in cream.
Fish	All white fish, e.g. cod, sole, ling, plaice. Mussels, oyster, scallops, clams. Cooked by low fat cooking methods. Oily fish, e.g. herring, mackerel, salmon, sardines, kipper.	1–2 servings weekly 120–200 g (cooked) High risk When possible eat 200–400 g fish twice/week (1–2 servings as oily fish 50–100 g/serving.)	Fish fried in suitable oil (oil should not be heated to smoke point or re-used) once per fortnight; avoid using fat in cooking if on a weight-reducing diet. Average serving of shrimp or squid no more than once a fortnight.	Fish roe. Fried especially deep-fried fish and seafood

Table 20.8 (*Cont'd*)

Food	Advisable	Daily/weekly amounts, serving size, comments	May be eaten in moderation	Should be avoided or eaten rarely
Coloured vegetables and salad	All fresh and plain frozen vegetables. Salad vegetables. High risk: Aim for total coloured vegetable intake of 400 g or more/day: raw or plainly cooked.	At least 3–4 servings daily. 1 serving = ½ cup cooked vegetables 1 cup raw green vegetables or salad 1 tomato or carrot	Try and have coloured vegetables with 2 meals each day. Aim to have half of the dinner plate taken up with plainly cooked or raw coloured vegetables or salad.	Vegetables roasted or fried in fat, or cooked in cream. Salads with standard salad cream, mayonnaise, cream or cream cheese dressings.
Legumes (rinse if using beans canned in salt/sugar)	Peas, beans of all kinds, e.g. haricot, red kidney, butter beans, lentils, chick peas are particularly high in 'soluble fibre' and should be eaten regularly.	At least 3–5 servings weekly. 1 cup cooked dried beans, chickpeas, lentils, dahl ½ cup tempeh or tofu 1 glass fortified soy milk (250 ml)	Falafel—baked or cooked in a very little suitable oil Baked samosa.	Deep fried falafel, samosa. Vegetarian dishes in cream sauce.
Starchy vegetables	Jacket or boiled potatoes, eat skins wherever possible. Corn, parsnip, yams, sweet potato.	1 serving or less daily to replace bread or grain products. 1 small potato ½ kumara ½ cup corn ⅓ cup yams ½ parsnip	Reduced-fat (< 5%), oven-baked chips, roast potatoes cooked in a little suitable oil. Once a fortnight or less, roast coloured vegetables cooked in a little suitable oil.	Chips or roast potatoes cooked in unsuitable fat or oil. Deep-fried chips and other fried vegetables, potato crisps.
Fruit	Fresh fruit, dried fruit, unsweetened tinned fruit.	1 medium apple, pear, orange, nectarine small banana, kiwi fruit ½ cup stewed frozen or canned 2–3 small apricots or plums 10–15 grapes, cherries, strawberries 1 cup other berries 3 prunes, dates, figs, 1 tbsp raisins, sultanas 6–8 halves of dried apricots 180 ml 100% fruit juice	Fruit in light juice or natural juice, fruit in light syrup or heavy syrup, crystallized fruit. Restrict the latter two items if triglycerides raised and avoid if following a weight-reducing diet. Restrict fruit juice to 1 glass/day.	

Table 20.8 (*Cont'd*)

Food	Advisable	Daily/weekly amounts, serving size, comments	May be eaten in moderation	Should be avoided or eaten rarely
Cereal foods (choose breads and cereals with 450 mg/ 100 g sodium or less)	Wholemeal flour, wholemeal, especially wholegrain bread, wholegrain cereals, oatmeal, cornmeal, porridge oats, sweet corn, basmati rice, par-boiled rice, wholegrain rice, pasta and wholemeal pasta, crisp breads, oatcakes. Low-fat crackers.	Serving size: – 1 slice bread, 30 g other breads or ¹/₂ bread roll ¹/₂ cup pasta, ¹/₃ cup rice, ¹/₂ cup cooked porridge ²/₃ cup wheat cereal, cooked ¹/₃ cup muesli or 3 crisp bread Aim for 6–8 servings/day (3 servings wholegrain)	White flour, white bread, sugary breakfast cereals, commercial muesli, white rice and pasta, plain semi-sweet biscuits, higher-fat crackers. Naan bread without added butter or oil.	Fancy breads, croissants, brioches, savoury cheese biscuits, bought pastry. Egg noodles, pasta made with eggs.
Nuts and seeds	If not overweight or if overweight but able to substitute nuts for other fats, a regular intake can be beneficial. Use plain unsalted nuts, not roasted in other fats.	High risk; recommendation-30 g/day 5–7 times/week. All others at least 3 times/week if at all possible.	Almonds, brazil nuts (3–5/day only), pine nuts, cashews, hazelnuts, macadamias, pistachios peanuts, pecans, walnuts. Sunflower seeds, pumpkin seeds, linseed/flax seed (Up to 12% flaxseed can safely be used as an ingredient in food), sesame seeds, Tahini.	Coconut Salted nuts, nuts cooked in other fats or oils.
Made-up dishes/ deserts	Low-fat puddings, e.g. jelly, sorbet, skimmed-milk puddings, low-fat yoghurt, low-fat sauces, low-fat frozen yoghurt.	1 small tub reduced-fat ice cream or frozen yoghurt	Cakes, pastry, puddings, biscuits and sauces made with suitable margarine or oil. Low-fat or soy-based frozen desserts ('ice cream'). If following a weight-reducing diet, choose foods mainly from the 'Advisable' column.	Cakes and pastry, and biscuits made with saturated fats. All puddings, made with butter, or cream, cream sauces. Deep-fried snacks, dairy ice cream.
Drinks	Tea, coffee, mineral water, slim-line or sugar-free soft drinks, unsweetened fruit juice. Clear soup, homemade vegetable soup.	Limit sweet soft drinks to 1 glass/day or less. Avoid high-calorie drinks between meals.	Sweet soft drinks, low-fat malted drinks or low-fat drinking chocolate and fortified chocolate drinks occasionally. Meat soups, packet soups (avoid if on low-salt diet).	Coffee or hot chocolate made with cream, full-fat malted milk drinks, drinking chocolate.

Table 20.8 (*Cont'd*)

Food	Advisable	Daily/weekly amounts, serving size, comments	May be eaten in moderation	Should be avoided or eaten rarely
	'Cream' soups made with skimmed milk. Milky coffee and low-fat chocolate made with skimmed milk.		Alcohol (no more than 1–2 drinks for women, 2–3 drinks for men). Avoid alcohol and sugary drinks if triglycerides raised or if following a weight-reducing diet.	Cream soups made with full-fat milk and cream.
Sweets, sauces and spreads	If on a weight-reduction diet, use sugar-free sweeteners	Limit to 1–3 servings/day or less. 1 tbsp jam, syrup, honey, marmalade, sugar 2 fruit slice biscuits 1 sweet	Sweet pickles and chutney, jam, honey, marmalade, syrup, marzipan, lemon curd (made without eggs and butter), boiled sweets, pastilles, sugar, peppermints, wine gums. If triglycerides are raised or if following a weight-reducing diet, choose foods mainly from the 'Advisable' column.	Chocolate spreads, Christmas mincemeat containing suet. Toffees, fudge, butterscotch, chocolate, coconut bars.
Snacks/salty foods	Avoid high-salt foods and snacks	If using added salt, use iodized salt	Limit high-salt foods to one serving/week. 30 g serving lean ham, pastrami 20–30 g cheese (limit under dairy foods) 50 g canned or smoked salmon or tuna 30 g other smoked fish/sardines 1 tbsp meat and fish pastes 1 tsp paté	Salt-coated snacks, highly salted. Savoury snacks or potato crisps. Stock cubes, stock powder, gravy mix, yeast spreads, soy sauce, Worcester sauce.
Spreads/dressings/sauces/spices	Herbs, spices, mustard, pepper, vinegar, low-fat dressings, e.g. lemon or low-fat yoghurt. Low-fat vegetable-based sauces.		Low-calorie salad dressing or low-calorie mayonnaise, bottled sauces, French dressing. If on a weight-reducing diet, choose foods mainly from the 'Advisable' column.	Standard salad cream, mayonnaise, cream or cream cheese dressings.

Tables prepared by Dr Alexandra Chisholm, Research Dietitian, Department of Human Nutrition, University of Otago, Dunedin, New Zealand

FURTHER READING

1. Armstrong, B.K., Mann, J.I., Adelstein, A.M., and Eskin, F. (1975) Commodity consumption and ischaemic heart disease mortality with special reference to dietary practices. *J Chron Dis*, **28**, 455–69.

2. Ascherio, A., Rimm, E.B., Giovannucci, E.L., *et al.* (1996) Dietary fat and risk of coronary heart disease in men: cohort follow-up study in the USA. *Br Med J*, **313**, 84–90.

3. Burr, M.L., Gilbert, J.F., Holliday, R.M., *et al.* (1989) Effects of changes in fat, fish and fibre intakes on death and myocardial reinfarction: Diet and Reinfarction Trial (DART). *Lancet*, ii, 757–61.

4. Dayton, S., Pearce, M.L., Hashimoto, S., *et al.* (1969) A controlled trial of a diet high in unsaturated fat in preventing complications of atherosclerosis. *Circulation*, **39/40** (Suppl. II), 1–63.

5. de Lorgeril, M., Renaud, S., Mamelle, N., *et al.* (1994) Mediterranean α-linolenic acid-rich diet in secondary prevention of coronary heart disease. *Lancet*, **343**, 1454–9.

6. Elliott, P., Stamler, J., Nichols, R., *et al.* (1996) Intersalt revisited: Further analysis of 24 hour-sodium excretion and blood pressure within and across populations. *BMJ*, **312**, 1249–53.

7. GISSI (1999) Dietary supplementation with n-3 polyunsaturated fatty acids and vitamin E after myocardial infarction. *Lancet*, **354**, 447–55.

8. Hertog, M.L., Feskens, E.J.M., Hollman, P.C.H., Katan, M.B., and Kromhout, D. (1993) Dietary antioxidant flavonoids and risk of coronary heart disease. *Lancet*, **342**, 1007–17.

9. Hjermann, I., Byer, K., Holme, I., *et al.* (1981) Effect of diet and smoking intervention on the incidence of coronary heart disease. *Lancet*, ii, 1303–10.

10. Keys, A., Menotti, A., Karvonen, M.J., *et al.* (1986) The diet and 15-year death rate in the Seven Countries Study. *Am J Epidemiol*, **124**, 903–15.

11. Knekt, P., Ritz, J., Pereira, M.A., *et al.* (2004) Antioxidant vitamins and coronary heart disease: A pooled analysis of cohorts. *Amer Clin Nutr*, **80**, 1508–20.

12. Law, M.R., Frost, C.D., and Wald, N.J. (1991) By how much does dietary salt reduction lower blood pressure? Analysis of data from trials of salt reduction. *Br Med J*, **302**, 819–24.

13. Liu, S., Manson, J.E., Stampfer, M.J., *et al.* (2000) Wholegrain consumption and risk of ischemic stroke in women: A prospective study. *J Am Med Ass*, **284**, 1534–40.

14. Mann, J.I., Appleby, P.N., Key, T.J., and Thorogood, M. (1997) Dietary determinants of ischaemic heart disease in health conscious individuals. *Heart*, **78**, 450–5.

15. Margetts, B.M., Beilin, L.J., Vandongen, R., and Armstrong, B.K. (1986) Vegetarian diet in mild hypertension: A randomized controlled trial. *Br Med J*, **293**, 1468–71.

16. Mensink, R.P., Zoch, P.L., Kester, A.D., and Katan, M.B. (2003) Effects of dietary fatty acids and carbohydrates on the ratio of serum total to HDL cholesterol and on serum lipids and apolipoproteins: A meta-analysis of 60 controlled trials. *Am J Clin Nutr*, **77**, 1146–55.

17. Ordovas, J.M. (2004) The quest for cardiovascular health in the genomic era: nutrigenetics and plasma lipoproteins. *Proc Nutr Soc*, **63**, 145–52.

18. Rimm, E.B., Ascherio, A., Giovannucci, E., *et al.* (1996) *J Am Med Assoc*, **275**, 447–51.

19. Robinson, S.M., Barker, D.J. (2002) Coronary heart disease: A disorder of growth. *Proc Nutr Soc*, **61**, 537–42.

20. Sacks, F.M., Svetkey, L.P., Vollmer, W.M., *et al.* (2001) Effects on blood pressure of reduced dietary sodium and the Dietary Approaches to Stop Hypertension (DASH) Diet. *N Eng J Med*, **344**, 3–10.

21. Scientific Advisory Committee on Nutrition (2003) *Salt and health*. The Stationary Office, London.

22. Stampfer, M.J., and Rimm, E.B. (1995) Epidemiological evidence for vitamin E in prevention of cardiovascular disease. *Am J Clin Nutr*, **62**, 1365S–1369S.

23. Strassullo, P., Scalfi, L., Branca, F., *et al.* (2004) Nutrition prevention of ischaemic stroke: present knowledge, limitations and future perspectives. *Nutr Metab Cardiovasc Dis*, **14**, 97–114.

24. The Heart Outcomes Prevention Evaluation Study Investigators (HOPE) (2000) Vitamin E supplementation and cardiovascular events in high-risk patients. *N Engl J Med*, **342**, 154–60.

25. Truswell, A.S. (2002) Cereal grains and coronary heart disease. *Eur J Clin Nutr*, **56**, 1–14.

26. WHO/FAO (2003) *Diet, nutrition and the prevention of chronic diseases*. WHO Technical Report Series 916. Geneva, World Health Organization.

21 Nutrition and cancer

Martin Wiseman

21.1 General epidemiology of cancer

Worldwide, some 13% of deaths are caused by cancer, but there is marked variation. For instance, cancers account for 5% of deaths in Africa, but about one-quarter of deaths in industrialized nations. In England in 2000, 24% of deaths in males and 28% in females were due to cancers, second only to cardiovascular diseases.

For the commonest cancers, age is a major determinant of risk. Adult cancers tend to be rare below the age of 40, with a marked increase after 65 years (Fig. 21.1). Therefore, as life expectancy increases in many regions of the globe, cancers can be expected to become more common, with attendant social and economic costs. Current approaches to controlling cancer focus on screening to detect cancers at an early stage, and surgical, chemotherapeutic and radiotherapeutic management of existing clinical disease. However, screening is an appropriate option for only some cancers, due to inadequacies in screening methods or lack of evidence of efficacy or of safety of interventions. Equally, treatments can be remarkably successful for some cancers (such as testicular cancer), but for many, and the most frequent, cancers (lung, breast, colon, cervix, stomach) they are often only incompletely effective, especially if the disease is advanced at diagnosis. In addition, screening for and management of existing cancers are expensive options, not always available to lower-income nations.

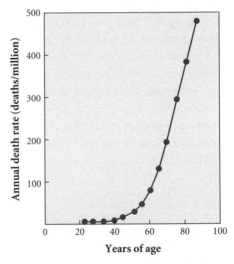

Fig. 21.1 Rates of colon cancer rise steeply with age compatible with multistep, time-dependent tumour progression.

Consequently, it will become increasingly important to identify means of primary prevention as a major thrust in controlling the burden of cancer worldwide. Rational approaches to primary prevention rely on a sound understanding of cause of disease, and understanding the causes of cancers is therefore an essential prerequisite.

The incidence of specific cancers varies markedly between different geographical regions (Table 21.1).

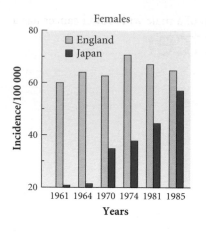

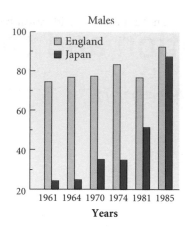

Fig. 21.2 Colorectal cancer incidence in women and men aged 55–60 in Miyagi, Japan and Birmingham, England.

Source: Parkin, D.M. Muir, C.S. Whelan, S.L., *et al.* (1992) *Cancer incidence in five continents*. Vol. I – VI. IARC, Lyon.

For instance, age-standardized rates for nasopharyngeal cancer are around 100 times higher in regions of China than in Western industrialized nations, for colon cancer 20 times higher in the USA than in India, and for breast cancer they are seven times higher in the USA than in non-Jews in Israel (WCRF, 1997). Table 21.1 shows the commonest cancers (excluding skin) in higher-income compared with lower-income countries. Furthermore, these geographical variations are not static. For example, in Japan, colorectal cancer was extremely rare in the 1960s, but by 1985, rates had risen to become comparable with those in Western industrialized nations (Fig. 21.2).

Worldwide, stomach cancer rates have fallen steeply over the last half century. In addition, cancer rates may change when populations migrate. The low rates of breast and colon cancer, and high rates of stomach cancer, that were typical of the Miyagi region of Japan were transformed amongst migrants from this population to Hawaii to resemble the local rates, with high incidence of colon and breast cancer and lower rates of stomach cancer, within one to two generations (Fig. 21.3).

The marked plasticity of these variations is amongst the strongest evidence for a major environmental determination for the patterns and rates of the common

Table 21.1 Common sites of cancer (listed in rank order) in developed countries and developing countries[a]

Developed countries	Developing countries
Lung	Cervix
Large bowel	Stomach
Breast	Mouth
Stomach	Oesophagus
Prostate	Breast
Bladder	Lung

[a]Skin cancers are not included because of difficulties involved in estimating incidence. The most serious of these, malignant melanoma, is more common in some countries, especially where fair-skinned people have a high exposure to sunlight (e.g. Australia, New Zealand, and South Africa).

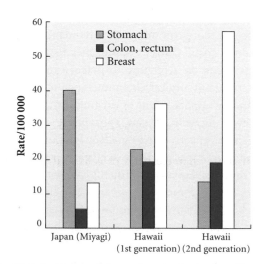

Fig. 21.3 Incidence of stomach, colon/rectum and breast cancers in Japanese women by generation in Japan and Hawaii, 1968–1977.

adult cancers, though childhood cancers do not appear to show the same effect. Twin studies also suggest that inherited genetic factors in general contribute only a small proportion to cancer risk, in the absence of uncommon germline mutations in specific genes, such as *BRCA1* and *BRCA2* for breast cancer. For instance, the identical twin of a male with bowel cancer has a 9% probability of developing the same cancer. Several studies over the last two decades have implicated food and nutrition as key environmental determinants of cancer risk, with estimates of their contribution varying between 25% and 40%, on average.

21.2 Biology of cancer

Cancer is a disease characterized by the development of a population of cells that have escaped normal regulation of growth, replication and differentiation and which invades surrounding or distant tissues. The maintenance of cellular and tissue integrity over a lifetime relies upon a tightly regulated series of processes, from cell division and DNA replication, through growth and differentiation, to programmed cell death (apoptosis). Cancer develops when a clone of abnormal cells acquires the ability to escape that regulation. At root, cancer results from abnormal cellular function, and these abnormalities are the result of mutations—alterations in the nucleotide structure of DNA—which are most commonly acquired during life (somatic mutations). Nevertheless, in a few rare but important cases, such as familial polyposis coli, the abnormalities may be inherited (germline mutations).

The normal cell cycle incorporates several critical points that determine the future for that cell—whether to replicate, to terminally differentiate or to undergo apoptosis. The cellular environment including its nutrient environment is an important determinant of the progress of the cell cycle. Cell division and DNA replication offer opportunities for errors to occur, resulting in mutation. Increasing elucidation of the regulation of cell division has enhanced understanding of those characteristics of cells that determine their behaviour, in particular whether or not they develop into an invasive tumour. An average human adult contains some 10^{10} cells, and over a lifetime will produce around 10^{16} cells, so perhaps the most remarkable phenomenon is the fact that abnormalities of these processes are not more common.

A developing body of evidence has led to an increasingly sophisticated understanding of the nature of the cellular characteristics that lead to cancer, and of the processes that influence them. Cancer cells display specific characteristics that confer particular capabilities, which are not present in normal cells; taken together these account for their abnormal behaviour. These abnormal capabilities influence aspects of cell growth, replication and differentiation, as well as the way cells interact with their neighbouring cells and the extracellular environment.

Six of these phenotypic characteristics have been termed the 'hallmarks of cancer' and they are the basis for the abnormal behaviour of cells that leads to cancer. The six capabilities that characterize cancer cells but not normal cells are:

- Self-sufficiency in growth signals
- Insensitivity to antigrowth signals
- Evasion of apoptosis
- Limitless replicative potential
- Sustained angiogenesis
- Tissue invasion and metastasis

Cells usually respond both to stimulatory and to inhibitory external growth signals, but cancer cells develop autonomy in growth that escapes the normal control mechanisms. Normal cells after a number of divisions usually undergo programmed cell death (apoptosis), a process that appears to protect the structural and functional integrity of cells and tissues, but cancer cells do not display this. On the contrary, the usual process whereby cells fail to divide further following a certain number of cell divisions is also disrupted, and abnormalities in the function of telomeres (at the ends of DNA strands) appear to allow clones of cells to develop immortality through continuing division. Finally, the relations of cells with their external environment are altered. While normal cells closely constrain vascular development in growing tissues through secretion of chemoactive substances, cancer cells continue to promote unconstrained angiogenesis, thus allowing the development of a tumour mass. The several processes that ensure the controlled interaction between neighbouring cells is also lost, allowing a clone of cells with a selective growth advantage to exploit that by invading neighbouring tissues and eventually spreading to distant sites. Alone, each abnormality will not be sufficient to cause cancer, but together these characteristics are required for cells to behave as cancers. Each represents a phenotypic abnormality that results from genetic mutation due to DNA damage, which has been acquired during the life of the cell or passed on from a parent cell. Each capability represents a complex set of functions, and may result from one mutation, or from a combination of mutations. Equally, a single mutation might contribute to more than one abnormal capability (Fig. 21.4). A cell has to accumulate all of these characteristics in order to generate the clone of cells that becomes a clinical cancer in a process of serial accumulation of DNA mutation leading to phenotypic abnormalities, in no special chronological

sequence. This is a development from the previous model, which suggested three distinct chronological elements of initiation, promotion and progression, based on studies of experimentally induced cancer using carcinogenic agents. It is estimated that the accumulation of sufficient genetic damage leading to clinically apparent tumours typically occurs over a period of one to two decades. This multistep time-dependent model is supported by the non-linear, exponential increase in cancer with age (Fig. 21.1).

Table 21.2 lists the main known causes of cancers. These may exert their effects directly, for instance by causing DNA damage and mutation (e.g. ionizing radiation) or indirectly by promoting cell replication. The process of cell division and replication is itself a critically vulnerable time for DNA to accumulate and pass on errors to subsequent generations of cells. Factors that promote cell division therefore expose more cells to any environmental causes of cancer, whether nutritional or otherwise, and so increase the likelihood of mutation. Common factors that promote cell division include inflammation, especially chronic inflammation, and exposure to growth factors such as insulin-like growth factors (IGFs) or sex hormones, which promote growth in specifically sensitive tissues. Nutrition may further influence

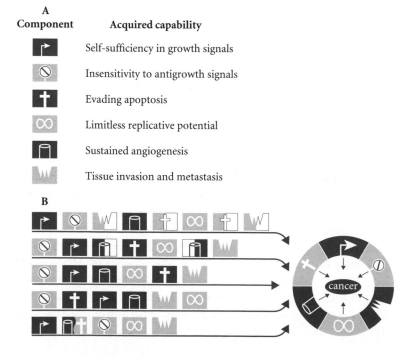

A

Component   **Acquired capability**

Self-sufficiency in growth signals

Insensitivity to antigrowth signals

Evading apoptosis

Limitless replicative potential

Sustained angiogenesis

Tissue invasion and metastasis

B

Fig. 21.4 The six capabilities needed for a cell to become cancerous can be acquired through different patterns of mutation. Five different possible pathways that all culminate in acquisition of these six characteristics by a cell are shown schematically. Each phenotypic capability may follow a single mutation, but may also result from two separate mutations. In contrast, a single mutation may cause (or contribute to) one (or more than one) phenotypic abnormality. For instance, in the eight-step pathway, two mutations are required each for tissue invasion and metastasis, and for evading apoptosis, whereas the other pathways require only one. In the five-step pathway, evading apoptosis and sustained angiogenesis both arise from one mutation.

Table 21.2 Factors increasing cancer risk

Environmental
Carcinogenic chemicals
Occupational
Food contamination
Smoking
Pollution
Infectious agents
Viruses (e.g. human papilloma virus, Epstein–Barr virus)
Bacteria (e.g. *Helicobacter pylori*)
Fungi (e.g. *Aspergillus* spp. producing mycotoxin)
Ionizing radiation
Exogenous hormones, e.g. growth factors
Intrinsic
Inherited germline mutations
Endogenous hormones, e.g. growth factors
Inflammation

the intracellular environment directly, for instance by altering the concentration of specific nutrients involved in the regulation of the cell cycle. It may also contribute indirectly by influencing these general processes of inflammation or growth factors.

Nutritional factors that influence the intracellular environment directly or indirectly therefore have potential to affect various aspects of the cell cycle, including abnormalities in DNA replication, and so also the likelihood of mutation. However, phenotypic expression depends on more than simply the genetic code based on the nucleotide sequence in DNA, which is altered by mutation. So-called epigenetic effects (those that result in altered gene expression without a change in the nucleotide sequence of DNA) may also have a profound impact on cellular phenotype. Alterations in histone (the protein core around which DNA helices are wound) can influence the overall stability of the genome, and DNH methylation can influence the expression of particular genes.

Therefore, nutritional factors that influence cell-cycle processes have potential for affecting the likelihood that a cell may eventually become cancerous, though the complexities of the processes make it likely that any impact will be the result of the interplay among many different influences.

21.3 Cause and prevention

A *cause* of any disease is any usual exposure that, if removed, reduces the likelihood of the disease developing, or its severity. Most conditions do not have a single cause, but are the result of an interaction among many causal factors. A factor that alone can result in a disease is a called a *sufficient* cause; if more than one factor is required, these are termed *contributory* causes; if a disease cannot occur in the absence of a factor, it is termed a *necessary* cause. Cancer is a condition that generally has several contributory causes. A key focus of research is to identify those factors or combinations of factors that are either necessary or sufficient for the development of cancer.

Controlled trials offer a robust way of testing causation directly by altering exposure in an experimental setting, so that, in well-designed studies, the outcomes can be attributed with confidence to the intervention applied. However, because there are many likely nutritional exposures of interest, and they are likely to interact, both amongst themselves and with other non-nutritional factors, conducting trials that both are well designed and encompass an appropriate range of exposures is usually impractical. Furthermore, trials are unlikely to take place over more than a small part of the many years during which the process of cancer development occurs. Consequently, well-designed trials exploring the causes of cancer tend to use high-risk individuals because they are more likely to progress to measurable outcomes, and to do so in a shorter time, than subjects drawn from the general population. Also, the exposures employed as interventions tend to be single nutrients given as supplements, often at unusually high doses, although some true diet intervention trials have been conducted. Finally, it is difficult either to conduct trials of diet in a truly blinded fashion, or to achieve sufficient sustained dietary change to differentiate between intervention and control groups. This means that, while positive results from such trials can be informative, negative results must be interpreted with caution.

Much of the evidence on the relationship between nutrition and cancer comes from observational epidemiology. These studies have the advantage that they can explore the relationship between hard outcomes and typical exposures in representative populations, but the lack of experimental design means that they are subject to confounding. Confounding distorts the apparent association between an exposure and outcome due to the effect of a third factor, which itself is a cause of the outcome but is also associated with the exposure. This means that by itself an association found between any nutritional factor and cancer in observational epidemiological studies cannot be assumed to be a causal one, although there are characteristics of the data that help to judge the likelihood of whether any such association is truly causal (such as the size of the effect, or whether there is a dose–response effect). There are broadly two main types of epidemiological studies of individuals —prospective studies (often in cohorts of people followed up for many years), which record exposures such as diet or physical activity prior to diagnosis; and retrospective studies (often case–control), which record past exposure after diagnosis. It has become clear that, at least for diet and physical activity, retro-

spective assessments even in otherwise well-designed studies are subject to serious recall bias, making interpretation of data from them difficult.

In addition, as well as trials and epidemiology, there is a considerable body of evidence drawn from laboratory experiments, much of it on animals or *in vitro* work on isolated tissues or cell lines. Although the direct relevance of much of this work to human cancer is remote, some types of experimental evidence are valuable contributors to understanding the mechanisms that might underpin observed associations in humans, particularly the more recent development of genetic manipulation (e.g. knockout models).

Consequently, in relation to causation of cancer, no single type of study can be regarded as paramount, and interpretation needs to embrace a consideration of several different sources of evidence.

The term *prevention* is often taken to mean complete avoidance of an outcome. However, it can equally be applied to delay in its appearance (so deferring any adverse outcome, possibly beyond the natural lifespan), or to reduction in risk in an individual, which translates to reduction in incidence in a population. In the latter case, an intervention that lowered incidence of an event from 50% to 25% will truly have prevented half the events, although it may never be possible to identify those particular individuals who would otherwise have been affected in the absence of the intervention. In the case of cancer, which has several contributory causes and probably no single necessary cause, interventions on some of them would not be expected to completely prevent cancer, but to reduce the likelihood of its occurrence or defer its appearance—this is also prevention.

21.4 Causes of cancer

There are several established classes of factors that are known to increase risk of developing cancer, due to increasing the likelihood of acquiring mutations in DNA that contribute to the cellular dysregulation characteristic of cancer (Table 21.2). Some factors may directly damage DNA as certain viruses or carcinogenic chemicals do, and others may promote replica-

tion and so increase the opportunity for other factors to operate, such as growth factors or inflammation (see section 21.2).

Nutritional factors may operate either directly through one or more of these mechanisms, or may interact with them, either reducing or enhancing their effects.

21.5 Nutrition and cancer

There is some evidence for a link between nutrition and most adult cancers. In addition, nutritional factors may show effects at more than one cancer site. The main relationships between the principal adult cancers and foods, food components, physical activity and obesity are set out together with known other causes in Table 21.3.

Because most evidence derives from observational epidemiology and from laboratory data on mechanisms, with only a few clinical trials, which are often difficult to interpret, the confidence of the conclusions on causal nutritional factors varies. In general, the confidence is greater for foods or food groups than for individual food components, because of the difficulty of excluding confounding by other food components. Similarly, direct anthropometric measures provide more reliable information than questionnaire-derived data. The number of nutritional factors listed in the table is lower than appears in some other reviews because only those factors judged to be convincingly or probably causal factors have been highlighted. There is a plethora of food components for which a body of evidence exists, but which is inconclusive or limited either by the amount, nature or quality of evidence. The judgement is personal, but based on authoritative texts (see Further Reading). Box 21.1 illustrates and explains the results of a meta-analysis of the observational studies that have examined the relationship between waist circumference and postmenopausal breast cancer. This approach, together with laboratory data on mechanisms, form the basis of much of our knowledge regarding the lifestyle-related determinants of cancer.

21.5.1 Foods, beverages and cancer

Vegetables and fruits This broad category embraces a wide variety of different plant foods that might

---

BOX 21.1 www.oxfordtextbooks.co.uk/orc/mann3e/

Go to the url above to see a forest plot showing the results of a meta-analysis of observational studies of the relationship between waist circumference and postmenopausal breast cancer.

The columns describe the study identifier, the numbers of cases and controls in those with smaller and larger waists, the weight that the study contributed to the statistical analysis, based on factors such as the size of the study and the numbers of cases, and the relative risk with 95% confidence intervals.

The square boxes represent the relative risk for each study and the size of the box is proportional to the weight. The vertical line is the line of no effect. Where the relative risk is less than 1, that is, lower risk with a smaller waist, the box is to the left of the line, and where greater than 1, to the right. The lines through each box represent the 95% confidence intervals. Under each section is a diamond representing the combined summary estimate with 95% confidence intervals. The

text to the left describes the statistical calculation of heterogeneity.

The different sections show results for cohort studies and case–control studies separately, first when adjusted for known confounders, and secondly when not so adjusted. The final section is a subgroup analysis cohort data in studies where it was possible to exclude the use of hormone replacement therapy.

This analysis shows a highly statistically significantly lower risk of postmenopausal breast cancer with smaller waist circumference from cohort studies. The risk is 39% lower (relative risk 0.61) in those with a waist circumference below compared with above the cut-off. Case–control studies do not show this effect, possibly due to recall bias or reverse causation. Low heterogeneity and the facts both that adjustment for confounders made little difference to the effect, and that the effect was maintained in those who had not had hormone replacement therapy, suggest that the association is robust.

Table 21.3 Associations between nutritional factors and common cancer sites. Other known causes of the cancers are also listed

Cancer site	Known causes	Nutritional factors decreasing risk	Nutritional factors increasing risk	Nutritional factors under investigation
Bladder	Tobacco smoking			
Breast		Physical activity ↓	Alcohol ↑↑ Greater growth in early life ↑ Obesity (postmenopausal) ↑↑	
Cervix	Human papilloma virus			Folate ↓
Colorectum		Fish and poultry ↓ Vegetables ↓ Physical activity ↓ Non-starch polysaccharide (dietary fibre) ↓	Processed and red meat ↑ Obesity ↑↑	Calcium ↓
Endometrium			Obesity ↑↑	
Gallbladder	Gallstones		Obesity ↑	
Kidney	Cigarette smoking		Obesity ↑↑	
Liver	Hepatitis (viral, alcoholic)		Aflatoxin ↑↑ Alcohol ↑	
Lung	Tobacco smoking, radon	Fruits ↓↓ Vegetables ↓ Physical activity ↓	High-dose β-carotene supplements ↑↑	
Mouth, larynx and pharynx	Tobacco smoking		Alcohol ↑↑	
Nasopharynx	Epstein–Barr virus		Cantonese-style salted fish ↑	
Oesophagus	Tobacco smoking		Obesity (adenocarcinoma) ↑↑ Hot drinks? (maté) ↑	
Ovary				
Pancreas	Tobacco smoking	Physical activity ↓	Obesity ↑↑	
Prostate		Selenium ↓		Tomatoes/lycopene ↓ Vitamin E ↓ Animal products ↑
Stomach	*Helicobacter pylori*	Fruit and vegetables ↓	High salt intake ↑	
Skin	Ionizing radiation			
Testis				

↑↑: Convincingly causal nutritional factor increases risk; ↑: probably causal nutritional factor increases risk.
↓↓: Convincingly causal nutritional factor decreases risk; ↓: probably causal nutritional factor decreases risk.

influence cancer risk. Much of the evidence is derived from case–control studies but in general prospective cohort data and the few intervention trials have been less impressive. Therefore, interpretation needs to be cautious. Table 21.3 indicates that risk of colorectal, stomach and lung cancers has been found to be lower amongst people with relatively high intakes of vegetables and fruits than among those consuming small quantities. There are several possible mechanisms that might underlie such associations.

Botanically there is no clear distinction between the category of fruit (the seed-bearing parts of plants) and vegetables (a dietary description relating to the way foods are included as part of the diet). Many vegetables are, in fact, botanically fruits (e.g. courgettes, aubergines). Although there are compositional similarities within the group, different vegetables and fruits may have very different composition in relation to their micronutrient or non-nutrient composition. Even for a single type of vegetable or fruit, composition may vary several fold with variety, season and growing conditions.

Components of vegetables and fruits that are relevant to their possible role in influencing cancer risk include the following:

- *Non-starch polysaccharide/dietary fibre* can be fermented by the colonic flora to produce butyrate, which helps to maintain normal differentiation of colonocytes. It may reduce dietary energy density, which may aid energy balance, and it decreases colonic transit time, which may reduce the contact of colonic epithelium with carcinogens (see below).

- *Vitamins C and E and carotenoids* may act as antioxidants to prevent oxidative and possibly other damage to DNA, lipids or proteins. Vitamin C may prevent formation of nitrosocompounds, which might be important for stomach cancer.

- *Glucosinolates* are found in brassica vegetables. They are enzymatically transformed by myrosinase released when the plant cells are damaged into *isothiocyanates*. These stimulate hepatic phase 2 enzymes, which conjugate and help excrete carcinogens. The effect of brassica vegetables in lung cancer is greatest in people who do not have an enzyme that eliminates isothiocyanates, making the association more likely to be causal.

- *Flavonoids, including phytoestrogens* from soy and other legumes have several antioxidant and potentially anti-oestrogenic actions.

- *Folate* is essential for normal DNA metabolism and for regulating gene expression.

- *Sulphur compounds* from allium species (onions, garlic, etc.) have been shown in experimental studies to demonstrate anticancer potential, but more robust evidence in humans is lacking.

Meat, fish, poultry and dairy These animal products are important sources of several nutrients, but higher intakes, typical of higher-income countries, have been linked with certain cancers. Processed and red meats have been linked to increased risk of colorectal cancer, while fish and poultry show an inverse association. Caution needs to be applied in interpretation as definitions of 'processed meat' vary from country to country.

Dietary components associated with animal products that are relevant to their possible role in cancer include the following:

- *Iron* is abundant in meat and meat products as haem, in which form it is more easily assimilated than in the inorganic form in vegetables. Evidence for the proposal that iron might increase risk of colorectal cancer through its action, in its free form, as a pro-oxidant is not convincing. There is some evidence that cooked meat protein can form heterocyclic amines, which might increase colorectal cancer risk, but this remains speculative. It appears that haem, rather than the iron *per se*, from meat and meat products is susceptible to endogenous nitrosation by bacterial flora in the colon, and these *N*-nitrosocompounds can increase the likelihood of neoplastic change. This effect is not shared by fish or poultry.

- *Calcium* is principally found in milk and dairy products in higher-income Western countries, but in many parts of the world these are not a major part of the diet. There is preliminary evidence from epidemiological studies in Western countries, and from trials of a few years duration on recurrence of adenomas (necessary precursors of cancer though not all progress), that calcium might reduce risk of colorectal cancer, possibly by forming insoluble soaps and limiting any carcinogenic effect of free fatty acids or bile salts.

- *Vitamin D* is mainly found in animal products but is also derived from endogenous formation in the skin. As well as its role in calcium and bone metabolism, vitamin D is an important modulator of cell differentiation and communication. It has been proposed that the strong effect of latitude on prostate cancer risk might be mediated by vitamin D status, but this is not supported by epidemiological studies.

- *Total fat* may be derived from both animal and vegetable sources, but the predominant sources of fat in high-income countries are animal products. Ecological studies suggest higher rates of breast cancer with higher fat intakes, but large prospective cohorts predominantly from the USA have been negative. At the time of writing, preliminary results of a large intervention study have suggested that the intervention, which reduced fat intake but also had other effects (e.g. reduced meat, increased fruit and vegetables, weight loss) modestly reduced risk of recurrent breast cancer in postmenopausal women. It is not clear whether any effect is due to the total fat itself or the proportions and amounts of different fatty acids (see below), or to other aspects of diet or lifestyle. A definitive conclusion is not currently possible.

- *Fatty acids* may have specific effects on cancer causation. In animal models, a relatively high intake of linoleic acid (around 12% of energy) seems to promote tumour progression, and this effect may be countered by increasing n-3 fatty acid intake. Specific mechanisms have not been identified.

Starchy staples In most parts of the world, starchy staples are the predominant energy source, but this is less so in high-income countries. The amount and type of starchy food consumed has been proposed as a major factor in determining global cancer patterns.

Factors associated with starchy foods that are relevant to any effect on cancer include:

- *Non-starch polysaccharide (dietary fibre) and resistant starch*. They have long been implicated as protective factors against colorectal cancer. However, because of difficulties of definition, the precise role that undigestible plant components play is not fully resolved. Nevertheless, there is good epidemiological evidence that higher dietary fibre intakes are associated with lower risk of colorectal cancer. Both non-starch polysaccharide and resistant starch escape digestion in the small bowel and provide substrate for the colonic flora, which ferment them to release short-chain fatty acids, including butyrate, which helps to maintain the integrity of the colonocyte DNA. In addition, fibre increases stool bulk and decreases transit time, both of which may reduce the opportunity for colonocytes to be in contact with faecal carcinogens. Short-term trials using certain forms of dietary fibre supplements have not shown an effect on adenoma recurrence but it is not clear whether these experimental results can be extrapolated more generally.

More recently, studies have explored the links between wholegrain cereals and cancer risk, but due to variation in definition, these are difficult to interpret. Any mechanisms underlying observed effects are likely to include the role of dietary fibre, intake of which is intimately associated with whole grains.

Selenium intake in populations is determined by its concentration in the soil, and where this is high, cereal products are the major source. Rich sources include nuts (especially brazil nuts), shellfish and meat. Selenium is an important cofactor for several enzymes including glutathione peroxidase, which is a major antioxidant. A trial found unexpectedly that prostate cancer (not a prior stated outcome) was markedly reduced after selenium supplementation, particularly in men with lower selenium status. Epidemiology is inconsistent. Trials in progress are expected to allow a more definitive conclusion.

Salt The main cause of stomach cancer is agreed to be infection with *Helicobacter pylori*. High salt intake appears to interact with this to influence risk. Stomach cancer rates are highest in those parts of the world with the highest salt intakes, e.g. China, Japan. In all countries, there has been a marked decline in stomach cancer rates over the last 50 years, attributed in part to lower salt intakes with increased use of other preservative methods. High salt intake increases risk of atrophic gastritis, which not only may render the stomach more susceptible to *H. pylori* infection, but also increases the susceptibility of the mucosa to neoplastic change once infection is established.

There is also strong evidence that Cantonese-style so-called salted fish increases risk of nasopharyngeal cancer, especially when consumed in childhood. The term 'salted fish' is misleading as this form of fish, while certainly salty, is only partly preserved and is partly putrefied. The presence of *N*-nitrosocompounds in fish resulting from the putrefaction is thought to account for the effect.

Alcohol Alcohol is classed as a carcinogen by the World Health Organization (WHO) International Agency for Research on Cancer. Higher consumption of alcohol increases risk of cancers of the mouth, larynx and pharynx, where it acts synergistically with tobacco smoking. It also increases risk of breast cancer, with no apparent threshold for an effect. Heavy alcohol consumption can lead to cirrhosis of the liver, which itself increases risk of liver cancer, irrespective of cause. It is less clear that alcohol *per se* has a specific effect. The main cause of hepatitis and cirrhosis worldwide is hepatitis C, though in high-income countries alcohol remains a major cause.

21.5.2 Energy balance, obesity, physical activity, growth and cancer

Energy Energy restriction is amongst the most consistent and powerful means of reducing cancer in experimental animals. So long as nutrient demands are otherwise met, energy-restricted animals have lower age-specific cancer incidence and prolonged life. It is not straightforward to extrapolate these findings to free-living humans, but clearly energy metabolism is implicated in modulating cancer risk in whole-body systems.

Obesity Obesity shows one of the most consistent epidemiological associations with cancer, and increases risk of cancers of the colorectum, breast (in post-menopausal women), endometrium, kidney, oeso-phagus (adenocarcinoma) and gallbladder. Obesity has several metabolic effects that may account for its effects on cancer risk. Obesity increases insulin resistance and plasma concentrations of insulin, reduces binding proteins for IGFs, and also influences the sex hormone axes. It is also a pro-inflammatory state. Many of these effects are reversed by weight loss.

Physical activity The level of physical activity is a major modifiable determinant of energy expenditure, and so of risk of obesity. Increasingly, physical activity is also recognized as an independent modulator of cancer risk. Higher levels of physical activity are associated with lower risk of cancers of the breast, colorectum, pancreas and lung. Physical activity has several metabolic effects that are relevant to cancer risk. Increasing activity increases insulin sensitivity and reduces insulin levels, increases concentrations of binding proteins for IGFs, and influences the sex hormone axes in both men and women. Higher levels of activity decrease colonic transit time.

Growth Increasingly it is recognized that adult health and susceptibility to disease is influenced not only by genetic background and contemporary environmental exposures (including diet) but also by events occurring from conception onward, which may influence development at critical stages of maturation resulting in permanent alterations. This so-called programming has been best described in relation to cardiovascular disease, but there is evidence for an effect in cancer, though it has so far not been studied in depth. It has long been known that taller women, and earlier menarche, are associated with higher breast cancer risk. It is now thought that this represents an effect of permanent alteration of the IGF axis, manifest by greater early growth. It is likely that the causal component is lifelong exposure to higher levels of growth factors. The secondary effect of early menarche is to increase lifetime exposure to oestrogens, which may have an independent effect.

21.5.3 Contaminants, cooking and dietary supplements and cancer

Worldwide, food and drink contamination remains a serious problem. High levels of arsenic in drinking water, for instance in Bangladesh, and aflatoxin contamination of grain, for instance in China and Africa, are the principal known contaminants associated with cancer.

Aflatoxin is a toxin and known carcinogen resulting from fungal infestation of grain stored in warm, humid conditions typical of subtropical regions of Asia, especially China and Thailand, and in parts of Africa, where its consumption is associated with liver cancer. Recent work that relates its effect on liver cancer risk to genetic differences in the ability to metabolize it add weight to the likelihood of this association being causal.

Cooking produces chemical effects in proteins and carbohydrates that might have adverse effects. The high-temperature frying of starchy carbohydrates produces significant quantities of acrylamide, a known carcinogen. In addition, charring of meat as in barbecuing produces polycyclic aromatic hydrocarbons and heterocyclic amines that have been shown to have carcinogenic potential in laboratory animals. However, there is no epidemiological evidence to suggest that the carcinogenic potential of these processes and substances is actually realized in free-living humans.

Dietary supplements For practical reasons, intervention studies of diet and cancer usually use purified supplements of micronutrients rather than attempting to achieve sustained dietary change. This methodology has the advantage of providing robust answers, but the disadvantage of being difficult to extrapolate to the usual free-living situation. In general, with the exception of selenium in relation to prostate cancer and calcium in relation to colorectal cancer (see above), dietary supplementation has failed to demonstrate effects over the short term on cancer risk. The possible reasons for this include a true lack of effect, a failure to address any more complex interactions, inappropriate dose or form of the nutrient, and timing or duration of the intervention. Consequently, the knowledge gained from negative outcomes of such trials is limited.

21.5.4 Nutrition in the management of cancer

This section is not concerned with interventions over the acute stage but rather in the stable situations before or after therapeutic interventions. The relevant question in the context of nutrition interventions in people with cancer is one of efficacy: does this intervention influence outcome in people who have already had a diagnosis of cancer? Outcome may refer to survival, to rate of recurrence, or progression of a cancer, or to development of a new cancer, or to quality of life. Given that the population is easily defined and that outcomes are likely to occur in a relatively short time, randomized controlled trials are an appropriate tool to offer a 'best' answer, especially as retrospective observational data are particularly likely to suffer from several forms of bias in this clinical setting.

Unfortunately, few trials have been reported, and those are mainly small, and with diverse interventions and outcome measures. Thus, it is difficult to be confident about what might be an appropriate, safe and effective nutrition intervention in people with cancer.

The largest study in this situation (the Women's Intervention Nutrition Study) has released preliminary results. The study was aimed at reducing fat intake in postmenopausal women who had completed their treatment for breast cancer. Preliminary reports indicate a small but statistically and clinially meaningful reduction in recurrence of breast cancer, although it is clear that the intervention resulted in many changes other than in fat consumption, including an increase in fruit and vegetable consumption.

There is some prospective observational evidence that obesity at or prior to diagnosis may lead to lower survival. However, there are several stages between baseline and outcome (times to diagnosis, to treatment and post-treatment) and this makes the information difficult to interpret.

Overall, the evidence is weak but suggests that women with breast cancer might benefit from a conventional, balanced diet rich in vegetables and fruits, low in fat, especially saturated fat, and from increasing physical activity and avoiding obesity and overweight.

There is insufficient evidence to make recommendations in respect of other cancers. It cannot be assumed that the response to particular dietary patterns or specific nutrients in cancer patients, whose nutritional demands may differ from normal, would be similar to healthy people.

21.6 Recommendations

Several authoritative reviews have made recommendations for the prevention of cancer through food, nutrition and physical activity (COMA, 1998; WCRF, 1997; WHO, 2003). The most recent from the WHO (2003) are set out in Table 21.4. Notably, these recommendations for cancer prevention are consonant with recommendations for other chronic disease, in particular cardiovascular disease.

Broadly, the recommendations from WHO are similar to those in the earlier reports. Although recommendations on alcohol were outside the remit of the Committee on Medical Aspects of Food Policy (COMA), the Committee on Carcinogenicity of the UK Department of Health did make a similar recommendation. COMA's recommendation on physical activity was embedded in one for obesity prevention. Because COMA's remit was to the UK, it made no recommendations relating to aflatoxin, Cantonese-style salted fish or scalding drinks. In other respects, their recommendations were similar, though COMA

Table 21.4 Recommendations for the prevention of cancer through food, nutrition and physical activity (WHO, 2003).

Maintain weight (among adults) such that body mass index (BMI) is in the range of 18.5–24.9 kg/m^2 and avoid weight gain (> 5 kg) during adult life

Maintain regular physical activity. The primary goal should be to perform physical activity on most days of the week; 60 minutes per day of moderate-intensity activity, such as walking, may be needed to maintain healthy body weight in otherwise sedentary people. More vigorous activity, such as fast walking, may give some additional benefits for cancer prevention

Consumption of alcoholic beverages is not recommended: if consumed, do not exceed 2 units per day

Chinese-style fermented salted fish should only be consumed in moderation, especially during childhood. Overall consumption of salt-preserved foods and salt should be moderate

Minimize exposure to aflatoxin in foods

Have a diet that includes at least 400 g/day of total fruits and vegetables

Those who are not vegetarian are advised to moderate consumption of preserved meat (e.g. sausages, salami, bacon, ham)

Do not consume foods or drinks when they are at a very hot (scalding hot) temperature did make a specific recommendation against the use of β-carotene supplements, and a general caution against the use of other high-dose purified micronutrient supplements.

The World Cancer Research Fund (WCRF, 1997) also made similar recommendations, but cautioned specifically against excess total fat and salt, and charring of food. WCRF, like COMA, cautioned against the use of dietary supplements to achieve nutritional protection against cancer.

The similarity of the conclusions and recommendations from these differently constituted groups adds to the robustness of their interpretations.

21.7 Conclusions

There is considerable epidemiological, clinical and laboratory evidence for an impact of nutrition including physical activity on risk of developing many adult cancers. For methodological reasons, identifying specific links depends on judgement of several different types of evidence, but reasonably firm conclusions can be drawn, as exemplified by the consistent recommendations of authoritative bodies. In contrast, there is as yet little evidence for the effect of nutrition on outcome in people with cancer.

Most cancers will have several contributory causes. The inherent methodological complexities mean that the precise roles of different foods, nutrients and other food components will be unlikely to be fully elucidated in the near future. Although much remains to be learned, a substantial improvement in public health could already be achieved by applying current knowledge.

FURTHER READING

1. **COMA (Committee on Medical Aspects of Food and Nutrition Policy)** (1998) *Nutritional aspects of the development of cancer*. London, The Stationery Office.

2. **Doll, R., and Peto, R.** (1981) The causes of cancer: quantitative estimates of avoidable risks of cancer in the United States today. *J Nat Cancer Inst*, **66**, 1191–1308.

3. **Hanahan, D., and Weinberg, R.** (2000) The hallmarks of cancer. *Cell*, **100**, 57–70.

4. **International Agency for Research on Cancer** (2002) *Weight control and physical activity*. Lyon, IARC Press.

5. **International Agency for Research on Cancer** (2003) *Fruit and vegetables*. Lyon, IARC Press.

6. **International Agency for Research on Cancer** (2004) *World Cancer Report*. Lyon, IARC Press.

7. **Key, T., Schatzkin, A., Willett, W., Allen, N., Spencer, E., and Travis, R.** (2004) Diet, nutrition and the prevention of cancer. *Publ Hlth Nutr*, **7**, 187–200.

8. **World Cancer Research Fund (WRCF)** (1997) *Food, Nutrition and the Prevention of Cancer. A global perspective*. Washington, DC, American Institute for Cancer Research.

9. **WHO** (2002) *World Health Report*. Geneva, World Health Organization.

10. **WHO** (2003) *Diet, nutrition and the prevention of chronic diseases*. WHO Technical Report, Series 916, Geneva, World Health Organization.

 To see topical and scientifically robust updates on nutrition associated with this textbook, and active web links to many of the journal articles in the Reference areas, please see the dedicated Online Resource Centre at www.oxfordtextbooks.co.uk/orc/mann3e/.

22 Diabetes mellitus and the metabolic syndrome

Jim Mann

Diabetes mellitus

Diabetes mellitus, a condition associated with loss of sugar in the urine, has been diagnosed by physicians for at least three millennia. Until the discovery of insulin in the 1920s, dietary treatment was all that could be offered to people with diabetes. Although dietary advice has altered over the years, reduction and sometimes near elimination of sugars and other carbohydrates formed the cornerstone of management for much of the time until the 1970s, when the merits of a diet low in carbohydrate, and consequentially high in fat, were questioned.

The term 'diabetes mellitus' is used to describe a group of conditions characterized by raised blood glucose levels (hyperglycaemia) resulting from an absolute or relative deficiency of insulin. In type 1 diabetes (T1DM), previously known as insulin-dependent diabetes, IDDM, there is destruction of the insulin-producing pancreatic islet β-cells usually resulting from an autoimmune process, and insulin treatment is essential to maintain life. In type 2 diabetes (T2DM), non-insulin-dependent diabetes (NIDDM), a key abnormality is resistance to the action of insulin, and in the early stages of the disease, insulin levels may actually be raised as the β-cells of the pancreas produce more insulin in an attempt to overcome the insulin resistance. In some patients with T2DM, the insulin-producing β-cells of the islets in the pancreas may show a degree of failure at some stage during the course of the disease process. Impaired glucose tolerance (IGT), impaired fasting glucose (IFG) and gestational diabetes (diabetes developing during pregnancy) may represent the earliest stages of T2DM. Hyperglycaemia may lead to glycosuria (glucose in the urine) when the renal threshold for glucose (level up to which glucose is reabsorbed in the renal tubules) is exceeded. Hyperglycaemia and glycosuria result in the classical symptoms of diabetes: polyuria (passing large quantities of urine), polydipsia (thirst), blurring of vision, increased susceptibility to infections and unintentional weight loss. The clinical features specific to the two major types are discussed below in section 22.2. Patients with T2DM are usually treated with 'lifestyle modification' therapy, with or without oral hypoglycaemic (blood glucose lowering) agents; insulin is not usually required.

22.1 Clinical features of diabetes

T1DM is invariably associated with marked symptoms of hyperglycaemia and often striking unintentional weight loss. If untreated, the absence of insulin leads to severe metabolic disturbances (ketoacidosis) during which the patient may become unconscious and which may be fatal without insulin treatment and correction of fluid and electrolyte imbalance. The diagnosis of T1DM is usually straightforward because blood glucose levels are markedly raised. In T2DM, symptoms are invariably less severe and ketoacidosis does not occur. IFG, IGT, gestational (pregnancy) diabetes (collectively sometimes known as pre-diabetes) and about half of all cases of T2DM are without symptoms. Diabetes is diagnosed if random venous plasma glucose is greater than 11.0 mmol/L or the fasting value is greater than 7 (two measurements are required if the person is asymptomatic). A glucose tolerance test (measurement of blood glucose fasting and 2 hours after a 75 g glucose load) may be required to diagnose the pre-diabetic states and those with borderline blood glucose levels (see Table 22.1).

Both types of diabetes may be associated with hypertension and a range of metabolic disturbances, which, together with the hyperglycaemia, help to explain the wide ranging complications of diabetes that account for much of the ill-health and premature death associated with diabetes. The complications result chiefly from the effects on the arterial and nervous systems. They include diabetic retinopathy, which may lead to blindness, diabetic nephropathy potentially resulting in kidney failure, foot ulceration, which may lead to gangrene, several different neurological conditions and cardiovascular disease (coronary heart disease and stroke), the most common causes of early death. Interestingly, coronary heart disease rates are similar in men and women with diabetes, whereas in the general population, women have appreciably lower rates than men.

Table 22.1 Venous plasma glucose levels for the diagnosis of diabetes, impaired glucose tolerance and impaired fasting glucose

	Fasting glucose (mmol/L)	2 hours after 75 g glucose (mmol/L)
Diabetes	> 7.0	> 11.0
Impaired fasting glucose	6.0–7.0	< 7.8
Impaired glucose tolerance	< 6.0	7.8–11.0
'Normal' glucose tolerance	< 6.0	< 7.8

22.2 Epidemiology and aetiology of type 2 diabetes

22.2.1 Epidemiology of type 2 diabetes

Diabetes has been recognized as a clinical entity for at least 3000 years. Worldwide, T2DM is overwhelmingly more common than T1DM. Thus, global statistics relating to 'diabetes' principally reflect frequencies of T2DM. Data relating to trends over time are not particularly reliable because diagnostic criteria have changed as have diagnostic facilities and rates of screening. These are clearly important determinants of prevalence rates, especially as so many cases are asymptomatic and may not be diagnosed until complications occur. Despite these reservations, there is no longer any doubt about the true world-wide increase in prevalence, resulting both from a tendency towards ageing populations (T2DM has been clearly shown to increase in frequency with age) and increased incidence at all ages. In the developed world in populations principally of European descent, the increase has been steady, with overall prevalence rates in adults over 20 years estimated to be around 6% and predicted to rise to over 8% by 2030. However, in some other population groups, there have been dramatic increases in prevalence associated either with migration or with a rapid change from a traditional (non-Western) lifestyle to increased consumption of energy-dense foods, high in fats and sugars, and reduced levels of physical activity—characteristics of the way of life in many Western countries. The American Pima Indians, Polynesians and Melanesians in the South Pacific, Australian Aboriginals and Asian Indian migrants to the UK and other countries are examples of populations in which the process of rapid acculturation has led to diabetes prevalence rates far higher than those observed in European populations. For example, amongst adult Maori, the indigenous people of New Zealand, almost half the adult population have been found to have an abnormality of carbohydrate metabolism. In some of these groups, T2DM, previously regarded as a disease of the middle-aged and elderly, has recently been diagnosed in teenagers and children. It has been predicted that by the year 2030 there are likely to be over 350 million adults worldwide with diabetes (mostly T2DM), with the greatest number of cases expected to be in China (25 million) and India (59 million). Thus, this condition may be regarded as one of the major epidemic diseases of the twenty-first century. Estimated numbers of people with diabetes are illustrated in Fig. 22.1.

22.2.2 Aetiology of type 2 diabetes and its complications

From the earliest times until recently, the sugary urine and raised levels of blood glucose have led to the assumption that an excessive intake of sucrose (table sugar) must be an important cause of the condition. While sugar may play a role, it is, on its own, not an important cause. A totally consistent observation in prospective as well as cross-sectional studies is the striking association between risk of T2DM and increasing obesity (Fig. 22.2), particularly when the excess body fat is centrally distributed, i.e. in association with a high waist circumference or high waist/hip ratio. (The significance of this ratio is discussed in Chapter 16.) It is also clear that there is a strong genetic component to this condition. The risk of developing T2DM is greatly increased when one or more close family members have the condition, although the precise mode of inheritance has not yet been resolved. It appears therefore that in predisposed populations or families, genetic and lifestyle factors combine to result in the development of

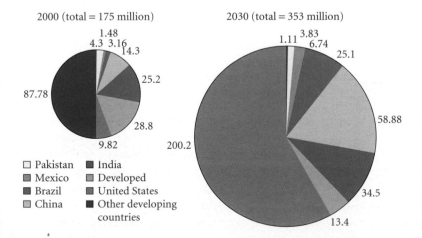

Fig. 22.1 Number of people with diabetes in 2000 and estimated for 2030.

Source: Yach, D. *et al.* (2006)

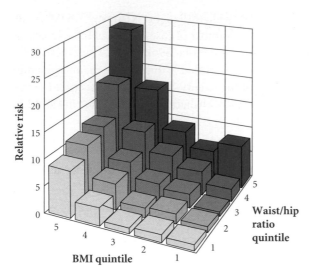

Fig. 22.2 Age-adjusted relative risk of incident diabetes according to quintiles of body mass index (BMI) and waist/hip ratio (Iowa Women's Health Study, 1986 to 1996). Cut points were 22.80, 24.87, 27.06 and 30.21 for BMI and 0.762, 0.805, 0.848 and 0.901 for waist/hip ratio.

Source: Folsom, A.R., Kushi, L.H., Anderson, K.E., *et al.* (2000) Association of general and abdominal obesity with multiple health outcomes in older women: The Iowa Women's Health Study. *Arch Intern Med*, **160**, 2117–28.

insulin resistance and consequently diabetes. The relative importance of genetic and lifestyle factors is well illustrated by diabetes rates in Pima Indians. Although rates amongst the American Pima Indians are amongst the highest in the world, a genetically similar group living in the mountainous regions of Mexico have relatively low rates. They still follow a traditional way of life unexposed to Western ways and diet and have a high level of physical activity.

There have been several attempts to implicate individual foods or nutrients as causal or protective factors in the aetiology of T2DM, but few of the hypotheses have stood the test of time. It is likely that more than one of the attributes that characterize the Western lifestyle (excessive intakes of energy-dense foods; relatively low intakes of vegetables, fruits and lightly processed cereal foods with intact cellular structure; inadequate physical activity) contribute to the aetiology. One very large prospective study involving health professionals in the USA has suggested that diets with a high glycaemic load and low cereal fibre content increase the risk of T2DM (Fig. 22.3). The glycaemic load provides an indication of both glycaemic index (GI) (see Chapter 2) and quantity of carbohydrate. A high intake of saturated fatty acids increases resistance to the action of insulin and is therefore likely to increase the risk of developing T2DM. Intrauterine growth retardation leading to babies born small for dates and prematurity have been suggested as risk factors for the development T2DM in later life. This appears to be especially the case when rapid catch-up growth occurs in infancy and childhood (fetal programming or 'Barker' hypothesis). The various lifestyle-related factors considered by the WHO/FAO Expert Consultation on Diet, Nutrition and the Prevention of Chronic Diseases (TR 916) believed to be convincingly or probably related to risk of developing T2DM are shown in Box 22.1.

Several complications of diabetes (e.g. retinopathy, nephropathy and neuropathy) appear to be a result of hyperglycaemia and other metabolic consequences of

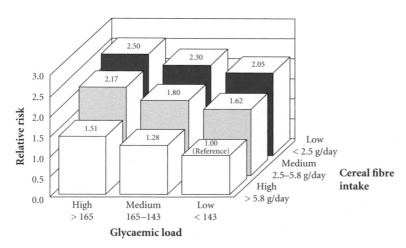

Fig. 22.3 Relative risk of type 2 diabetes mellitus by different levels of daily cereal fibre intake and glycaemic load.

Source: Salmeron, J., Manson, J.E., Stampfer, M.J., *et al.* (1997) Dietary Fiber, glycemic load, and risk of non-insulin-dependent diabetes mellitus in women. *J Am Med Assoc*, **277**, 472–7.

BOX 22.1 Summary of strength of evidence on lifestyle factors and risk of developing type 2 diabetes

Evidence	Decreased risk	Increased risk
Convincing	Voluntary weight loss in overweight and obese people Physical activity	Overweight and obesity Abdominal obesity Physical inactivity Maternal diabetes[a]
Probable	Non-starch polysaccharides	Saturated fats Intrauterine growth retardation
Possible	ω-3 fatty acids Low glycaemic index foods Exclusive breastfeeding[b]	Total fat intake *trans*-fatty acids
Insufficient	Vitamin E Chromium Magnesium Moderate alcohol	Excess alcohol

[a]Includes gestational diabetes.
[b]As a global public health recommendation, infants should be exclusively breastfed for the first 6 months of life to achieve optimal growth, development and health.
Source: WHO (2003) *Diet, Nutrition and the Prevention of Chronic Diseases*. WHO Technical Report Series 916.

Table 22.2 Risk factors for coronary heart disease (CHD) in people with type 2 diabetes

Risk factors that may be of particular relevance in type 2 diabetes	General CHD risk factors that are also relevant in type 2 diabetes
↑ Triglycerides and very-low-density lipoproteins	
↑ Small dense low-density lipoprotein particles	
↓ High-density lipoproteins	Hypertension
↑ Oxidation of low-density lipoprotein	Cigarette smoking
↑ Platelet aggregation	Obesity, especially when centrally distributed
↑ Plasminogen activator inhibitor	Physical inactivity
↑ Pro-insulin-like molecules	
Microalbuminuria	

↑: increased; ↓: decreased.

---

diabetes and hypertension. Diet plays a role in their prevention and treatment principally by helping to improve blood glucose control and lower blood pressure (see section 22.6). Cardiovascular disease, which is responsible for the greatest number of deaths and much non-fatal illness in people with T2DM, seems to be even more closely linked to dietary factors. There appear to be some risk factors for coronary heart disease (CHD) that are more important in people with diabetes than in the population at large (Table 22.2). They may help to explain the great excess of CHD in this condition. However, other important determinants of atherogenesis and thrombogenesis seem to be similar in those with and without diabetes. Many are diet-related (see Chapter 20). In countries with low CHD rates in the general population, CHD is also relatively infrequent in people with diabetes. Thus, a major focus of dietary recommendations for people with diabetes relates to the need to reduce cardiovascular risk.

22.3 Reducing the risk of type 2 diabetes

While the precise mechanisms by which genes and lifestyle interact to result in T2DM remain elusive, the geographic variation, rapid changes over time and dietary patterns related to risk suggest that lifestyle modification might help to prevent, or at least delay, the onset of T2DM in predisposed individuals. Randomized controlled trials in Finland, the USA and China confirm that this is indeed the case. The target interventions (Box 22.2) resulted in an approximately 60% reduction in rates of progression from IGT to T2DM over a 4-year follow-up period in both the Finnish and the US study. Of particular interest is the fact that in the Finnish study remarkably few of those individuals who complied with at least four of the five target interventions progressed from IGT to T2DM (see Fig. 22.4). Similar lifestyle interventions have been shown to increase insulin sensitivity in insulin-resistant individuals prior to the development of IGT or diabetes. These observations suggest that in groups or populations with high rates of diabetes, it is

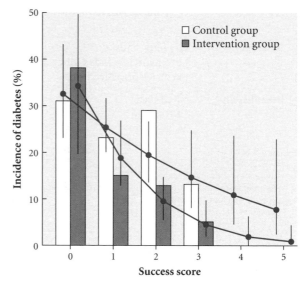

No. with diabetes/Total no.

Intervention group	5/13	10/66	9/69	2/38	0/25	0/24
Control group		15/48	25/107	14/48	2/15	0/11	0/4

Fig. 22.4 Incidence of diabetes during follow-up, according to the success score. At the 1-year visit, each subject received a grade of 0 for each intervention goal that had not been achieved and a grade of 1 for each goal that had been achieved; the success score was computed as the sum of the grades. The association between the success score and the risk of diabetes, with 95% confidence intervals, was estimated by means of logistic regression analysis of the observed data. The curves show the model-based incidence of diabetes according to the success score as a continuous variable. The curve whose data points align with the white bars represents the model-based incidence for the control group, and the curve whose data points align with the shaded bars represents the model-based incidence for the intervention group.

Source: Tuomilehto *et al.* (2001).

BOX 22.2 Lifestyle modifications suggested to the intervention group in the Finnish Diabetes Prevention Study

- Weight loss of 5–7% initial body weight or a weight loss of 5–10 kg depending upon degree of obesity
- Reduce total and saturated fat by encouraging low-fat dairy and meat products
- Prefer unsaturated soft margarines and vegetables oils rich in monounsaturated fatty acids
- Increase wholegrains, vegetables and fruit
- Physical activity, at least moderate intensity for a minimum of 30 minutes daily

Source: Tuomilehto *et al.* (2001).

> **BOX 22.3** Specific recommendations for reducing the risk of type 2 diabetes
>
> - Prevention/treatment of overweight and obesity, particularly in high-risk groups
> - Maintaining an optimum BMI, i.e. at the lower end of the normal range. For the adult population, this means maintaining a mean BMI in the range 21–23 kg/m² and avoiding weight gain (> 5 kg) in adult life
> - Voluntary weight reduction in overweight or obese individuals with impaired glucose tolerance (although screening for such individuals may not be cost-effective in many countries)
>
> - Practising an endurance activity at moderate or greater level of intensity (e.g. brisk walking) for 1 hour or more per day on most days per week
> - Ensuring that saturated fat intake does not exceed 10% of total energy and for high-risk groups, this should be < 7% of total energy
> - Achieving adequate intakes of non-starch polysaccharides through regular consumption of wholegrain cereals, legumes, fruits and vegetables (a minimum daily intake of 20 g is recommended)
>
> *Source*: WHO (2003) *Diet, Nutrition and the Prevention of Chronic Diseases*. WHO Technical Report Series 916.

appropriate to screen high-risk individuals (in particular those with central adiposity, a family history of diabetes and those with other cardiovascular risk factors) so that preventive measures may be started in those with pre-diabetes and treatment initiated in those who have already developed the disease. In addition, population-based advice to increase physical activity and to adopt appropriate dietary measures to reduce overweight and obesity will be essential for primary prevention and reducing the epidemic proportions of the disease. The fetal programming hypothesis has led to the reinforcement of the importance of appropriate maternal nutrition as a means of reducing the risk of T2DM, but the strength of evidence regarding the influencing of growth in infancy and childhood by manipulating dietary intake (see section 22.3.2) is regarded as insufficient to justify recommendations. The specific recommendations for reducing the risk of T2DM, according to the WHO/FAO Technical Consultation TR916, are shown in Box 22.3.

22.4 Epidemiology and aetiology of type 1 diabetes

The frequency of T1DM also shows marked geographic variation. For example the incidence rates of childhood diabetes (under 15 years) in Europe, ranges from 3.2 cases per 100 000 per year in Macedonia to 40.2 per 100 000 per year in parts of Finland.

In many countries, there have been considerable increases in incidence in recent years. As an example, the increase in incidence in children aged less than 10 in Norway is shown in Fig. 22.5. Although the total number of cases in all countries is appreciably lower than the number of cases of T2DM, the proportional increase has been comparable or greater in many countries. The frequency does not exactly parallel that of T2DM and there is no clear explanation for the variation from one country to another or the change over time. Genetic factors are important in T1DM although only about 10% of people with the condition have a clear family history. It is not clear what triggers the autoimmune process that leads to the destruction of the pancreatic islet β- cells. Various nutritional factors have been suggested but there is reasonable evidence for only one of these. Several epidemiological studies suggest that the early introduction of cow's milk into the diet of infants is associated with an increased risk of developing T1DM later in life, but the extent to which breast milk is protective and cow's milk detrimental remains to be established. The importance of infant nutrition as a risk factor for T1DM and the mechanism by which it might operate are far from clear. It is possible that

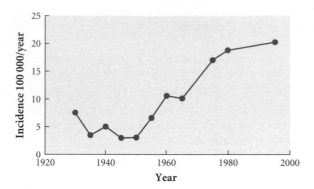

Fig. 22.5 Incidence of diabetes in children under age 10 years in Norway, 1925–1995.

Source: Gale, E. (2002) The rise of childhood type 1 diabetes in the 20th century. *Diabetes*, **51**, 3353–61.

cow's milk protein might be immunogenic in susceptible individuals. Several immunosuppressive drugs have been suggested as potentially useful means of reducing the risk of T1DM but these drugs have side effects and none has been demonstrated to be of benefit in randomized controlled trials. Clinical trials involving various infant dietary regimens have also been suggested.

As with T2DM, many of the complications of T1DM are associated with unsatisfactory metabolic control, and cardiovascular disease in people with T1DM is associated with risk factors similar to those in the general population. In the aetiology of kidney damage (nephropathy), a high intake of protein, especially animal protein, may be associated, but the evidence is not conclusive.

22.5 Lifestyle treatments for diabetes

All people with T1DM require insulin replacement treatment. For them, the goals of lifestyle and dietary advice are to minimize short-term fluctuations in blood glucose and especially to reduce the risk of hypoglycaemia by balancing injected insulin with carbohydrate-containing food and physical activity (Box 22.4). Dietary modification also helps to reduce the risk of long-term complications by helping to achieve optimal blood glucose control and satisfactory levels of blood pressure, blood lipids and other risk factors influenced by diet.

Dietary modification is the cornerstone of treatment for people with T2DM and many of those who manage to comply with dietary advice will show improvement in the metabolic abnormalities associated with this condition to the extent that oral hypoglycaemic drugs (Box 22.5) and insulin are not required. Even when drug treatment is required, attention to diet may further improve blood glucose control and modify cardiovascular risk factors in a way that might be expected to reduce CHD risk.

The principles of dietary advice for people with T1DM and T2DM are similar to those recommended for entire populations at high risk of CHD and this means that there is no need for people with diabetes to have meals that differ from those of the rest of the family. Evidence-based dietary recommendations for people with diabetes have been issued in most countries; the most widely quoted are those of the American Diabetes Association (ADA) and the Nutrition Study Group of the European Association for the Study of Diabetes (EASD). The two sets of recommendations are broadly comparable and are summarized in Table 22.3. The evidence for the benefit of implementing the recommendations derives principally from trials in which dietary manipulations have been shown to improve glycaemic control or level of risk factors, which have in turn been shown to influence clinical outcome in people with diabetes.

Recent dietary recommendations have tended to be less rigid than those in the past and acknowledge that quality of life of the individual must be taken into account when defining nutritional objectives. Healthcare providers are encouraged to achieve a balance between the attempts to achieve optimal control of blood glucose and risk factors and the wellbeing of the patient. However, increasingly 'carbohydrate counting' is being introduced as a means of matching injected insulin with carbohydrate intake and improving glycaemic control in T1DM (see section 22.6.4). This approach is more flexible than the traditional method of prescribing 'carbohydrate portions' since

BOX 22.4 Balancing injected insulin with carbohydrate-containing food

All those with T1DM require subcutaneous insulin, usually injected by means of an insulin 'pen' two or four times per day. Some people with T2DM also require injected insulin when the pancreatic β-cells are unable to secrete sufficient insulin. The most frequently used insulin regimens are (a) twice daily injections of a mixture of quick-acting (soluble) and longer-acting (isophane) insulins and (b) soluble insulin, administered shortly before or with the three main meals, and isophane insulin before going to bed. Older forms of soluble insulin need to be injected 15–30 minutes before meals to achieve optimum effects. Recently available insulin analogues are more rapidly acting and can be injected immediately before or even after meals, followed by longer-acting insulin before bed time. Carbohydrate-containing food must be consumed at times of peak insulin action to avoid hypoglycaemia (low blood glucose) and slowly released carbohydrate (see sections 22.6.4 and 22.6.5) at night before going to bed to avoid hypoglycaemia during the night. Insulin dose and type can be adjusted to adapt to preferred quantity and timing of carbohydrate-containing meals and snacks. Some patients with T1DM use insulin pumps, which deliver a continuous supply of small amounts of soluble insulin, boosted at meal times, to reproduce as closely as possible normal insulin secretion.

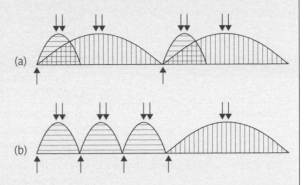

(a) ↑ = injection of insulin mixture containing soluble (≡) and isophane (⦀) insulins before breakfast and before evening meal.
(b) ↑ = injection of soluble (≡) insulin before main meals and isophane (⦀) before bed. ↓↓ = Breakfast, lunch, evening meal and bed time snack to provide available carbohydrate at times of peak insulin activity.

BOX 22.5 Oral hypoglyaemic medications. If dietary modification is unable to achieve target blood glucose levels in patients with T2DM, oral hypoglycaemic agents may be prescribed. Several different classes of drugs are available

Drug class	Examples	Comment
Biguanide	Metformin	Reduces gluconeogenesis and glycogenolysis and improves uptake and utilization of insulin Very widely used in overweight patients
Sulphonylureas	Glipizide Glyclazide	Stimulates insulin secretion May be used alone or in conjunction with metformin
Thiazolidinediones	Pioglitazone Rosiglitazone	Insulin sensitizer Relatively new agents

it permits altering insulin dose on the basis of the quantity of carbohydrate consumed. Carbohydrate portions were formerly prescribed in fixed quantities to match prescribed amounts of injected insulin.

Lifestyle treatments should be adapted to the needs of individuals and may change with time. The recommendations given below are those of the EASD; they are broadly comparable with those of the ADA.

Table 22.3 Key aspects of the current recommendations for diabetic diet and lifestyle

Dietary energy and body weight	Achieve and/or maintain BMI of 18.5–25 Diet and exercise important
Dietary fat	Saturated plus *trans*-unsaturated fatty acids: < 10% total energy, < 8% if low-density lipoprotein raised Polyunsaturated fatty acids: < 10% total energy Monounsaturated fatty acids: 10–20% total energy Total fat: < 35% total energy (if overweight < 30%) Oily fish, soybean and rapeseed oil, nuts and green leafy vegetables to provide ω-3 fatty acids Cholesterol: < 300 g/day
Carbohydrate	Total carbohydrate: 45–60% total energy, influenced by metabolic characteristics Vegetables, fruits, legumes and cereal-derived foods preferred

Dietary fibre and glycaemic index	Naturally occurring foods rich in dietary fibre are encouraged
	Ideally dietary fibre intake should be more than 40 g/day (or
	  20 g/1000 kcal/day), half soluble (lesser amounts also beneficial)
	Five servings/day of fibre-rich vegetables and fruit and four or more
	  servings of legumes/week help to provide minimum requirements
	Cereal-based foods should be wholegrain and high in fibre
	Carbohydrate-rich low-glycaemic-index foods are suitable choices,
	  provided other attributes are appropriate

Sucrose and other free sugars	If desired and blood glucose levels are satisfactory, free sugars up to
	  50 g/day may be incorporated into the diet
	Total free sugars should not exceed 10%, total energy (less for those
	  who are overweight)

Protein and renal disease	Total protein intake at lower end of normal range (0.8 g/kg/day) for type 1 patients with established nephropathy For all others, protein should provide 10–20% total energy
Vitamins, antioxidant nutrients, minerals and trace elements	Increase foods rich in tocopherols, carotenoids, vitamin C and flavonoids, trace elements and other vitamins Fruits, vegetables, wholegrains rather than supplements recommended Restrict sodium to less than 6 g/day

Alcohol	Up to 10 g for women and 20 g for men per day is acceptable for most
	  people with diabetes who choose to drink alcohol
	Special precautions apply to those on insulin or sulphonylureas, those
	  who are overweight and those with hypertriglyceridaemia

Special 'diabetic' or foods, functional foods and supplements	Non-alcoholic beverages sweetened with non-nutritive sweeteners
	  are useful
	Other special foods not encouraged
	No particular merit of fructose and other 'special' nutritive sweeteners
	  over sucrose

Families	Most recommendations suitable for whole family

Source: Derived from the 2004 recommendations of the Nutrition Study Group of the European Association for the Study of Diabetes. Mann *et al.* (2004).

22.5.1 Energy balance and body weight

The key recommendation for those who are overweight (BMI > 25 kg/m^2) is that calorie intake should be reduced and energy expenditure increased so that the BMI moves towards the recommended range (18.5–25 kg/m^2). Prevention of weight regain is an important aim once weight loss has been achieved. For those who are overweight or obese, reducing energy-dense foods (those high in fats and free sugars) is usually sufficient to achieve weight loss, prescription of precise energy requirements only being necessary for those unable to achieve the desired weight reduction. Even modest weight reduction (a loss of less than 10% body weight) in the overweight or obese improves insulin sensitivity, glycaemic control, body lipids, blood pressure and other cardiovascular risk factors. Weight loss may reduce or even eliminate the need for hypoglycaemic drug therapy in T2DM and lead to a reduction of insulin dose and improved glycaemic control in T1DM. The reduced life expectancy of overweight people with diabetes is improved in those who lose weight.

22.5.2 Protein

Protein intake in most Western populations ranges between 10 and 20% total energy, corresponding to 0.8–2.0 g/kg body weight. In patients with T1DM and evidence of established nephropathy, protein intakes should be at the lower end of this range (0.8 g/kg body weight/day). Such restriction has been shown to reduce the risk of end-stage renal failure or death when compared in randomized controlled trials with more usual intakes (1.2 g/kg/day). The evidence for appreciably reducing protein intake is less convincing for T2DM patients with established nephropathy or for T1DM or T2DM patients with microalbuminuria (incipient nephropathy). However, in those with no nephropathy or microalbuminuria it is suggested that protein intake not exceed 20% total energy since there is evidence that beyond this level of intake renal function may deteriorate, especially in the presence of hypertension or poor glycaemic control.

22.5.3 Dietary fat

The striking association between saturated and *trans*-unsaturated fatty acids and CHD justify their restriction to less than 10% total energy, or less than 8% if low-density lipoprotein (LDL) is raised.

The wide range of acceptable intakes of *cis*-monounsaturated fatty acids (10–20% total energy) reflects their beneficial effect when compared with saturated fatty acids or low fibre, high glycaemic index, carbohydrate-containing foods on lipids, lipoproteins and insulin sensitivity. The range also permits a more flexible approach to the selection of food choices and dietary patterns (see section 22.6.10) provided total fat intake does not exceed 35% total energy or 30% in the overweight or obese. The reasons for recommending an upper level of intake for total fat include the potential to increase insulin resistance at higher levels and the high energy density associated with high fat intakes. ω-6 polyunsaturated fatty acids facilitate LDL lowering, but intakes should be limited to 10% or less total energy because of an increased risk of lipid oxidation or reduction in high-density lipoprotein (HDL) associated with higher levels of intake. The optimal ratio of ω-3 to ω-6 polyunsaturated acids is unknown but ω-3 fatty acids are essential and have a number of potentially beneficial effects in terms of reducing cardiovascular risk. Regular intakes of oily fish, rapeseed (canola) or soybean oil, nuts and some green leafy vegetables ensure adequate intakes. Modest restriction of cholesterol to less than 300 mg/day (further reduction if LDL is raised) is based on the adverse effects of large quantities on LDL (particularly in the presence of relatively high intakes of saturated fatty acids) and evidence from some prospective studies that substantial intakes are related to increased risk of cardiovascular disease.

22.5.4 Carbohydrate

The recommended range of intakes, 45–60% total energy, is based on the limits for fat and protein and the acceptability in terms of glycaemic control and risk factor status across the wide range. However, the nature of the carbohydrate is important, especially with intakes at the upper end of the range. Vegetables, legumes, intact fruits and wholegrain cereals are always the preferred carbohydrate sources because of their favourable effect on glycaemic control and their potential for reducing cardiovascular risk. High intakes of starchy or highly processed foods with a high glycaemic index (see Table 2.3) often may give poor glycaemic control, increased triglycerides and low levels of HDL. Thus, metabolic characteristics, as well as personal preferences, determine the level of intake. Those with dyslipidaemia (high triglycerides, low HDL) and poor glycaemic control may be more satisfactorily controlled in terms of their metabolic derangement, on intakes at the lower end of the range, and most of their carbohydrate-containing foods should be rich in dietary fibre and have a low glycaemic index. For those on tablets to lower blood glucose or insulin, timing and dosage of medication should match quantity, nature and timing of carbohydrate intake. Failure to do so may result in symptoms of hypoglycaemia and reduce the potential to achieve good blood glucose control. Prescribing and measuring precise quantities of carbohydrate often helps to improve glycaemic control, especially in those on insulin. Measurement of glucose on a finger-prick blood sample at home by the patient, using one of the many meters now available, provides the opportunity for people with diabetes to adjust insulin dose as well as amount and type of carbohydrate to achieve the best possible blood glucose control.

22.5.5 Dietary fibre and glycaemic index

Randomized controlled trials have shown the potential of naturally occurring foods, rich in dietary fibre, especially soluble forms, to improve glycaemic control and lipid profile in patients with T1DM and T2DM, hence the recommendation to encourage such foods and a fibre intake of 40 g or more (or 20 g/1000 kcal) daily. About half the dietary fibre should be soluble. Five or more servings per day of fibre-rich vegetables and fruit and four or more servings of legumes per week help to provide minimum requirements for fibre intake, when most cereal-based foods are wholegrain-fibre-rich. Beneficial effects are also obtained with lower, and for some, more acceptable amounts.

Diets rich in low-glycaemic-index foods have also been shown to produce improved glycaemic control, especially in patients with T2DM (see Chapter 2). Most (but not all) of such foods are high in dietary fibre. Low-glycaemic-index foods are therefore suitable food choices for people with diabetes. However, there are some important limitations to the use of glycaemic index. Foods high in fat and sugars generally have a low glycaemic index, yet they may be energy dense and include inappropriate fat sources and are therefore poor food choices for people with diabetes. Thus, glycaemic index concept is only meaningful when used to classify predominantly carbohydrate-containing food and when comparing foods within a comparable food group (e.g. breads, fruits, pasta and rice). The idea must be interpreted in relation to energy content and content of other macronutrients.

22.5.6 Sucrose and other free sugars

When incorporated in modest amounts (50 g/day) into diets of appropriate macronutrient composition and energy content, sucrose appears not to be associated with any measurable untoward clinical or metabolic effect, hence the recommendation that such modest amounts of free sugars might be included in a diabetic dietary prescription. As for the general population, it is advised that total free sugars do not exceed 10% total energy, though more restrictive advice concerning free sugars may be useful for those needing to lose weight.

22.5.7 Antioxidant nutrients, vitamins, minerals and trace elements

Foods naturally rich in dietary antioxidants (tocopherols, carotenoids, vitamin C, flavonoids), trace elements and other vitamins are encouraged. Daily consumption of a range of vegetables, fruits, wholegrain breads and cereals should provide adequate intakes of vitamins and antioxidant nutrients and there is currently no evidence that dietary supplements confer benefit. Given the tendency towards high levels of blood pressure in people with diabetes, restriction of salt intake to less then 6 g/day is advised, with further restriction considered appropriate for those with elevated blood pressure levels.

22.5.8 Alcohol

A limited amount of information tends to confirm that people with T2DM, like adults in the general population, who have a moderate intake of alcoholic drinks may have a reduced risk of CHD. On the other hand, alcohol may be a relevant source of energy in those who are overweight and may be associated with raised levels of blood pressure, increased triglycerides and an increased risk of hypoglycaemia, especially in insulin-treated individuals or those on some oral hypoglycaemic agents. Thus, it is recommended that moderate use of alcohol (up to 10 g/day for women and 20 g/day for men) is acceptable rather than beneficial for those with diabetes who choose to drink alcohol. When alcohol is taken by those on insulin, it is essential that it be taken with carbohydrate-containing food in order to avoid the risk of potentially profound and prolonged hypoglycaemia. Alcohol should be limited by those who are overweight, hypertensive or hypertrygly-ceridaemic. Abstention is advised for women who are pregnant and those with a history of alcohol abuse or pancreatitis, appreciable hypertriglyceridaemia and advanced neuropathy.

22.5.9 Diabetic foods, functional foods and supplements

Foods advertised as being of particular benefit for people with diabetes ('diabetic' foods) are generally sucrose free but may nevertheless be high in fructose or other nutritive sweeteners and sometimes also fat. These have no substantial advantages over sucrose-containing foods for people with diabetes and should not be encouraged. Non-nutritive sweeteners (e.g. aspartame) may be useful, especially in drinks. Many functional foods and supplements are currently also being promoted for diabetes management or for reducing the risk of diabetes or its complications. These include fibre-enriched products and margarines containing plant sterols or stanols and supplements

containing various dietary fibres, ω-3 fatty acids, minerals, trace elements and some herbs. Several of these products have not been tested in long-term clinical trials and are therefore not recommended at present.

22.5.10 Translating nutritional principles into practice

Many medical practitioners do not have the training or the time to help people with diabetes translate the nutrition principles described here into practice. Dietitians or appropriately trained nutritionists play a key role in translating these general principles into specific advice for individuals. The high intakes of total and saturated fat by people with diabetes in Europe (Fig. 22.6) provide an indication of the extent of dietary change required by many. The wide

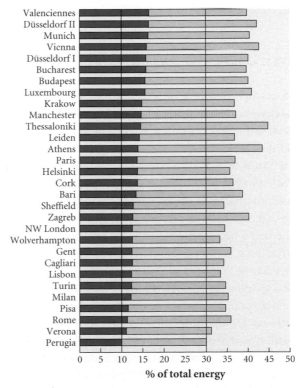

Fig. 22.6 Intake of total (■) and saturated (■) fatty acids as proportion of total dietary intake, calculated from 4-day diet records. Data from European centres participating in the EURODIAB study.

Source: Toeller, M., Klischan, A., Heitkamp, G. *et al.* (1996) Nutritional intake of 2868 IDDM patients from 30 centres in Europe. *Diabetologia*, **39**, 929–39.

ranges of acceptable intake for monounsaturated fatty acids and carbohydrates enable the nutrient recommendations to be translated into a variety of dietary patterns. The importance of increased physical activity as well as dietary advice for those who are overweight cannot be overemphasized. Behaviour modification techniques and various special lifestyle programmes can be of considerable value. Ongoing encouragement and reinforcement of lifestyle changes are essential, and one-off advice is rarely adequate.

22.6 Families and communities

Individual compliance with dietary advice is improved if the general aspects of advice are understood by the family and are of potential benefit to them. In view of the strong genetic component to T2DM, the possibility that lifestyle changes might reduce the risk of developing the condition and that the dietary principles are similar to those that reduce CHD risk, it seems perfectly reasonable to suggest that foods and meals that are suitable for people with diabetes are appropriate for their families. In countries with high rates of T2DM, community programmes are needed but, as with CHD prevention, appropriate food labelling and availability of appropriate foods at reasonable cost are essential components of such initiatives. In both families and communities, avoidance and treatment of overweight and obesity provide the best means of reducing diabetes risk. There is at present insufficient evidence to justify programmes aimed at identifying people at risk of T1DM.

Metabolic syndrome

Resistance to the action of insulin, an important underlying abnormality in T2DM, is also associated with a range of additional clinical and metabolic abnormalities (Box 22.6) that are often seen in association with T2DM, IGT or IFG, but may also occur with normal blood glucose levels. Several national and international organizations have suggested sets of diagnostic criteria for what has become known as the metabolic syndrome (Box 22.7). The validity of describing this constellation of abnormalities as a 'syndrome' has been questioned on the grounds that the criteria are clearly arbitrary and its causes ill understood. Nevertheless, its existence does help to define a group of individuals who are at high risk of cardiovascular disease and of developing T2DM if they have not already done so. As many as one quarter (and in some instances appreciably more) of all adults in many affluent and some developing countries will fit the criteria set by the WHO and the US National Cholesterol Education Programme (NCEP). However, this figure is appreciably greater if the criteria suggested by the International Diabetes Federation are implemented. Lifestyle-related risk factors are identical to those described for T2DM as are the measures for prevention and treatment. Lifestyle modification

---

BOX 22.6 Clinical and metabolic features other than hyperglycaemia associated with insulin resistance

- Central obesity
- Raised blood pressure
- Dyslipidaemia
  - increased triglyceride
  - low HDL
  - predominance of small dense LDL particles
- Increased uric acid and gout
- Increased plasminogen activator inhibitor (PAI-1)
- NASH (non-alcoholic steatohepatitis)
- Endothelial dysfunction
- Increased proinflammatory cytokines
- Increased homocysteine

BOX 22.7 Diagnostic criteria suggested for the metabolic syndrome by different international organizations

WHO (1999)	NCEP, ATP111 (2001)	IDF (2005)
Hyperglycaemia or insulin resistance Plus two or more of:	Three of more of:	Central obesity: Waist (ethnic specific) Europeans ≥ 94 cm (M), ≥ 80 cm (F) South Asians/Chinese ≥ 90 cm (M), ≥ 80 cm (F)
Obesity: W/H > 0.9 (M), 0.85 (F) or BMI > 30 kg/m²	Central obesity: Waist > 102 cm (M), 88 cm (F) Fasting glucose ≥ 6.1 mmol/L	Plus two of: Fasting glucose ≥ 5.6 mmol/L
Dyslipidaemia: Triglyceride ≥ 1.7 mmol/L or HDL < 0.9 mmol/L (M), 1.0 mmol/L (F)	Hypertriglyceridaemia: Triglyceride ≥ 1.7 mmol/L Low HDL < 1.0 mmol/L (M), 1.3 mmol/L (F)	Treated dyslipidacmia: Raised triglyceride ≥ 1.7 mmol/L Reduced HDL ≥ 1.03 mmol/L (M), ≥ 1.29 mmol/L (F)
Hypertension: Blood pressure ≥ 140/90 mmHg	Hypertension: Blood pressure ≥ 135/85 mmHg or treatment	Treated hypertension: Raised blood pressure: > 130 systolic or > 85 diastolic
Microalbuminuria		

ATP = adult treatment panel; BMI = body mass index; F = female; HDL = high-density lipoprotein; IDF = International Diabetes Federation; LDL = low-density lipoprotein; M = male; NCEP = National Cholesterol Education Programme; W/H = waist/hip ratio; WHO = World Heath Organization.

---

is the pivotal component of management since weight loss associated with increased physical activity and the appropriate dietary measures offers the only means of favourably influencing the broad range of abnormalities associated with the syndrome.

FURTHER READING

1. **Alberti, K.G.M.M., and Zimmet, P.Z.** (1998) Definition, diagnosis and classification of diabetes mellitus and its complications. *Diabet Med*, **15**, 539–53.

2. **American Diabetes Association (ADA)** (2000) Clinical practice recommendations. *Diabet Care*, **23** (Suppl. 1), S1–S112.

3. **Chandalia, M., Garg, A., Lutjohann, D.,** *et al.* (2000) Beneficial effects of high dietary fiber intake in patients with type 2 diabetes mellitus. *N Engl J Med*, **342**, 1392–8.

4. **Chan, J.M., Rimm, E.B., Colditz, G.A.,** *et al.* (1994) Obesity, fat distribution and weight gain as risk factors for clinical diabetes in men. *Diabet Care*, **17**, 961–9.

5. **Garg, A.** (1994) High monounsaturated fat diet for diabetic patients. *Diabet Care*, **17**, 242–6.

6. **Ha, T.K.K., and Lean, M.E.J.** (1998) Technical review: Recommendations for the nutritional management of patients with diabetes mellitus. *Eur J Clin Nutr*, **52**, 467–81.

7. **Jarvi, A.E., Karlström, B.E., Grandfeldt, Y.E.,** *et al.* (1999) Improved glycaemic control and lipid profile and normalized fibrinolytic activity in a low-glycaemic index diet in type 2 diabetic patients. *Diabet Care*, **22**, 10–18.

8. **Mann, J.** (2000) Stemming the tide of diabetes. *Lancet*, **356**, 1454–5.

9. **Mann, J.** (2001) Editorial: Dietary fibre and diabetes revised. *Eur J Clin Nutr*, **55**, 919–21.

10. **Mann, J.I., De Leeuw, I., Hermansen, K.,** *et al.* (2004) Evidence-based nutritional approaches to the treatment and prevention of diabetes mellitus. *Nutr Metab Cardiovasc Dis*, **14**, 373–94.

11. **Salmeron, J., Ascherio, A., Rimm, E.B.,** *et al.* (1997) Dietary fibre, glycaemic load and risk of NIDDM in men. *Diabet Care*, **20**, 545–50.

12. **Stumvoll, M., Goldstein, B., and van Haeften, T.** (2005) Type 2 diabetes: principles of pathogenesis and therapy. *Lancet*, **365**, 1333–46.

13. **Tuomilehto, M.D., Lindstrom, M.S., Eriksson, J.G.,** *et al.* (2001) Prevention of type 2 diabetes mellitus by changes in lifestyle among subjects with impaired glucose tolerance. *New Engl J Med*, **344**, 1343–50.

14. **Vessby, B., Uusitupa, M., Hermansen, K.,** *et al.* (2001) Substituting dietary saturated for monounsaturated fat impairs insulin sensitivity in healthy men and women: the KANWU Study. *Diabetologia*, **44**, 312–9.

15. **Yach, D., Struckler, D., and Brownell, K.D.** (2006) Epidemiologic and economic consequence of the global epidemics of obesity and diabetes. *Nat Med*, **12**, 62–6.

 To see topical and scientifically robust updates on nutrition associated with this textbook, and active web links to many of the journal articles in the Reference areas, please see the dedicated Online Resource Centre at www.oxfordtextbooks.co.uk/orc/mann3e/.

23 The eating disorders: anorexia nervosa, bulimia nervosa and EDNOS

Hannah Turner and Robert Peveler

For many years the term 'eating disorders' has been taken to include two principal conditions, anorexia nervosa (AN) and bulimia nervosa (BN). However, it is now recognized that a significant proportion of patients seen in routine clinical practice present with a syndrome that falls short of the 'full-blown' AN or BN, which is usually termed 'eating disorder not otherwise specified' (EDNOS). Thus, there is now some debate about the threshold of 'clinical' eating disorders. Although descriptions of AN date back to 1873, BN was not described as a clinical disorder until 1979. The term EDNOS has only been in use since 1980. Eating disorders are a significant cause of physical and psychosocial morbidity, particularly among female adolescents and young adult women.

23.1 Definitions

23.1.1 Anorexia nervosa

The diagnostic criteria for AN (as given in the fourth edition of the *Diagnostic and Statistical Manual of Mental Disorders* (DSM-IV)) are shown in Table 23.1. The first is the maintenance of body weight at least 15% below that expected for age and height (body mass index, BMI < 17.5 kg/m^2). Weight loss is commonly achieved through extreme dietary restriction, although a subgroup of patients will also engage in other weight loss behaviours such as compulsive and driven exercise, self-induced vomiting and laxative misuse. The second feature is a characteristic set of attitudes and values concerning shape and weight. Patients often experience intense feelings of fatness, as well as extreme fear of loss of control over eating and weight gain. They express a level of dissatisfaction with their body weight and shape that far exceeds that typically seen in the general population, and they tend to judge their self-worth almost solely in terms of their weight, shape and ability to control their food intake. The third diagnostic feature is amenorrhoea (in postmenarchal females who are not taking an oral contraceptive), and both men and women may report loss of sex drive.

23.1.2 Bulimia nervosa

The DSM-IV diagnostic criteria for BN are also shown in Table 23.1. The first is recurrent episodes of binge eating during which an objectively large amount of food is consumed, with associated loss of perceived control of eating. The second feature is the use of compensatory behaviours designed to prevent weight gain. These include dietary restriction, self-induced vomiting, misuse of laxatives or diuretics

Table 23.1 Diagnostic criteria for anorexia nervosa, bulimia nervosa and EDNOS

Anorexia nervosa
A refusal to maintain body weight at or above a minimally normal weight for age and height (e.g. weight loss leading to a maintenance of body weight less than 85% of that expected, or failure to make expected weight gain during period of growth, leading to body weight less than 85% of that expected)
Intense fear of gaining weight or becoming fat, even though underweight
Disturbance in the way in which one's body weight or shape is experienced, undue influence of body weight or shape on self-evaluation, or denial of the seriousness of the current low body weight
In postmenarchal females, amenorrhea (i.e. the absence of at least three consecutive cycles)
Bulimia nervosa
Recurrent episodes of binge eating. An episode of binge eating is characterized by (1) eating, in a discrete period of time (e.g. within any 2-hour period), an amount of food that is definitely larger than most people would eat during a similar period of time and under similar circumstances; and (2) a sense of lack of control over eating during the episode
Recurrent inappropriate compensatory behaviour in order to prevent weight gain, such as: self-induced vomiting; misuse of laxatives, diuretics, enemas or other medications; fasting or excessive exercise
The binge eating and inappropriate compensatory behaviours both occur, on average, at least twice a week for 3 months
Self-evaluation is unduly influenced by body shape and weight
The disturbance does not occur exclusively during episodes of anorexia nervosa
Examples of EDNOS include:
All the criteria for anorexia nervosa are met except that the individual's current weight is in the normal range, or, for females, regular menstruation continues
All of the criteria for bulimia nervosa are met, except that the binge eating and inappropriate compensatory mechanisms occur at a lower frequency than that required for a full diagnosis
Use of inappropriate compensatory behaviours by an individual of normal body weight after eating small amounts of food
Repeatedly chewing and spitting out, but not swallowing, large amounts of food
Binge-eating disorder

and excessive exercise. The third feature is the same set of attitudes and values seen in AN, with self-worth being determined almost exclusively on the basis of weight, shape and ability to control food intake. Although most people with BN are within the normal weight range, a proportion will have a history of AN. Where BN occurs in the context of AN, the latter diagnosis takes precedence.

23.2 Epidemiology

About 1 in 250 females and 1 in 2000 males will experience AN, most often in adolescence and young adulthood. About five times that number will suffer from BN. In community studies, prevalence rates of BN have been estimated at between 0.5% and 1.0% in young women. AN is less common, with prevalence estimated at 0.3% in young women. The prevalence of EDNOS remains unclear, although reports suggest it is the most common presentation seen in clinical practice.

23.3 Anorexia nervosa

23.3.1 Development of the disorder

The onset of AN is usually in adolescence, although cases of prepubertal and adult onset have been reported. The disorder typically starts with an episode of dieting although the path into this behaviour can vary. For some, natural bodily changes that accompany puberty, or a negative weight-related or shape-related comment from another person, may lead to a conscious decision to diet. For others, an episode of physical illness with associated weight loss, such as glandular fever, may lead to more intentional dietary restriction. Commonly occurring in the context of low self-worth, positive feedback in the form of attention from others initially serves to reinforce dieting behaviour and further weight loss. Patients with AN often report a sense of euphoria at being in control of their weight. For others, it brings feelings of success and a fleeting sense of superiority at achieving something few in the general population can accomplish.

23.3.2 Clinical features

As dieting intensifies, so weight falls and the physiological and psychological effects of starvation develop. Behaviours around food become increasingly rigid and deceptive, and the range of acceptable foods slowly diminishes. Foods that are viewed as fattening are typically avoided and vegetarianism is common. The average energy intake is in the region of 600–900 kcal/day, with the proportion of energy derived from fat being particularly low. Mineral intake is also low, although mineral deficiencies are rare. It is possible that zinc deficiency may contribute to the maintenance of the disorder through an effect on appetite and taste. However, true 'anorexia' is rare in so far as most patients report feeling persistently hungry. A proportion will feel driven to engage in excessive exercise, leading to further weight loss. Some will also engage in other forms of weight-control behaviour, such as self-induced vomiting or laxative misuse. A minority of patients will intermittently lose control over their eating and binge, although the amounts consumed tend not to be large.

Reduction in food intake is accompanied by a number of cognitive changes. Many will view either their body, or particular parts, as being bigger than their true size, and this is typically accompanied by an intense dislike or loathing of the body or body part. Cognitive rumination about weight and shape becomes all-consuming and an increasing amount of time is given to thinking about food. Over time, general functioning becomes increasingly impaired, interest in other areas of life diminishes, and day-to-day routines become characterized by social withdrawal and isolation. Depression, irritability and anxiety are common, as are obsessional features. Typically, all features get worse with further weight loss. Chronic presentations may also be accompanied by thoughts of hopelessness and suicide.

Physical health AN is associated with a range of physical abnormalities, many of which are now believed to be secondary to disturbed patterns of eating and low weight. Although patients often present

Food Diary

		Place	*	V/L	Comments
		Kitchen			Feel OK
12 pm	Salad of lettuce, cucumber and tomato 3 crab sticks 1 cracker Black coffee	Lounge			Worried that I've eaten too much
2 pm	Apple Glass of water	Kitchen			
6 pm	Steamed vegetables 1/2 piece of chicken	Lounge			Feel full + bloated Worried that my weight will go up tomorrow

* = binge, V = vomiting, L = laxatives

Fig. 23.1 Example of a food diary of a patient with anorexia nervosa.

with few physical complaints, further enquiry often reveals heightened sensitivity to cold and a variety of gastrointestinal symptoms including constipation, fullness after eating, bloatedness and vague abdominal pains. Other symptoms include restlessness, lack of energy, low sexual appetite, early morning wakening and dizziness on standing. In postmenarchal females who are not taking an oral contraceptive, amenorrhoea is often present, with infertility posing a concern for many women. On examination, patients are typically emaciated and underweight. Those with a prepubertal onset may be short in stature and show failure of breast development. Often there is fine downy hair (lanugo) on the back, arms and side of the face. The skin tends to be dry and the hands and feet cold. Blood pressure and pulse are low and there may be dependent oedema. The findings on investigation are shown in Table 23.2.

23.3.3 Aetiology

Predisposing factors AN is a complex illness that develops over time, often as a result of multiple influ-

ences. Dieting appears to be a general risk factor, although only a small percentage of those who diet go on to develop a clinical eating disorder. This suggests the importance of other aetiological factors. Other risk factors identified in the literature include a history of obesity, and premorbid characteristics such as long-standing low self-esteem and perfectionism. Patients with AN are often high achievers who have an intense need to be accepted by others. Family relationships are often disturbed, although it remains unclear as to whether this is a cause or consequence of the eating disorder or both. A history of eating disorders and depression are also commonly seen within patients' families, and genetic studies have shown a significant linkage on chromosome 1 for restricting AN.

Maintaining factors As weight loss continues, so the physical and psychological sequelae of starvation become more prominent, some of which perpetuate the disorder. For example, delayed gastric emptying results in fullness even after eating small amounts of food, a situation that can fuel concern about uncontrollable weight gain. Weight loss may initially be

Table 23.2 Anorexia nervosa and bulimia nervosa: common abnormalities on investigation

Anorexia nervosa	Bulimia nervosa
Endocrine	*Endocrine*
Low levels of female sex hormones (luteinizing hormone, follicle-stimulating hormone and oestradiol)	Electrolyte disturbance, especially hypokalaemia, in those who vomit frequently or misuse large quantities of laxatives or diuretics
Low triiodothyronine (T_3) level but normal levels of thyroxine (T_4) and thyroid-stimulating hormone	*Gastrointestinal*
Raised growth hormone and cortisol levels	Prolonged digestion
Cardiovascular	Oesophageal damage and/or irritation of the oesophagus and/or pharynx due to contact with gastric acids
Low blood pressure (especially postural)	Perforation of upper digestive tract, oesophagus or stomach
Bradycardia	Abdominal pain and distension
Other arrhythmias	Hypertrophy of salivary glands
Haematological	*Cardiovascular*
Slightly lowered white cell count	Cardiac arrhythmias
Anaemia (normocytic normochromic)	*Other findings*
Low erythrocyte sedimentation rate	Dental erosion—gastric acids may cause deterioration of tooth enamel (perimolysis)
Other metabolic abnormalities	Hand callouses
Raised blood cholesterol	Blood in vomit
Increased serum carotene	Sore throat
Low blood sugar	Fatigue
Dehydration	Nausea
Electrolyte disturbance (in those who vomit frequently or misuse large quantities of laxatives or diuretics), especially hypokalaemia	Weight gain
Other findings	Hypertrophy of salivary glands (especially parotids)
Skeletal abnormalities (raised rate of osteopenia with risk of fractures)	
Delayed gastric emptying and prolonged gastrointestinal transit time	
Enlarged cerebral ventricles and external cerebrovascular fluid spaces ('pseudoatrophy')	

accompanied by positive feedback from others, but over the course of time, social withdrawal can lead to isolation from peers. Controlling food intake can lead to a powerful sense of self-control and often serves to enhance self-esteem. Those with AN can also hold a powerful position with the family.

23.3.4 Assessment

A large proportion of people with AN are ambivalent about seeking treatment and many will have been persuaded to seek help by concerned relatives or friends. Thus, assessment forms a crucial part of the treatment process. Assessment should cover psychological, social and physical needs, as well as assessment of risk to self and others. Where possible, the diagnosis should be made using a standardized diagnostic instrument, such as the Structured Clinical Interview for DSM-IV (SCID-I). No physical tests are required to make the diagnosis, and unless there are positive reasons to suspect the presence of another physical condition, no tests are required to exclude other medical disorders, when it is apparent that weight loss is self-induced.

A proportion of patients will present in a general medical setting and will report physical symptoms such as gastrointestinal symptoms, amenorrhoea or infertility. However, once it is been established that weight loss has been self-induced, a diagnosis of AN can be explored. All patients with AN should have a thorough physical examination. Those who vomit frequently or misuse significant quantities of laxatives or diuretics should have their electrolytes checked. Given the increased risk of osteoporosis, it can be useful to conduct a DEXA scan (dual energy X-ray absorptiometry) to assess bone density in patients who have been underweight for an extended period of time. It may also be helpful to conduct a pelvic ultrasound to assess ovarian and uterine maturity in those with persisting amenorrhea.

23.3.5 Management

There are three aspects to the management of AN. The first is to help patients to recognize that they have an illness. Acceptance and motivation to change are crucial given the recalcitrant nature of the illness. The second goal is the normalization of eating habits and weight restoration. Due to the risk of re-feeding syndrome, calorie intake should be increased gradually and it may be necessary to monitor phosphate levels during this initial phase. Weight gain may be achieved through outpatient, day-patient or inpatient treatment, and is typically facilitated through providing a combination of nutritional advice and psychological support. Drugs have almost no role, although dietary supplements can be of value in assisting weight restoration. The third aspect involves addressing patients' over-evaluation of weight and shape, their extreme control over eating patterns and underlying psychosocial functioning. These aspects of treatment are typically addressed in specialized treatments such as family therapy, cognitive behaviour therapy or cognitive analytic therapy.

23.3.6 Course and outcome

Response to treatment varies widely. For those who are willing and able to change, the illness duration can be relatively short. However, for others it can become a chronic problem commonly characterized by a resistance to change despite a wish to recover. Although there are few consistent predictors of outcome, a long history and late onset have both been associated with a poor prognosis. Low weight and a history of premorbid psychosocial problems also tend to be associated with a poor outcome.

Long-term follow-up studies indicate that at 6-year follow-up, 55% had no eating disorder, 27% continued with AN, 10% had BN, 2% were classified with EDNOS and 6% were deceased. AN is associated with increased mortality, the standardized mortality ratio over the first 10 years after presentation showing a tenfold increased risk. Most deaths are either a direct result of medical complications or due to suicide. The mortality rate appears to be the highest for those presenting with lower weight during their illness and for those presenting between 20 and 29 years of age.

23.4 Bulimia nervosa

23.4.1 Clinical features

As in AN, those with BN tend to judge their self-worth almost exclusively on the basis of their weight and shape and their ability to control their food intake. They also use extreme forms of weight control, such as fasting and self-induced vomiting. However, people with BN tend to lie within the normal weight range, and they regularly engage in episodes of 'binge eating'. Binges will vary in size; they typically involve the consumption of 2000 kcal or more and tend to consist of foods the person is attempting to avoid. Patients typically become stuck in a vicious cycle of dietary restriction, bingeing and purging, and are plagued by a constant fear of weight gain. This cycle invariably has a detrimental impact on other areas of functioning, such as work and social relationships, and it can have significant financial implications, leading some to steal money or food from others. People with BN tend to 'value' their symptoms less compared with those with AN and often binge and purge in secret.

Evidence suggests that a significant proportion of people with BN have difficulty regulating their emotions, and for many bingeing may serve as a form of emotional regulation: a means of reducing the intensity of emotions when they become intolerable. Many also have impulse control problems and a history of interpersonal difficulties. A subgroup will also present with comorbid depression and/or borderline personality disorder, and many of these will engage in a range of self-destructive behaviours such as cutting, overdosing and substance misuse, with the dominant behaviour changing over time.

Physical health Physical complications most commonly associated with BN include irregular or absent menstruation, weakness and lethargy, vague abdominal pains and toothache. On examination, appearance is usually unremarkable. Parotid gland enlargement may be present and there may be significant erosion of the dental enamel, particularly on the lingual surface of the upper front teeth. The most important abnormality on investigation is the electrolyte disturbance that

Food Diary

Time	Food and drink consumed	Place	*	V/L	Comments
9 am	Black coffee	Kitchen			Feel OK — today is going to be a good day
1 pm	Ham and Salad sandwich	Office desk			So far so good
6 pm	2 cheese rolls	Kitchen			Ate whilst preparing dinner—wish I hadn't but know I'll bring it up later
6:30 pm	Lasagne and garlic bread	Kitchen	*	V	Shouldn't have had seconds
7 pm	Bowl of cereal 2 bowls of ice-cream Chocolate bar 2 slices of toast Bottle of coke (small)	Lounge " " " "	*	V	Feel horrible — can't believe I lost control after being so good at work

* = binge, V = vomiting, L = laxatives

Fig. 23.2 Example food diary for a patient with bulimia nervosa.

is encountered in those who vomit frequently and in those who take large quantities of laxatives or diuretics. Clinically serious electrolyte disturbance may require treatment with potassium supplements until the eating disorder has been resolved.

23.4.2 Aetiology

Although many patients with BN will report a history of AN, a number of factors have been identified that preferentially increase the risk of BN. These include childhood and parental obesity, early menarche and parental alcoholism. A history of trauma, including childhood sexual abuse (CSA) has also been associated with BN. However, while the rate of CSA in patients with BN is higher than that amongst matched subjects in the general population, it is not higher than that found amongst young women with other psychiatric disorders. This suggests it may serve as a general risk factor for psychiatric disorder rather than for BN *per se*.

23.4.3 Assessment

Many patients with BN feel too guilty and ashamed of their illness to ask for help, and often live with their disorder for years before seeking treatment. As with AN, they may present complaining of physical symptoms such as gastrointestinal or gynaecological symptoms. The lack of clear markers can make diagnosis difficult and highlights the importance of conducting a thorough assessment.

Those with BN typically present with a loss of control over their eating that is characterized by frequent episodes of binge eating and compensatory behaviours. Assessment and diagnosis is often relatively straightforward although chaotic eating patterns can sometimes make it difficult to establish the presence of discrete episodes of binge eating. As with AN, no physical tests are needed to establish the diagnosis. However, the electrolytes should be checked of all those who vomit frequently or misuse large quantities of laxatives or diuretics.

23.4.5 Management

Most patients with BN can be treated on an outpatient basis. Cognitive behavioural therapy (CBT) represents the most extensively researched and validated psychological therapy for BN. CBT is a time-limited intervention that focuses on modifying disturbed eating habits and addressing the overvaluation of shape and weight. An alternative treatment is interpersonal psychotherapy (IPT), an intervention that targets interpersonal problems rather than eating patterns *per se*. Both treatments can be administered on an outpatient basis. A subset of patients will respond well to less intensive behavioural interventions, such as guided self-help programmes, although this is unlikely to be sufficient for the majority. Antidepressant drugs have been shown to have an antibulimic effect, leading to a rapid decline in the frequency of binge eating and purging and an improvement in mood. However, the effect is not as great as that obtained with CBT and evidence suggests that improvements are not maintained.

23.4.5 Course and outcome

Relatively little is known about the long-term course and outcome of BN. Outcome studies conducted to date suggest that at best only 50% of those who receive CBT are likely to be free from their symptoms at follow-up, 20% can expect to continue with a full diagnosis, while the remaining 30% will experience episodes of relapse or will continue with a subclinical form. Evidence has also shown IPT to be equally as effective as CBT at 18-month follow-up.

23.5 EDNOS

Although recent findings suggest that EDNOS is commonly seen in clinical practice, this group of patients has less often been the focus of research and thus their characteristics remain poorly described. However, a number of subgroups have been suggested (see Table 23.1). For example, a proportion present with all the key features of BN but fail to fulfil the diagnostic criteria relating to frequency of occurrence of behavioural symptoms. Others may present with all the diagnostic features of AN but (in the case of women) may continue to menstruate at a BMI of 17.5 or below. It has also been documented that a subgroup with AN are aware that they are underweight and do not experience feelings of fatness. However, the most well-recognized subgroup is those with binge-eating disorder. These patients present with all the characteristic features of BN but do not engage in compensatory behaviours. Other key characteristics include eating much more rapidly than normal, eating until feeling uncomfortably full, eating large amounts of food when not feeling physic-

ally hungry, and feeling disgusted with oneself or very guilty after overeating. Binge-eating disorder is commonly associated with obesity and it affects between 5% and 10% of obese patients seeking weight-loss treatment. Modified versions of the standard treatments for BN have been developed for use with those presenting with binge-eating disorder, and it is recommended that these interventions are used where appropriate. However, with the exception of binge-eating disorder, no clinical trials have been conducted on those presenting with EDNOS. Thus, it is currently recommended that therapists treat these patients following the principles suggested for the eating disorder that the eating problem most closely resembles.

23.6 Eating disorders and comorbidity

A number of other high-risk groups have also been identified. These include those presenting with an eating disorder and type 1 diabetes mellitus (T1DM), and athletes with eating disorders. In relation to the former, it has been suggested that full and subclinical eating disorders may be more common among those with T1DM compared with aged-matched peers. Patients with T1DM may adopt the underuse or omission of insulin as a means of weight control, and it has been shown that even relatively short periods of impaired metabolic control can lead to increased risk of the physical complications associated with diabetes, such as retinopathy, nephropathy or neuropathy, as well as increased mortality. There is little primary research concerning the treatment of diabetic patients with an eating disorder and advice is therefore based on guidelines provided for the treatment of non-diabetic patients. However, the

coexistence of diabetes with an eating disorder invariably complicates psychological interventions and thus the clinical management of this group remains a challenge.

Female athletes have also been identified as a group at increased risk of developing disturbed eating and associated problems. Pressure to conform to a sport-specific 'ideal' in disciplines such as distance running, gymnastics and figure skating may lead a proportion to diet in order to improve performance. In order to capture the risks associated with eating disorders in athletes, terms such as 'anorexia athletica' and the 'female athlete triad' have been developed, the latter referring to the following three conditions: disordered eating, amenorrhea and osteoporosis. Identifying disordered eating among athletes must include the identification and assessment of a wide range of weight-control behaviours.

Summary

Although traditionally equated with AN and BN, it is now recognized that a significant proportion of the eating-disorder population present with EDNOS. Eating disorders are associated with significant psychological and physical complications. While many of these features will remit with weight restoration and/or cessation of weight-control behaviours, those presenting with a chronic course may experience long-term complications such as osteoporosis and infertility. The co-occurrence of subclinical disordered eating and conditions such as T1DM is also associated with significant physical morbidity and mortality. Patients with eating disorders present in a range of clinical settings and thus careful assessment is crucial for accurate identification and diagnosis. Comprehensive treatment requires the management of both physical and psychological aspects of the illness. While a proportion of patients will recover, a minority will present with an unremitting pattern of symptoms that may require longer-term management.

FURTHER READING

1. **American Dietetic Association** (2001) Position of the American Dietetic Association: Nutrition intervention in the treatment of anorexia nervosa, bulimia nervosa, and eating disorder not otherwise specified (EDNOS). *J Amer Diet Assoc*, **101**, 810–19.

2. **Birmingham, C.L., and Beumont, P.J.V.** (2004) Medical management of eating disorders: a practical handbook for healthcare professionals. Cambridge, Cambridge University Press.

3. **Fairburn, C.G., and Brownell, K.D.** (2002) *Eating disorders and obesity: A comprehensive handbook*, 2nd edition. New York, Guilford Press.

4. **Fairburn, C.G., and Harrison, P.J.** (2003) Eating disorders. *Lancet*, **361**, 40–16.

5. **National Collaborating Centre for Mental Health** (2004) *Core interventions in the treatment and management of anorexia nervosa, bulimia nervosa and related eating disorders*. London, British Psychological Society.

6. **Palmer** (2000) *Helping people with eating disorders: a clinical guide to assessment and treatment*. London, Wiley.

7. **Treasure, J., Schmidt, U., and van Furth, E.** (2003) *Handbook of eating disorders*, 2nd edition. London, Wiley.

 To see topical and scientifically robust updates on nutrition associated with this textbook, and active web links to many of the journal articles in the Reference areas, please see the dedicated Online Resource Centre at www.oxfordtextbooks.co.uk/orc/mann3e/.

PART 4

Foods

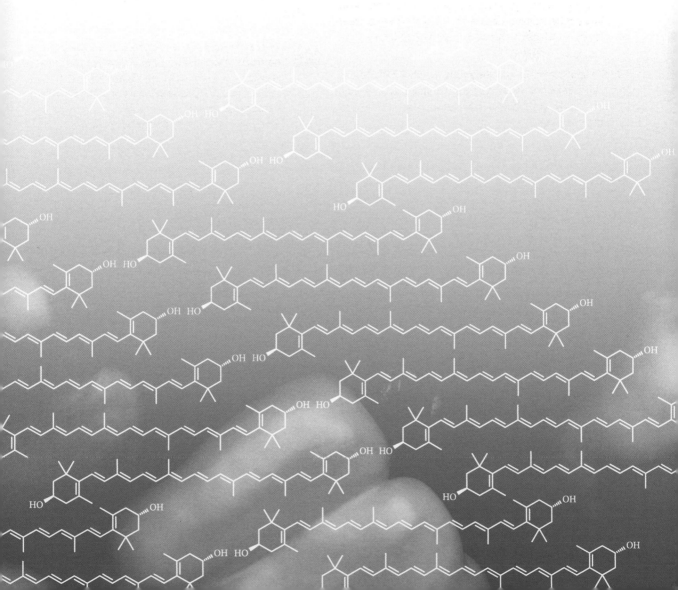

24 Food groups

24.1 Breads and cereals

Trish Griffiths

Cereals, the 'seeds of civilization', have constituted much of the food eaten by humans for thousands of years. It was not until the nomadic hunter-gatherers learned to farm crops that permanent settlements arose. Cultivation of wheat can be traced back to about 7000 BC in the Euphrates valley, while cultivation of rice dates back to around 3000 BC in China and shortly after in India. Maize (corn) was first cultivated about 5000 BC in Mexico. Food patterns were, and still are, most often built around a cereal. Wheat and barley were the staple foods of ancient Egypt, Greece, and Rome; rice in India and Southern China; maize, the staple of the early Americans; oats and rye staples in the colder regions of Europe and millets (including sorghum) were important in Africa and parts of Asia. Early breads were made from crude flours produced by pounding grains with a stone. Water was then added and the dough baked to a flat bread. Leavened bread dates back to Egypt in about 2000 BC.

Wheat, rice and maize are currently the predominant cereals in terms of both the land devoted to them and their consumption. Wheat covers more of the earth's surface than any other crop, largely having replaced rye, barley and oats in Northern Europe, and increasingly replacing sorghum and millet in Africa. About 50% of the food protein available on the globe is derived from cereals, with consumption greatest in the developing countries (providing two-thirds of energy and protein). With increasing income, cereal consumption tends to decrease, while the intake of animal products and refined carbohydrates increases.

Broadly speaking, the nutritional value of different cereal grains is essentially similar, with some variation due to genetic factors and environmental conditions such as soil type and temperature (Table 24.1). Cereals are an important source of energy, providing between 1400 and 1600 kJ per 100 g of whole cereal. Cereals provide starch and dietary fibre (soluble and insoluble), which together comprise 70–77% of the grain. Grains usually are processed and cooked so that the starch is digestible. Protein accounts for 6–15% of the grain and the limiting amino acid is lysine, with maize additionally low in tryptophan. Gluten is the major protein in wheat and rye and oryzenin the major protein in rice. All cereals are low in fat, oats have more; most of the fat is polyunsaturated. Whole grains are a good source of thiamin, their germ is rich in vitamin E and they contain significant amounts of minerals especially potassium, phosphorus, magnesium, iron and zinc plus selenium,

Table 24.1 Nutrient content of grains

Nutrient	Nutrients per 100 g (raw grains)				
	Wheat[a]	Brown rice[b]	Maize[b]	Millet[b]	Oats[b]
Water (g)	11.0	12.0	13.8	11.8	8.3
Protein (g)	12.6	7.5	9.0	10.0	15.0
Fat (g)	2.7	1.9	3.9	2.9	7.0
Carbohydrate (g)	72.4	77.4	72.2	72.9	69
Thiamin (mg)	0.5	0.34	0.37	0.73	0.6
Niacin (mg)	6.1	4.7	2.2	2.3	1.0
Calcium (mg)	35.0	32.0	22.0	20.0	53.0
Iron (mg)	3.7	1.6	2.1	6.8	4.5

[a]Based on Bread Research Institute of Australia Inc.
[b]Based on Lorenz, K.J., and Kulp, K. (eds) (1991) *Handbook of cereal science and technology*. New York, Marcel Dekker.

copper and manganese. The net contribution of cereals to mineral intake may be less than anticipated because phytate in the outer bran layers binds some minerals and inhibits their absorption. Bioavailability of minerals is better from refined products but because the mineral content is less, overall more minerals will be provided by whole grains. During fermentation, as in bread making, the enzyme phytase is produced, which breaks down phytate.

Wholegrain cereals are rich in fibre and 'bioactive' components, including antioxidants (especially phenolics), phyto-oestrogens (lignans), phytosterols, vitamins, minerals and trace elements. Epidemiological studies suggest consumption of whole grains is associated with reduced risk of chronic diseases and this is thought to be due to their content of bioactives.

24.1.1 Processing of cereal grains for human consumption

Wheat requires some processing to increase its digestibility. This is achieved by milling, which involves a series of grinding and sifting steps to produce flour. The nutritional value of flour varies with the extrac-

tion rate (the number of parts by weight of flour produced after milling 100 parts of grain). Starch and protein are in the endosperm so are reduced little by this processing. Typically, fibre, vitamins and minerals are concentrated in the outer bran and aleurone layers of grains and the extent to which these layers are removed during milling determines the nutrient content of flour. White flour has a lower micronutrient content than wholemeal but white flour products such as bread still make a significant contribution to the diet. In many industrial countries, cereal products are fortified with added vitamins or minerals (e.g. thiamin, niacin, calcium, iron). The protein content and 'hardness' of wheat determines how it is used. Hard high-protein wheat is most suitable for bread; soft low-protein wheats are most suitable for biscuits and extra-hard durum wheat is used almost, exclusively to make pasta. In addition to flour, milling produces bran, germ, and semolina. Bread, one of the most widely eaten foods in the world, is the major product made from wheat flour. White, wholemeal and mixed grain breads are popular in Western countries; flatbreads are common in the Middle East and steamed breads in China. Gluten (used predominantly by the baking industry) and wheat starch are also products of wheat processing.

Rice is the staple food of over half the world's population. After harvesting, paddy rice is cleaned and de-hulled but the bran layer is retained to produce brown rice. Alternatively, the brown rice can be further milled and polished to give white rice. Brown rice has a higher protein, mineral and vitamin content than milled rice but also has a higher content of phytate and fibre. The practice of extensive abrasive polishing of rice is of concern in many Asian nations where the majority of food eaten is rice and loss of nutrients like protein, thiamin and iron becomes critical. The practice of parboiling rice before milling is encouraged as this results in an inward migration of water-soluble vitamins (including thiamin) to the endosperm. The process of rice enrichment may also improve nutrient intake. This involves mixing the ordinary white rice in a fixed proportion with rice that has been treated with a vitamin mixture and often iron. Lastly, 'Golden rice' is a new strain of rice genetically modified to produce β-carotene in the grain (which the body turns into vitamin A). It was developed in an attempt to reduce vitamin A deficiency and childhood blindness in developing countries. It remains controversial because of its genetically modified status—and the β-carotene content is quite small. In developed countries, people have been enticed to eat more rice by a range of novel products such as rice cakes, rice bran, rice noodles and rice crackers.

Maize (corn) may be either dry milled (the protein and starch fractions are not separated) or wet milled (the protein and starch are separated). Dry milling produces grits, meals, flour and hominy feed, while wet milling yields starch, dextrose, corn syrup solids and glucose. Immature maize is often eaten fresh as a vegetable, i.e. sweet corn. Maize kernels also can be frozen or canned. Maize is used in the production of corn meals, corn flour, corn chips, tacos and tortillas and consumption of these foods is no longer confined to Mexico. In African countries, maize is widely consumed as a porridge, either a stiff porridge (ugali) or thin gruel (uji) which can also be used as the basis for alcoholic or non-alcoholic beverages. Maize is also processed to make flaked breakfast cereals (corn flakes). While maize contains little niacin or its amino

acid precursor, tryptophan, the traditional Central American cooking method (using a lime cooking step) for tortillas increases the availability of niacin and apparently prevents widespread pellagra in populations relying on maize tortillas as a staple food.

Oats are processed by steaming or kiln-drying before de-hulling. The resultant 'groats' can be cut to produce a coarse meal, which is steamed, then rolled to make oat flakes, or granulated to produce a fine oat meal. Oats are generally eaten as a breakfast cereal (porridge or muesli). Consumption of oat bran became popular because of the cholesterol-lowering properties of its soluble fibre. However, the amounts usually consumed often have only a minor effect.

Barley is used in the form of pearled grains for soups, flour for flatbreads and ground grain for porridge. Barley flour is generally milled by conventional roller milling as used for wheat. Malted barley is important in the brewing (for making beer and some whiskies) and baking industries and is also used in making vinegar and for flavouring breakfast cereals.

Rye is milled in a similar fashion to wheat. Cracked rye is used for porridge and other breakfast cereals and rye flour can be baked into bread, pumpernickel and crispbreads.

Millet is a name given to a group of cereals that includes sorghum. These are consumed in Africa, parts of India, Pakistan and China. The grains are pounded into flour and mixed with water to make porridge. In Ethiopia, finely ground millet grains are left to ferment slightly before being baked into flatbreads called injera.

While it has been common practice to highly refine cereals such as wheat and rice, there appear to be significant benefits from eating more wholegrain foods. In addition to their higher nutrient content, consumption of wholegrains is associated with protection from coronary heart disease, ischaemic stroke and type 2 diabetes and with bowel health. These foods have more slowly digested carbohydrate, which is useful in the control of blood glucose in people with diabetes (lower glycaemic index).

FURTHER READING

1. **Juliano, B.** (1993) *Rice in human nutrition. Food and Nutrition Series No. 26*. Rome, IRRI and FAO.

2. **Montonen, J., Knekt, P., Jarvinen, R., Aromaa, A., and Reunanen, A.** (2003) Whole grain and fibre intake and the incidence of type 2 diabetes. *Am J Clin Nutr*, **77**, 622–29.

3. **Slavin, J.** (2003) Why whole grains are protective: biological mechanisms. *Proc Nutrition Society (UK)*, **62**, 129–34.

4. **Time Magazine** (2000) This rice could save a million kids a year (beta-carotene enriched rice). *Time Magazine* 7 August 2000.

5. **Truswell, A.S.** (2002) Cereal grains and coronary heart disease (review). *Eur J Clin Nutr*, **56**, 1–14.

24.2 Legumes

Sue Munro

Legumes are the edible seed from the *Leguminosae* family (*Fabaceae*) and include dried peas, beans, soya beans, lentils and dhal. Peanuts are also legumes. Cultivated since earliest civilizations, legumes were often considered an inferior food eaten by peasants, described as being 'poor man's meat'. They never assumed the importance of a staple food as did the cereal crops of wheat, rice, maize or barley. Yet, they played an important synergistic role with staple foods both in meeting nutritional requirements and fertilizing the soil.

The cereal-and-bean combination is a feature of many cuisines. Mexicans eat kidney beans and tortillas, Indians top their rice with dhal, the Chinese enjoy soy products with rice, those in the Middle East combine lentils with rice, while the English put baked beans on toast. The ratio of quantities of cereal and beans consumed is similar between cuisines, with cereal foods assuming the role of staple, the main source of energy, and the legumes used as accompaniments.

Of all foods, legumes most adequately meet the recommended dietary guidelines for healthful eating. They are high in carbohydrate and dietary fibre, mostly low in fat, and supply adequate protein while being a good source of vitamins and minerals. Cooked legumes contain about 6–9% protein, about twice as much protein as in cereal foods. The exceptions are soybeans and peanuts, which contain 14% and 24% respectively, when cooked. The limiting amino acids of legumes are the sulphur-containing methionine and cysteine but, being rich in lysine, legume proteins are well complemented by cereals. Reports suggest that the amount of indispensable amino acids in soy protein products is sufficient to meet protein requirements for normal human growth and development. Soy protein has been shown to have a beneficial role in the control of blood lipids.

Legumes provide 10–13 g of carbohydrate that is the slowly digested type, and 6–9 g of fibre per 100 g of cooked beans. Some of the fibre is soluble fibre, which might lower blood cholesterol. Legumes also contain oligosaccharides, which escape digestion in the gut to be fermented by bacteria in the large bowel. This is responsible for the abdominal discomfort and flatulence often experienced and is perhaps the factor limiting consumption. However, these compounds may have beneficial effects for gastrointestinal health. Legumes are low in fat (~ 2.5%) but soybeans and peanuts contain 8% and 47% fat, respectively. This fat is mostly monounsaturated or polyunsaturated. Soybeans contain the ω-3 fatty acid, α-linolenic acid.

Legumes supply vitamins and minerals including thiamin, niacin, iron, zinc, calcium and magnesium (Table 24.2). Soybeans contain the phyto-oestrogens isoflavones and lignans. They may have a role to play in the prevention of certain cancers and coronary heart disease. It is reported that phyto-oestrogens may be a useful treatment for menopausal symptoms including maintenance of bone density. There are, however, several substances in uncooked legumes that inhibit their nutritional quality. Most of these toxic substances are destroyed or inactivated by normal cooking or processing.

Table 24.2 Nutrient content of legumes

Nutrient	Nutrients per 100 g cooked beans
Protein (g)	6.2 (cannelini) to 24.7 (peanuts)
Fat (g)	0.4 (lentils) to 7.7 (soybeans)
Carbohydrate (g)	1.4 (soybeans) to 12.6 (haricot beans)
Dietary fibre (g)	3.7 (lentils) to 8.8 (haricot beans)
Thiamin (mg)	0.6 (lima beans) to 0.79 (peanuts)
Riboflavin (mg)	Trace (kidney beans) to 0.7 (soybeans)
Niacin equivalents (mg)	1.6 (lima beans) to 19.8 (peanuts)
Calcium (mg)	13.0 (split peas) to 76.0 (soybeans)
Iron (mg)	1.1 (split peas) to 2.2 (soybeans)
Zinc (mg)	0.6 (split peas) to 1.6 (soybeans)

Source: English, R., and Lewis, J. (1990) *The composition of foods Australia*. Canberra, Australian Government Publishing Service.

Trypsin inhibitors may reduce the effectiveness of the digestive process; haemagglutinins appear to reduce the efficiency of absorption of digestive products; phytate binds metals, like zinc and iron, decreasing their absorption; goitrogens interrupt the absorption of iodine. Apart from antinutrient toxins, other substances in beans can cause specific diseases. *Lathyrus sativus* is drought-resistant but can precipitate lathyrism (a neurological disorder that occurs in India) when consumed in large amounts. Broad beans may result in favism, a haemolytic anaemia, in individuals of Mediterranean descent who are genetically susceptible to this disease. Some legumes contain toxic cyanide and alkaloids. Peanuts are common food allergens and can cause anaphylaxis (Chapter 32). Peanuts are susceptible to *Aspergillus* mould, which produces aflatoxin, a potent liver carcinogen. Careful storage and monitoring are essential to avoid this contamination.

24.2.1 Products from the basic food

Uncooked dried legumes are virtually indigestible, tasteless and too hard to eat anyway. Processing is essential to make beans edible and improve the nutritional quality and digestibility of the bean. Cooking and processing inactivates most antinutrients and toxins. Germination and fermentation improve the nutritional quality of the bean resulting in increases in vitamin C, niacin, riboflavin and thiamin, and vitamin E content.

There are distinct differences in preparation between the East and West. In India and some parts of Africa, raw legumes are milled to remove fibrous seed coats. Cotyledons are split along natural cleavage lines to form two split peas or dhal. Then the peas or beans are boiled, roasted, fermented, germinated or ground into flour or paste, as required. In Western countries and South America and much of Africa, the seeds are soaked and cooked for long periods of time to inactivate toxic substances and improve digestibility. The beans are either eaten whole, puréed and fried or made into cakes. In Asia, various methods of processing the soybean have evolved, along with its cultivation. Immature beans are eaten whole in salads, vegetable dishes or soups; mature soybeans are not usually eaten as whole beans but rather processed into curd, cheese, sauces, pastes, or sprouted as a vegetable.

Today, peanuts and soybeans account for most of the legume products. Soybeans are made into a range of products, including soy protein concentrates or isolates, extrusion-textured products, soy flour, soy milk and tofu. Many soy products are used in manufactured food products, including bread and baked goods, processed meat products, soy ice-cream, sauces and low-fat spreads. Peanuts are made into butters and used in confectionery and baked goods.

FURTHER READING

1. **FAO** (1989) *Utilization of tropical foods: tropical beans. Food and Nutrition Paper 47/4*. Rome, Food and Agricultural Organization.

2. **Messina, M. (ed.)** (2000) Proceedings of the third international symposium on the role of soy in preventing and treating chronic disease. *J Nutr*, **130**, 653S–711S.

3. **McGee, H.** (2004) Legumes: beans and peas. In: McGee, H. *On food and cooking. The science and lore of the kitchen*, 2nd edition. New York, Scribner, pp. 483–501.

24.3 Nuts and seeds

Margaret Allman-Farinelli

Nuts and seeds have been valued for their oils as much as for a food in itself and were an important source of nutrients and energy since the earliest civilizations. Traditional cuisines have utilized the locally grown nuts and seeds for both savoury and sweet dishes. In recent years, there has been much interest in the nutritional properties of nuts that promote health. Today, nuts and seeds are processed for their oil, ground into pastes, used as ingredients in baked goods, or eaten raw or roasted as snack foods.

Common types of nuts include almonds, walnuts, pecans, cashews, brazil nuts, macadamias, hazelnuts and pistachios. Sunflower, sesame and pumpkin seeds are the most common seeds eaten as foods. Caraway and poppy seeds are used as seasonings.

Nuts and seeds have similar nutritional qualities; their low water content and high content of energy, protein, vitamins and minerals makes them nutritious foods (Table 24.3). The energy content of nuts is mostly due to their high fat content. The fat in nuts

Table 24.3 Nutrient content of raw nuts and seeds

Nutrient	Nutrients per 100 g cooked beans
Protein (g)	2.0 (chestnuts) to 24.4 (pumpkin seeds)
Fat (g)	2.7 (chestnuts) to 77.6 (macadamias)
Carbohydrate (g)	3.1 (brazil nuts) to 36.6 (chestnuts)
Dietary fibre[a] (g)	1.9 (pine nuts) to 7.9 (sesame seeds)
Thiamin (mg)	0.11 (Barcelona nuts) to 0.93 (sesame seeds)
Riboflavin (mg)	0.06 (macadamias) to 0.75 (almonds)
Niacin equivalents (mg)	0.9 (chestnuts) to 9.1 (sunflower seeds)
Calcium (mg)	11.0 (pine nuts) to 670.0 (sesame seeds)
Iron (mg)	1.6 (macadamias) to 10.4 (sesame seeds)
Zinc (mg)	0.5 (chestnuts) to 6.6 (soybeans)

[a]Englyst method (see section 27.2.4).
Source: Holland, B., Unwin, I.D., and Buss, D.H. (1992) *Fruit and nuts*. First supplement to: *McCance and Widdowson's: The composition of foods*, 5th edition. London, Royal Society of Chemistry, MAFF.

varies in both quantity and type. Chestnuts are low in fat, but other nuts contain from 45% to 75% fat. The majority of nuts contain unsaturated fatty acids, either monounsaturated (e.g. macadamia) or poly-unsaturated. Walnuts are rich in ω-6 polyunsaturated fatty acids but also a good source of ω-3 linolenic acid. The protein content of nuts ranges from 2% to 25%; lysine is the limiting amino acid. They are good sources of dietary fibre, B vitamins (thiamin, riboflavin and niacin), vitamin E, and iron, zinc, magnesium, potassium and calcium.

Several epidemiological studies indicate that people eating nuts four or five times per week may have a lower risk of coronary heart disease. The constituents likely to confer these benefits are the amino acid arginine, vitamin E and/or unsaturated fat. There is a danger here of confounding. Nuts make up only a small percentage of the total diet. Studies have also indicated that people regularly consuming nuts have either the same or a lower body weight than those not eating nuts. Thus, nuts are a useful addition to the diet for most people. However, an estimated 1% of people are allergic to tree nuts or peanuts.

FURTHER READING

1. **Albert, V.M., Gaziano, J.M., Willett, W.C., and Manson, J.E.** (2002) Nut consumption and decreased risk of sudden death in the Physician's Health Study. *Arch Int Med*, **162**, 1382–87.
2. **Hu, F.B., Stampfer, M.J., Manson, J.E., *et al*.** (1998) Frequent nut consumption and risk of coronary heart disease in women: prospective cohort study. *Br Med J*, **317**, 1341–45.
3. **Sabate, J.** (1999) Nut consumption, vegetarian diets, ischaemic heart disease risk, and all cause mortality: evidence from epidemiologic studies. *Am J Clin Nutr*, **70** (Suppl. 3), 500S–503S.
4. **Sicherer, S.H., Munoz-Furlong, A., and Sampson, H.A.** (2003) Prevalence of peanut and tree nut allergy in the USA determined by means of a random-digit dial telephone survey: a 5-year follow-up study. *J Allergy Clin Immunol*, **112**, 1203–1207.

24.4 Fruit

Stewart Truswell

In its strict botanical sense, a 'fruit' is the fleshy or dry ripened ovary of a plant enclosing the seed and so includes corn grains, bean pods, tomatoes, olives, cucumbers, and almonds and pecans (in their shells). We usually restrict the term 'fruit' to mean the ripened ovaries that are sweet and either succulent or pulpy and usually eaten as an appetizer or a dessert. Fresh fruits were formerly only available seasonally, but with technology and imports, many are available most of the year. Most of us eat more species in the fruit food group than in any other food group, for example, 30 or more species: some daily (e.g. apples, oranges, bananas) and others rarely (e.g. golden berries, elderberries, mulberries, loganberries, passion fruit).

Our ancestors originally ate fruits for their sweetness. They learned that those fruits that were not bitter were unlikely to be toxic. The sugar that makes them sweet provides energy and may be fructose and/or glucose and/or sucrose and others (such as sorbitol). Fruits generally provide useful amounts of potassium, vitamin C, carotenoids and folate (Table 24.4). Avocados are unusual because they have a high content of fat (mostly monounsaturated) and contain a 7-carbon sugar.

Fruits are preserved in jams by boiling with sugar; the pectin (soluble dietary fibre) they contain makes a gel. Some fruits are dried: especially grapes, plums, dates, bananas and apricots (dried fruits have lost the vitamin C).

Quite large amounts of some fruits, especially citrus and apples, are consumed in the form of fruit juices, which contain most of the nutrients but less of the fibre, and give less satiety.

Grapes are high in sugar (glucose), which makes crushed grapes a good substrate for fermentation into wine; apples are fermented to make cider.

Most fruits taste somewhat sour, because they contain organic acids such as citric, malic, tartaric,

Table 24.4 Nutrient content of raw fruits

Nutrient	Nutrients per 100 g cooked beans
Protein (g)	0.3 (apples) to 2.6 (passionfruit)
Fat (g)	trace (most) to 19.3 (avocado)
Sugars (g)	trace (olive) to 20.9 (bananas)
Dietary fibre (g)	0.1 (watermelon) to 3.8 (kumquat)
β-Carotene (mg)	5.0 (lemon) to 1800 (mango)
Vitamin C (mg)	3.0 (durian) to 230 (guava)
Folate (mg)	3.0 (grapes) to 34 (blackberries)
Vitamin B_6 (mg)	0.02 (gooseberries) to 0.29 (banana)
Vitamin E (mg)	0.2 (strawberries) to 2.4 (blackberries)
Potassium (mg)	88.0 (watermelon) to 400 (banana)

Source: Holland, B., Unwin, I.D., and Buss, D.H. (1992) *Fruit and nuts*. First supplement to: *McCance and Widdowson's: The composition of foods*, 5th edition. London, Royal Society of Chemistry, MAFF.

ascorbic, and in some cases, benzoic or sorbic acids. Only citric and malic acids provide small amounts of energy in the mammalian body. Because of the sourness, sugar is added to some fruits to make them palatable.

Fruits contain other substances, not classical nutrients, which can be biologically active, for example flavonoids, salicylates and limonoids. Tiny amounts of many different natural esters, aldehydes and ketones contribute the distinctive volatile flavours of fruits (e.g. in an apple, 103 flavour compounds have been identified).

People have taken these other substances for granted. It was a surprise when Canadian pharmacologists discovered that grapefruit juice increases the blood concentrations of a number of commonly used potent drugs, for example, most statins and felodipine, by downregulation of cytochrome P450 3A4, which is involved in their first-pass metabolism. The active substances in grapefruit are probably naringin (a flavonoid) and 6′,7′-dihydrobergamottin.

People cannot live for long on fruits alone unless they include nuts. Fruits are inadequate in protein, sodium, calcium, iron and zinc. Nutritionists, however, look very favourably on fruit as part of a mixed diet and urge people to eat plenty of fruits each day. This is because they are low in energy, fat and sodium and make valuable contributions to the intakes of vitamin C, carotenoids, folate and dietary fibre. Numerous epidemiological studies have shown that people who eat above-average amounts of fruit and vegetables (intakes of these two food groups are usually recorded together) have below-average rates of heart disease and cancer. This may be partly because more fruit is eaten in more privileged sections of society, and partly because of the good things in fruits, such as antioxidant nutrients (vitamin C and carotenoids) or other substances yet to be fully elucidated.

There is little to be said about fruits on the negative side, except that in the orchard they are often sprayed with pesticide. These pesticides should have decomposed before sale but it is safer to wash fruits before eating. The seeds or stones of some fruits contain cyanogenic glycosides, which are potentially toxic.

FURTHER READING

1. Bailey, D.G., Malcolm, J., Arnold, O., and Spence, J.D. (1998) Grapefruit juice—drug interactions. *Br J Clin Pharmacol*, **46**, 101–10.

2. **Steffen, L.M.** (2006) Eat your fruit and vegetables. *Lancet*, **267**, 279–79.

3. **Strandhagen, E., Hansson, P.O., Boseaus, I., Isaksson, B., and Eriksson, J.H.** (2000) High fruit intake may reduce mortality among middle aged and elderly men. The study of men born in 1913. *Eur J Clin Nutr*, **54**, 337–41.

24.5 Vegetables
Soumela Amanatidis

Vegetables comprise any plant part, other than fruit, that is used as food. They include roots and tubers such as potatoes, taro, turnips, parsnips, carrots and yams, bulbs such as onions, stems like celery, leaves such as lettuce, cabbage and parsley, and flowers such as broccoli and cauliflower. Some fungi (e.g. mushrooms) are also consumed as vegetables. Zucchini, squash and tomatoes, although strictly fruits, are usually treated as vegetables by the consumer. Peas and beans are legumes but when immature and green are treated as vegetables. The nutritional composition and the usage pattern of the roots and tubers is somewhat different to that of the stems, leaves and flowers.

Potatoes have their origins in the New World, being staples of the Incas; other tubers such as yams and taro have been staple foods in the Pacific Islands for many years. Leafy vegetables were grown in monastery gardens during the Middle Ages. Today, most nations have cereal staples like rice or wheat but some countries have vegetable staples. Cassava is a staple energy source for about 200 million people in tropical countries. Potatoes, whether as potato chips, boiled or baked, or French fries, remain a much-consumed commodity in developed nations. While leafy vegetables are commonly eaten in developed countries, they are less popular in developing nations. It is estimated that in India there were 40 species of leaves grown 70 years ago, but that number has now diminished to about four.

Potatoes supply moderate amounts of protein in many people's diets. The biological value is good, with the limiting amino acid being methionine. Stem, bulb, leaf and flower vegetables usually provide smaller amounts of protein to the diet although their content may be similar. All vegetables contain negligible fat. Starch predominates in tubers, mainly amylopectin; the other vegetables contain sugars. Vegetables are a good source of dietary fibre. The fibre includes the soluble-type (e.g. pectin) but also insoluble fibre, like cellulose.

Green leafy vegetables have a very high water content and are exceptionally low in energy while relatively high in micronutrients, so in a weight-conscious community they are a good food choice. Some vegetables are rich in micronutrients: potatoes are a major source of vitamin C, carrots are exceptionally high in β-carotene and spinach is rich in folic acid. Dark-green leafy vegetables like spinach are a good source of lutein, and orange capsicums are a good source of zeaxanthin. These two carotenoids function in the macula lutea in the centre of the retina. Broccoli is relatively rich in calcium and spinach in iron, although neither is necessarily consumed in sufficient quantities to make a large contribution to the mineral intake. The other factor to consider is the bioavailability. Studies have shown that β-carotene from vegetables is more poorly absorbed than the pharmaceutical preparation. This is unfortunate because leaves are rich in β-carotene, and blindness from vitamin A deficiency remains a major public health risk in many developing countries. It is well established that the absorption of non-haem iron from vegetables is not as good as the haem form found in meat, but the presence of vitamin C will enhance non-haem iron absorption (Table 24.5).

Cooking reduces the vitamin C and folate content of vegetables, often by a considerable amount. Vegetables should be cooked, therefore, for the shortest possible time in a small amount of water. Apart from the well-recognized nutrients, vegetables contain a variety of substances that may be beneficial for health.

Table 24.5 Nutrient content of vegetables

Nutrient	Nutrients per 100 g cooked beans
Energy (kJ)	27.0 (lettuce) to 441.0 (taro)
Protein (g)	0.6 (celery) to 4.7 (broccoli)
Fat (g)	0.0 (Chinese cabbage) to 0.6 (pumpkin)
Carbohydrate (g)	0.4 (lettuce) to 30.4 (cassava)
Fibre (g)	0.8 (globe artichoke) to 4.0 (broccoli)
β-Carotene (mg)	0.0 (potato) to 10.35 (carrots)
Vitamin C (mg)	4.0 (lettuce) to 110.0 (brussels sprouts)
Calcium (mg)	4.0 (potato) to 82.0 (okra)
Iron (mg)	0.2 (pumpkin) to 3.2 (English spinach)
Flavonoids[a] (mg)	0.0 (spinach) to 35.3 (onion)

[a]Hertog, M.G.L., Hollman, P.C.H., and Katan, M.B. (1992) Intake of potentially anticarcinogenic flavonoids and their determinants in adults in the Netherlands. *J Agric Food Chem*, 41, 1242–46.
Source: English, R., and Lewis, J. (1990) *The composition of foods Australia*. Canberra, Australian Government Publishing Service.

Epidemiological studies indicate that vegetable consumption is associated with a lower prevalence of certain types of cancer like bowel, lung and stomach. Initially this was attributed to their high content of antioxidant vitamins (β-carotene) but randomized controlled trials with β-carotene were disappointing, and other constituents may be more important. Flavonoids like quercetin and kaempferol, found in onions and broccoli, and glucosinolates, found in cruciferous vegetables like broccoli and brussels sprouts, may protect against cancer. The flavonoids may also be cardioprotective because they function as antioxidants and may decrease platelet aggregation.

While eating vegetables is desirable, there are a few potential toxic effects. Potatoes, especially green ones, contain solanine, a neurotoxin, and this is harmful if excessive amounts are eaten. Sweet potatoes if infected with a certain fungus may contain furanoterpenes that cause lung disorders. Cassava contains cyanogenic glycosides, which liberate cyanide, but this is largely removed by peeling and cooking.

Vegetables are an enjoyable, nutritious food commodity. A number of major epidemiological studies

have led to the advice to consume five servings of vegetables and fruit per day. It seems to be generally agreed that the five servings can include one fruit juice, can include frozen and canned fruit or vegetables, and one serving of dried fruit, but presumably not potato chips. Whether the planet can provide all this fruit and vegetable for all people is another problem that will need to be addressed.

FURTHER READING

1. **Law, M.R., and Morris, J.K.** (1998) By how much does fruit and vegetable consumption reduce the risk of ischaemic heart disease? *Eur J Clin Nutr*, **52**, 549–56.

2. **Potter, J.D.** (2005) Vegetables, fruit and cancer. *Lancet*, **366**, 527–30.

3. **Tohill, B.C., Seymour, J., Serdula, M., Kettel-Khan, L., and Rolls, B.J.** (2004) What epidemiologic studies tell us about the relationship between fruit and vegetable consumption and body weight. *Nutr Rev*, **62**, 365–74.

4. **Williams, C.** (1995) Healthy eating: clarifying advice about fruit and vegetables. *Br Med J*, **310**, 1453–55.

24.6 Milk and milk products

Anita S. Lawrence

All mammals produce milk and man consumes a variety of milks from cows, sheep, goats, horses, reindeer, yaks, water buffalos and camels. Use of animals' milk as a food source presumably coincided with the domestication of animals around 10 000 years ago. Sheep and goats were domesticated first, probably about 8000–9000 BC. Cave paintings show that cows were domesticated by 4000 BC, and traces of cheeses have been found in Egyptian tombs dating back to 2000 BC. Hippocrates recommended milk as a health food and medicine about 400 BC.

Milk is the only food for the first few months of human life. Although human milk has several advantages for babies over cows' milk, it is clear that milk contains all the nutrients that a new growing mammal needs. After weaning, adult milk consumption varies in different parts of the world. In some regions adults consume milk regularly, in other regions they do not habitually consume it. In Western countries, a milk group of foods (milk and products) is one of the food groups recommended for health in nutrition education (see Chapter 36).

24.6.1 Composition

Milk is a good source of high-quality protein. It contains useful amounts of all of the indispensable amino acids. Milk protein is able to complement lysine-deficient protein foods such as wheat and maize. A small proportion of individuals are allergic to milk protein. Prevalence is highest in the first year of life, occurring in approximately 2% of infants. Of these, the great majority (approximately 90% of affected children) grow out of their milk allergy by 3 years of age.

Note: As the main type of milk consumed internationally is cows' milk, for the rest of this chapter the term 'milk' is used to denote cows' milk, unless it is preceded by the name of another animal.

Carbohydrate is present in cow's milk in the form of the disaccharide, lactose. Lactose is normally digested in the small intestine by the enzyme lactase. However, many individuals, particularly those originating from South-East Asia, the Middle East and parts of Africa, produce reduced levels of lactase after early childhood and some lactose passes to their

Table 24.6 Nutritional composition of cows' milk and milk products per typical portion

	Whole milk (250 mL)	Reduced-fat milk (250 mL)	Skimmed milk (250 mL)	Cheddar cheese (40 g)	Reduced-fat strawberry yogurt (200 g)
Energy (kJ)	678	510	360	672	696
Protein (g)	8.3	9.8	9.0	10.1	9.8
Fat (g)	9.5	3.5	0.3	13.5	1.8
Carbohydrate (g)	11.8	13.3	12.5	0.0	29.0
Vitamin A (µg) (RE)	120.8	36.3	0	158.6	16.0
Riboflavin (mg)	0.5	0.5	0.5	0.2	0.6
Calcium (mg)	285	343	308	312	320

RE, retinol equivalent.
Source: Australian Dairy Corporation, 1999.

colon undigested. Its fermentation can cause discomfort and diarrhoea.

Contrary to popular belief, individuals with lactose non-persistence can usually consume two cups of milk each day without any unpleasant symptoms, if they drink them with food at separate meal times. Also, lactose tolerance is improved by regular milk consumption.

The geographic distribution of lactose persistence into adulthood is genetically determined and matches the traditional distribution of dairy farming. Gene analysis indicates that selection occurred relatively recently in the last 5000–10 000 years. The high rate of lactase persistence can be explained by survival advantage associated with consuming dairy foods, the only source of lactose.

Whole, reduced-fat and skimmed milk typically contain 3.8%, 1.4% and less than 0.1% fat, respectively. Milk fat is a very complex natural fat, its triacylglycerols being synthesized from more than 400 different fatty acids. About one-quarter are monounsaturated and about two-thirds are saturated. Milk fat includes components thought to be beneficial for health including fat-soluble vitamins, rumenic acid (*cis*-9, *trans*-11 conjugated linoleic acid), vaccenic acid, sphingolipids and butyric acid.

Milk provides significant amounts of a range of vitamins, particularly vitamin B_{12}, riboflavin, folate and, if whole milk, vitamin A. It also contains traces of vitamin D, more if fortified, as in North America.

Milk and its products are generally the richest source of calcium in Western diets as they have a high calcium content per serving and the calcium is highly bioavailable. Few other foods provide the body with as much calcium per serving as dairy foods. Milk also supplies a wide range of other minerals, including phosphorus, magnesium, potassium, zinc, selenium, sodium and iodine but it is low in iron. As milk contains about 90% water, it is a useful vehicle for rehydration.

Goats' milk provides comparable nutrients to whole cows' milk but is a poor source of folate and riboflavin. Sheep's milk on the other hand contains more protein, fat and (most) vitamins and minerals than cows' milk; it is more nutrient energy-dense.

24.6.2 Processing

Milk is pasteurized to destroy disease-causing bacteria: heating to 72°C for 15 seconds and then cooling immediately is a commonly used method. It leads to small loses of nutrients but these are not nutritionally significant. Milk is available in different forms. In some countries, milk is drunk in a cultured form, e.g. as kefir or as cultured butter milk. Skimmed milks have (almost) all the fat taken out and so do not naturally contain the fat-soluble vitamins A (or D). Spray-dried powdered milk has its moisture removed. It is the basis of infant formulas after adjustments are made to 'humanize' it. Milk powder (often fortified with vitamin A) is a major commodity for feeding young children, imported by countries where there is insufficient local dairy supply.

A 200 g portion of reduced-fat *yoghurt* provides a similar range of nutrients to a 250 mL glass of reduced-fat milk but less lactose. (There is also a higher carbohydrate content if sugar is used to sweeten the yogurt.) In addition to the starter cultures, some types of yogurt contain probiotic organisms, which can survive the passage through the gastrointestine and have been shown to benefit gastrointestinal health.

Cheese is made using some or all of the following processes: standardization and pasteurization of the milk, addition of rennet (chymosin) and starter cultures, coagulation of the milk, cutting and stirring of the curd, heating, salting, hooping, pressing, maturing and wrapping. The added salt provides flavour, helps to inhibit the growth of spoilage microorganisms, regulates the structure and assists in the ripening process of the cheese.

Cheese is a concentrated source of many of the nutrients found in milk, but is much lower in lactose. A 40 g portion of cheese (e.g. Cheddar) provides about the same amounts of energy and calcium as a 250 mL glass of whole milk but more fat and protein, vitamin A and vitamin K_2. The sodium content varies widely according to the type of cheese; for example, cottage cheese and Cheddar cheese contain about 200 mg and 650 mg per 100 g, respectively. There are probably about 1000 different varieties of cheese but most are not mass produced and from the viewpoint of their nutritional composition they can be grouped. Twenty-five different types are shown in the British food tables.

Left to settle, the fat naturally present in milk rises to the top of the milk. *Cream* consists of about equal proportions of water and dairy fat. If cream is shaken, beaten or churned, it turns into butter and butter-milk. Butter consists of about 80% dairy fat.

24.6.3 Health aspects

A number of randomized controlled studies have demonstrated that increased consumption of milk or other calcium-rich dairy foods increases bone mass at one or more skeletal sites during growth and helps to reduce age-related bone loss in adulthood.

The 2005 Dietary Guidelines for Americans state 'Adults and children should not avoid milk and milk products because of concerns that these foods lead to weight gain'. Indeed, some observational studies and some tightly controlled clinical trials suggest that consumption of three daily serves of calcium-rich dairy foods may assist in the maintenance of a healthy weight and, when included in a reduced-calorie diet, increase weight and body fat loss.

Milk fat, butter and cream containing mostly saturated fatty acids (10% of the fat is myristic) tend to raise plasma low-density-lipoprotein cholesterol and total cholesterol. Yet in ten cohort epidemiological studies, milk drinking has not been associated with increased cardiovascular disease. Comparing cheese with butter (at the same dairy fat intake) in three separate sets of human experiments, the cheese raised plasma LDL cholesterol less than butter.

Collectively, the data from prospective cohort studies indicate that milk intake is associated with a reduced risk of colorectal cancer.

Milk is non-cariogenic (it neither promotes nor reduces the prevalence or incidence of dental caries), and cheese has cariostatic properties (it can help to reduce the risk of dental caries).

FURTHER READING

1. **Bersaglieri, T., Sabeti, P.C., Patterson, N.,** *et al.* (2004) Genetic signatures of strong recent positive selection at the lactase gene. *Am J Hum Genet*, **74**, 1111–20.

2. **Elwood, P.C., Pickering, J.E., Hughes, J., Fehily, A.M., and Ness, A.R.** (2004) Milk drinking, ischaemic heart disease and ischaemic stroke II. Evidence from cohort studies. *Eur J Clin Nutr*, **58**, 718–24.

3. **Miller, G.D., Jarvis, J.D., and McBean, L.D. (eds)** (1999) *Handbook of dairy foods and nutrition*. Florida, CRC Press.

4. **Nestel, P.J., Chronopoulos, A., and Cehun, M.** (2005) Dairy fat in cheese raises LDL-cholesterol less than in butter in mildly hypercholesterolaemic subjects. *Eur J Clin Nutr*, **59**, 1059–63.

24.7 Meat and poultry

Margaret Allman-Farinelli

There is evidence of primitive man hunting for animals from around 500 000 BC but it was not until the end of the last Ice Age (10 000–12 000 years ago) that humans began to domesticate animals along with the development of agriculture. The term 'meat' encompasses not only the muscle tissues but also organs like liver, kidneys and pancreas (termed offal). The major animals nowadays reared for human consumption are pigs, cattle and sheep, and birds like chicken and turkey. More unusual meats that are consumed include seals by the Eskimos, kangaroos in Australia, deer in Europe (venison), antelopes in Africa and guinea-pigs in South America.

Muscle meat is generally a good source of protein and minerals, while offal meats offer a rich source of vitamins. Muscle is rich in indispensable amino acids, particularly sulphur amino acids. The greater the proportion of muscle to connective tissue, the greater the digestibility of the protein and its biological value. The mineral content is high with potassium

Table 24.7 Nutrient content of meats

Nutrient	Nutrients per 100 g cooked meats			
	Beef (grilled steak)	Lamb (grilled chop)	Pork (grilled chop)	Chicken (roast, no skin)
Protein (g)	28.6	27.8	32.3	24.8
Fat (g)	6.0	12.3	10.7	5.4
Saturated fatty acids	2.5	5.9	3.8	1.6
Monounsaturated fatty acids	2.8	4.6	4.1	2.5
Polyunsaturated fatty acids	0.2	0.6	1.5	1.0
Carbohydrate (g)	0.0	0.0	0.0	0.0
Vitamin B_{12} (μg)	2	2	2	trace
Iron (mg)	3.5	2.1	1.2	0.8
Zinc (mg)	5.3	4.1	3.5	1.5

Source: Holland, B., Welch., A.A., Unwin, I.D., Buss, D.H., Paul, A.A., and Southgate, D.A.T. (1991) *McCance and Widdowson's: The composition of foods*, 5th edition. London, Royal Society of Chemistry, MAFF.

and phosphorus accounting for the largest proportion. Meat is a major source of readily available iron and zinc, and a good source of magnesium. Liver and kidney are richer in iron and zinc than muscle, and pig liver contains more than that from sheep or beef. The bioavailability of minerals from meat is superior to that from cereal and other plant foods. Meat provides a valuable source of thiamin, niacin and riboflavin, with pork higher in thiamin than the other meats. Organ meats contain more vitamins A and B_{12}, especially liver because this is where these vitamins are stored (Table 24.7). Liver is so rich in vitamin A that it is no longer advised for pregnant women because too much vitamin A is teratogenic.

In a number of Western countries, there has been a decline in the consumption of meat, especially red meat. One of the reasons is the perceived threat to good health. In the past, meats had a higher fat content. The fat was largely saturated and it is well known that saturated fat will raise plasma cholesterol. However, there is some question as to whether the major fatty acid constituents of meat, palmitic and stearic acids, will raise cholesterol. Animal producers have made large efforts over the past couple of decades to

breed leaner animals and butchers have been altering the type of cuts and trimming meats. This means that the fat content of lean meat is less than many consumers perceive. Meat also contains unsaturated fat including the very-long-chain fatty acid, arachidonic acid, which is a predominant polyunsaturated fatty acid in cell membranes. Humans can produce this from linoleic acid in vegetable oils, but an intake of preformed arachidonic acid may be important in pregnant and lactating women and the infant for optimal development of the infant brain and retina.

Meat is made into a range of products by curing (e.g. ham and bacon) and by the addition of cereals (e.g. sausages). There is some concern about the nitrate used to cure meat because the nitrites formed have been linked with nitrosamine and cancer in animals. However, the amount permitted to be used has been lowered to the minimum that prevents bacterial growth and we actually obtain more nitrites via conversion of nitrates from plant foods (which obtain it from the soil).

Nutritionists who have researched Paleolithic diets—which all humans lived on before the agricultural revolution—conclude that meats and offal on average provided a higher proportion of total dietary energy and nutrients for our ancestors than they do today, i.e. *Homo sapiens* evolved on a relatively high-meat diet.

Meat provides satiety and it appears to be useful in a low-calorie diet for weight reduction, for example, as part of the 'CSIRO total wellbeing diet'.

Meat has a short shelf-life and must be kept at low temperatures and be cooked adequately to prevent microbial growth. The mode of cooking may be important. Frying or grilling on a hot plate may lead to the development of heterocyclic amines shown to be mutagenic. However, it cannot necessarily be extrapolated that these cause cancer in humans. The relationship between red meat consumption and the development of cancer remains debatable. In the cohort epidemiological studies, any association of red meat with colorectal cancer is very small but processed meats seem to increase the relative risk. The most recent concern for meat eaters is the development of 'mad cow disease' (bovine spongiform encephalopathy) in British beef. The link between eating affected meat and neurological disease in man (Creutzfeldt–Jakob disease) has been difficult to understand but as a precaution millions of cattle were destroyed (Chapter 25).

Chicken and turkey meats are consumed in growing amounts in countries like the USA and Australasia. Much of this is because people are selecting 'white' meat over red meat because they believe it to be healthier. More exotic birds consumed include pigeon, pheasant and partridge. It is not only the muscle that is consumed but also parts like the feet (in China), the liver (goose paté) and even the head. Poultry is a good source of protein, with the fat content dependent on the individual bird; for example, turkey is leaner than chicken, which is leaner than goose or duck. Much of the fat is located just under the skin and can be removed easily. Like red meat, poultry is a good source of protein and minerals, including iron and zinc.

FURTHER READING

1. **Cordain, L., Brand Miller, J., Boyd Eaton, S., Mann, N., Holt, S.H.A., and Speth, J.D.** (2000) Plant-animal subsistence ratios and macronutrient energy estimations in world wide hunter-gatherer diets. *Am J Clin Nutr*, **71**, 682–92.

2. **Lawrie, R. (ed.)** (1998) *Lawrie's meat science*, 6th edition. Cambridge, Woodhead Publishing.

3. **Norat, T., Bingham, S., Ferrari, P., *et al*.** (2005) Meat, fish and colorectal cancer risk: the European prospective investigation into cancer and nutrition. *J Natl Cancer Inst*, **97**, 906–16.

4. **Truswell, A.S.** (2002) Meat consumption and cancer of the large bowel. *Eur J Clin Nutr*, **56**, S19–S24.

24.8 Fish and seafood

Samir Samman

Man has searched rivers, lakes and the seas for food since the earliest times. Today most fish are still caught in the oceans, rivers and lakes but some are produced under intensive farm conditions. Usually, the main edible parts are the flesh but other components, such as roe, are eaten also. Fish, like meat, contains protein of high biological value. The recent nutritional interest in fish, however, is the fat content, which ranges from 0.5% to 15%. It varies according to season and environmental factors such as water temperature. In canned fish, more of the fat may be contributed by the oil used in packaging or cooking than by the fish itself. Fish oils contain long-chain ω-3 polyunsaturated fatty acids, mainly eicosapentaenoic acid (EPA) and docosahexaenoic acid (DHA). Because of the highly polyunsaturated fats, fish decomposes rapidly.

There is very little carbohydrate in fish and quite small amounts of cholesterol (more in fish roe). It is not usually a good source of fat-soluble vitamins, such as vitamin E, but fish liver and whole-body fish like sardines provide vitamin D. Fish is, however, a source of vitamin B_6, B_{12}, riboflavin, folate and most

Table 24.8 Nutrient content of fish

Nutrient	Nutrients per 100 g raw edible portion
Protein (g)	11.2 (steamed plaice) to 23.8 (steamed halibut)
Fat (g)	0.6 (steamed haddock) to 13.0 (grilled herring)
Calcium (mg)	22.0 (baked cod) to 550 (sardines in oil, drained)
Iron (mg)	0.4 (baked cod) to 4.6 (sardines in tomato sauce)
Zinc (mg)	0.5 (baked cod) to 3.5 (anchovies)

Source: Holland, B., Welch., A.A., Unwin, I.D., Buss, D.H., Paul, A.A., and Southgate, D.A.T. (1991) *McCance and Widdowson's: The composition of foods*, 5th edition. London, Royal Society of Chemistry.

inorganic nutrients, notably iodine, selenium and fluoride. Calcium, although not found in high amounts in fish flesh, can be eaten as part of the edible soft bones (as in sardines). Sodium content is usually low, but as with fat it can be introduced as part of the processing (e.g. fish canned in brine).

Fish obtained from cold, clear, deep water are generally more flavoursome than those obtained from warm, muddy, shallow water. Sauces and garnishes are often used to enhance the flavour of fish, the cooking methods determined by the fish's fat content. Fatty fish, for example, salmon or mullet, is usually grilled or baked, whereas lean fish, for example, whiting or cod, is fried. Undercooked fish can present some problems such as tapeworms, which deplete vitamin B_{12}, and thiaminase, which destroys thiamin. Other potential hazards associated with the consumption of fish are: toxic metal contamination (such as by mercury), or tetradoxin poisoning (which is mainly associated with puffer fish), poisoning by dinoflagellates (*Ciguatera*) and bacterial spoilage, particularly in tuna. The major food authorities advise that pregnant women, women planning pregnancy and young children should limit their intake of large fish species at the top of the food chain or those that live a long time, as these may accumulate higher levels of mercury.

The health benefits of fish consumption are considerable. Long-term fish consumption may reduce death from heart disease. Fatty fish appears to be the most protective and benefits are most obvious in high-risk populations. These effects may be attributable to

the ω-3 fatty acids in the fatty-fish flesh, which can reduce the risk of dangerous arrhythmia and also reduce thrombotic tendency by an array of mechanisms. For individuals at high risk of coronary heart disease, the American Heart Association encourages increased intake of ω-3 polyunsaturated fatty acids up to 1 g of EPA and DHA per day from food sources and supplements. With the growth of the world population and increased size of fishing boats and nets, fish species in some seas have meanwhile been depleted of wild fish.

Shellfish are nowadays a luxury food for most people. They have similar nutritional characteristics to fish. The sterols they contain are not cholesterol, as was once thought. Oysters are rich in zinc. Some coastal societies notably the Japanese enjoy seaweeds, and green, brown and red algae ('vegetables from the sea'), often cultivated. They have a high iodine content.

FURTHER READING

1. He, K., Song, Y., Daviglus, M.L., *et al*. (2004) Accumulated evidence on fish consumption and coronary heart disease mortality: a meta-analysis of cohort studies. *Circulation*, **109**, 2705–11.

2. **Markmann, P., and Gronbaek, M.** (1999) Fish consumption and coronary heart disease mortality. A systematic review of prospective cohort studies. *Eur J Clin Nutr*, **53**, 585–90.

3. **Ruiter, A. (ed.)** (1995) *Fish and fishery products. Composition, nutritive properties and stability*. Wallingford UK, CAB International.

24.9 Eggs

Kim Bell-Anderson

For Harold McGee, 'the egg is one of the kitchen's marvels and one of nature's. . . . The cook can use eggs to generate such a variety of structures'. The egg is a convenient nutritional package providing high-biological-value protein, rich in essential amino acids, and is an excellent source of micronutrients (Table 24.9). Eggs have often been associated with raised cholesterol levels, however recent cohort studies suggest that consumption of up to one egg per day has little effect on serum cholesterol and only increases the risk of cardiovascular disease marginally in the normal, healthy population. It is still not clear if the risk is greater in individuals with hyperlipidaemia and/or type 2 diabetes.

An egg is an ideal source of nutrition for pregnant women as it supplies extra kilojoules, protein and important micronutrients such as iron, zinc, folate and vitamin B_{12}. Children benefit from eggs as a good source of riboflavin and zinc (often both are low in children's diets) and vitamin A, which is essential for growth and eye health. An egg makes a good centre of a meal for someone eating at home on their own. Egg allergy is more common in children under 2 years, with egg tolerance usually developing between the ages of 2 and 4 years. The egg white, which is mainly protein, is the main source of allergens.

Eggs are a bioavailable source of the antioxidants lutein and zeaxanthin which may help to maintain normal vision. Antioxidant (lutein)-enhanced eggs are available in some countries. Other 'designer' eggs may be enriched in vitamin C, selenium or ω-3 fatty acids. These changes are achieved by changing the hens' rations.

FURTHER READING

1. **Hu, F.B., Stampfer, M.J., Rimm, E.B.,** *et al*. (1999) A prospective study of egg consumption and risk of cardiovascular disease in men and women. *J Am Med Assoc*, **281**, 1387–94.

2. **McGee, H.** (2004) On food and cooking. *The science and lore of the kitchen*. New York, Scribner.

Table 24.9 Nutrient content and % recommended dietary intake (RDI) of one egg

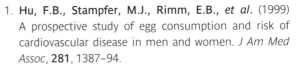

Nutrient	Per egg	% RDI	Nutrient	Per egg	% RDI
Energy (kJ)	267.0	3.0	Calcium (mg)	30.0	3.7
Protein (g)	5.8	11.5	Iron (mg)	0.7	
Fat (g)	4.5	6.5	Selenium (μg)	14.0	20.0
Saturated (g)	1.4	6.0	Riboflavin (mg)	0.2	10.0
Monounsaturated (g)	1.9		Niacin equ (mg)	1.6	16.0
Polyunsaturated (g)	0.45		Vitamin B_{12} (μg)	0.5	25.0
ω-3 (g)	0.05	2.0*	Folate (μg)	22.0	11.0
Cholesterol (mg)	168.0		Vitamin A (μg)	72.0	10.0
Carbohydrate (g)	0.15		Lutein + zeaxanthin (μg)	131.0	

Values are for one raw egg (large, shell excluded) 45 g.
*= % adequate intake recommendation.
Source: Natoli, S. (2004) *Nutritional and health benefits of eggs*, 2nd edition. Sydney, Australian Egg Corporation Ltd.

24.10 Fats and oils

Ron Bowrey

The type and amount of fats consumed today is very different from the days of the hunter-gatherer when lean animals were eaten and fat came from some seeds and nuts. It is necessary for the diet to provide the essential fatty acids, but in most developed countries obtaining sufficient amounts of fat is rarely a problem. Overconsumption of fats and oils, particularly saturated fat, is of far greater concern. The main sources of dietary fat are meats, dairy products, and vegetable oils and spreads and their associated products. During the past 30 years, the type of fat consumed has changed from predominantly animal sources like butter and lard towards vegetable-derived fats and oils. The knowledge that saturated fat is associated with raising blood cholesterol and risk of coronary heart disease has resulted in the emphasis on consumption of more unsaturated fats. Consumer demand has seen the development and production of new oils and margarines. However, the diet remains high in saturated fats because lifestyle changes have resulted in greater use of preprepared foods inside the home and food outside the home that are manufactured with saturated fats and oils.

The bulk of edible fats and oils is made up of triglycerides (i.e. three fatty acids on a glycerol backbone). The predominant fatty acid present in the oil or fat will determine whether it is classified as a saturated, monounsaturated or polyunsaturated fat (see Table 24.10). Hence, canola, which has oleic acid as its major fatty acid, is called a monounsaturate, safflower with linoleic acid as the predominant fatty acid is a polyunsaturate, and butter is a saturate. Fats and oils also contribute fat-soluble vitamins to the diet especially vitamin E and vitamin D in margarines. Table 24.11 lists the minor constituents of fats and oils.

Animal fats are usually obtained by a process called rendering. This involves heating or steaming to remove the adipose tissue from the animal carcass. These fats

Table 24.10 Fatty acid composition of common fats and oils

Fat/oil	Saturates (%)	Monounsaturates (%)	Polyunsaturates (%)
Butter fat	64	33[a]	3
Canola	7	63	30
Coconut	91	7	2
Cottonseed	26	22	51
Olive	14	76	10
Palm	51	39	10
Peanut	19	45	36
Safflower	9	14	77
Soybean oil	15	23	62
Sunflower (high oelic)	10	85	5
Sunflower	11	23	66
Tallow	50	47[a]	3

[a]Tallow and butter fat contain about 5% *trans* fatty acids and appear as monounsaturates in this table.

Table 24.11 Minor constituents of fats and oils

Fat/oil	Minor constituents
Monoglycerides and diglycerides	One or two fatty acids esterified to glycerol
Free fatty acids	Not combined with any other molecule
Phospholipids	Also known as phosphatides
Sterols	Phytosterols (in plant oils), cholesterol (in animal fats)
Tocopherols	Vitamin E (antioxidant) compounds
Carotenoids	Yellow red colours
Chlorophyll	Green pigment
Vitamins	Vitamin E and perhaps A and D

are most commonly obtained from pigs (lard) and cattle (tallow). After rendering they may contain residual amounts of free fatty acids, water and protein, all of which must be removed for a high-quality product. Fats and oils derived from animal sources contain cholesterol and are usually high in saturated fat.

Vegetable oils and fats are obtained from a wide variety of plants. They can be obtained from seeds (canola (rapeseed), sunflower, cottonseed, safflower and palm), legumes (soybean and peanuts), fruits (olive) and nuts (almond and walnut). Vegetable oils are pressed from seeds or nuts and then the unwanted components, such as colour pigments, phosphatides and free fatty acids, are usually removed. Solvent extraction may also be used to remove residual fat from the meal. Further processing or refining is usually required when specific sensory properties or functions are required. This produces a clear, high-quality oil that is suitable for use as an ingredient, for frying, salad dressings, mayonnaise, and the production of margarine and shortenings. Most crushing of seeds, nuts and fruits requires a cooking stage prior to pressing to increase oil yields. A cold-pressed oil has this step omitted and the temperature during pressing is controlled. Cold-pressed oils tend to have stronger flavours and odours, which may be desirable in certain foods, but there is little nutritional difference between the two types. Close attention is paid to minimizing the loss of vitamin E during the extraction process.

Margarine is a water-in-oil emulsion produced from vegetable oils (liquid at ambient temperature) and fat (solid or semi-solid 'hard' fraction). The hard fraction is essential to give solidity to the margarine and is produced by interesterification. An older process termed hydrogenation is used less commonly now as it produces *trans* fatty acids. By blending interesterified fats with liquid oils in varying proportions, the functional and nutritional properties can be altered. Water, skimmed-milk powder, salt, lecithin emulsifiers, colours, flavours and vitamins are added to the blend. Margarine spreads containing approximately 40% less fat are becoming popular (as reduced-energy products). These products have the spreading and organoleptic properties of full-fat products but should not be used for cooking or baking because of their high water content.

Other commodities based around fats and oils include animal and vegetable shortenings (with no water, salt or milk) used by the baking industry and frying oils (stable to heat and moisture) for domestic, small-scale food outlets and large-scale food production. Salad dressings and mayonnaises are oil-in-water emulsions. Mayonnaise is about 80% oil, which is 'winterized' to prevent crystal formation upon refrigeration that would break the emulsion. For baking and frying, saturated fats such as palm oil and coconut oil and tallow and lard are still commonly used because they provide the sensory and functional properties that are required, as well as being stable. The way a biscuit melts in the mouth is important, and also a more saturated oil avoids the problem of oxidation producing off-flavours. Newer products such as high-oleic sunflower oil and blends of vegetable and hydrogenated vegetable fat are now finding their way into the baking and frying sector of the food industry.

FURTHER READING

1. **FAO/WHO** (1994) *Fats and oils in human nutrition.* Report of a Joint Expert Consultation. Rome, Food and Agricultural Organization.

2. **Gunstone, F.D. (ed.)** (2004) *Chemistry of oils and fats.* Oxford, Blackwell.

24.11 Fat replacers
Stewart Truswell

The push to produce low-fat and fat-free products becomes stronger as the consumers in developed nations battle obesity and heart disease. Fat replacers are ingredients that recreate the attributes of fat without providing the dietary energy. The success of fat replacement in foods is dependent on the ability to recreate the texture, mouthfeel, appearance and flavour of the original food. Fat mimetics replace the mouthfeel and texture of fats but do not possess all of the physical and chemical properties. Fat substitutes, however, resemble the triglyceride structure and can be used to replace fat on a gram-for-gram basis (Table 24.12).

Fat mimetics may be based on starch, cellulose or protein, or may be hydrophilic colloids. Starch may be modified by acid or enzymic hydrolysis to yield smaller polymers like maltodextrin or β-glucan, or glucose may be polymerized to give polydextrose. Cellulose may be modified to microcrystalline aggregates. Protein-based products include those made from skimmed milk and egg whites, which are micro-

Table 24.12 Examples of fat replacers

Mimetics	Name
Starch-based	Starch hydrolysis product (SHP) N-Oil (National Starch and Chemical Corp., Bridgewater, NJ) Maltrin M040 Maltodextrin (Grain Processing Corp., Muscatine, IA)
Gums	Carrageenan (Carrageenan Marketing Corp., Santa Ana, CA) Gum arabic Alginates
Polysaccharide-based	Cellulose (microcrystalline, modified) Fibercel (α-Beta Technologies, Cambridge, MA) Oatrim (Rhône Poulenc, Cranbury, NJ)
Protein-based	Simplesse (NutraSweet Co., Skokie, IL) Dairylite (John Labatt Ltd, Ault Foods London, Canada)
Synthetic 'triglyceride-like' substitutes	Caprenin (Procter and Gamble, Cincinnati, OH; Grinsted Products, Kansas City, MO) Dailkyldihexadeclymalonate (DDM) (Frito-Lay Inc., Dallas, TX) Olestra sucrose polyester (Proctor and Gamble, Cincinnati, OH)

particulated. Hydrocolloids and gums will provide mouthfeel, juiciness and thickening. All the mimetics are soluble or dispersible in the water phase and will retain moisture. They cannot be used to replace oil for frying because they may denature and burn or will not melt. Applications of mimetics include their use in ice cream, frozen desserts, confectionery, salad dressings, cheese spreads, dairy-type foods and baked goods.

Fat substitutes have the same functionality as fat. Synthetic substitutes are either resistant or partially resistant to the action of lipase in the gut and hence contribute nil or a lower energy content. The best known is sucrose polyester ('Olestra'), which consists of a sugar backbone with fatty acids esterified to the sugar. They have the potential to replace fat in a wide variety of foods including fried foods like potato chips and snack food. Some caution needs to be exercised because diarrhoea or malabsorption of soluble vitamins may occur with excessive consumption.

FURTHER READING

1. **Truswell, A.S.** (1995) Dietary fat. Some aspects of nutrition and health and product development. Brussels, ILSI Europe.

24.12 Herbs and spices
Kim Bell-Anderson

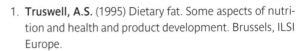

The supply of exotic spices such as cinnamon, mace and nutmeg to sixteenth and seventeenth century Europe from Asia did much more than contribute distinct flavours to the creation of new food cultures —it helped to define sea routes across the globe. The quest for spices from Asia and America played a major role in shaping the European exploration of the world.

Spices are defined as parts of dried seed, bark or root. The definition of herbs used for culinary purposes is the fresh or dried leaves of a plant; in herbal medicine the term more loosely includes any part of a plant that contributes savoury, aromatic or medicinal properties.

As well as adding distinctive flavour to food and drink, herbs and spices have traditionally been used for spiritual fulfilment and for their medicinal qualities. Before the development of synthetic drugs in the nineteenth century, herbs were the major ingredient in medicines; even now plant extracts are present in many prescription drugs.

Herbs and spices impart overwhelming flavour and aroma to food due to the fusion of volatile chemicals concentrated within the plants. The major chemical families from which these aroma compounds are derived are the terpenes and the phenolics. Terpenes are extremely volatile and reactive molecules, which often contribute to the first flavour or aroma we detect, and quickly dissipate upon heating. Phenolics contribute a more persistent flavour and are more likely to be found in spices. Some spices are valued not for their aroma but for their pungency, which imparts an irritating sensation that is pleasurable. The chemicals responsible include thiocyanates, found in mustards, ginger, horseradish and wasabi; and alkylamides, for example capsaicin, found in chilli.

Herbs and spices typically contribute minimally to nutrient intake, although some may be a significant source of calcium and iron (e.g. parsley) if eaten in large enough quantities. They are also rich in phosphorus, manganese and zinc. Fresh herbs contain substantial amounts of β-carotene and vitamin C, although drying and grinding of herbs will reduce their content. The health-promoting properties of herbs and spices can be mainly attributed to their active phytochemical content, in particular the phenolics and terpenes. Terpenes have been shown to help reduce the body's production of DNA-damaging molecules. Phenolics are powerful antioxidants, and high antioxidant activity has been reported in oregano, sage, peppermint, thyme, bay leaf, dill, rosemary, turmeric, cloves, allspice, cinnamon and marjoram (50–100 mmol/100 g). Consumption of 1 g of these herbs and spices could make a relevant contribution (> 1 mmol) to the dietary intake of antioxidants.

The American National Cancer Institute has recognized some commonly used herbs as having anticarcinogenic qualities. These include basil, mint, oregano, rosemary, sage, thyme, turmeric, ginger, liquorice root, caraway, coriander, cumin, dill, parsley and tarragon. Turmeric is highly valued for its active ingredient curcumin, which has been shown to suppress the development of tumours in the stomach, breast, lung and skin. Curcumin is also known for its anti-inflammatory properties in humans.

Other physiological effects of herbs and spices include hypocholesterolaemia and hypolipidaemia (fenugreek, garlic), anticoagulant, antiemetic (ginger) and immune-stimulating (liquorice).

There are thousands of active phytochemicals in herbs and spices and there is little information known about the bioavailability and bioactivity of these compounds. Furthermore, the concentrations of these chemicals are subject to seasonal variation, species variety and agricultural processes. It should also be noted that some herbs and spices may be toxic in high amounts.

Seasoning meals with a generous amount of herbs and spices to enhance flavour and increase the appeal and consumption of nutritious foods is a useful means of promoting health, protecting against chronic disease and reducing our reliance on salt as a flavour enhancer.

FURTHER READING

1. **Craig, W.J.** (1999) Health-promoting properties of common herbs. *Am J Clin Nutr*, **70**, 491S–99S.

2. **Greenberg, S., and Ortiz, E.L.** (1983) *The spice of life*. London, Mermaid Books/Channel 4 TV.

3. **McGee, H.** (2004) *McGee on Food and Cooking*. Great Britain, Hodder and Stoughton.

24.13 Food processing
Stewart Truswell

All the foods we eat are living matter, made of cells that contain enzymes, and many foods, especially those of animal origin, are inhabited by microorganisms. Hence food processing is necessary to prevent food decaying and to keep it safe for consumption. Food processing destroys the growth of microorganisms, including pathogens like *Salmonella* and *Listeria*, and will inactivate autolytic enzymes and some natural toxins (e.g. trypsin inhibitors). The storage life of the food is increased, which means that it can be grown some distance from the point of consumption. This enables us to benefit from economies of scale by growing large quantities of food on the most suitable land. Not all processing involves food preservation; some also improves the appearance and flavour of foods, and convenience. One of the major considerations of modern consumers is the ease and speed with which a meal can be prepared, and more meals are now consumed away from the home. Food processing is essential to meet these consumer needs.

24.13.1 Methods of food processing

Many methods involve *reduction of water content* so that microorganisms cannot grow and autolytic enzymes are inhibited. One of the earliest methods of food preservation used was drying. The ancient Greeks sun-dried grapes to produce raisins, which lasted longer than the fresh fruits because of their low water content. In addition to sun drying and smoking of foods, modern technology includes tunnel drying, spray drying and freeze drying of food to make milk powders, egg powders and coffee powders.

Freezing, while not removing the water, changes it into a form that is unavailable for normal enzyme functions, and the low temperature decreases both bacterial growth and enzyme activity. Addition of salt (as in salting of fish) or inclusion of sugar (as in jams) also prevents bacterial growth because of their osmotic effects.

Heat is used in several ways to prevent food spoilage and microbial growth. Pasteurization of milk by heating to 72°C for 15 seconds destroys pathogenic organisms. Blanching of food (75–95°C for 1 to 8 minutes) before freezing and canning inactivates autolytic enzymes. Canned and sealed foods are sterilized by the application of heat.

Many fruits and vegetables are foods with particularly short shelf-lives. If people are to meet the recommendations made by various health authorities to increase fruit and vegetable consumption, some processing is essential. Fresh fruits need to be harvested and stored using modern technology to increase year-round availability and distribution around the globe. Bananas are picked before they are ripe and shipped and stored at a *controlled temperature* until they are ripened by exposure to ethylene gas (which is naturally given off during ripening of bananas). Californian oranges may be consumed in New Zealand and New Zealand kiwi fruit in California when local production ceases seasonally.

Other food-processing methods include *milling* and *pressing*. Most cereal products such as wheat, maize and rice are subjected to varying amounts of crushing with metal rollers and sieving to separate coarse and fine components, which eventually produces the different flours and brans. *Pressing* is used to crush the juice from fruits like grapes and to press edible oils from oilseeds like canola and sunflower seeds.

Packaging and refrigeration also assist in preventing spoilage of food. Sealing sterilized foods in cans or vacuum packs prevents microbial growth because oxygen is unavailable. Refrigeration retards the multiplication of microorganisms (although some will still reproduce at 4°C).

Food irradiation is a newer technique that can be applied to foods, the flavour of which would be altered by heating (e.g. spices and strawberries). However, the employment of irradiation is an emotive issue (though food that has been irradiated is *not* radioactive) and the practice is restricted by legislation in many countries at present. Food irradiation also can be used to inhibit sprouting of potatoes, delay the ripening of fruits, and kill insect pests in fruit, grains or spices, reduce or eliminate food spoilage organisms and reduce microorganisms on meats and seafoods.

24.13.2 Food additives (see Table 24.13)

Chemical *preservatives* may be added to specific foods to prevent bacterial growth. Examples include benzoic acid, propionic acid, sorbic acid and sodium metabisulphite. *Antioxidants* may be added to slow the oxidation of oils and fats, preventing rancidity. *Fermentation* of products will produce acid or alcohol, both of which inhibit autolytic enzymes and bacterial growth.

Other food processing includes the addition of chemicals to provide a variety of functions. Additives such as *emulsifiers* keep the oil and aqueous phases together in mayonnaises and sauces. *Humectants* prevent food from drying out (e.g. glycerol in cake frostings). *Thickeners* may be added to sauces or jams to improve texture. *Anticaking agents* may be added to ensure that powdered foods do not become lumpy (e.g. flavoured coffee mixes). *Food acids* may be used for flavour or to adjust the pH for preservation reasons.

Some foods have their organoleptic properties enhanced by the addition of *colours* and *flavours*. About half of the colours used are from natural sources (e.g. β-carotene).

Artificial sweeteners are used to replace sugars and reduce the energy content of foods because they provide no calories. They have an intense sweet taste but some have other lesser tastes (e.g. bitter) and a better effect is often achieved by combining two different sweeteners. Saccharine and cyclamate break down with heat so they cannot be ingredient(s) before a food is cooked. All these sweeteners have been researched and monitored for safety; diabetics can consume relatively large amounts. Aspartame is a dipeptide of phenylalanine and aspartic acid. It should be avoided (it must be on the label) by people with phenylketonuria.

Flavours are usually a 'trade secret' so that the names of individual flavours are not declared on the label. However, in most developed nations, food

Table 24.13 Some common food additives, the code number used in the European Union and other countries and one of the foods or drinks to which it is added

Food additive	Code number	Foods
Preservatives		
Benzoic acid	210	Fruit juices
Lactic acid	270	White bread
Fumaric acid	297	Confectionery
Propionic acid	280	Bread
Sodium metabisulphite	223	Wine
Sorbic acid	200	Cheesecake
Antioxidants		
Ascorbic acid	300	Stock cubes
Butylated hydroxyanisole	320	Ice cream
Propyl gallate	310	Gelatin desserts
α-Tocopherols	307	Oils
Emulsifiers		
Lecithins	322	Chocolate
Mono- and diglycerides of fatty acids	471	Potato crisps
Humectants		
Glycerol	422	Pastilles
Sorbitol	420	Chewing gum
Thickeners		
Alginic acid	400	Ice cream
Guar gum	412	Salad dressings
Methyl cellulose	461	Jelly
Pectin	440	Jams
Xanthan gum	415	Bottled sauces
Anticaking agents		
Magnesium carbonate	504	Icing sugar
Food acids		
Acetic acid	260	Tomato ketchup
Citric acid	330	Marmalades
Malic acid	296	Canned tomatoes

Table 24.13 (*cont'd*)

Food additive	Code number	Foods
Colours		
β-Carotene	160a	Margarines
Canthaxanthin	161g	Biscuits
Curcumin	100	Curry powder
Erythrosine	127	Glacé cherries
Artificial sweeteners		
Saccharine	954	Tea and coffee
Cyclamate	952	Tea and coffee
Aspartame	951	Soft drinks
Acesulphame K	950	Baked goods

legislation only permits those that have been shown to be safe. In the USA they are known as GRAS, meaning 'generally regarded as safe'.

Other types of food additive are *vitamins* or *minerals*. Some foods may have their micronutrient content restored (e.g. the thiamin removed with the bran during milling of flour is replaced), while other food may be fortified (for example, foods are being fortified with folic acid because of the difficulty for women of childbearing age to obtain adequate amounts in the diet). Vitamins may be added to a food that becomes a replacement for a food in which the vitamin naturally occurs; such an example is margarine to which vitamin A and D are added, both occurring in butter.

24.13.3 Safety aspects of food additives

A series of strict tests must be conducted before a food additive is permitted. The Food and Agriculture Organization/World Health Organization (FAO/WHO) have a joint expert committee on food additives (JECFA) and most countries have an expert body that prepares food legislation, for example the US Food and Drug Administration (FDA), the European Scientific Committee for Food, and the food authority of Australia and New Zealand (Foods Standards Australia New Zealand, FSANZ). The acute toxicity of the additive must be tested in both male and female animals in a minimum of three species and distribution of the compound in the body is assayed. Short-term feeding trials are conducted in at least two species of animal (only one can be a rodent) and reproduction is studied over two generations. After this, both mutagenicity and carcinogenicity are tested for in bacteria and tissue culture. Effects of food additives in humans are continually reviewed. It is not sufficiently realized that the most likely toxic substances in our foods are naturally occurring ones rather than food additives. Additives are the most thoroughly monitored and tested of all chemicals in the food supply chain (see also Chapter 25).

24.13.4 Effects of food processing on nutrient content

Some nutrient losses will occur during processing but domestic cooking also results in appreciable losses of vitamins and leaching of minerals. Most labile of the vitamins are vitamin C and folate, which are unstable with heat, although low pH will protect vitamin C (Table 24.14). The losses during processing by the food industry are standardized and easily quantified, unlike those in domestic kitchens. In some cases, the nutrient content may be greater when using a processed food than preparing it from the raw product in a domestic kitchen.

24.13.5 Conclusion

Food processing allows an abundant, year-round pathogen-free food supply. No pregnant woman would debate the importance of pasteurization of milk to remove bacteria that could cause miscarriage. Some nutrient losses are inevitable upon processing but they are not usually sizeable. The impact of nutrient loss will be dependent on the overall composition of the diet (e.g. milling and polishing of rice would only precipitate thiamin deficiency in those people who eat nothing else). If it were not for processing, the food would be unavailable for consumption throughout the year and the nutrient may be missed altogether.

Table 24.14 The effect of freezing and boiling on vitamin C content of selected vegetables

Food	Vitamin C mg/100 g
Brussels sprouts (raw)	115
Brussels sprouts (boiled)	60
Brussels sprouts (frozen, boiled)	69
Peas (boiled)	16
Peas (frozen, boiled)	12

Source: Food Standards Agency (2002) *McCance and Widdowson's, the composition of foods*, 6th Summary Edition. Royal Society of Chemistry, Cambridge.

FURTHER READING

1. **Coultate, T.P.** (2002) *Food: The chemistry of its components*, 4th edition. York, UK, Royal Society of Chemistry.

2. **International Food Information Service** (2005) *Dictionary of food science and technology*. Oxford, Blackwell.

3. **FAO/IAEA/WHO** (1999) *High dose irradiation: wholesomeness of food irradiated with doses above 10 kGy*. Report of a Joint Study Group. WHO Technical Report Series 890. Geneva, World Health Organization.

 To see topical and scientifically robust updates on nutrition associated with this textbook, and active web links to many of the journal articles in the Reference areas, please see the dedicated Online Resource Centre at www.oxfordtextbooks.co.uk/orc/mann3e/.

25 Food toxicity and safety

Peter Williams

Until recently, eating food in modern industrialized countries has usually been regarded as a low-risk activity, but several highly publicized food safety scares have raised consumer concerns about the safety of our food supplies (Table 25.1).

Very few of the foods that we commonly eat have been subject to any toxicological testing and yet they are generally accepted as being safe to eat. However,

Table 25.1 A chronology of recent food scares

1986	First cases of 'mad cow' disease in Britain
1990	Benzene in Perrier mineral water in France
1996	*Salmonella* in peanut butter in Australia
1997	Contagious swine fever in The Netherlands
1999	Contaminated Coca-Cola in Belgium
1999	Pollen from genetically modified maize reported to kill Monarch butterflies
2001	Foot-and-mouth disease all over Europe
2002	Acrylamide found in starchy foods cooked at high temperature
2003	Outbreak of bird flu in Asian poultry
2004	Warnings about mercury in shark, mackerel and swordfish in the USA

all chemicals, including those naturally found in foods, are toxic at some dose. Laboratory animals can be killed by feeding them glucose or salt at very high doses, and some nutrients such as vitamin A and selenium are hazardous at intakes only a few times greater than normal human requirements. Even very common foods such as pepper have demonstrated carcinogenic activity. Toxicity testing of a food or ingredient can tell us what the likely adverse effects are and at what level of consumption they may occur, but by itself this does not tell us whether it is safe to eat in normally consumed amounts.

'Risk' is the probability that the substance will produce injury under defined conditions of exposure. The concept of risk takes into account the dose and length of exposure as well as the toxicity of a particular chemical, and is a better guide to the safety of a food. For example, although it is well known that potatoes contain solanine—a poisonous alkaloid—at normal levels of consumption eating potatoes as they are normally prepared is not a risk to health; in other words, the solanine in potatoes is toxic but not usually hazardous.

Consequently, any attempt to examine the safety of the food supply should not be based on the question 'Is this food or ingredient toxic?' (the answer is always 'yes') but rather by finding out if eating this substance in normal amounts is likely to increase the risk of illness significantly—i.e. 'Is it safe?'

25.1 Hazardous substances in food

Three general classes of hazards are found in foods: (1) microbial or environmental *contaminants*, (2) naturally occurring toxic *constituents*, and (3) those resulting from intentional food *additives* or *novel foods or ingredients*. The most dangerous contaminants are those produced by infestations of bacteria or moulds in food, which can produce toxins that remain in the food even after the biological source has been destroyed. Other contaminants, such as pesticide residues or heavy metals, are usually well controlled in modern food supplies but can be significant hazards in particular localities. Naturally occurring toxic constituents can be considered normal and unavoidable. They are usually present in doses

Table 25.2 Potential hazard in foods

Hazards	Examples
Microbial contamination	
Pathogenic bacteria	Toxins from *Clostridium botulinum*
Mycotoxins	Aflatoxin from mould on peanuts
Environmental contamination	
Heavy metals and mineral	Arsenic and mercury in fish
Criminal adulteration	Aniline in olive oil
Packaging migration	PVC from plastics
Industrial pollution	Polychlorinated biphenyls, radioactive fallout
Changes during cooking or processing	Carcinogens produced in burnt meat
Natural toxins	
Inherent toxins	Cyanide in cassava
Produced by abnormal conditions	Ciguatera poisoning from fish
Enzyme inhibitors	Protease inhibitors in legumes
Antivitamins	Avidin in raw egg white
Mineral-binding agents	Goitrogens in brassica vegetables
Agricultural residues	
Pesticides	DDT
Hormones	Bovine somatotrophin
Intentional food additives	
Artificial sweeteners	Cyclamate
Preservatives	Sodium nitrite

DDT = dichloro-diphenyl-trichloroethane; PVC = polyvinyl chloride.

that are too small to produce harmful effects when foods are eaten normally, except in the cases of atypical consumers who may be allergic to individual ingredients. Food additives or novel foods are generally the least dangerous hazards because their toxicology is well studied and the conditions of use are tightly controlled. Table 25.2 summarizes the types of hazardous substances that may be present in food.

The US Food and Drug Administration (FDA) has ranked the relative importance of health hazards associated with food in the following descending order of seriousness:

1. Microbiological contamination
2. Inappropriate eating habits
3. Environmental contamination
4. Natural toxic constituents
5. Pesticide residues
6. Food additives

This list is very different from that found in public opinion polls, which show that most people rate food additives as one of their major concerns about the safety of the food supply.

25.2 Microbial contamination

25.2.1 Pathogenic bacteria

Outbreaks of acute gastroenteritis caused by microbial pathogens are usually called food poisoning. They can be caused by foodborne intoxication—where microbes in food produce a toxin that produces the symptom—or foodborne infection—where the symptoms are caused by the activity of live bacterial cells multiplying in the gastrointestinal system. Table 25.3 lists the most common bacterial causes of food poisoning, in order of the rapidity of onset of symptoms. In general, the intoxications have a more rapid onset.

The most important pathogens are *Clostridium botulinum*, *Staphylococcus aureus*, *Salmonella* species and *Clostridium perfringens*. The last three organisms account for about 70–80% of all reported outbreaks of foodborne illness, but there are many others, as well as some viral and protozoan agents. The four most frequently identified factors contributing to food poisoning incidents are improper cooling of food (44%), lapses of 12 hours or more between preparing and eating (23%), contamination by food handlers (18%) and contaminated raw foods or ingredients (16%).

The reported incidence and cost of foodborne illness in most countries is increasing, although it is difficult to measure this exactly. Collection of data on foodborne illness is notoriously difficult, relying on medical practitioners to report cases to a central authority. It is estimated that less than 1% of cases are captured in existing notification schemes. Some of the reasons for increasing rates of foodborne illness are: new and emerging pathogens, changes in the food supply (including more intensive animal husbandry and longer-shelf-life fresh-chilled products), ageing populations, and a greater proportion of food eaten away from home. Around 60–80% of foodborne illness arises from the food service industry.

25.2.2 Control of food poisoning

The trend in all countries today is to require more formal training of all food handlers and the development of food safety plans wherever food is prepared and served to the public, based on the principles of Hazard Analysis of Critical Control Points (HACCP). HACCP is a preventative approach to quality control, developed in the USA to ensure the safety of astronauts' food in space. HACCP is now used worldwide in all segments of food production, from primary production, to food manufacture and food service settings. It is based on seven principles, namely:

1. Identify all potential *hazards* at each step in the food chain and possible preventative actions (hazard analysis).

2. Determine the *critical* points in the operation where the hazards must be controlled (risk assessment).

Table 25.3 Common bacterial food-poisoning organisms

Organism	Symptoms	Time after food	Typical food sources
Toxins			
Staphylococcus aureus	Vomiting, diarrhoea, abdominal pain	1–6 hours (mean 2–3 hours)	Custard and cream-filled baked goods, cold meats
Clostridium perfringens	Diarrhoea, severe pain, nausea	8–24 hours (mean 8–15 hours)	Meat products that are incompletely cooked or reheated
Bacillus cereus	(a) Nausea, vomiting (b) Abdominal pain, watery diarrhoea	(a) 1–5 hours (b) 6–16 hours (mean 10–12 hours)	Rice dishes, vegetables, sauces, puddings
Clostridium botulinum	Dry mouth, difficulty swallowing and speaking, double vision, difficulty breathing Often fatal	2 hours–8 days (mean 12–36 hours)	Home-canned foods (usually meat and vegetables), inadequately processed smoked meats
Infections			
Vibrio parahaemolyticus	Diarrhoea, abdominal cramp, nausea, headache, vomiting	4–96 hours (mean 12 hours)	Fish, crustaceans
Salmonella spp.	Diarrhoea, fever, nausea, vomiting	8–72 hours (mean 12–36 hours)	Undercooked poultry, reheated food, cream-filled pastries
Yersinia enterocolytica	Fever, abdominal pain, diarrhoea	24–36 hours	Raw and cooked pork and beef
Escherichia coli	Fever, cramps, nausea, diarrhoea	8–44 hours (mean 26 hours)	Faecal-contaminated food or water
Shigella spp.	Diarrhoea, bloody stools with mucus, fever	1–7 days (mean 1–3 days)	Faecal-contaminated food
Campylobacter jejuni	Fever, abdominal pain, diarrhoea	1–10 days (mean 2–5 days)	Raw milk, poultry, eggs, meat
Listeria monocytogenes	Septic abortion, septicaemia, meningitis, encephalitis. Often fatal	1–7 weeks	Milk, dairy products, raw meat, poultry, eggs, vegetables, salads, seafood

3. Establish *limits* at each critical control point. Examples of control procedures are washing hands, sanitizing food-preparation surfaces and tools, cooking food to a specific temperature and maximum food storage times.

4. Set up procedures to *monitor* each critical control point.

5. Plan the *corrective actions* to be taken if a critical limit is exceeded.

Table 25.4 An example of six steps from a HAACP plan for chilled chicken salad

	STEP 1 Growing and harvesting	STEP 2 Raw material processing	STEP 3 Supply storage temperatures	STEP 4 Ingredient assembly	STEP 5 Bagging	STEP 6 Labelling
Hazard	Chemicals Antibiotics	Chemical Microbiological	Microbiological	Microbiological	Microbiological	Incorrect dates Traceability
Control	Raw material specifications	Certified supplier	Raw material specifications	Temperature control specs	Correct seal settings	Legible, correctly dated and coded
Limit	Regulatory approved residues	Free of pathogens and foreign material	Chicken < −12°C Vegetables < 4°C	Food < 4°C	Upper tolerance limit on sealer	Use proper labels
Monitoring	Certificate of compliance	Monitor supplier HACCP program	Check coolroom records daily	Check temperature once per shift	Check setting every 15 minutes	Each batch at changeover
Action if limit exceeded	Reject lot	Reject as supplier	Investigate time/temp abuse	Report to supervisor	Examine all packages	Destroy incorrect labels
Responsibility	Receiving operator	Purchaser	Store person	Cook	Seal inspector	Packer

Source: Adapted from Microbiology and Food Safety Committee of the National Food Processors Association (1993) HACCP implementation: A generic model for chilled foods. *J Food Prot*, **56**, 1077.

6. Establish a *recording system* to document performance of the process.

7. *Verify* that the HACCP process is working.

Table 25.4 outlines an example of some parts of a HACCP plan for a commercial food product sold as ready-to-eat.

25.2.3 Mycotoxins

Moulds (or fungi) are capable of producing a wide variety of chemicals that are biologically active. Humans have used some of these as effective antibiotics, but there are also a number of diseases resulting from accidental exposure to fungal products that contaminate food. Some examples are as follows.

Aflatoxins These are a group of closely related compounds from the common *Aspergillus* fungus species that are highly toxic and carcinogenic, causing liver damage. They are stable to heat and survive most forms of food processing. Aflatoxin contamination can occur whenever environmental conditions are suitable for mould growth, but the problem is more common in tropical and semi-tropical regions. Aflatoxins were first recognized in the 1960s in peanuts. On a worldwide basis, maize is the most important food contaminated with aflatoxin.

Patulin is an antibiotic that is produced by the mould *Penicillium caviforme*. It has been implicated as a possible carcinogen from one study in rats but other studies have not confirmed this. Patulin in primarily associated with the apple-rotting fungus and so apple juices and some baked goods with fruit can contain patulin.

Fumonisins are carcinogenic mycotoxins from the *Fusarium* fungus associated with maize. There were first characterized in 1988 and are known to be potent inhibitors of sphingolipid synthesis. Ingestion of fumonisin-affected maize has been associated with outbreaks of diseases in horses and pigs and has been shown to be carcinogenic in rats. In 1990 it was reported that use of mouldy maize with high levels of fumonisins to make beer in the Transkei of South Africa was associated with a very high incidence of oesophageal cancer.

25.2.4 New foodborne diseases

Three of the most serious food pathogens today (*Campylobacter*, *Listeria* and enterohaemorrhagic *E. coli*) were unrecognized as causes of illness 20 years ago. Some of the more important new organisms are described here.

Campylobacter jejuni was a well-known bacterium in veterinary medicine before it was identified as a human, pathogen in 1973. It is now recognized as one of the most important causes of gastroenteritis in humans, of similar importance to *Salmonella*. It is present in the flesh of cattle, sheep, pigs and poultry, and can be introduced wherever raw meat is handled.

Listeria monocytogenes is a bacterium widely distributed in nature but is unusual in that it grows at refrigeration temperatures (down to 0°C). Listeriosis can cause abortions, as well as death, in the elderly and those with compromised immune systems, such as people with AIDS. *Listeria* has been linked to the consumption of contaminated paté, milk, soft cheese and undercooked chicken, and is often found in preprepared chilled food.

Escherichia coli O157:H7 is a bacterium that can damage the cells of the colon, leading to bloody diarrhoea and abdominal cramps. Raw or under-cooked hamburger meat was a major vehicle of transmission in a number of well-publicized outbreaks in the USA in 1993 and contaminated metwurst was responsible for a major outbreak of illness in Australia in 1995.

Salmonella typhimurium became a major pathogen in the UK in the 1990s due to the emergence of multidrug-resistant strains. As well as being highly virulent, it can survive at low pH and be infectious in very low numbers.

Norwalk virus is found in the faeces of humans. Illness is caused by poor personal hygiene among infected food handlers. Symptoms include nausea, vomiting, diarrhoea, abdominal pain and fever. Because it is a virus, it does not reproduce in food, but remains active until the food is eaten.

'Mad cow disease' (or BSE, bovine spongiform encephalopathy) is a slowly progressive and ultimately fatal neurological disorder of adult cattle that results from infection by an unique transmission agent called a prion. Prions are not well understood but seem to be modified forms of normal cell-surface proteins. BSE was first confirmed in Britain in 1986, but has now spread to cattle in other countries of Europe, Japan and North America. It is now accepted that the same infective agent is also responsible for variant Creutzfeldt–Jakob disease (vCJD), a fatal disease of humans, mostly affecting young adults. The disease causes mental changes such as memory loss and slurred speech, followed by muscle twitching, confusion, fits and unconsciousness. By July 2005, there were 150 definite cases of vCJD in the UK, with the possible size of the epidemic estimated at over 100 000 cases. Three principal controls have been put in place to keep infected meat out of the food chain: banning slaughter of beef aged over 30 months (before the age at which BSE typically develops), removing parts of the body with the highest levels of infection (e.g. nervous and bone tissue), and banning feeding of meat and bonemeal to any farmed livestock. Milk and gelatine products from beef do not appear to be affected.

25.3 Environmental contamination

25.3.1 Heavy metals and minerals

Selenium is one of the most toxic essential trace elements. The level of selenium in foods usually reflects the levels in the soil. In a few high-selenium areas, such as North Dakota and parts of China, excessive selenium intake has been associated with gastrointestinal disturbances and skin discoloration. In China in the early 1960s, selenium intoxication affected up to 50% of the population in certain villages, with brittle hair, skin lesions and neurological disturbances seen as the main symptoms.

Mercury Fish can contain 10–500 mg/kg of organic mercury, and even higher levels when mercury wastes are released into lake waters. Serious poisonings from mercury in fish have occurred in Japan, the most famous being that in Minamata Bay (from 1953 to 1960). Another example of widespread mercury intoxication occurred in Iraq in 1971–1972 as a result of bread made from wheat treated with mercury-based pesticides. Most countries have now established maximum permitted levels on mercury in fish in the range of 0.4–1.0 mg/kg.

Cadmium This toxic element accumulates in biological systems. Chronic exposure at excessive levels can lead to irreversible kidney failure. Plants readily take up cadmium from the soil, and there has been a slow increase in the cadmium levels in soils due to the use of phosphate fertilizers and the affect of air and water pollution. The average food-based cadmium intake is now approximately 10–50 µg/day, which is approaching the provisional tolerable weekly intake of 7 µg/kg/week. Measures to control cadmium contamination include controls on waste disposal and developing new crops that accumulate less cadmium.

25.3.2 Criminal adulteration

Modern food regulations began in the nineteenth century when there were widespread examples of adulteration of foods to increase profits. Milk was diluted with water, cocoa with sawdust; some operators preserved milk with formaldehyde and butter with borax. Today the standards of the food industry are much higher and risks from illegal adulteration are rare. However, there are still some notorious instances. For example, in Spain in 1981 there was an outbreak of an apparently new disease characterized by fever, rashes and respiratory problems. Many thousands were hospitalized and over 100 people died. The agent responsible was identified as cooking oil that had been fraudulently sold as pure olive oil; in fact it was mostly rapeseed oil, intended for industrial use, and contaminated with aniline.

25.3.3 Packaging migration

The materials used to package food can sometimes result in contamination of the food itself. At one time, the lead used in the solder of metal cans was a significant source of contamination of infant formulae, but this problem has been eliminated by the introduction of non-soldered cans. Polyvinyl chloride (PVC), the parent compound for many polymers used in food packaging materials, has been detected in a variety of products stored in PVC containers. Although there is some evidence that PVC is carcinogenic in humans, the level of exposure from this route is very low and not regarded as a significant risk to health.

25.3.4 Industrial pollution

Throughout the industrial era, many potentially hazardous substances have been released into the environment and are now widely distributed in the food chain. Among the most important are the polychlorinated biphenyls (PCBs). PCB is a generic term for a wide range of highly stable derivatives of biphenyl that have been used in a vast number of products, including plastics, paints and lubricants. Although manufacture has now ceased, their stability and lipid solubility has meant that they accumulate in fatty tissue and they have become widespread, particularly in seafood. They can be found at low levels now even in human milk. The health effects of PCBs are not well established, although they are thought to be mild carcinogens. In one incident, in Japan in 1978, when rice oil was contaminated with 2000–3000 p.p.m. PCB, growth retardation occurred in young children and the fetuses of exposed mothers.

25.3.5 Radioactive fallout

The most important dangerous radioisotopes in fallout are strontium-90 and caesium-137, with half-lives of 28 and 30 years. Strontium is absorbed and metabolized like calcium and stored in bones. Because it is concentrated in milk, it is particularly dangerous for infants and children. Since the Nuclear Test Ban Treaty of 1963, the level of radioactive contamination from atmospheric dust has markedly declined, but accidental exposure can still occur, such as that after the Chernobyl disaster, and lead to dangerous food contamination over widespread areas.

25.3.6 Changes during cooking or processing

Food is frequently exposed to high temperatures during cooking. In roasting and frying, localized areas of food may be subjected to temperatures that lead to carbonization and under these circumstances any organic substance is likely to give rise to carcinogens. The major compounds are polycyclic aromatic hydrocarbons, produced mainly by burning of fats, and heterocyclic amines produced from amino acids. Char-broiling or barbecuing is particularly likely to lead to carcinogen formation.

Acrylamide In 2002, the Swedish National Food Authority announced that the chemical acrylamide could be found in starch-containing foods cooked at high temperatures, such as fried or roasted potato products and bread. At high levels, acrylamide is known to be toxic to the nervous system and may cause genetic damage, but epidemiological studies show no link between current acrylamide intake levels from food and any increase in disease. The World Health Organization (WHO) is currently coordinating research to clarify the risk further.

Irradiation This can be used to sterilize foods, control microbial spoilage, eradicate insect infestations and inhibit undesired sprouting. Despite the great potential of the technology, there has been substantial opposition from consumer groups concerned about the process producing toxic chemicals in foods. Extensive studies have shown the products formed are no different from those produced in normal cooking and over 1300 studies have consistently found no adverse effects from feeding irradiated food to animals or humans. Food irradiation is approved by the WHO and currently more than 30 countries have approved some form of use.

25.4 Natural toxins

Many plant species contain hazardous levels of toxic constituents. Intoxications from poisonous plants usually result from the misidentification of plants by individuals harvesting their own foods, but many ordinary foods that we consume also contain potential toxicants at less harmful levels. Toxins occurring naturally in foods are not subject to regulatory control and many would not receive approval if they were proposed as new food additives.

25.4.1 Inherent natural toxins

There are many examples of potentially dangerous toxins in natural food products: cyanogenic glycosides in plants such as almond kernels, cassava and sorghum; alkaloids in herbal teas and comfrey; lathyrus toxin in chickpeas. In Japan, the puffer fish, which contains a potentially fatal neurotoxin called tetrodotoxin, is considered a delicacy and it is consumed to produce a tingling sensation. However, natural toxicants are a generally accepted hazard because the foods that contain them have been eaten in traditional diets for many generations. We are protected from their harmful effects in three ways: avoidance, removal and detoxification.

First, traditional knowledge has been passed down to us about which foods are safe and which are not. Thus, we know it is safe to eat certain mushrooms and not others. Secondly, traditional food-preparation methods have evolved to reduce the harmful effects of natural toxins. Specialist chefs prepare puffer fish to remove the parts with the highest toxin concentration. People in South America and Africa use complex chopping and washing procedures in their preparation of cassava that removes much of the cyanide naturally found in the raw product. Thirdly, the body has numerous detoxification systems, mainly enzymes in the liver, to deal with the toxins that we do ingest. So we can still happily eat nutmeg and sassafras, even though they both contain the naturally occurring carcinogen safrole.

25.4.2 Abnormal conditions of the animal or plant used for food

Some foods only become hazardous during particular conditions of growth or storage.

Ciguatera poisoning This serious human intoxication is caused by eating contaminated fish. It results in gastrointestinal disorders, neurological problems and, in severe cases, death. There are over 400 species of fish that may become ciguatoxic, but almost all of the two dozen or so fatal cases annually are attributable to barracuda. The poisoning is particularly insidious because it can occur in fish that are normally safe to eat. The precise nature of the intoxication is not yet known but most likely occurs when certain tropical and subtropical fish have been feeding on dinoflagellates that produce toxins that accumulate in the flesh of the fish.

Paralytic shellfish poisoning It has been known for many centuries that shellfish can occasionally become toxic. Symptoms include numbness of the lips and fingertips and ascending paralysis, which can lead to death within 24 hours. Paralytic shellfish poisoning, which primarily involves mussels and clams, is also associated with the growth of dinoflagellates in the water. When the dinoflagellates are undergoing periods of rapid growth ('blooms' or 'red tides') in areas where the shellfish are growing, the toxin saxitoxin accumulates to hazardous levels in the shellfish's hepatopancreas. The toxin cannot be removed by washing or destroyed by heat.

Glycoalkaloids in potatoes Solanine is one of a range of heat-stable glycoalkaloid compounds found in the green parts of the potato plant that are toxic above concentrations of 20 mg/100 g. In normal peeled potatoes there is about 7 mg solanine/100 g. Solanine synthesis can be induced by exposing the tubers to light so that they go green, and also by simple mechanical injury. In very green potatoes, the levels can reach up to 100 mg/100 g. These glycoalkaloids possess anticholinesterase activity, which can produce gastrointestinal and neurological disorders, and deaths have occasionally been reported from consumption of excessive amounts of green potatoes.

25.4.3 Enzyme inhibitors

Protease Inhibitors Substances that inhibit digestive enzymes are widespread in many legume species, and trypsin inhibitors are found in oats and maize as well as brussels sprouts, onion and beetroot. These inhibitors are proteins, and therefore are denatured and inactivated by cooking. Thus for humans these substances are not a problem, although feeding raw legumes to animals can result in pancreatic enlargement.

25.4.4 Antivitamins

One of the best known antivitamins is the biotin-binding protein, avidin, in raw egg white. Biotin deficiency induced by eating raw egg white is rare because biotin is well provided in most human diets. The few cases that have been reported involved abnormally large amounts of raw egg white, so the occasional raw egg is perfectly safe. Avidin is inactivated when heated.

Other antivitamins, such as the pyridoxine antagonist amino-D-proline in flax seeds, the antithiamin compound caffeic acid found in bracken fern, and a tocopherol oxidase in raw soybeans, are only of importance in animal feeding.

25.4.5 Mineral-binding agents

Goitrogens   There are a number of glucosinolate and thiocyanate compounds found in foods that interfere with normal utilization of iodine by the thyroid gland and which can result in goitres. Goitrogens are widely distributed in cruciferous vegetables such as cabbage, brussels sprouts and broccoli. The average intake of glucosinolates from vegetables in the UK is 76 mg/day and clinical studies have found that intakes of 100–400 mg/day may reduce the uptake of iodine by the thyroid. There is no evidence that normal consumption of these foods by humans is in any way harmful, but it is possible that eating large amounts of brassica plants might contribute to a higher incidence of goitre in areas of the world where dietary iodine intake is low.

Phytate   In wholemeal cereals, this can bind minerals and make them less available for absorption. In leavened bread, phytases in the yeast break down the phytate, but in some parts of the Middle East, where unleavened bread is a dietary staple, phytate has been reported to be the cause of zinc deficiency.

Oxalate   Certain plants, including rhubarb, spinach, beetroot and tea, contain relatively high levels of oxalate. Oxalate can combine with calcium to form an insoluble complex in the gut that is poorly absorbed and high intakes can lower plasma calcium levels. Kidney damage and convulsions can accompany oxalate poisoning. However, the average diet supplies only 70–150 mg oxalate per day, which could theoretically bind 30–70 mg calcium. Since calcium intakes are usually ten times this amount, there is no good evidence that food oxalates normally have any detrimental effect on mineral balance.

Tannins (polyphenols)   These are present in tea, coffee and cocoa as well as broad beans. Tannins inhibit the absorption of iron; in Egypt, in children with low iron intakes, regular consumption of stewed beans has been associated with anaemia. High levels of tea consumption may contribute to low iron status in people with marginal iron intakes.

25.5 Agricultural residues

25.5.1 Pesticides

The most common agricultural chemicals found in foods are pesticides, albeit at very low levels. The chlorinated organic pesticides (such as DDT and chlordane) were among the first modern pesticides to be used. In general, they have low toxicity to mammals and are highly toxic to insects. However, they are very stable compounds that persist in soils. They are stored in the fat tissue of animals. Because of concern about their effect on the reproduction of certain birds and possible carcinogenic activity, the use of these compounds has been restricted. Surveys of foods show that the levels of organochlorine compounds have been in declining in recent years. Alternative insecticides now in use—such as organophosphates—do not accumulate in the environment. No food poisonings have ever been attributed to the proper use of insecticides on foods, but in 1997 there were 60 cases of food poisoning in India attributed to indiscriminate organophosphate spraying in a kitchen.

25.5.2 Fungicides and herbicides

Most fungicides and herbicides show very selective toxicity to their target plants and therefore present very little hazard to humans. In addition, most do not accumulate in the environment.

25.5.3 Hormones

The use of hormones such as bovine somatotrophin (BST) to improve yields of meat and milk, and to reduce the percentage of carcass fat, has been a subject of controversy in many countries. Although low levels of BST can be detected in the milk of treated cows, the hormones are inactive in humans even when injected and, because they are proteins, are digested and inactivated in the stomach when consumed in food. The US FDA approved the commercial use of BST in 1993, and later reviews by Canadian authorities and Codex Alimentarius have agreed that there are no health risks to humans. However, in the EU, BST use is not permitted on animal welfare grounds. It likely that a number of other biotechnological hormones will be approved in the future.

25.6 Intentional food additives

25.6.1 Approval process for food additives

Each country has its own legislation to control the approval of additives in foods, but most follow the same general principles that are used by the two main international bodies of experts organized by WHO and the FAO: the Joint Expert Committee on Food Additives (JECFA) and the Codex Alimentarius Committee on Food Additives and Contaminants. The aim of the evaluation of a food additive is to establish an acceptable daily intake (ADI). The ADI is usually expressed in mg/kg body weight and is defined as the amount of a chemical that might be ingested daily, even over a lifetime, without appreciable risk to the consumer. The evaluation process consists of a number of steps, as follows:

1. Toxicity testing is carried out in experimental animals, usually mice and rats, but other species may also be employed. Three types of testing are performed: (a) acute toxicity studies at high doses to determine the range of possible toxic effects of the chemical, (b) short-term feeding trials at various doses, and (c) long-term studies of 2 years or more to examine the effect of lifetime exposures over several generations.

2. From the feeding trials, the level of additive at which observed health effects do not appear in the animals is determined. This is called the 'no observed effect level' (NOEL).

3. The lowest NOEL is divided by a safety factor to derive a level of exposure that is regarded as acceptable for human exposure—the ADI. Most commonly, a safety factor of 100 times is used, but for some substances factors of up to 1000 have been used. This safety factor allows for possible differences in susceptibility to the additive between experimental animals and humans and also the differences in sensitivity of individual people.

Not all additives have been evaluated for safety using modern testing procedures. Some additives have been used for many years without apparent harm and in the USA, ingredients not evaluated by prescribed testing procedures have been classified as 'generally recognized as safe' (GRAS). This list includes commonly used ingredients such as salt and sugar, seasonings and many food flavourings.

While the 100-fold safety factor is accepted for most additives, in the USA, the Delaney Clause prohibits the use in *any* amount of substances known to cause cancer in animals or humans. When the bill was introduced in 1958, chemicals could be detected down to 100 parts per billion; anything less was considered zero. Improved analytical techniques can now detect substances at parts per trillion, and it has been argued that the trivial risk from such minute quantities should be put into perspective against the benefits of additives in improving the quality, quantity and convenience of the modern food supply. The US FDA has now changed the interpretation of the clause so that if a food additive increases the chance of developing cancer over a lifetime by less than one case per million of cancer, the threat is considered too small to be of concern.

Table 25.5 Rankings of possible carcinogenic hazards

Daily human exposure	Carcinogen and dose per 70 kg person	Index of possible hazard (HERP, %)
Natural dietary toxins		
Wine (250 mL)	Ethyl alcohol, 30 mL	4.7
Basil (1 g of dried leaf)	Estragole, 3.8 mg	0.1
Peanut butter (32 g/one sandwich)	Aflatoxin, 64 ng	0.03
Cooked bacon (100 g)	Dimethylnitrosamine, 0.3 μg	0.003
Food additives		
Diet cola (1 can)	Saccharin, 95 mg	0.06
Pesticides		
DDE/DDT (daily diet intake)	DDE, 2.2 μg	0.0003
EDB (daily diet intake)	EDB, 0.42 μg	0.0004

Source: Reprinted with permission from Ames, B.N., Magaw, R., and Gold, L.S. (1987) Ranking of possible carcinogenic hazards. *Science*, **236**, 271–80. *Science Copyright 1987. American Association for the Advancement of Science.*

Ames has ranked the level of carcinogenic risk associated with a variety of chemicals we may be commonly exposed to. The Human Exposure/Rodent Potency Index (HERP) expresses the typical human intakes as a percentage of the dose required to produce tumours in 50% of rodents. The values in Table 25.5 show that the HERP (i.e. the risk) for the alcohol in a glass of wine is almost 100 times higher than that from the aflatoxins in a peanut butter sandwich or the saccharin in a can of diet cola, and more than 10 000 times the hazard from the residues of the pesticide ethylene dibromide (EDB). That the risks from wine appear more acceptable to most consumers seems to relate to the fact that benefit is easily perceived, that wine is seen as 'natural' and because the risk is voluntary. Although the risks from other additives and contaminants may be far smaller, they arouse suspicion because they are risks that people generally cannot control.

25.6.2 Artificial sweeteners

Saccharin This is one of the oldest artificial sweeteners, having been used in foods since the last century. Studies in rats have linked high doses (7.5% of the diet by weight) of saccharin with bladder cancer, and because of this there have been attempts to ban its use in human foods. However, at lower doses, such as 1%, no adverse effects are found and large epidemiological studies of diabetics who have had lifetime exposure to saccharin have found no increased incidence of cancer in humans.

Cyclamate Dietary cyclamate appears to promote bladder cancer and induce testicular atrophy in rats, although carcinogenicity testing in mice, dogs and primates has been negative. The US FDA banned the food use of cyclamate in 1969, but in over 50 other countries it is still a permitted sweetener, and there is no good evidence from mutagenicity testing or epidemiological studies that it is a health risk to humans.

Aspartame Aspartame is a dipeptide of two amino acids, phenylalanine and aspartic acid. Aspartame is metabolized to phenylalanine and therefore carries a risk for people with phenylketonuria, but for the normal population it is an extremely safe sweetener that is digested like any other protein.

25.6.3 Preservatives

Preservatives are used in foods as antioxidants and to prevent the growth of bacteria and fungi. Most pose no toxicological problems, but a few have generated some concerns.

Sodium nitrite This is used as an antimicrobial preservative. It is very effective in preventing the growth of *Clostridium botulinum* as well as acting as a colour-fixing agent (to preserve the red colour) in cured meat products like bacon and ham. Nitrite reacts with secondary amines in foods to produce *N*-nitroso derivatives, many of which are carcinogenic. However, the risk to human health from dietary nitrite is difficult to assess. While food additive nitrites are significant, a substantial amount is also produced by bacterial reduction from naturally occurring nitrate in vegetables. In recent years, manufacturers have worked to reduce the levels of nitrite used in cured meats, and have added agents such as ascorbic acid, which help to prevent the formation of nitrosamines in the stomach.

Sulphur dioxide Sulphur dioxide and its salts (sulphites) are commonly used as inhibitors of enzymic browning, dough conditioners, antimicrobials and antioxidants. Although sulphites have been used for many centuries, with no adverse effect for most consumers, 1–2% of asthmatics are sensitive to sulphites, and in those individuals the reaction can be fatal.

25.6.4 Colours and flavours

All colours and flavours approved for use in foods are rigorously evaluated before being approved for use.

Red No. 2 (Amaranth) In the early 1970s, data from Russian studies raised questions about the safety of Red No. 2. The FDA Toxicology Advisory Committee evaluated numerous reports and decided there was no evidence of a hazard, but they concluded that feeding it at a high dosage results in a statistically significant increase in malignant tumours in female rats. The FDA ultimately decided to ban the colour, but it is still found in foods in Canada and Europe.

Tartrazine (E102) Food sensitivity to tartrazine can be experienced by a small number of individuals, but claims related to clinical problems such as asthma and hyperactivity are not well supported by scientific studies. Tartrazine is still a permitted additive, but its presence has to be declared in ingredient lists so sensitive individuals can avoid it.

Monosodium glutamate (MSG) The flavour enhancer MSG is a sodium salt of glutamic acid, one of the most common amino acids. It is present in virtually all foods and found in high levels in tomatoes, mushrooms, broccoli, peas, cheese and soy sauce. 'Chinese restaurant' syndrome has been claimed to be caused by foods with a lot of added MSG, but most controlled studies have not demonstrated this effect.

25.7 Novel foods

Technology now allows the development of many new ingredients or whole foods that do not have a history of traditional use in the human food supply. Many of these novel foods have been developed to have improved nutritional quality. Recent examples include genetically modified foods, artificial fat substitutes for energy-reduced foods, new algal sources of ω-3 fatty acids, and phytosterols to reduce cholesterol.

25.7.1 Approval process for novel foods

There are significant practical difficulties in assessing the long-term safety of modified whole foods or ingredients. Unlike additives, which can be fed at very high doses to assess their toxic effects, it is not possible to feed large amounts of one single food to animals without making their diet nutritionally unbalanced. Animals also prefer a mixture of foods and are likely to refuse to eat if offered a single food in large amounts. These difficulties, and welfare concerns about the use of animal studies that were unlikely to result in meaningful information, led to the development of the concept of 'substantial equivalence', particularly for the assessment of genetically modified (GM) foods. This type of assessment does not quantify the safety or risk of a food, but aims to determine whether novel foods are as safe as traditional counterparts. Some have called for the 'precautionary principle' (that potential unknown risks should be taken into account) be applied to assessments of novel foods, but most countries limit their rigorous assessments to established scientific evidence.

For GM foods, the process involves assessment and comparison of a wide range of factors including:

- source and nature of any new protein;
- stability of any genetic changes;
- potential toxicity of the new protein;
- levels of naturally occurring and newly introduced allergens;
- nutritional composition;
- levels of antinutrients;
- ability of the food to support normal growth and wellbeing; and
- potential unintended environmental consequences.

25.7.2 Genetically modified foods

Genetic modification using modern biotechnology now allows specific individual genes to be identified, copied and transferred into other organisms in a much more direct and controlled way. The most obvious difference from traditional breeding is that genetic modification allows transfer of genetic material between species, to produce transgenic organisms. For example, genes for the enzyme chymosin from beef have been inserted into yeast to allow them to be grown commercially in fermentation tanks, and the chymosin from these GM organisms has now widely replaced natural rennet from animals in cheese making. Genetic modification can also allow individual genes to be switched on or off; for example, the gene that controls fruit softening can be repressed to maintain a higher solids content in tomatoes designed for use in tomato paste.

It is estimated that 75 million hectares of transgenic crops were planted in 2006. Production of GM crops is primarily in the USA, with significant growth in Argentina, Canada and China. Together, these four countries account for over 83% of total global transgenic production. Most of these plants have been modified for agricultural purposes: herbicide-tolerant soy and canola, and insect-resistant corn and cotton now make up the bulk of those crops in North America. Many future uses are planned that will bring more direct consumer benefits: oils with improved fatty acid profiles, rice with improved levels of vitamins, nuts with lower levels of allergens, potatoes that absorb less fat during frying, and even milk products containing vaccines. However, concern has been expressed about the environmental impacts and safety of these novel foods, in particular with relation to the issues of allergenicity, toxicity of transgenic food and possible transfer of antibiotic resistance.

Allergens can be transferred into GM foods. When genes from brazil nuts were introduced into soybeans to increase the levels of sulphur-rich amino acids, testing showed that allergenic nut protein was also transferred to the soy, and the company did not pursue development of the product. A widely reported study on GM potatoes suggested that they damaged rat organs and depressed their immune systems, but later studies have disputed those results. Some transgenic plants have incorporated a specific toxin from the bacterium *Bacillus thuringiensis*, Bt. This crystal protein has been well studied and is specific for butterflies and moths—it is not toxic to other species.

Genetic modification usually requires the introduction of the selected gene together with a marker gene. The marker genes are often antibiotic resistance genes that allow selection of the plants that have successfully integrated the new selected gene. Many have expressed concern that when the modified food is eaten the resistance gene might be transferred to bacteria in the gut and acquire resistance to clinically useful antibiotics. Although it has been estimated that the chances of this occurring are extremely small, the use of this method is now being phased out.

Most countries have now established stringent approval processes for GM foods, including mandatory labelling to inform consumers when foods include GM-modified ingredients. Assessments to date have usually found GM foods to be as safe as their normal counterparts and there are likely to be increasing numbers of GM foods in the marketplace in the future.

25.7.3 Fat substitutes

There are a number of fat substitutes now in use, including Simplesse (microcapsules of milk proteins or egg white), Splendid (derived from pectin) and N-oil (derived from tapioca). In the US, Olestra is a mixture of heat-stable sugar polyesters that are not digested and yield no energy; it has been controversial because it can reduce the absorption of fat-soluble vitamins. The FDA approved the use of Olestra in a limited range of foods in 1996, but required the addition of vitamins A, D and K as well as further monitoring of the health impacts and warning labelling (that it may cause abdominal cramping and loose stools). In 2003, after a scientific review of several post-market studies, the FDA concluded that the warning statement was no longer warranted. Olestra is not yet approved in the UK, Europe or Australasia.

25.7.4 Phytosterols

In many countries, plant sterols are now approved to be added to a range of foods to help lower blood cholesterol. They work by reducing the absorption of cholesterol from the gut, but have a side effect of also lowering absorption of carotenoids. A typical daily dose of 2–3 g/day can reduce serum β-carotene levels by 20–25%. Safety reviews have concluded that since there is no evidence of reduction in serum retinol levels, this effect is not a significant health concern and that advice to maintain adequate fruit and vegetable intakes can ensure adequate carotene intakes.

25.8 Regulatory agencies

Although all regulators use similar processes to evaluate scientific evidence and assess the safety of foods, the management of food safety legislation varies among countries.

The Codex Alimentarius Commission (Codex) was created in 1963 by the Food and Agriculture Organization (FAO) and the WHO to develop international standards, guidelines and codes of practice related to food composition and safety, with the aim of harmonizing food regulations among countries. Over 165 countries are members of Codex. While not legally binding on individual countries, Codex standards are very influential and form benchmarks for key World Trade Organization agreements such as those on the Application of Sanitary and Phytosanitary Measures and Technical Barriers to Trade, which make it increasingly difficult for countries to adopt food standards that are significantly different from Codex.

In the USA, the FDA develops standards for food composition, quality and safety, as well as being responsible for approval of therapeutic drugs and cosmetics. It also has food inspection and monitoring responsibilities nationally. The work of the FDA, such as the GRAS listings, is influential internationally because of the high quality and resourcing of the many expert scientific staff.

In Australasia, the binational authority—Foods Standards Australia New Zealand—sets standards for all manufactured foods for both countries, including standards for additives and contaminants and assesses the safety of novel foods. Primary food production and food service safety standards are set separately in each country. In Australia, compliance is the responsibility of individual State governments, not the national body standard-setting agency.

In Britain, an independent food safety watchdog—the Food Standards Agency (FSA)—was established in 2000 to protect the public's health and consumer interests after concerns raised by the BSE outbreak. The FSA provides advice and information to the public and Government on food safety from farm to fork, nutrition and diet. It also protects consumers through effective food enforcement and monitoring.

In Europe, the European Food Safety Authority (EFSA) was created in 2002 to provide independent scientific advice on all matters linked to food and feed safety. EFSA principally deals with requests for risk assessments from the European Commission, Parliament and Council and plans to take on a wider brief from other European institutions in the near future.

One of the key roles of all regulatory agencies is risk assessment and management.

Risk assessment is a scientific process consisting of four steps:

1. Hazard identification (biological, chemical or physical agents capable of causing adverse health effects).

2. Hazard characterization (qualitative and quantitative evaluation of the hazards—in including dose–response effects).

3. Exposure assessment (the likely intake of the risk factor from food, taking into account typical dietary patterns).

4. Risk characterization (estimating the probability and severity of potential adverse effects).

Risk management Risk management is the process of weighing policy options in the light of the risk assessment results and selecting appropriate control measures. Control options can include prohibiting certain substances in foods entirely (some carcinogenic herbs, for example), setting maximum permitted levels in foods (e.g. additives, or agricultural residues), through the development of codes of good manufacturing practice, labelling requirements (e.g. warnings about allergens) or by public education about safe use of foods (e.g. in relation to mercury in fish).

Risk communication Risk communication is the process of making the risk management information comprehensible to food producers, policy makers and consumers.

25.9 Summary

Despite the many potential health risks associated with foods, in practice the degree of risk associated with the modern food supply is extremely low. The lifespan of humans in Western countries is steadily increasing and age-specific death rates for most cancers that might be associated with food ingredients are either decreasing or stable. By far the most important hazards of significance are those from biological agents: pathogenic bacteria, viruses, fungi and a few toxic seafoods. All of these hazards are avoidable by following established food-handling practices. The other categories of hazard (contaminants and additives) are closely monitored and regulated and represent only a theoretical risk to most consumers. The development of novel foods and ingredients provides new challenges for traditional safety assessment processes and as the food supply becomes increasing global, food regulations about food safety are becoming more harmonized internationally.

FURTHER READING

1. **Branen, A.L., Davidson, P.M., Salminen, S., and Thorngate, J.H.** (eds) (2002) *Food Additives*, 2nd edition. New York, Marcel Dekker.

2. **Bryan, F.L.** (1992) *Hazard analysis critical control point evaluations. A guide to identifying hazards and assessing risks associated with food preparation and storage*. Geneva, World Health Organization.

3. **Cliver, D.O., and Rieman, H.P.** (eds) (2002) *Foodborne diseases*, 2nd edition. San Diego, Academic Press.

4. Committee on Comparative Toxicity of Naturally Occurring Carcinogens, National Research Council (1996) *Carcinogens and anticarcinogens in the human diet. A comparison of naturally occurring and synthetic substances*. Washington, DC, National Academy Press.

5. Food Standards Australia New Zealand (2005) *Safety assessment of genetically modified foods*. Canberra, FSANZ.

6. Institute of Medicine and National Research Council (2004) *Safety of genetically engineered foods. Approaches to assessing the unintended health effects*. Washington, DC, National Academies Press.

7. Omaye, S.T. (2004) *Food and nutritional toxicology*. Boca Raton, FL, CRC Press.

8. Schmidt, R.H., and Rodrick, G.E. (eds) (2003) *Food safety handbook*. Hoboken, NJ, John Wiley.

9. WHO (1994) *Safety and nutritional adequacy of irradiated food*. Geneva, World Health Organization.

USEFUL WEBSITES

Key food safety websites:

World Health Organization: http://www.who.int/foodsafety/en/

US Food and Drug Administration: http://www.cfsan.fda.gov/list.html/

European Food Safety Authority: http://www.efsa.eu.int/

Australian Food Safety Centre of Excellence: http://www.foodsafetycentre.com.au/

 To see topical and scientifically robust updates on nutrition associated with this textbook, and active web links to many of the journal articles in the Reference areas, please see the dedicated Online Resource Centre at www.oxfordtextbooks.co.uk/orc/mann3e/.

Functional foods

Martijn B. Katan

This textbook teaches you who needs to eat which nutrients and in what amounts. But translating this knowledge into foods and meals is no simple task. Armies, hospitals and nursing homes employ dietitians to translate nutritional recommendations into diets and meals, so that soldiers, patients and residents receive the nutrients they need, and in the right amounts. However, most people do not have access to a dietitian. Also, the variety of food keeps increasing, as does the number of potentially beneficial food ingredients. And last but not least, many persons—whether healthy or sick—would like to decide for themselves which foods are good for them, without the advice of a professional.

All this has created a market for new foods that promises to increase the wellbeing or health of the consumer. Functional foods are part of that market. This chapter reviews typical functional foods, their ingredients, and their efficacy in improving health. It will also review health claims and their regulation—or lack of regulation.

26.1 What is a functional food?

The definition of a functional food is a contentious issue. The International Food Information Council, which is supported primarily by food, beverage and agricultural industries, defines functional foods as 'foods that provide health benefits beyond basic nutrition'. That definition is unsatisfactory because it leaves the status of foods without a brand name (such as fruits, vegetables or low-fat cheese) up in the air. Even tap water would meet this definition because a liberal intake of water prevents cystitis, kidney and bladder stones, and possibly bladder cancer, but no one would call tap water a functional food.

A more concrete definition is provided by the Institute of Medicine of the US National Academy of Sciences. The Institute of Medicine defines functional

---

BOX 26.1 Competing definitions for functional foods

Industry
Foods that provide a health benefit beyond basic nutrition

Institute of Medicine
Foods in which the concentrations of one or more ingredients have been manipulated or modified to enhance their contribution to a healthful diet

This chapter
Branded foods that claim explicitly or implicitly to improve health or wellbeing

foods as 'those foods in which the concentrations of one or more ingredients have been manipulated or modified to enhance their contribution to a healthful diet'. Functional foods are indeed specifically created to promote health, but the Institute of Medicine definition still omits one aspect that is central to functional foods—namely the commercial aspect. In the reality of the marketplace, the term 'functional foods' is almost exclusively attached to branded products that claim or suggest to improve health.

Therefore, functional food is defined here as:

> A branded food that claims explicitly or implicitly to improve health or wellbeing.

An example may clarify the central role of branding and health claims. Polyunsaturated oils such as sunflower or soybean oil reduce plasma cholesterol and the risk of coronary heart disease, but few people would call a generic bottle of sunflower oil a functional food. However, if a manufacturer developed a proprietary brand of sunflower oil and marketed it with a cholesterol claim, then that oil could well be called a functional food. Box 26.2 emphasizes the role of marketing in creating a functional food.

BOX 26.2 Functional foods have four layers

1. The active ingredient (e.g. plant sterols)
2. The food matrix (e.g. orange juice, yoghurt, a cookie, chocolate, margarine)
3. The package with the health claim or health suggestions
4. Other marketing efforts, including flyers, TV commercials and sponsored media coverage

---

The active ingredients of functional foods, such as vitamins, plant sterols, lactic acid bacteria or herbal extracts, can also be packaged into a capsule or tablet instead of a food, and such products are not called foods but dietary supplements. The terms 'nutraceutical' and 'nutriceutical' have been used both for foods and for supplements; there is no consensus on what these words mean. Some products are halfway between foods and supplements, e.g. candies or sweets with added vitamins.

26.2 Typical ingredients of functional foods

26.2.1 Established nutrients

Many functional foods employ ingredients that are also available from regular foods. You can get lycopene from special drinks and supplements, but the same lycopene is found in tomatoes or tomato ketchup. The newness of such functional foods is in the way in which known ingredients are incorporated into a palatable and attractive food that can be patented and marketed. That is also the benefit of functional foods from a nutritional point of view—they may provide nutrients in a form that is more attractive or convenient for the consumer than regular foods that contain the same nutrients. Thus, people who do not like to eat vegetables may be persuaded to buy vegetable drinks that supposedly provide the same benefits.

Table 26.1 lists established nutrients typically found in functional foods, and the quality of the evidence for the efficacy of these ingredients. Whether the food itself is efficacious also depends on the amount and form of the ingredient; thus, 'wholewheat cookies' may contain too little wheat bran to affect defecation, or the bran may have been ground to a powder, which is less active than coarse bran.

The health claims for some of these ingredients are well substantiated, as indicated by the '*Evidence*' column of the table. For other ingredients, the evidence is weaker.

Intakes of vitamins and minerals from functional foods, but especially from supplements, may be much higher than from regular foods, and the adverse effects of such high intakes are a cause for concern. For example, megadoses of vitamin B_6 cause peripheral

Table 26.1 Examples of established nutrients that are used as functional food ingredients, and the evidence for the efficacy of these ingredients in maintaining health and preventing disease. Whether the food itself is efficacious depends on the amount and bioavailability of the ingredients

Ingredient	Examples of products	Health claim	Strength of evidence in humans
Folic acid	Cereals	Protects against neural tube defects	++
Dietary fibre	Drinks	Relieves constipation	++
Low in sodium	Drinks, soups	Reduces blood pressure	++
Unsaturated fatty acids	Spreads, cookies	Reduces risk of heart disease	++
Sugar alcohols	Chewing gum	Reduce caries risk	++
Soluble fibre from whole oats or *Psyllium* husk	Cereals, cookies	Reduces cholesterol and risk of heart disease	++ For cholesterol reduction
Soy protein	Drinks, bars	Reduces cholesterol and risk of heart disease	+ For cholesterol lowering
Calcium	Cereals, fruit juices, milk products, spreads	Protects against osteoporosis, helps maintain bone density	+ For consumers with a low calcium intake
Folic acid, vitamin B_6 (pyridoxine)	Cereals	Decreases homocysteine and risk of cardiovascular disease	++ For homocysteine − For cardiovascular disease
Vitamin E	Supplements	Antioxidant; prevents cardiovascular disease	+ For observational studies − − For clinical trials
Zinc	Sweets, lozenges	Prevention/cure of common cold	+ −
Vitamin C	Drinks, sweets	Protects against cardiovascular disease	+ − In observational studies − − In clinical trials

Evidence was graded according to the Australia New Zealand Food Authority criteria for levels and kinds of evidence for public health nutrition. The evidence consisted of randomized trials in humans, unless indicated otherwise.
++ = Proven efficacy: consistent effect seen in multiple high-quality studies; + = reasonable evidence for efficacy: effect seen in a limited number of studies, or some inconsistency between studies; + − = evidence for no effect: absence of an effect evident from a limited number of studies; − − = proven not to work: absence of an effect evident in multiple high-quality studies.
Source: References may be found in Katan and De Roos (2004)

neuropathy, and some authors have listed concerns over excessive intakes of calcium.

26.2.2 Novel ingredients

Table 26.2 lists some more novel or exotic ingredients of functional foods. Most of the claims for benefits of novel or 'exotic' ingredients have not been substantiated in clinical trials. However, a few have been well

investigated and show some promise, such as the following examples.

Sterols and stanols Margarines and other foods can be enriched with plant stanols or sterols, which lower low-density lipoprotein (LDL)-cholesterol. The effect on LDL has been documented in many well-controlled trials in humans, and no major adverse effects have been noted. However, long-term safety

Table 26.2 Newer functional food ingredients and their efficacy

Ingredient	Product examples	Health effect or claim	Evidence in humans
Plant stanols and sterols	Margarine, yoghurt, cereal bars	Lower cholesterol and risk of coronary heart disease	++ For LDL-cholesterol lowering No data on coronary heart disease
Lactobacillus GG bacteria	Yoghurt	Reduce diarrhoea	+ For rotavirus-induced diarrhoea in infants + For antibiotic-induced infections
Lactobacillus GG bacteria	Yoghurt	Reduce risk of early atopic disease	+− Results of trials contradictory
Other 'probiotic' live bacteria, plus fermentable sugars ('prebiotics')	Yoghurt	Enhance immunity	+− Some effects on biomarkers but none on disease
Isoflavones (phyto-estrogens)	Soy products	Reduce menopausal symptoms, osteoporosis, cardiovascular disease	+− Little evidence from clinical trials
Catechins	Tea	Reduce cardiovascular risk	+− Some epidemiological evidence No trial data
Conjugated linoleic acid (CLA)	Supplements (small amounts occur naturally in milk, beef and lamb)	Reduces body weight, protects against cancer	− Minimal effects on body weight in humans Some evidence for adverse effects on insulin resistance

++ = proven efficacy: consistent effect seen in multiple high-quality studies; + = reasonable evidence for efficacy: effect seen in a limited number of studies, or some inconsistency between studies; +− = equivocal data; − = evidence for no effect: absence of an effect evident from a limited number of studies.

and clinical efficacy have not been evaluated in clinical trials of the size and duration customary for new drugs. Some regulatory agencies have voiced concerns about the proliferation of foods with stanols and sterols, and have put limits on their intakes.

Pre- and probiotics Probiotics are viable bacteria that survive passage through the gastrointestinal tract and exert beneficial effects on the consumer. Probiotic bacteria provide a novel approach to diet and health and, unlike most food ingredients, probiotics can be patented because each bacterial strain is unique. That makes probiotics attractive to industry, but documented beneficial effects of probiotics are still scarce.

Some foods with lactic acid bacteria may reduce the severity of certain types of diarrhoea, but results of trials of probiotics and atopic eczema are contradictory, and there is little evidence for other claimed effects including cancer prevention and lowering of serum cholesterol. Prebiotics are non-digestible carbohydrates that selectively stimulate growth of beneficial bacteria. Inulin and fructo-oligosaccharides are examples of compounds marketed as prebiotics. Health effects of prebiotics appear to be limited to improved bowel function; no adequate scientific support exists for other proposed health effects such as cancer prevention, lipid lowering and prevention of diarrhoeal diseases.

Polyphenols High intakes of tea rich in catechins and other flavonoid polyphenols have been associated with a reduced risk of coronary heart disease. A clinical trial to evaluate these effects would seem feasible but has not been done. Whether polyphenols explain the so-called 'French paradox' (see Box 6.4) is questionable, as foods typically eaten in France are not particularly rich in polyphenols. For example, red wine and olive oil are lower in phenolic compounds than tea or coffee.

26.2.3 Herbs and herbal extracts

Herbal ingredients are used both in supplements and in foods, but amounts in foods are much lower. Safety is a concern, as exemplified by herbal teas with *Aristolochia*, which causes renal cancer, and products with *ephedra*, which causes hypertension, strokes and seizures. The efficacy of herbal supplements is hotly debated, but most of the popular herbal remedies have not been shown to be safe and effective by pharmaceutical standards.

26.3 How to prove efficacy and safety

26.3.1 Types of evidence—food versus pharma

The health benefits of a functional food should be supported by solid scientific evidence. But should we require the same level of evidence for functional foods as for new drugs?

This author believes not, because pharmaceutical research produces *new* molecules while nutrition deals with molecules that have been eaten for many centuries. Associations between diet and disease provide important clues about efficacy and safety, and such epidemiological studies are a vital source of evidence for diet that is not available for drugs. However, epidemiology has its limitations, and therefore other types of research need to be combined with epidemiology to show that a functional food is effective —and safe. Table 26.3 lists the types of research applied in nutrition, and their strengths and weaknesses.

26.3.2 Cell studies

A true understanding of the effect of a nutrient on health requires insights at the molecular level, and such comprehension remains the ultimate goal of nutrition science. However, as phrased by Willett (1998) 'our understanding of biologic mechanisms remains far too incomplete to predict confidently the ultimate consequences of eating a particular food or nutrient' and therefore cell and molecular studies

cannot by themselves establish efficacy and safety of a food ingredient.

26.3.3 Animal research

Animal feeding trials have been a prime source of knowledge about nutrition and health, from the thiamin-deficient chickens that helped Eijkman and Grijns to discover the cause of beri-beri (Chapter 12), down to recent findings on the anti-arrhythmogenic effects of n-3 polyunsaturated fatty acids in marmosets. However, the existence of such an effect in animals does not prove that the same effect exists in humans, because animal 'models' are often expressly constructed to reflect a hypothetical effect of a nutrient on a disease. For instance, a mouse strain may be made sensitive to a nutrient by deleting a gene or by giving it drugs. The nutrient will be effective in this model because that is what it was built to do, but extrapolation to man is uncertain.

26.3.4 Hereditary diseases

The role of a metabolite or pathway in disease causation can often be deduced by studying genetic polymorphisms that produce unusual levels of the metabolite in people who carry a certain mutation. Such 'Mendelian randomization' studies (Davey Smith *et al.*, 2005) do not suffer from the confounding that plagues conventional epidemiology, because

Table 26.3 Types of research used to investigate the relation between diet and disease, and the strengths and weaknesses of the various approaches

Type	Strengths	Limitations
(Sub)cellular studies	Mechanistic insights	Extrapolation to entire human organism uncertain
Animal feeding trials	Long-term Hard endpoints Show cause and effect	Extrapolation to humans uncertain Conditions often extreme and unphysiological
Hereditary diseases	Human Long-term Hard endpoints Show cause and effect	Mutation may act through other paths than the one of interest (pleiotropic mutations) Effects involved are often extreme
Randomized trials with surrogate endpoints	Human Controlled Show cause and effect	Short duration Validity of surrogate endpoints uncertain
Epidemiologic observations	Long-term Hard endpoints Applicable to general populations	Confounding Associations do not prove causality
Randomized clinical trials	Hard endpoints Show cause and effect	Duration sometimes too short Selected groups

such genetic variants usually do not cause people to smoke, exercise or eat differently. An example is familial hypercholesterolaemia—once the nature of the mutation in this disease was cleared up, the conclusion that high levels of LDL-cholesterol caused coronary heart disease became inescapable. However, even these 'experiments of nature' are not foolproof, because a mutation may act through another pathway than the one suspected, or through several pathways. Also, patients with inborn errors of metabolism often represent extremes, and extrapolation to milder conditions is not automatically justified.

26.3.5 Trials with surrogate endpoints

Trials with surrogate endpoints measure the effect of diet on an intermediate disease marker such as blood pressure or insulin sensitivity. Such trials are valuable because they allow causal conclusions about the effects of diet in humans. However, even established markers can lead us astray. For instance, high-carbohydrate, low-fat diets lower total serum cholesterol, and this was long equated with lowering of the risk of coronary heart disease. The distinction between 'bad' and 'good' cholesterol came only later, and then it became clear that high-carbohydrate, low-fat diets lower both the harmful LDL and the beneficial high-density lipoprotein (HDL)-cholesterol. If both are taken into account, the predicted effect on coronary heart disease risk becomes nil.

Thus, even changes in established markers cannot be automatically equated with changes in the disease that they predict. Also, there are few validated markers outside the cardiovascular field; thus, one can measure the effect of diet on hundreds of variables involved in immune response, but the relevance of each of them to prevention of infection is uncertain. Therefore, we still need experiments in which disease and death are outcome variables.

26.3.6 Observational epidemiology

Epidemiology is the prime source of information on the effects of foods on disease, but an epidemiological association is not enough to prove causality unless the association is very strong, and, unfortunately, relative risks in nutritional epidemiology are typically weak. When associations are weak, confounding becomes a problem; someone who eats lots of vegetables may also exercise more, smoke less and do other healthy things, and even the best computer programs cannot completely separate these factors. When epidemiological findings are consistent with other forms of evidence, a causal link becomes more probable. That is why a causal role of *trans* fat in heart disease is highly likely; the association between *trans* fatty acids intake and coronary heart disease in epidemiological studies is corroborated by the adverse effects of *trans* fatty acids on blood lipids in metabolic trials.

Selective publication and 'data-dredging' is also a problem in epidemiology, because hundreds of associations may be tested but only the 'statistically significant' ones may get published. The validity of such selected associations is much more doubtful than suggested by the *P*-values. Therefore, associations should be observed in multiple cohorts, preferably from different societies.

26.3.7 Randomized clinical trials

Randomization eliminates confounding. Therefore, randomized clinical trials with hard endpoints—disease and death—are the gold standard in biomedical research, and they offer a level of confidence that no other type of research can match.

Randomized clinical trials also have their weaknesses. Chief of these is that they last too short a time. Many benefits of diet may not be reaped within the 3–5 years of a randomized clinical trial, and a negative outcome is thus less than definitive, especially if contradicted by the outcomes of observational epidemiological studies.

26.3.8 Conclusion

The costs of establishing properly that a functional food promotes health is huge, and understandably there is pressure from industry to adopt *in vitro*; and 'functional' tests as substitutes for more expensive and lengthy studies. However, the history of β-carotene—which seemed to prevent cancer *in vitro*; but actually may have caused cancer in clinical trials—shows the risks of relying on soft evidence. If nutrition is to hold its own in an increasingly pharmacized world we will need strict standards of evidence.

26.4 Health claims

Functional foods are more expensive than 'ordinary' foods, and the price is justified by the claimed beneficial effect on health. Unlike taste or convenience, the health effect of a food cannot be perceived directly by the consumer, which is why it is communicated in the form of a health claim.

26.4.1 Soft and hard claims

The demands of the market put pressure on manufacturers to document health claims rapidly without the excessive costs of proving that a food really prevents disease. The alternative preferred by many food producers is a claim for a 'functional' effect. The 'function' can be a surrogate marker for disease, but it can also be something as simple as showing that an added ingredient reaches the circulation, thus: 'Vitamin C is an essential nutrient. Product 'X' increases the level of vitamin C in your bloodstream'. Even though such 'function' claims are legally distinct from health claims, they can still be used to suggest an effect on health. The reason is that consumers do not recognize the subtle legal distinctions between soft and hard claims; to them the phrases 'rich in calcium' and 'prevents fractures' mean essentially the same (Williams, 2005). The message that every claim tries to convey is:

'Buy this product. It will make you healthier and feel better.' Present regulations offer producers room for suggestive claims, competition forces them to exploit this room, and a whole industry has sprung up of consultants, seminars and conferences that teach food manufacturers how to express unsubstantiated health effects of foods without breaking the law.

26.4.2 Health claims and the law

The trustworthiness of health claims is largely dependent on government regulation. Such regulations differ among countries. Many countries do not allow 'medical' claims that refer explicitly to a disease, though some do; thus, stanol and sterol margarines are allowed to claim a beneficial effect on heart disease in the USA, but in Europe they are only allowed to claim cholesterol reduction, and heart disease cannot be mentioned. Governments consider this important, but consumers usually miss the legal distinctions. To them 'lowers cholesterol' implies 'lowers heart disease'.

Consumers often assume that claims on foods have been approved by government authorities, but present legislation in many countries does not require that the health benefits claimed or suggested by functional foods are supported by proper scientific evidence. As a result there is now a plethora of foods that carry a suggestion of a health benefit that has not been proven scientifically.

If supervision is lacking, the integrity of scientific information becomes threatened. One example of this is selective publication. Some industrial sponsors may prefer to keep studies secret when the outcome does not support a health effect (Fig. 26.1). As a result the scientific literature will offer a biased view of what a food or ingredient really does. This explains why meta-analyses of small studies may show beneficial effects while large studies do not; small negative studies may end up in a drawer, but large studies are usually published, even if the results are negative.

Proper legislation is essential to the emergence of evidence-based functional foods. If a claim is true, then manufacturers should be free to advertise it even

(a)

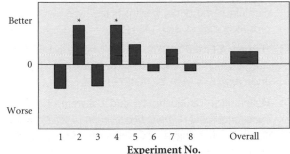

Overall estimate of the health effect of a food ingredient if all studies have been published

(b)

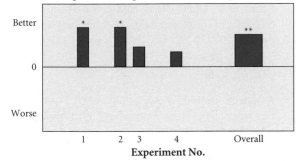

Overall estimate of the health effect of a food ingredient if negative studies are not published

Fig. 26.1 Hypothetical representation of the effect of publication bias on the perceived health effect of a food ingredient. The vertical axis plots the effect of a food ingredient on some risk indicator for disease. Each bar represents the mean outcome of one experiment. All experiments measured the effect of the same ingredient on the same risk factor; the differences between outcomes are due to chance and biological variability. (a) If all experiments are published, then the mean overall effect in a meta-analysis would be small and not significantly different form zero. (b) If experiments with nil or negative outcomes are kept secret, then the mean overall effect in a meta-analysis becomes significant, and the effect of the ingredient appears favourable. $* = P < 0.05$; $** = P < 0.01$.

if it is a medical claim; and if a claim or suggestion is untrue, it should be suppressed by law.

FURTHER READING

1. Aggett, P.J., Antoine, J.M., Asp, N.G., *et al.* (2005) PASSCLAIM: Consensus on criteria. *Eur J Nutr*, **44** (Suppl. 1), 15–30.

2. **Davey Smith, G., Ebrahim, S., Lewis, S., Hansell, A.L., Palmer, L.J., and Burton, P.R.** (2005) Genetic epidemiology and public health: hope, hype, and future prospects. *Lancet*, **366**, 1484–98.

3. **Harper, A.E. (ed.)** (2000) Physiologically active food components. Proceedings of the 17th Ross Conference. *Am J Clin Nutr*, **71**, 1647S–1743S.

4. **Heller, I.R., Taniguchi, Y., and Lobstein, T.** (1999) *Functional foods—Public health boon or 21st century quackery?* Washington, DC, Center for Science in the Public Interest.

5. **Jacobson, M.F., and Silverglade, B.** (1999) Functional foods: health boon or quackery? *Br Med J*, **319**, 205–6.

6. **Katan, M.B., and De Roos, N.M.** (2004) Promises and problems of functional foods. *Crit Rev Food Sci Nutr*, **44**, 369–77.

7. **Katan, M.B.** (2004) Editorial: Health claims for functional foods. *Br Med J*, **328**, 180–1.

8. **American Dietetic Association** (1999) Position of the American Dietetic Association: functional foods. *J Am Diet Assoc*, **99**, 278–85.

9. **Willett, W.C.** (1998) *Nutritional epidemiology*, 2nd edition. New York, Oxford University Press.

10. **Williams, P.** (2005) Consumer understanding and use of health claims for foods. *Nutr Rev*, **63**, 256–64.

USEFUL WEBSITES

Overview of the scientific evidence required to substantiate health claims for foods: http://europe.ilsi.org/passclaim/docs/PASSCLAIMConsensusonCriteria.pdf/

Critical look at functional food regulations in Japan, the USA, and the UK from the consumer's point of view: http://www.cspinet.org/reports/functional_foods/index.html/

 To see topical and scientifically robust updates on nutrition associated with this textbook, and active web links to many of the journal articles in the Reference areas, please see the dedicated Online Resource Centre at www.oxfordtextbooks.co.uk/orc/mann3e/.

Editor's note

Food Standards in Australia and New Zealand allows 'general-level claims' on foods, about what is in the food, or any vague general health effect of the food, provided that the food company holds satisfactory evidence. But 'high-level health claims' about a serious disease (or a biomarker of serious disease such as blood pressure) must be approved by the Authority, which has an independent scientific advisory group.

Only four high-level health claims were allowed as at mid-2006, involving:

• Folate and neural tube defects
• Salt and blood pressure
• Saturated or *trans* fat and LDL cholesterol
• Calcium with or without vitamin D and bone mineral density

PART 5

Nutritional assessment

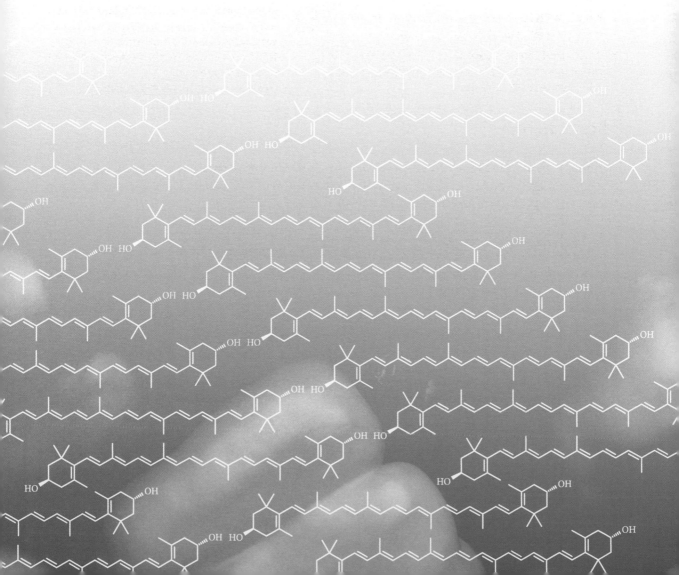

27 Food analysis, food composition tables and databases

Philippa Lyons-Wall

Food composition tables or databases are designed to describe the composition of the foods in the country of origin. They contain data on foods eaten on a regular basis by the population and generally include some less widely consumed foods that are unique to the culture or eaten on special occasions. The values for nutrient and non-nutrient constituents are based on chemical analyses, sometimes performed by the compiler of the tables (or databases) or in an associated laboratory. Some food composition values may be 'borrowed' from a major overseas food table, or represent estimated averages from reports in the literature. Alternatively, they may be imputed from analytical values existing for a similar food or derived from the ingredients of a mixed food. The origins of the nutrient composition values should be specified, although in practice this is not always done. The UK food composition tables (*McCance and Widdowson's: The composition of foods*) and the US data (*USDA Handbook, No. 8*) are widely used reference sources. The US data are also available as a nutrient database at the USDA internet site, which is updated regularly.

When compiling food composition data, there are two important considerations. First, food items must be relevant; sampling of an individual food should be representative of the types commonly consumed by the population on a year-round, nationwide basis, and pertinent to the current food supply. Secondly, the food composition data must be of high quality; analyses of the foods should be conducted in a rigorous, scientific environment so that values are precise and accurate. Well-established food composition tables have evolved over many years and often combine old and new analytical methods from a variety of different sources. Clear and detailed documentation of sampling and analytical procedures at all stages is as critical as the choice of the analytical procedure itself, so that compilers of tables faced with the challenge of inevitable changes in the food supply can continue to evaluate the relevance of the item and quality of the data.

27.1 Sampling

How does one sample foods that are truly representative of a particular food item? Does the analyst just go out to the corner shop nearest the laboratory and buy some food or try to include the varieties of that food across the nation? Foods are ultimately based on parts of plants or animals that vary naturally according to many factors. For example, varieties of sweet potato differ widely in β-carotene content according to whether the flesh is orange, yellow or white in colour. Seasonal variation can markedly influence water and vitamin content, and fruits and vegetables tend to increase their concentration of sugars as they ripen, a process that is highly temperature dependent. Fat depots in animal foods are also extremely variable according to degree of exercise, type of feed and age of the animal. Guidelines for sampling protocols that take these variations into account are detailed by Greenfield and Southgate (2003). In general, the greater the natural variation in a particular food the larger the number of samples required. National food production figures may also indicate the types of foods most widely consumed and therefore most representative of the population.

When the food arrives in the laboratory for analysis, it must first be unambiguously identified with both scientific and local names. Full descriptions are required for the part of the animal or plant used, and its stage of maturity, size, shape and form (see Table 27.1). Any cooking or processing methods used in preparing the item must be documented and the edible portion must be carefully separated from inedible refuse. Analyses may then proceed in one of two directions. Individual samples of the same food from different locations can be analysed separately in order to provide information on the variation between samples as well as their average nutrient content. This approach, however, may be a luxury that many laboratories cannot afford. Alternatively, a composite sample can be prepared by pooling several individual subsamples of a food from many locations to give a single sample for analyses. Often, a weighting scheme is used to ensure that those varieties and/or locations where the food item is consumed more frequently are proportionately represented in the final composite. Whether derived from an individual or composite sample, the edible portion must be homogenized or

Table 27.1 INFOODS guidelines for describing foods

Name and identification	Name of food in national language of the country
	Name in local language or dialect
	Nearest equivalent name in English, French or Spanish
	Country or area in which sample of food was obtained
	Food group and code in database used in the country
	Food group and code for food in regional nutrient database
	Codex Alimentarius or INFOODS food indexing group
Description	Food source (common and scientific name)
	Variety, breed, strain
	Part of plant or animal
	Manufacturer's name and address
	Other ingredients (including additives)
	Food processing and/or preparation
	Preservation method
	Degree of cooking
	Agricultural production conditions
	Maturity or ripeness
	Storage conditions
	Grade
	Container and food contact surface
	Physical state, shape or form
	Colour

Source: Truswell, A.S., Bateson, D.J., Madafiglio, K.C., Pennington, J.A.T., Rand, W.M., and Klensin, J.C. (1991) INFOODS guidelines for describing foods: a systematic approach to describing foods to facilitate international exchange of food composition data. *J Food Comp Anal*, **4**, 18–38. Available online at http://www.fao.org/infoods/

ground thoroughly to ensure that the aliquot taken for analysis is representative of the original sample. For trace minerals, it is also important that the sample is not exposed to adventitious sources of contamination during the collection, homogenization, sample preparation and analytical stages. Similarly, care must be taken that vitamins and other susceptible organic components are not degraded by air or light, for example.

27.2 Analysis

The ultimate aim of food tables or databases is to provide nutrient information on food components that are of nutritional importance to the health of the population, over their lifetime and in different disease states (Table 27.2). Some of the more common methods used to analyse food components are described below. It is important to document the accuracy and precision of all analytical methods and to use reference materials of a similar matrix to the food sample and certified for the nutrient of interest. Reference materials can be obtained from the US National Institute for Standards and Technology, Washington, DC, and the International Atomic Energy Agency, Vienna.

27.2.1 Moisture

Moisture (water) is the first component to be analysed in a food, and it is probably the single most important piece of food composition data. Underestimation of water content will lead to an overestimation of other components that are subsequently determined in the dried food. Water can be gained or lost during the cooking process, with changes in the apparent content of an array of nutrients, as well as energy. Water content is an important preliminary consideration when comparing the nutrient content of similar items in tables from different countries, as may happen if a specific food is not available in the local database. Furthermore, a high moisture content, typical of many fresh fruits and vegetables, indicates a low-energy value while the reverse is true for items of low-moisture content.

The moisture content in foods is determined by simply evaporating off the water and calculating the difference in weight at the beginning and end. Different methods are used. Water may be driven off in

Table 27.2 Food components of nutritional importance

Basic components[a]
Moisture
Energy
Protein, fat and carbohydrate
Up to 13 vitamins, and 10 or more minerals or trace elements

More detailed profiles[b]
Fatty acid profile (up to 20 fatty acids)
Amino acid profile (around 18 amino acids)
Carbohydrate components (sugars, starches)
Dietary fibre and components (soluble, insoluble)
Alcohol

Optional components[c]
Cholesterol
Vitamin A-inactive carotenoids (lycopene, lutein, zeaxanthin and others)
Organic acids (malic, citric, lactic, formic, oxalic, salicylic acids)
Biologically active components (e.g. flavonoids and isoflavonoids)
Glycaemic index

[a]Essential for growth and maintenance of body tissues and always listed in food tables.
[b]Useful for research into diet and disease risk and usually included in well-established tables.
[c]Not essential nutrients but may influence nutritional status indirectly by exerting physiological effects. Not routinely listed in food tables but may be cited in appendix sections.

Table 27.3 Sample calculations of protein content from nitrogen

Item (100 g)	Total nitrogen (g)		Conversion factor[a]		Protein (g)
Rump steak	3.02	×	6.25	=	18.9
White rice	1.23	×	5.95	=	7.3

[a]Conversion factors for converting nitrogen in foods to protein: milk and milk products, 6.38; eggs, meat, fish, 6.25; rice, 5.95; barley, oats, rye, whole wheat, 5.83; soybeans, 5.71; peanuts, brazil nuts, 5.46; almonds, 5.18.

an oven at temperatures around its boiling point, provided the sample itself does not decompose or oxidize or contain other volatiles that would contribute to the weight loss. Alternatively, evaporation can be achieved at lower temperatures by vacuum drying under reduced pressure, or by freeze-drying. In practice, a wide range of methods varying in temperature, time interval and sample preparation have evolved to optimize this apparently simple process.

27.2.2 Protein and amino acids

Protein in foods is determined indirectly by measuring the content of amino-nitrogen, an essential constituent of the amino acid units that combine to form proteins. For the amino-nitrogen assay, the food sample is digested in hot concentrated sulphuric acid to convert the nitrogen into ammonium ion, which is then quantified by either distillation and titration in the classic *Kjeldahl method* or by *spectrophotometric analysis*. The protein content in the original food is then estimated by multiplying the total nitrogen value by specific conversion factors for different foods as shown in Table 27.3. Alternatively, the general conversion factor of 6.25 is used because nitrogen is assumed to represent about 16% of the protein content.

From a nutritional viewpoint, the importance of a particular dietary protein lies in its ability to sustain growth or replenish tissues, functions that depend more on the quality of the protein (or pattern of content of indispensable amino acids) than the total amount (see Chapter 4). Gelatin, for example, is a food that comprises over 80% protein, one of the

highest values listed in food composition tables, yet as the sole protein source it cannot sustain life no matter how much is eaten because it is deficient in the indispensable amino acid tryptophan. *Amino acids* are measured by hydrolysing the protein with strong acid or alkali to break down the peptide bonds, followed by separation and measurement of the free amino acids using ion-exchange chromatography. Food tables may list the amino acid composition of major foods in addition to the total amount of protein, either in the main tables or in an appendix. The profile of indispensable amino acids can then be compared with that of a reference protein, such as hen's egg (a protein known to be utilized very efficiently) for adults, or human milk for babies, to develop a measure of the protein quality, referred to as the amino acid score or chemical score. Table 27.4 shows the indispensable amino acids in two common food proteins compared with those in hen's egg.

27.2.3 Fat

A characteristic property of fats is their solubility in organic solvents such as *n*-hexane, petroleum ether or chloroform. Estimation of fat in foods involves extraction with one of these solvents followed by evaporation of the solvent and weighing of the final fat residue.

The accuracy of this estimation depends on the type of fat as well as the mix of other components in the food. The traditional *Soxhlet method* tended to underestimate fat that was bound to other food components such as protein. To overcome this problem, the sample is now predigested in concentrated

Table 27.4 Content of indispensable amino acids in food proteins (mg amino acid per g of protein)

	Hen's egg	Cheese	Wheat flour
Isoleucine	54	67	42
Leucine	86	98	71
Lysine	70	74	20[a]
Methionine + cysteine	57	32	31
Phenylalanine + tyrosine	93	102	79
Threonine	47	37	28
Tryptophan	17	14	11
Valine	66	72	42

The nutritive value of a dietary protein can be estimated by comparing its pattern of indispensable amino acids with those in a reference protein such as hen's egg. The amino acid score is the content of the most limiting (inadequate) amino acid, as a percentage of the reference value for this amino acid.

[a]For wheat flour, the most limiting amino acid is lysine and the amino acid score is 20/70 or 28%. In real life, however, wheat flour (as bread) is frequently eaten with another protein (e.g. cheese) that has even more lysine than egg, so the amino acid score of whole meals is usually much higher than for individual foods. The limiting amino acid in an equal mixture of wheat and cheese protein is methionine + cysteine and the amino acid score is 55%.

acid or alcoholic ammonia to release the bound portion before extraction. The fat residue may be further analysed in various ways. Thin-layer chromatography can separate the fat into lipid classes including triglycerides, phospholipids and sterols. If lipids are hydrolysed to liberate their fatty acids, these can be separated by gas–liquid chromatography. Fatty acid profiles of major foods are provided in several comprehensive food tables such as *USDA Handbook, No. 8* and the New Zealand Food Composition Tables. Total saturated fatty acids (including branched-chain acids), monounsaturated (*cis* and *trans* together) and polyunsaturated fatty acids are given in a supplement to the UK's *McCance and Widdowson's: The composition of foods*.

The presentation of the fat content of foods differs among food tables. In addition to providing the total fat content, compilers may sum the individual fatty acids into groups: polyunsaturated, monounsaturated and saturated, and list each class separately, or they may present these as a ratio of polyunsaturated and monounsaturated fatty acids to that of saturated fatty acids, termed the PMS ratio. Alternatively, they may list each fatty acid according to its chain length and degree of saturation. The PMS ratio provides a crude estimate of overall atherogenic risk; the higher the proportion of unsaturates, the more favourable the ratio. For research purposes, however, the content of individual fatty acids is more useful because each may exert independent effects. (Chapters 3 and 20 discuss further the role of individual fatty acids in health and disease.)

27.2.4 Carbohydrates

Food composition tables vary widely in the methods used to measure carbohydrate. One approach is to estimate 'by difference', which defines carbohydrate as the difference between 100 and the sum of the weight percentages for protein, fat, water and ash. However, inaccuracies arise using this approach because of the summation of the errors in estimating these four constituents. In addition, such values are of limited use because they do not distinguish between different carbohydrates, especially those that are available to the body (i.e. digested, absorbed and utilized) and those that are unavailable. More accurate methods quantify the available and unavailable carbohydrate by direct measurements.

Available carbohydrate includes sugars (monosaccharides and disaccharides) and starches and dextrins (which are polysaccharides). Individual sugars can be extracted with aqueous alcohol and measured by high-performance liquid chromatography or using specific enzymatic colorimetric tests. Starches and dextrins, which are glucose polymers, are measured in the same way after an initial hydrolysis step to liberate free glucose. Food tables that report carbohydrate by direct analysis may list the monosaccharide equivalents because this is the form in which the carbohydrate is estimated. To obtain the actual values for disaccharides and starch (polysaccharide) in the food, these values should be divided by 1.05 and 1.10, respectively. A published database is also available for the glycaemic index (GI), which ranks carbohydrate-containing foods according to the degree of rise in blood glucose immediately after the food is consumed, compared with that of a standard food—either glucose or white bread (Foster-Powell *et al.*, 2002). The GI data are derived from studies in which human subjects are fed a range of carbohydrate-containing foods, and therefore provide a qualitative biological rather than quantitative chemical measure of carbohydrate intake.

Unavailable carbohydrate or dietary fibre is the mixture of plant components that are resistant to digestive enzymes in the human small bowel. The chemical diversity of fibre makes it a very challenging and elusive component to analyse in the laboratory. Accordingly, a number of methods have evolved. All begin with the defatted, dried food sample but each method measures a different chemical fraction. The *Englyst method* is the most sensitive and perhaps the most useful from a nutritional perspective because it can distinguish between soluble and insoluble fibres, both of which have physiologically distinct effects in the body in relation to chronic diseases such as diabetes, heart disease and cancer. In the Englyst method, starch is initially removed by digestion with strong amylases and then the constituent sugars of dietary fibre are measured directly after acid hydrolysis to produce the free sugars. This yields estimates of both soluble (pectin, gums, mucilages and hemicelluloses) and insoluble (cellulose and other hemicelluloses) fibre components, collectively called non-starch polysaccharides (NSPs). Lignin escapes detection because it is not a carbohydrate but a polymeric phenolic compound. The older *Southgate method* gives a higher value for dietary fibre content as it measures lignin, as well as NSPs.

Other methods are less precise because they measure fibre 'by difference' but they involve less analytical work so are more economical. In the widely used procedure of the *Association of Official Analytical Chemists* (AOAC), developed by Prosky *et al.* (1984),

starch is first removed by enzymatic hydrolysis and the undigested residue is weighed, analysed for nitrogen and then ashed. Protein and ash contents are then subtracted from the residue weight. *Van Soest's neutral detergent fibre* method measures only the insoluble cellulose and lignin, and not the soluble fibre; hence, this method underestimates total dietary fibre. The *crude fibre* method is the least accurate, involving rigorous treatment with boiling acid and alkali, which removes much of the dietary fibre itself.

A further complication in the analysis of dietary fibre is the recognition that a variable but small proportion of the dietary starch found in beans, wholegrains, potatoes (especially if eaten cold) or unripe bananas is not completely digested and is unavailable to the body for absorption. This starch, termed 'resistant starch', escapes digestion because it is physically inaccessible to the enzymes and, instead, it is probably fermented in the colon, thus behaving like soluble dietary fibre. Current values for dietary fibre in food tables do not include separate values for resistant starch, although the AOAC and Southgate methods include some of the resistant starch in the fibre value.

Different analytical methods can result in several-fold variations in the estimate of fibre for the same item, as shown in Table 27.5. Most food tables, however, are internally consistent in their choice of analytical method(s) and these should be stated clearly in the introductory section or in the main tables alongside the nutrient values. Special care should be taken when comparing carbohydrate values from different food composition tables. For reasons outlined above, values from those tables in which total carbohydrate is analysed by difference (i.e. including dietary fibre) are not compatible with others in which carbohydrate constituents are analysed directly.

27.2.5 Energy

The total energy of a food is measured by *bomb calorimetry* in which a sample of the food is burned with oxygen in a sealed chamber until completely oxidized. The heat released corresponds to the chemical or gross energy of the food. Food energy is

Table 27.5 Dietary fibre content of dried red kidney beans estimated by five different methods

Method	Fibre content (g/100 g)	Fibre components
Englyst[a]	15.7	Soluble + insoluble fibre (not lignin or resistant starch)
Southgate[a]	23.4	Soluble + insoluble fibre, lignin
AOAC (Prosky and Asp)[b]	21.5	Soluble + insoluble fibre, lignin
Neutral detergent fibre (Van Soest)[c]	10.4	Insoluble fibre only
Crude fibre[c]	6.2	Part of the insoluble fibre

Note: Red kidney beans contain both soluble and insoluble dietary fibre. AOAC, Southgate, and Englyst methods measure total dietary fibre, but Englyst fibre is lower because it does not measure lignin or resistant starch. Neutral detergent fibre is lower because it does not measure soluble fibre.

Sources:

[a]Holland, B., Welch, A.A., Unwin, I.D., Buss, D.H., Paul, A.A., and Southgate, D.A.T. (1991) *McCance and Widdowson's: The composition of foods*, 5th edition. Cambridge, Royal Society of Chemistry.

[b]English, R., and Lewis, J. (1991) *Nutritional values of Australian foods*. Canberra, Australian Government Publishing Service.

[c]USDA (1986) *Composition of foods: legumes and legume products*. Handbook Nos 8–16. Washington, DC, US Department of Agriculture.

reported in kilojoules (kJ) or kilocalories (kcal), where 1 kJ = 0.24 kcal or 1 kcal = 4.187 kJ. When a food is eaten, however, the energy-yielding components, protein, fat, carbohydrate and (where present) alcohol, are oxidized by enzymatic processes within the body to provide energy, but not with 100% efficiency. Some energy is lost into the faeces as not all food components are fully absorbed from the digestive tract. Further energy is lost into urine since dietary protein, unlike carbohydrate and fat, is not completely oxidized by the body and its excretory product, urea, still retains some of the chemical energy from the original protein. The eminent American physiologist Atwater measured the energy losses into faeces and urine by a series of meticulous experiments in humans fed a mixture of foods. In his experiments, 92% of protein, 95% of fat and 97% of carbohydrate were absorbed by the body, but for every gram of protein ingested, about one-quarter of its gross energy was lost into the urine.

Atwater's experiments, conducted at the turn of the nineteenth century, represent landmark studies from which the energy content of foods in today's food composition tables are derived. Atwater developed a system of four conversion factors, which represent the energy available in (1) protein (17 kJ/g, 4 kcal/g); (2) fat (37 kJ/g, 9 kcal/g); (3) carbohydrate (16 kJ/g, 4 kcal/g); and (4) alcohol (29 kJ/g, 7 kcal/g), taking into account the estimated energy losses into faeces and urine. The value is slightly higher for starch (due to lower hydration) than that given for all carbohydrates and slightly lower for sugars. These factors provide values for food energy as it is utilized by the body (i.e. metabolizable energy). The energy content of each food is calculated by first multiplying the weight of each component by its Atwater conversion factor, and secondly, summing the energy from each component to give a grand total for the food, as shown in Table 27.6. Note that the total weight of each nutrient is obtained by direct analysis of the food, as described previously (also see Chapter 5).

The biggest variable is the carbohydrate value and whether this includes fibre, because Atwater factors are applied to the total carbohydrate content irrespective of whether this is analysed directly or by difference. In practice, the value for energy is somewhere between the two extremes of 16 kcal/g for available carbohydrate and 0 kJ/g for unavailable carbohydrate.

Table 27.6 Calculation of metabolizable energy content in raw soy bean using Atwater conversion factors

Component	Weight (g/100 g)		Atwater factor (kJ (kcal)/g)		Energy content (kJ (kcal)/100 g)
Water	8	—	—	=	—
Protein	31	×	17 (4)	=	527 (124)
Fat	20	×	37 (9)	=	740 (180)
Available carbohydrate	7	×	16 (4)	=	112 (28)
Dietary fibre	20	—	Not included	=	—

Note: The energy content of individual components is then summed to given a grand total of 1379 kJ/100 g or 332 kcal/100 g.

This is because a proportion of dietary fibre is fermented in the colon to short-chain fatty acids, which can be absorbed from the large bowel and oxidized for energy. Livesey (1991) has estimated that about half the dietary fibre can be utilized by the body in this way and proposed an average energy conversion factor of 8 kJ/g (2 kcal/g) for unavailable carbohydrates, about half the value for available carbohydrate. Values in food tables do not usually incorporate estimates of the energy from fibre.

The energy conversion factors used today vary somewhat from Atwater's original factors. The German, British, Australian and New Zealand food composition tables, for example, apply the same four factors to all foods, whereas the US and East Asian tables use a range of slightly differing conversion factors, rather lower for components in plant foods than in animal foods, reflecting Atwater's initial observation that the energy from plants was less available. The conversion factors selected to calculate energy should be specified in the introduction or appendix section of all food composition tables and the reader is referred to these for more in-depth information.

27.2.6 Inorganic nutrients and vitamins

The range of inorganic nutrients in foods including calcium, iron, magnesium, zinc, copper, manganese, potassium and sodium can be determined by *flame atomic absorption spectrophotometry* (AAS), a method whereby a solution of the ashed or acid-digested food sample is sprayed into the flame of an atomic absorption spectrophotometer and quantified by the degree of absorption at a specified wavelength. For selenium, direct AAS with a Zeeman background correction is required. Graphite-furnace AAS is used for analysing the ultratrace elements, such as chromium, nickel and manganese. Alternatively, all the minerals can be measured in the one sample using inductively coupled plasma spectrophotometry or X-ray fluorescence. Minerals are a very stable component of foods and these procedures can be highly accurate provided any interfering substances such as plant pigments or organic constituents have first been removed. This is achieved by reducing the food sample to a dry ash by thorough heating in a muffle furnace, or by breaking down and oxidizing the organic components by wet ashing with boiling concentrated acids. For trace element analysis, precautions must be used to avoid adventitious contamination by the use of ultrapure acids, acid-washed glassware, plastic materials for sample preparation and analysis, and high-grade deionized water.

In contrast to the minerals, many of the vitamins in foods are not very stable. Riboflavin and vitamin A are sensitive to light; thiamin, folate and vitamin C are sensitive to heat, and vitamin E to oxidation. Vitamins are either analysed by the traditional but more time-consuming microbiological methods or by newer, faster chemical techniques. *Microbiological assays* are conducted with a culture of organisms that have a specific growth requirement for the particular vitamin. The assumption is made, however, that the micro organism reacts in the same way as the human organism. Such methods are available for a wide range of B vitamins including thiamin, niacin, riboflavin, vitamins B_6 and B_{12}, folate, biotin and pantothenate, and have the advantage of estimating the total biological potential of the vitamin. Alternative chemical methods, such as *high-performance liquid chromatography* (HPLC), can be used for most of the vitamins. They require an initial extraction step to remove other components in the food, but are useful for separating and quantifying different chemical forms of the vitamin. It should be borne in mind that many of the existing values for vitamins, as well as minerals, in food tables were obtained with older, less specific colorimetric methods that may now be obsolete.

Values in food composition tables represent the total content of each mineral or vitamin in the food and do not address the complex problem of bioavailability, defined as the proportion of a nutrient that is actually absorbed from the food and utilized. When a vitamin exists in two or more forms that are utilized differently in the body, some food composition tables tabulate each form separately. Vitamin A, for example, has two major components obtained from quite different food sources, preformed vitamin A (retinol), which is found in many animal products, and the provitamin A carotenoids derived from plants. The compiler may further attempt to calculate the overall potency of the vitamin in the body by summing the different forms, taking into account their relative biological activities. Some of the assumptions and calculations made in food tables regarding the different forms of niacin, folate and vitamins A, C, D and E are shown in Table 27.7.

27.2.7 Non-nutrient biologically active constituents

In addition to the nutrient components, such as protein, fat, carbohydrate, vitamins and minerals, plant foods in particular contain an abundant array of chemical constituents or 'phytochemicals'. Examples of nutritional importance include the flavonoids, isoflavonoids and non-vitamin A carotenoids. Although not classed as essential nutrients in terms of preventing a specific nutritional deficiency, these constituents are biologically active in the body and are thought to contribute to optimal health and longevity (see Chapter 15).

Phytochemicals occur in relatively small mg or μg quantities per 100 g food. While precise HPLC assays are available for quantification, it is often difficult to estimate levels in foods accurately. For example, the concentration of isoflavonoids in soybeans, a rich natural source, shows up to sixfold variation. This reflects genetic differences and also the fact that isoflavonoids, unlike more stable structural components, such as proteins, are part of the plant's natural response to stress. Insect infestations or climatic considerations including low temperature and high soil moisture can trigger dramatic increases in isoflavonoid content. This natural variability means that the isoflavonoid content in the same variety of soybean or soy product available in local retail outlets could vary several fold between different batches. Despite certain limitations, the identification and quantification of biologically active substances in plants is an area of intense current research. Databases for isoflavonoids and a range of other special-interest constituents have been collated by the Nutrient Data Laboratory at the US Department of Agriculture, and are available at the USDA internet site (http://www.ars.usda.gov/ba/bhnrc/ndl).

27.3 Compilation of food composition data

Compilation of food composition data either in the form of tables or computerized databases is a very large task. It requires painstaking inspection of a wide range of sources that use a variety of sampling and analytical procedures. Data analysed outside the compiler's laboratory must frequently be traced back

Table 27.7 Presentation of different vitamin forms in food composition tables

Vitamin	Main forms	Unit of total vitamin activity
Niacin[a]	1. Preformed in foods (nicotinic acid + nicotamide) 2. Derived from tryptophan	Niacin equivalents (NE)
Folate[b]	1. Food folates 2. Folic acid supplements	Dietary folate equivalents (DFE)
Vitamin A[c]	1. Retinol 2. Provitamin A carotenoids	Retinol equivalents (RE) or Retinol activity equivalents (RAE)
Vitamin C[d]	1. Ascorbic acid 2. Dehydroascorbic acid	Vitamin C
Vitamin D[e]	1. Vitamin D (cholecalciferol) 2. 25-Hydroxyvitamin D	Total vitamin D activity
Vitamin E[f]	1. Tocopherols ($\alpha, \beta, \gamma, \delta$) 2. Tocotrienols ($\alpha, \beta, \gamma, \delta$)	α-Tocopherol equivalents

[a]Because approximately 1% of protein is tryptophan and 1/60th tryptophan is converted to niacin in the body:
NE (mg) = preformed niacin (mg) + dietary protein (g) × 0.16.
[b]Bioavailability of folate from food is about 50% from foods, 85% from fortified foods or as a supplement (consumed with food) or 100% as a supplement (on an empty stomach) (institute of medicine, 2000):
1 µg DFE = 1 µg food folate = 0.6 µg folic acid (taken with meals) = 0.5 µg folic acid (on empty stomach).
[c]Vitamin A can be expressed as RE, where β-carotene has one-sixth the activity of retinol and other carotenoids have one-twelfth the activity of retinol. To acknowledge lower reported availability from vegetable sources, some databases (e.g. USDA, 2006) now express vitamin A as RAE, where β-carotene has only one-twelfth the activity of retinol (Institute of Medicine, 2000):
RAE(µg) = retinol (µg) + β-carotene (µg)/12 + (α-carotene + β-cryptoxanthin (µg)/24.
[d]Both forms have equal activity and are summed to give total vitamin C.
[e]Vitamin D in food is measured as natural cholecalciferol (or ergocalciferol) and 25-hydroxyvitamin D (an active circulating form in animals, and hence meats), which has about five times the activity of cholecalciferol (Food Standards Agency, 2002):
Total vitamin D activity = sum of cholecalciferol + 5 × 25-hydroxycholecalciferol (in meats).
[f]α-Tocopherol is the most abundant form with over twice the activity of other tocopherols and tocotrienols. Activities of individual vitamin forms are cited in: Food Standards Agency (2002).

to its source and any items without clear documentation discarded because there is no way to evaluate their quality. Values from different sources must be compared and statistical calculations made to provide a meaningful average for the nutrient content of a food. As food patterns within a population are constantly changing and evolving, data must also be scrutinized to determine its relevance in the current food supply.

Not only should data be accurate and relevant, but also the format must be clear so that the user may easily understand the data. Food items are listed alphabetically and usually grouped according to food sources with similar nutritional properties (e.g. vegetables, fruits, grains, meats and dairy products); or by product use (e.g. snacks, desserts and breakfast cereals). In cases where foods are collected or prepared with inedible matter, the percentage edible portion, sometimes expressed indirectly as percentage refuse, is also given. However, irrespective of the proportion of edible matter or the accustomed serving size, nutrient values for items are always presented in terms of 100 g edible portions. Consequently, this does not include the core or stone in fruit, or the bones in meat and chicken, but it does include optional materials such as certain vegetable skins and trimmable meat fat, unless specified otherwise. Most food tables cite both scientific and local names for each item, and some specify the number of food items analysed, and whether a single or composite sample was used for analysis. Rarely do tables include the natural variation around the mean value but rather provide a single mean representative value. The German (Souci *et al.*, 2006) and the United States (USDA, 2006) tables are exceptions, citing the range (i.e. highest and lowest values known) or the standard error of the mean, respectively, in addition to the mean value.

Ideally, food composition tables or databases should include analyses for all food components of nutritional relevance to the potential user, whether this be a dietitian prescribing advice to a client, a research worker investigating certain nutrients in relation to disease risk, or a food manufacturer seeking accurate nutrient information on their products for the purposes of marketing and food legislation. In practice, however, inclusion is determined more by the analytical resources and public health priorities of the country concerned. Nevertheless, a wealth of analytical and descriptive information on food habits and customs already exists within different cultures. Yet, many of these data are not widely accessible outside the country, often because local names are idiosyncratic or culture-specific making it difficult to identify the food. In this regard, the INFOODS guidelines (Table 27.1) were established to ensure foods are named and described in a standardized manner with a view to facilitating interchange of food composition data at the international level.

FURTHER READING

1. **Agricultural Research Service** (2006) *USDA National Nutrient database for standard reference, release 19, Nutrient data laboratory*. US Department of Agriculture.

2. **Burlingame, B.A., Milligan, G.C., Spriggs, T.W., and Athar, N.** (1997) *The concise New Zealand food composition tables*, 3rd edition. Palmerston North NZ, Institute for Crop and Food Research.

3. **Food Standards Agency** (2002) *McCance and Widdowson: The composition of foods*, 6th edition. Cambridge, Royal Society of Chemistry.

4. **Foster-Powell, K., Holt, S.H.A., and Brand-Miller, J.C.** (2002) International table of glycaemic index and glycaemic load values. *Am J Clin Nutr*, **76**, 5–56.

5. **Greenfield, H., and Southgate, D.A.T.** (2003) *Food composition data. Production, management and use*, 2nd edition. Rome, Food and Agricultural Organization.

6. **Livesey, G.** (1991) Calculating the energy values of foods: towards new empirical formulae based on diets with varied intakes of unavailable complex carbohydrates. *Eur J Clin Nutr*, **45**, 1–12.

7. **Institute of Medicine** (2000) Dietary reference intakes: applications in dietary assessment. Washington, DC, The National Academics Press.

8. **Prosky, L., Asp, N.G., Furda, I., De Vries, J.W., Schweizer, T.F., and Harland, B.F.** (1984) Determination of total dietary fibre in foods, food products and total diets: Interlaboratory study. *J Assoc Off Anal Chem*, **67**, 1044–52.

9. **Souci, S.W., Fachmann, W., and Kraut, H.** (2006) *Food composition and nutrition tables*, 7th edition. Stuttgart, Medpharm Scientific Publishers.

10. **Wu Leung, T., Bukum, R.R., Chang, EH., Rao, M.N., and Polacchi, W.** (1972) *Food composition tables for use in East Asia*. FAO, Rome.

USEFUL WEBSITES

http://www.sfk-online.net/cgi-bin/sfkstart.mysql/

US Department of Agriculture. Home Page, http://www.nal.usda.gov/fnic.foodcomp.

 To see topical and scientifically robust updates on nutrition associated with this textbook, and active web links to many of the journal articles in the Reference areas, please see the dedicated Online Resource Centre at www.oxfordtextbooks.co.uk/orc/mann3e/.

28 Dietary assessment

Sheila Bingham

28.1 Introduction

Dietary assessment is one of the specialized interests of nutritionists, used in surveillance of populations, clinical assessment, experimental research and nutritional epidemiology. It has become of particular importance with the realization that nutrition plays a major role in the aetiology of common chronic diseases such as obesity, diabetes, heart disease and cancer. As these diseases have a long onset, and nutritional factors interact with gene variants in influencing risk, very large populations must be studied prospectively over prolonged periods of time in order to assess the magnitude of nutritional factors in the aetiology of these diseases. Accumulated evidence can then be used as a basis for public health and clinical advice for the prevention of these conditions. However, a major problem until recently has been the conflict between the need for accuracy to establish exactly where an individual lies within the overall distribution of foods and nutrients, and the logistics of doing so when very large populations required for epidemiological studies are investigated.

28.2 Population estimates

Population estimates are needed for surveillance, for example, to assess intakes of a particular food or nutrient in relation to reference nutrient intakes (RNIs). Such information would also be used during emergencies when food is in short supply, to make recommendations concerning usual diet, and in considering the case for fortification of foods on a national basis. Population estimates of dietary intake have also been compared with disease rates in different countries or populations or within the same country over time to identify clues as to possible nutritional causes of the disease.

Typically the 24-hour recall (see section 28.3) is used in *national nutrition surveys*. This is appropriate provided that it can be assured that this or indeed any other individual method yields unbiased estimates of the usual mean intake of that population. In addition, population estimates may be derived from food balance sheets, household food surveys and, potentially, supermarket records.

Food balance sheets are based on national statistics of food produced, imported and exported with factors for wastage included. The Food and Agricultural Organization (FAO) of the United Nations

---

BOX 28.1 National nutrition surveys

National nutrition surveys estimate food intake of individuals and add some examination to assess nutritional status, which may include blood tests. Examples are NHANES in the USA, National Diet and Nutrition Surveys in the UK, National Nutrition Surveys in Australia (1995) and the National Nutrition Survey in New Zealand (1997). They have all been somewhat different. They are looking for low intakes of some nutrients on the one hand and overweight/obesity on the other. They also want information about food usage as a basis for formulating and evaluating health policy and regulatory needs. The food intake method used has to be a 24-hour recall or food record because of the need to know the exact types of food people are eating. Food intake results from national nutrition surveys should give average individual intakes of foods and of nutrients of different age and sex subgroups at the time of the survey. Though subjects sampled in these surveys are intended to represent the nation, the results report the food and nutrient intake of individuals.

BOX 28.2 Food consumption at the national level

Food consumption at the national level is also called food moving into consumption, food disappearance data and apparent food consumption. The food supply is calculated from estimates of domestic food production plus imports, minus exports. Potential food diverted for farm animal feed, non-food industrial use and wastage at wholesale level are subtracted. The total is divided by the estimated population each year. These statistics are useful for monitoring changes in consumption of commodities and comparing countries' food habits. FAO food balance sheets are based on these statistics and available each year from some 175 countries. For many countries, these are the only regular measures of food intakes. However these are macro figures. The calorie and nutrient numbers are around 25% (or more) above what individuals actually eat and drink, because there is wastage of food in homes and catering establishments, and food is fed to tourists and pets. They give no idea of distribution of food resources among regions, socioeconomic groups, or within the family.

(http://faostat.fao.org/faostat) collates these and they have been used extensively for population comparisons, linking for example population estimates of fat and cardiovascular disease rates, and population estimates of meat and fat and bowel and breast cancer rates.

Household surveys are records kept by the householder of all food available to the family over 1 week, and the total food entering the household is divided by the number of people living there. This approach has been used in the UK in the National Food Survey, which has been running continuously for over 50 years as a combined food consumption and expenditure survey and which in recent years has taken into account food eaten away from home (http://statistics.defra.gov.uk/esg/publications/nfs). From this, regional comparisons and secular trends

in consumption are available, for example the recent trend towards a lower saturated fat composition of the diet in the UK.

Potentially, computerized supermarket records of sales or loyalty cards could be used to obtain regional information on nutritional consumption (Robertson *et al.*, 2004).

When using data derived from food balance sheets or household surveys, it is not possible to compare the intake of food or nutrients in different age and sex groups with differential trends in disease incidence or risk factors, nor for individual data to be assessed. This is because the findings relating to, for example, children, the elderly or males and females cannot be separated out from the overall population average data.

28.3 Individual methods

Several methods are available for measuring the dietary intake of individuals. They generally consist either of the collation of observations from a number of separate days' investigations, as in records, checklists and 24-hour recalls, or attempts to obtain average intake by asking about the usual frequency of food consumption, as in the diet history and food frequency questionnaires (FFQs). In all methods of dietary assessment, some estimate of the quantity of food consumed is required and, for the determination of nutrient or other food component intake, either an appropriate description that can be matched with an entry in the food tables or an aliquot for chemical analysis. Each of the methods is described briefly below and further details regarding equipment, protocols, uses and limitations are available in the references in the further reading list. Detailed examples of methods used in particular studies are shown on the web sites given.

28.3.1 Food records

Food records involve subjects being taught to describe and either weigh or estimate the amount of food immediately before eating and to record leftovers. Records are generally completed by the participant on sheets or booklets, which, in the case of estimated records, may include photographs to facilitate estimation of portion size. Cups, spoons and rulers may be provided to aid accurate description. Verbal records, with descriptions of amounts recorded on tape cassettes, have also been used, as have records incorporating bar codes from purchased foods. As this method is a record kept at the time of eating and does not involve participants attempting to remember if or how often a food has been eaten, it is generally regarded as providing the most reliable information regarding the dietary intake of individuals, provided sufficient days' observations are collected on each individual (see section 28.5.2). In the past, it has been used for the purpose of validating other methods of dietary assessment but this approach is now recognized

---

> **BOX 28.3 Estimating individual food intake**
>
> Basically, four types of method are used to estimate individual food intakes:
>
> - **Dietary history** 'What do you eat on a typical day and how does your food intake vary?' This requires a skilled and patient interviewer. Food models, cups, plates and spoons are used to estimate portion sizes
>
> - **24-hour recall** 'Tell me everything you had to eat and drink in the last 24 hours.' This is less subject to wishful thinking about what the subject feels they ought to have eaten. The weakness is that yesterday may have been an unusual day; 24-hour recalls can, however, be repeated
>
> - **Food diary or record** 'Please write down (and describe) everything you eat and drink (and estimate the amount) for the next 3 (4 or 7) days.' Amounts are usually recorded in household measures, but for more accuracy subjects can be provided with quick reading scales to weigh food before it goes on the plate (and any leftovers).
>
> - **Food frequency questionnaire** 'Do you eat meat/fish/bread/milk, etc. on average more than once a day, two or three times a week, once a week, once a month, etc.?' (usually filling in 100 to 150 lines on a questionnaire form). (See Fig. 28.2).

---

to underestimate the extent of measurement error (see section 28.5.6). Respondent burden is higher than with other methods but the approach has been used in multicentre cross-sectional comparisons of representative population samples in which instructions to participants have been standardized among different centres (e.g. the Key's study of coronary heart disease (see Chapter 20) and other epidemiological settings such as the very large prospective studies of diet and health, for example a study of 25 000 people in EPIC Norfolk (see http://www.srl.cam.ac.uk/epic/nutmethod). Figure 28.1 shows an example from this website. Weighed records have also been used in

| DATE | 2 | 3 | 1 | 0 | 1 | 9 | 9 | 3 | DAY OF WEEK | SATURDAY |

BEFORE BREAKFAST

Food/Drink	Description and Preparation	Amount
Orange Squash	Robinsons whole orange–sweetened	1 Glass

BREAKFAST

Food/Drink	Description and Preparation	Amount
Beef Patty with onion	Homebaked cold Salt added	3a
Tea	Typhoo	1 Cup
Milk	S/Skimmed	1 Dessertspoon
Sugar	White	$1\frac{1}{2}$ Teaspoon

MID MORNING – between breakfast time and lunch time

Food/Drink	Description and Preparation	Amount
Coffee	Maxwell House, Instant $\frac{1}{2}$ Water/$\frac{1}{2}$ S/Skimmed milk	1 Mug
Sugar	White	$1\frac{1}{2}$ Teaspoons
Cake	Homemade Date Cake	16a

LUNCH

Food/Drink	Description and Preparation	Amount
Gammon Steak	Microwaved	6oz
Chips	Deep Fried in Oil (Crisp & Dry)	7a
Peas	Birds Eye (Frozen)	12a
Bread	Local Bakery White unsliced	$\frac{1}{2}$ Slice $\frac{1}{2}$ Thick
Apple Pie	Homemade	3β
Sugar	White—sprinkled on	1 Teaspoon
Custard	Birds—made with S/Skimmed milk	Small Fruit Dish

TEA – between lunch time and the evening meal

Food/Drink	Description and Preparation	Amount
Tea	Typhoo—tea bag	1 Mug
Milk	S/Skimmed	1 Dessertspoon
Sugar	White	$1\frac{1}{2}$ Teaspoons
Biscuit	Chocolate Digestive Fox's	1

Fig. 28.1 Example of a food diary.

Source: Reproduced with permission from EPIC Norfolk (http://www.srl.cam.ac.uk/).

surveillance procedures; for example, records from representative population samples have been routinely obtained by the UK Government National Diet and Nutrition Survey (http://www.food.gov.uk/science).

28.3.2 Twenty-four-hour recalls

This method is also a report of daily habits, but interviewed or written information about the previous day's intake, the 24-hour recall, is obtained. The participant has to remember the actual foods consumed, and give information on portion weights from memory. Some information may be forgotten and descriptions of portion size are more difficult to supply, though the interviewers will often use food models or photographs as memory aids and to assist in quantifying portion size. Although the 24-hour recall may consist of a very simple written list completed by the participant, most 24-hour recalls have several stages or multiple passes, in which data are checked and verified by a skilled interviewer, and each recall may take about 40 minutes. The respondent burden for a single 24-hour recall is less than for several days of food records and the method is typically used for determining average usual intakes of a large population or group, e.g. in national nutrition surveys. For details of methods used in the USA NHANES survey, see http://www.cdc.gov/nchs/about/major/nhanes/index.htm. For individual dietary assessments, multiple 24-hour recalls may be needed, with a subsequent increase in respondent burden, depending on the level of precision required and nutrient to be studied (see section 28.5).

28.3.3 Food frequency questionnaires (FFQs)

FFQs are designed to assess long-term habits, over months or years, and may either comprise a relatively small list of foods that are the major sources of a limited group of nutrients of interest, or a longer list if a full dietary assessment is required. Participants usually complete the FFQ themselves, generally after receiving the FFQ in the post with detailed instruc-

tions regarding completion of the questionnaire. The length of the list of foods generally does not exceed 150 items. Various methods to assess portion sizes may be used, for example fitting average portion weights derived from other data to the respondents' chosen food and frequency selections. To assess the frequency of food consumption, accompanying the food list is a multiple response grid in which respondents attempt to estimate how often selected foods are eaten. Up to ten categories ranging from never or once a month or less, to six times per day is a usual format. Figure 28.2 shows an example of a FFQ taken from http://www.srl.cam.ac.uk/epic/nutmethod. Because responses are standardized, FFQs can be analysed in comparatively short periods of time so that large numbers of individuals can be investigated relatively inexpensively. The FFQ has been widely used in large epidemiological cohort studies to identify food patterns associated with inadequate intakes of nutrients and descriptive information on usual intakes of foods and to classify participants according to quantiles of intake of nutrients and disease incidence in each quantile examined. However, there are emerging doubts about the ability of FFQs to detect associations between diet and disease using this method (Kristal *et al.*, 2005).

28.3.4 Diet histories

The diet history is usually conducted by trained interviewers who record a 24-hour recall followed by more detailed information on usual foods consumed, portion sizes, recipes and frequency of food consumption over the recent past. This method is less commonly used in epidemiological research due to the necessity for face-to-face interviews of up to 90 minutes, and consequent costs, but it is the most frequently used method for the assessment of diet by dietitians in the clinical context.

28.3.5 Checklists

The checklist is a record, to be completed for 7 days or more. However, the checklist method is a printed list of representative foods in which participants are

PLEASE PUT A TICK (✓) ON EVERY LINE

FOODS AND AMOUNTS	AVERAGE USE LAST YEAR								
DRINKS	Never or less than once/month	1–3 per month	Once a week	2–4 per week	5–6 per week	Once a day	2–3 per day	4–5 per day	6+ per day
Tea (cup)								✓	
Coffee, instant or ground (cup)						✓			
Coffee, decaffeinated (cup)	✓								
Coffee whitener, eg. Coffee-mate (teaspoon)	✓								
Cocoa, hot chocolate (cup)						✓			
Horlicks, Ovaltine (cup)	✓								
Wine (glass)	✓								
Beer, lager or cider (half pint)	✓								
Port, sherry, vermouth, liqueurs (glass)	✓								
Spirits, eg. gin, brandy, whisky, vodka (single)	✓								
Low calorie or diet fizzy soft drinks (glass)	✓								
Fizzy soft drinks, eg. Coca cola, lemonade (glass)						✓			
Pure fruit juice (100%) e.g. orange, apple juice (glass)	✓								
Fruit squash or cordial (glass)							✓		
FRUIT (1 fruit or medium serving) **For very seasonal fruits such as strawberries, please estimate your average use when the fruit is in season**									
Apples				✓					
Pears				✓					
Oranges, satsumas, mandarins		✓							
Grapefruit	✓								
Bananas			✓						
Grapes			✓						
Melon	✓								
Peaches, plums, apricots				✓					
Strawberries, raspberries, kiwi fruit						✓			
Tinned fruit		✓							
Dried fruit, eg. raisins, prunes	✓								
	Never or less than once/month	1–3 per month	Once a week	2–4 per week	5–6 per week	Once a day	2–3 per day	4–5 per day	6+ per day

Please check that you have a tick (✓) on EVERY line

Fig. 28.2 Example of a food frequency questionnaire. This is one of several different pages that have to be filled in.

Source: Reproduced with permission from EPIC Norfolk (http://www.srl.cam.ac.uk/).

asked to check off at the end of each day which foods they have eaten. This means that participants do not have to estimate how often the food is eaten, thus avoiding problems in the estimation of the frequency of food consumption that occur in the FFQs. Like the FFQs however, the foods can be precoded for rapid data entry and computerized linkage to food tables. In one published version, the checklist took the form of a booklet, which comprised one page of instructions, one of an example and seven pages (one for each day over 1 week) of the checklist. When selecting foods, participants were asked to count half for a small portion and two for a large portion. A space was left to record foods not present on the printed list, but otherwise the list was precoded for nutrient analysis. The list of 160 foods was that used for a FFQ and, where possible, 'units' (slices, cups, etc.) were specified (Bingham *et al.*, 1994). This method has been developed more recently (Lillegaard and Andersen, 2005).

28.3.6 Precise weighing

If there is inadequate food table information, 'precise weighing' may be necessary, for example if food composition tables with values for cooked foods are not available or if exposure to phytochemicals and contaminants are being investigated. Raw ingredients, the cooked food, meal or snack, plus the individual portions must all be weighed, and aliquots for chemical analysis may also be necessary. This method is very labour-intensive compared with the records outlined above and it is usual for skilled field-workers to carry out this survey, rather than the subjects themselves (Bingham, 1987).

28.3.7 Retrospective assessment

Methods that are designed to assess recent past diet (the 24-hour recall, FFQs and diet history) can in theory also be used to assess distant past diet, for example in case–control investigations where dietary habits before the onset of symptoms (and possible change in diet) are required. However, there is evidence to suggest that individuals cannot remember past diet and instead report present diet (Friedenreich *et al.*, 1992). This may introduce bias into case–control studies if dietary habits have changed as a result of the symptoms of the disease in question. For this reason, more weight is placed on results of prospective studies than retrospective case–control studies in nutritional epidemiology.

28.4 Calculation of nutrient intake

Once the primary data concerning foods consumed are obtained, the information is converted to nutrient intake using tables of food composition. In the past, this was generally done manually, perhaps with the assistance of a calculator, and the information obtained was generally restricted to a narrow range of nutrients, for example energy and macronutrient consumption. Computerized databases of food composition revolutionized the amount of information that could be obtained, but in some data entry systems the matching of the description of the food consumed to the correct computer code has to be done manually, which leads to errors. In present-day surveys, necessitated partly by the growth in the variety of foods consumed, this procedure is now usually entirely computerized usually by the investigators themselves. Programs are more expensive to run and develop for record or 24-hour recall methods than for FFQs since at least 150 000 different food items are available in westernized food supplies, all of which require estimation of portion size and individual computer coding (see http://www.srl.cam.ac.uk/epic/nutmethod/). Furthermore, most investigators will incorporate some means of calculating nutrient intake from individual recipes used in home cooking since these can have a marked effect on some nutrients, for example on specific fatty acids. The checklist and FFQ methods require much simpler methods and considerably less coding time by the investigator, although much information on actual foods consumed is lost.

28.5 Measurement error in dietary assessments

Methods of measuring diet are associated with both random and systematic error. Both types of error can arise in the assessment of portion size, daily variation, frequency of food consumption and failure to report usual diet, either due to changes in habits while taking part in an investigation, or misreporting of food choice or amount. Error may also result from the use of food tables.

28.5.1 Assessment of portion size

Information about the weight of food consumed may be obtained either by asking subjects to weigh out individual items of food onto the plate as it is being served (weighed records), or portions of food are described in terms of household measures, volume models, photographs, average portions, units or pack sizes (estimated records, diet histories and 24-hour recalls). Errors are reduced when weights are obtained, but participants need to be given a set of scales accurate to 1–2 g with a capacity of 2 kg. Digital scales are now usually used and have replaced spring balances used in older surveys. Participants need instruction on the use of the scales, and on the detail of information required, including description of recipes used (see Further reading). Estimated records are much easier for participants to complete but conversion of descriptions of food into weights requires considerable investment by the investigator, and may necessitate the determination of density of separate foods, as well as a detailed database of weights of foods equivalent to the photographs, models, package sizes and household measures used. On balance, there appears to be little or no systematic bias in group averages of nutrients obtained by records with estimates of food, compared with group averages obtained by weighed dietary records. Nevertheless, despite the absence of overall bias in a population, the estimation of portion size rather than direct weighing is associated with imprecision at the individual level. In general, this is in the order of 50% (coefficient of variation) for foods, but less, about

20%, for nutrients, probably due to cancellation of error from the use of food tables. Models and photographs may incur less error in the estimation of portion weights, at least when compared with estimations from household measures and dimensions.

28.5.2 Daily variation

Individuals do not consume the same food from day to day and substantial error is introduced when diet is assessed from a single day's dietary investigation in records or 24-hour recalls. Thus, daily variation is one of the main factors in reducing precision of individual estimates in either of these methods of assessing diet. The variability from day to day is closely related to the nutrient under study. The early descriptions of record techniques specified that subjects should be observed for 7 days and this practice has been followed for over 60 years. Nevertheless, when only the average intake of a group of individuals is required for cross-sectional studies, it is difficult to justify gathering this amount of data, even for the more variable nutrients such as cholesterol or polyunsaturated fatty acids. A 1-day record or 24-hour recall collected from a large number of subjects may suffice for the assessment of group means, although it is generally more useful to undertake the assessment on at least two days in order to be able to estimate the within-subject component error.

Seven days is generally accepted as the minimum length of time required to gain precision in observations on each individual, although shorter periods of time with correction for the within-subject component error are under investigation. The actual number of records required to classify individuals in any specific population according to quantiles of nutrient intake will depend on the ratio of the average within-person daily variation and the between-person variation. Thus, whereas a 7-day record is probably sufficient to classify into thirds of the distribution for energy and energy-yielding nutrients, longer periods are necessary for items such as some vitamins and minerals, and cholesterol.

28.5.3 Frequency of food consumption

Overestimation, compared with records of food consumption, particularly of vegetables but also of energy and energy-yielding nutrients is a usual finding with FFQs. The cause of this is uncertain, but may result from the use of lists. Restriction of the choice of food into a comparatively short list of around 150 foods or fewer, means that error associated with estimation of amounts of single items is more likely to be biased than when the full variety of foods is analysed, as occurs, for example, in a 24-hour recall or record of food consumption. Participants using the FFQ may also have difficulty in choosing the correct category of how often food is consumed, so that overestimation occurs of the number of times foods are eaten over a defined period of time. FFQs routinely overestimate intake of fruits and vegetables.

28.5.4 Under-reporting

The term under-reporting particularly applies to methods that attempt to assess total energy intake. This problem has been demonstrated by comparing the group average intake of energy from diet assessment methods with group energy expenditure estimated from body weight, or, more accurately, the doubly labelled water technique (see below). Under-reporting has been documented with all methods of dietary assessment, including 24-hour recalls, weighed records, diet histories and FFQs designed to assess total diet. Overweight individuals in particular are likely to under-report the amount they eat. Table 28.1 is an example showing that some but not all nutrients and foods are under-reported: Protein, sugars and fat, and foods such as cakes and sweets, tend to be under-reported but nutrients such as carotene, non-starch polysaccharides and vitamin C, and vegetables are not.

The problem of under-reporting is particularly difficult when mean intakes are to be compared with reference nutrient intakes for surveillance and clinical

Table 28.1 Mean (standard error, SE) intakes of energy and macronutrients expressed as reported and after energy adjustment in individuals who under-reported dietary intake and those who did not, as judged by the urine to dietary nitrogen ratio

Nutrient	Valid records $n = 126$ (mean (SE))	Under-reporters $n = 33$ (mean (SE))	P
Reported intakes			
MJ	8.14 (0.04)	6.65 (0.23)	< 0.001
Protein (g)	71 (0.2)	60 (1.7)	< 0.001
Fat (g)	80 (0.3)	62 (2.5)	< 0.001
Carbohydrate (g)	231 (4.3)	191 (8.2)	< 0.001
Energy adjusted intakes			
Protein (g)	69 (0.8)	67 (1.4)	> 0.05
Fat (g)	77 (0.9)	75 (0.9)	> 0.05
Carbohydrate (g)	223 (2.7)	225 (4.0)	> 0.05

work, or amounts of nutrients eaten by a different population or group (such as obese compared with lean individuals). Cut-offs based on estimated energy expenditure calculated from body weight have been devised but they are imprecise when used in the absence of information on energy expenditure. Ideally, all dietary studies should include independent measures of validity (see section 29.6 and Black, 2000).

28.5.5 Energy adjustment

Energy adjustment can be carried out by a variety of methods including expressing results for nutrients as a percentage of the total energy, or using regression techniques (Willett, 1997). One reason for attempting to correct for energy intake in dietary assessments is to reduce extraneous variation from the general correlation of nutrients with total energy intake, brought about by differences in body size and hence (in sedentary populations) energy expenditure. In addition, the correlation between results from one method and another is sometimes improved by energy adjustment. Furthermore, although there are significant differences in absolute macronutrient intake between individuals who give valid records and those who do not, these differences are substantially reduced after energy adjustment, although the overall mean within a population is not altered. Table 28.1 shows reported and energy adjusted intakes of fat, carbohydrate and protein in a group of women. Differences between under-reporters and those who gave valid records were no longer significant after energy adjustment.

The effect of energy adjustment depends on the correlation between the nutrient concerned and energy intake, and also on the correlation between the errors of measurement for these two quantities. The latter is heavily dependent on the dietary method used. Hence, the relation between nutrient intakes derived from FFQs and weighed records can be much improved by energy adjustment, but to a lesser extent between nutrient intakes derived from weighed records and 24-hour recalls. Energy adjustment is inappropriate (and without effect) if there are zero correlations between energy intake and the nutrient concerned, for example in the case of some vitamins. More details of techniques for energy adjustment are given in Willett (1997).

28.5.6 Effects of measurement error

Measurement error is a serious problem in dietary assessment. The effect of measurement error may be to introduce bias, so that, for example, group mean intakes may be over-or underestimated when population intakes are investigated for comparison against recommended levels (see section 28.5.4). In epidemiological research, individuals may be misclassified in the distribution of nutritional intakes so that a null or attenuated relationship may be obtained and the true effect between diet and disease missed. For example, in a prospective study relating diet to breast cancer risk, diet was assessed using both a FFQ and a detailed 7-day diary of food and drink in 13 070 women in 1993–1997. By 2002, there were 168 incident breast cancer cases for analysis. When their baseline dietary intake was compared with matched controls (four for each of the breast cancer cases), the hazard ratio for breast cancer for each quintile increase of energy-adjusted fat was strongly associated with saturated fat intake measured using the food diary (1.219 (95% CI 1.061–1.401), $P = 0.005$). However, with saturated fat measured using the FFQ, the comparable ratio was 1.100 (0.941–1.285, $P = 0.229$) (Bingham *et al.*, 2003).

Different methods of dietary assessment have different types of error structure, so that the magnitude of the error varies according to the method and may not always be predictable in different populations. In large prospective epidemiological studies, it is now common practice to correct for measurement error in the assessment of relative risk by regression calibration when the correction factors are derived by comparison of the method in use, such as a FFQ, with a 'reference' method, such as a record. This 'relative validation' relies on the assumptions that errors in the reference instrument are not correlated with both 'true' intake and errors in the method in use. However, errors associated with the method under investigation may be correlated with those of the reference method, so that correction for regression dilution is substantially underestimated (Day *et al.*, 2001; Schatzkin *et al.*, 2003). For example, an individual who under-reports using one dietary assessment method such as a food record will also do so with another such as a FFQ. The use of biomarkers (see below) has therefore superseded relative validity studies between one method and another.

28.6 Biomarkers

The presence of measurement errors has generated much controversy and discussion as to the most 'accurate' method of dietary investigation. Numerous 'relative validation' studies, comparing results of one dietary assessment method with another, presumed more accurate, on the same individuals have been conducted. However, all traditional methods, even weighed records, rely on food consumption as reported by the individuals. True estimates of food consumption can only be obtained by actually observing the activities of participants, or by developing some other independent way of assessing food intake. This has become possible with the advent of biological markers in biological specimens, such as blood, urine or hair, that reflect intake sufficiently closely to act as objective indices of true intake (Bingham, 2002).

28.6.1 Types of biomarkers

There are four main classes of biomarkers used for assessment of the accuracy of dietary methods (Bingham, 2002). The most important are *recovery biomarkers*. These biomarkers have been tested under controlled conditions, usually in a metabolic suite, and have been shown to reflect an individual's intake of energy or of a particular nutrient with a high degree of accuracy. Thus, they provide a true gold standard against which another method of dietary assessment may be compared. Few such biomarkers of dietary intake have been identified; they include doubly labelled water as a measure of energy intake, used for example in the OPEN study (Schatzkin *et al.*, 2003) and markers of potassium and nitrogen in 24-hour urine collections (Bingham, 2002; Bingham *et al.*, 1995). A recent new category has been the *predictive*

biomarker of 24-hour urinary sucrose and fructose, which is closely correlated with intake of sugars, despite the very small fraction of intake that is present in urine collections (Tasevska *et al.*, 2005).

Several *concentration biomarkers* (including serum levels of some vitamins such as vitamin C and carotenoids) are available to compare with estimates of dietary intake. Concentration biomarkers cannot be related directly to absolute levels of intake but concentrations do correlate with intakes of corresponding foods or nutrients, although correlation coefficients are much lower (usually equal to less than 0.6) than that expected for recovery biomarkers. Results from a dietary intake method that agreed most closely with these biomarkers would be expected to yield more reliable estimates of intake than one that did not. Finally, *replacement biomarkers* may be used if databases of food composition for certain items are not available or considered to be inaccurate, for example iodine, aflatoxins and phyto-oestrogens. As it is not usually possible to measure added salt or salt used in cooking, and as a consequence salt intake cannot be measured by dietary methods, 24-hour urine sodium is also an example of a replacement biomarker.

28.6.2 Validation of dietary methods with biomarkers

Biomarkers have been used to validate methods used for dietary assessments in both large-scale epidemiological studies designed to establish the nutritional aetiology of non-communicable diseases and in national nutrition surveys intended to evaluate population nutrient intakes. For example, in the UK

National Diet and Nutrition Survey, pilot studies were carried out before the main survey in order to compare intakes of energy from the dietary assessment method and energy expenditure from doubly labelled water (see http://www.food.gov.uk/science/101717/ndnsdocuments/ndnsappendices). In the USA, doubly labelled water has been used to assess 24-hour recalls and FFQ methods used in epidemiological studies (Schatzkin *et al.*, 2003). To assess the validity of several different methods of dietary assessment in UK cohorts of the EPIC study, 160 women were asked to complete 16 days of weighed-food records over 1 year, as four repeated 4-day records. The volunteers were also asked to provide eight 24-hour urine collections, as four repeated 2-day collections, and completeness of the urine collections was assessed using a specially developed marker. Correlations were greater ($r = 0.7$) between the biomarker 24-hour urine nitrogen and estimates of nitrogen intake from records than from estimates of intake from other methods including FFQs ($r = 0.4$). A similar pattern was evident with the urinary potassium biomarker (Bingham *et al.*, 1995). This study showed that the 7-day food diary was associated with less measurement error and, consequently, estimates of diet from the 7-day food diary as well as a FFQ were obtained in the full cohort of 25 000 people (Black, 2000; Bingham *et al.*, 2001).

28.6.3 Calibration

Another way to reduce measurement error is to increase the heterogeneity of the population and pool results from different populations with diverse dietary practices so that it becomes easier to correctly classify intake of individuals in the distribution of food and nutrient intake. This was the approach adopted in the largest epidemiological study of diet, cancer, genetic factors and health in the European Prospective Investigation of Cancer (EPIC). However, as diet was measured by country-specific questionnaires designed to capture local dietary habits and to provide high compliance, it was also necessary to calibrate results. A second dietary measurement was taken from an 8% random sample (36 000 individuals) of the cohort using a computerized 24-hour diet recall method (EPIC SOFT) in order to calibrate the questionnaires. A total of 1103 volunteers of both genders from 12 centres also provided complete 24-hour urines for biomarker analysis, and the high, sex-partial Spearman correlation of 0.72 between mean urinary and dietary nitrogen suggests that confidence can be placed in the validity of the calibration method used. When dietary intake was related to disease risk, calibration of the main method against the more detailed method strengthened associations considerably. Examples of the effect of calibration include the reduced risk of colorectal cancer associated with dietary fibre consumption, and increased risk associated with red and processed meat consumption (Bingham and Riboli, 2004; Norat *et al.*, 2005).

Conclusion

Dietary assessment methods are used to evaluate nutrient intakes for research and surveillance and in clinical assessment. However, in all situations, accurate and reliable data on the food intake of free-living individuals are required. Many lessons about the ability to obtain accurate data have been learnt from incorporating appropriate statistical, biomarker and epidemiological techniques into nutritional assessment. Use of biomarkers has shown that substantial attenuation of diet effects and loss of statistical power can occur in epidemiological studies in homogeneous populations when relatively inaccurate methods of dietary assessment are used. There has even been a recent suggestion that FFQs should be abandoned in large epidemiological studies (Kristal *et al.*, 2005). Attenuation and loss of power, together with genetic variation in response, could account for the inability of existing studies to show causal links between diet and chronic disease. Caution in the interpretation of null results from the epidemiological literature on diet and disease is now being exercised and this will also be the case in other types of research and in clinical studies. Some of this measurement error can be overcome by studying populations whose dietary habits are more heterogeneous than single populations, but biomarker studies suggest that improved, more detailed methods of dietary assessment will be necessary if further causal associations between diet and disease are to be established with any degree of certainty in future investigations.

FURTHER READING

1. **Bingham, S.A.** (1987) The dietary assessment of individuals: methods, accuracy, new techniques and recommendations. *Nutr Abstracts Rev*, **57**, 705–42.

2. **Bingham, S.A.** (2002) Biomarkers in nutritional epidemiology: Key note lecture. *Publ Hlth Nutr*, **5**, 821–28.

3. **Bingham, S.A., Cassidy, A., Cole, T.,** *et al.* (1995) Validation of weighed records and other methods of dietary assessment using the 24-hour urine nitrogen technique and other biological markers. *Br J Nutr*, **73**, 531–50.

4. **Bingham, S.A., Gill, C., Welch, A.** *et al.* (1994) Comparison of dietary assessment methods in nutritional epidemiology. *Br J Nutr*, **72**, 619–42.

5. **Bingham, S.A., Luben, R., Welch, A.,** *et al.* (2003) Fat and breast cancer: are imprecise methods obscuring a relationship? Report from the EPIC Norfolk prospective cohort study. *Lancet*, **362**, 212–14.

6. **Bingham, S., and Riboli, E.** (2004) Is diet important in cancer pathogenesis? The European Prospective Investigation of Cancer (EPIC). *Nat Rev Canc*, **4**, 206–15.

7. **Bingham, S.A., Welch, A., McTaggart, A.,** *et al.* (2001) Nutritional methods in the European Prospective Investigation of cancer in Norfolk. *Publ Hlth Nutr*, **4**, 847–58.

8. **Black, A.E.** (2000) The sensitivity and specificity of the Goldberg cut-off for EI: BMR for identifying diet reports of poor validity. *Eur J Clin Nutr*, **54**, 395–404.

9. **Day, N.E., McKeown, N., Wong, M.Y.,** *et al.* (2001) Epidemiological assessment of diet: a comparison of a 7-day diary with a food frequency questionnaire using urinary markers of nitrogen, potassium and sodium. *Int J Epidemiol*, **30**, 309–17.

10. **Friedenreich, C.M., Slimani, N., and Riboli, E.** (1992) Measurement of past diet: Review of previous and proposed methods. *Epidemiol Rev*, **14**, 177–96.

11. **Gibson, R.S.** (2005) *Principles of nutritional assessment* (2nd edition). New York, Oxford University Press.

12. **Kristal, A.R., Peters, U., and Potter, J.D.** (2005) Is it time to abandon the food frequency questionnaire? *Canc Epidemiol Biomarkers Prevent*, **14**, 2862–28.

13. **Lillegaard, I.T., and Andersen, L.F.** (2005) Validation of a pre-coded food diary with energy expenditure, comparison of under-reporters versus acceptable reporters. *Br J Nutr*, **94**, 998–1003.

14. **Margetts, B.M., and Nelson, M.** (1997) *Design concepts in nutritional epidemiology*, 2nd edition. Oxford, Oxford Medical Publications.

15. **Norat, T., Bingham, S., Ferrari, P.,** *et al.* (2005) Meat, fish, and colorectal cancer risk: The European Prospective Investigation into Cancer and Nutrition. *J Natl Canc Inst*, **97**, 906–16.

16. **Robertson, C., Best, N., Diamond, J., and Elliott, P.** (2004) Tracing ingestion of 'novel' foods in UK diets for possible health surveillance—a feasibility study. *Publ Hlth Nutr*, **7**, 345–52.

17. **Schatzkin, A., Kipnis, V., Carroll, R.J.,** *et al.* (2003) A comparison of a food frequency questionnaire with a 24-hour recall for use in an epidemiological cohort study: results from the biomarker-based OPEN study. *Int J Epidemiol*, **32**, 1054–62.

18. **Tasevska, N., Runswick, S.A., McTaggart, A.,** *et al.* (2005) Urinary sugars as biomarkers for sugars consumption. *Canc Epidemiol Biomarkers Prevent*, **14**, 1287–94.

19. **Willett, W.** (1997) *Nutritional epidemiology*, 2nd edition. New York, Oxford University Press.

USEFUL WEBSITES

http://www.cdc.gov/nchs/about/major/nhanes/index.htm/

http://www.food.gov.uk/science/101717/ndnsdocuments/ndnsappendices

http://faostat.fao.org/faostat

http://www.srl.cam.ac.uk/epic/nutmethod/

http://www.srl.cam.ac.uk/epic/nutmethod/

http://www.srl.cam.ac.uk/epic/nutmethod/

http://statistics.defra.gov.uk/esg/publications/nfs/

29 Assessment of nutritional status and biomarkers

Stewart Truswell

29.1 Nutritional status versus dietary intake

Dietary intake estimation, described in the preceding chapter, cannot always prove that an individual or community is well nourished or poorly nourished —or overnourished. This has to be confirmed or established by one or more methods of examination.

Food intake can be distorted by intrusion of investigators; intake over a day or a few days may not represent intake over time. It is difficult to relate mixed dishes to lines in the food tables. Nutrients in food tables are only averages, often from another country and an earlier time. Not all nutrients are in the food tables. Nutrient reference intakes (recommended dietary intakes) may not be enough for everyone, especially if they have an illness. Then is an intake below the recommended dietary intake serious or covered by safety factors? Health professionals cannot rely on the history of quantity and type of food when assessing a patient's state of nourishment. You cannot diagnose obesity, overnutrition, from someone's dietary history, and undernourished people may not be able to tell you what they have and have not eaten for a variety of reasons.

Food intake measurement—really estimation— is ultimately *subjective*. It depends on the memory, cooperation and honesty of individuals. Assessment of nutritional status is, by contrast, ultimately *objective*. A person's weight, height and chemical concentration in blood or urine is measured by an outside observer and if a second and third observer repeats the measurement, they should obtain about the same result.

BOX 29.1

Nourish—verb, from the Latin *nutrire* meaning to feed, foster, or cherish.

- To bring up, rear, nurture a child, an animal.
- To promote the growth of, tend or cultivate plants.
- To sustain a person (or living thing) with food or proper nutriment.
- To supply (a thing) with whatever is necessary for growth, formation or proper condition.
- To cherish or nurse (a feeling) in one's heart or mind.
- To maintain, encourage, strengthen (one's heart, mind, etc.) in or with something.

From *The Shorter Oxford English Dictionary*.

29.2 Uses of nutritional assessment

29.2.1 Evolution of assessment methods: looking for malnutrition

The scientific methods of assessing nutritional status were put together after World War II when there was widespread malnutrition across Europe. They were used to detect people who were poorly nourished. Nutrition surveys were done in communities considered at risk by nutrition specialists from Britain and North America.

In the 1950s, these methods were applied in the rest of the world, especially in less-developed countries (where kwashiorkor (Chapter 18) was re-discovered in 1952). The US Interdepartmental Committee for Nutrition in National Defence carried out surveys of military personnel and civilians between 1956 and 1967 in 26 countries that had alliances with the USA, each as a separate operation with its own report. The standardized methods for the nutritional surveys: national food supply, sampling, clinical examination, biochemical studies and dietary data, were published in a manual in 1963. This enabled investigators to compare results between communities, to plan applied nutrition programmes and to advise on national food and nutrition policy.

In the same year, the WHO Expert Committee on Medical Assessment of Nutritional Status commissioned Derek Jelliffe to prepare a standard guide for nutrition surveys everywhere in the world. He consulted 25 top nutrition experts in various countries and wrote a WHO monograph, *The assessment of the nutritional status of the community (with special reference to field surveys in developing regions of the world)* in 1966. This classic of nutrition literature is the foundation of examining people systematically to see whether they are malnourished.

Since the 1960s, the biggest change is that most of the 50 clinical signs of malnutrition in Jelliffe's book are little used today. They are rare in industrial countries, require experienced medical personnel to diagnose and many have other causes as well as malnutrition. Pallor (= anaemia), oedema, sore lips, inflamed tongue and enlarged liver can all be due to poor nutrition, but other causes are more common in most countries. A small number of clinical signs are important in nutrition work but it depends where you are. Hair changes of kwashiorkor in a toddler suggest protein deficiency in deprived parts of Africa but not in the developed world. Bitôt's spots or the skin changes of pellagra are reliable signs of vitamin A deficiency or niacin deficiency, respectively, in places where these deficiencies are known to occur and when observed by an experienced clinician. Thyroid enlargement in teenagers (likely to be endemic goitre from iodine deficiency) and mottled teeth (likely to indicate mild excess of fluoride in early life) are reliable signs of nutritional status and so are some of the signs of rickets (enlarged radial epiphysis, beading of costochondral junction).

The two main types of methods used today for nutritional assessment are anthropometry, measuring weights and heights and other body measurements, and biochemical tests, usually on blood, sometimes on urine. These are described in detail in sections 18.3 and 18.4. Professional staff have to be trained and paid to do accurate anthropometry and each particular biochemical measurement has a cost so nutritional assessments can only be done where there is sufficient funding.

29.2.2 Parenteral and enteral nutrition (see Chapter 40)

Modern formulae for total parenteral nutrition, including balanced amino acids and safe intravenous lipid preparation, have been available and approved since 1977. Special nutrition support teams have been set up in major hospitals and there are international societies for the nutritional speciality of enteral and parenteral nutrition (ASPEN in America, ESPEN in Europe). For assessing and monitoring hospital patients' nutritional status, clinical teams use selections from the general methods for nutritional assessment. Rapid biochemical tests are available for monitoring but critically ill patients lying in bed with lines and tubes attached cannot be weighed so other anthropometric measurements have to be used.

29.2.3 Overnutrition

With the increase of overweight and obesity in the last decade, there has naturally been a focus on reliable and accessible indicators of the amount and effects of a person's excess accumulated calories. The two established simple anthropometric measures are (1) body mass index (BMI) where:

$$BMI = \frac{weight}{height^2} \text{ (see section 29.3.3)}$$

where weight is in kg and height is in metres and (2) waist circumference (either alone or expressed against hip circumference). Reference numbers have been derived for different ages and nations for BMI and for men and women (for the waist measurement). Along with these physical measurements, biochemical tests can indicate if overweight is accompanied by metabolic abnormalities. The most usual are plasma LDL and HDL-cholesterol, fasting triglycerides and fasting or postprandial glucose.

29.2.4 Biomarkers to check on, support or replace some food intake estimates

Some biochemical tests are increasingly being used for this purpose in human nutrition experiments and epidemiological studies. Not many are suitable but four good examples are given below.

- For checking protein intake (and hence roughly energy intake)—24-hour urinary nitrogen.
- To support change of type of fat—plasma fatty acid pattern, especially 18:2 ω-6.
- More reliable than estimating salt intake—24-hour urinary sodium.
- The only way to gauge iodine intake (because it varies greatly among foods)—urinary iodine.

29.3 Anthropometric assessment

The basic anthropometric measurements are simple, straightforward, inexpensive, safe and anyone can do them. For research purposes, weight and height are measured more precisely and for clinical work some other measurements are made.

29.3.1 Body mass (body weight)

In affluent communities, most people know their body weight and many weigh themselves regularly on an electronic bathroom scale. These are not as accurate as health professionals require in a clinic or consulting room. The best weighing machines are beam balances with non-detachable weights (Fig. 29.1), but these are bulky and difficult to move. They should stand on a level, hard surface and be checked with a known weight regularly. People should be weighed to the nearest 0.1 kg, wearing minimal clothing. If changes in body weight are being followed, the measurement should if possible be made at the same time of day because meals, drink, a full bladder and bowel action can all affect the reading. When people in a steady state are weighed repeatedly, the day-to-day fluctuation can be ±1.0 kg.

Nutritionists are very interested in the measurement of body weight and its interpretation, whether someone is overweight or underweight, and whether their weight is increasing or going down. They want as well to estimate what components inside the body make up the weight and the change in weight.

Figure 29.2 shows the different compartments in an average, healthy weight adult. About 20% of this average person is fat and the rest is fat-free mass. Women have more fat and less muscle than men. Of the fat-free mass, part is muscle (about 40% of total body weight), part is bones and the rest is all the

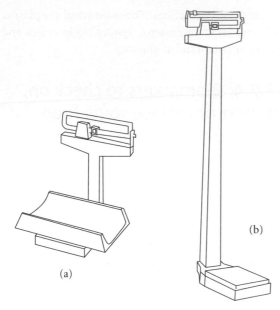

(b)

(a)

Fig. 29.1 Measurement of weight. (a) Paediatric scale for infants, and (b) beam balance for a child or adult.

Source: Gibson (2005).

other organs, in descending order of weight, skin, blood, gut, liver, brain, lungs, heart and so on. Chemically, the largest component is water, then there are about equal amounts of protein and fat (each around 20%) and the rest is bone mineral. In adults, weight gain is nearly all fat; weight loss from negative energy balance is of fat but some fat-free mass, i.e. protein is lost as well.

When total body mass has been measured, we need to judge whether it is in the healthy range or whether he/she is too thin or too fat. First, an adjustment has to be made for size. A lean giant must weigh more than a dwarf. Weight has to be considered in terms of height (or stature). Different indices have been proposed and tested. Of all the possibilities, weight/(height)^2 has been found the most generally useful (Cole, 1991) as a direct measure of over- or underweight. It only requires two measurements, weight and height, and a simple calculation. This BMI is expressed in kg (for weight) and metres (for height), i.e. in SI units. Quite different numbers would be obtained if height were in centimetres. The Belgian mathematician Quetelet first recommended this index.

29.3.2 Measurement of height (stature)

Height is more difficult to measure than weight. Consequently, people's heights are seldom measured and often not accurately remembered. For adults and children, a level floor and straight wall are needed (Fig. 29.3). The subject has to stand straight with buttocks, shoulders and back of the head touching the wall, with heels flat and together, shoulders relaxed, and arms hanging down. The head should be erect and look straight forward, the lower border of the orbit in line with the external auditory meatus (the Frankfurt plane). The headpiece (a metal bar or

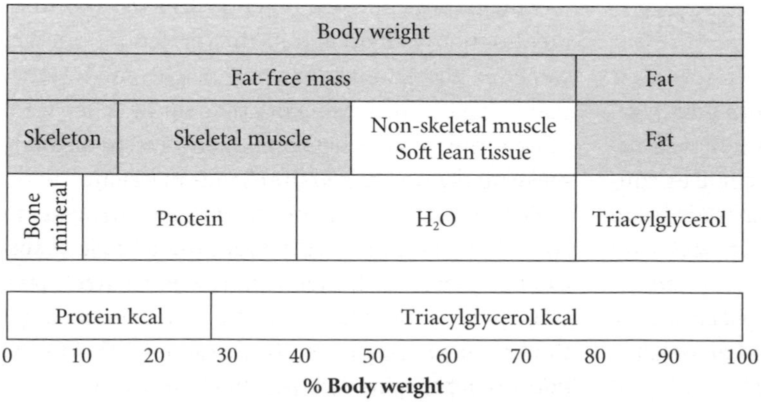

Body weight			
Fat-free mass			Fat
Skeleton	Skeletal muscle	Non-skeletal muscle Soft lean tissue	Fat
Bone mineral	Protein	H$_2$O	Triacylglycerol

Protein kcal	Triacylglycerol kcal

0   10   20   30   40   50   60   70   80   90   100

% Body weight

Fig. 29.2 Compartments of the body. Relationship between anthropometry (shaded), body composition and energy reserves.

Source: Heymsfield, S.B. (1984) Anthropometric assessment of adult protein-energy malnutrition. In: Wright, R.A., Heymsfield, S.B., and McManus, C.B. (eds) *Nutritional assessment*. Boston, Blackwell Scientific.

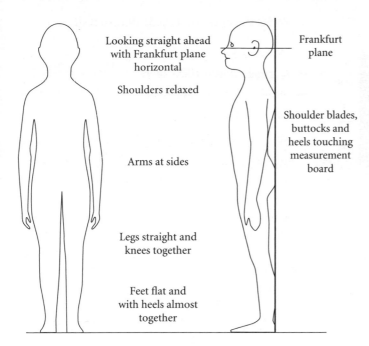

Fig. 29.3 Positioning of person for height measurement.

Source: Gibson, R.S. (2005) *Principles of nutritional assessment*. Oxford, Oxford University Press.

wooden block) is lowered gently, pressing down the hair. Ideally, this headpiece should be on a sliding scale but if a loose object is used, such as a firm book, this must be kept horizontal. In practice, two people can better manage an accurate reading. For research work, a specially designed stadiometer can be obtained. There is a circadian variation in height. People are taller in the morning by 1–2 cm. Then, during the day, the intervertebral discs get somewhat compressed.

For children that cannot yet stand properly, their length is best measured lying supine on a specially designed measuring board. Two examiners are needed to position the infant correctly and comfortably.

For adults who are deformed (e.g. with scoliosis) or bedridden, estimates of what their height would be if they could stand straight can be made from *knee height* or *arm span* (right fingertips outstretched to tips of left fingers) or *demispan* (from sternal notch to webspace between middle and ring fingers). These measurements are used in geriatrics. Equations to give estimated height differ for gender and ethnic group.

29.3.3 Interpretation of body mass index

WHO and government health departments of the major countries have all adopted BMI as the standard way of diagnosing overweight and obesity. With the same cut-offs for men and women, this is much simpler than the earlier tables of desirable weights for height, with different numbers for frame size and for gender. For those who are put off by, say,

$$65 \text{ (kg)} \div (1.73 \times 1.73 \text{ (metres))} \rightarrow 21.67$$

graphs like Fig. 29.4 are available.

Increased BMI indicates increased adiposity but the correlation is not of course 100%. People with broad frame and weight lifters (with big muscles) can have a high BMI for their present body fat. In older people (Chapter 34), muscle bulk declines and percentage of body fat increases. As BMI increases above 25, mortality increases gently at first and then (above BMI 30) more steeply (Fig. 29.5).

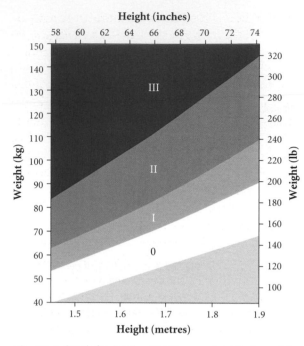

Fig. 29.4 Graph for reading BMI from weight (in kg or lb) and height (in metres or inches). Obesity grades I, II and III have a BMI (weight/height²) of 25–29.9, 30–40, and over 40, respectively.

Source: Garrow, J.S. (1981) *Treat obesity seriously*. Edinburgh, Churchill Livingstone.

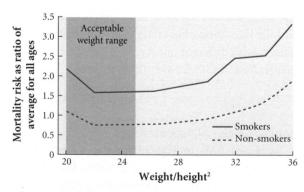

Fig. 29.5 Variations in mortality by weight among 750 000 US men and women.

Source: Lew, E.A. and Garfinkel, L. (1979) Variations in mortality by weight among 750,000 men and women. *J Chron Dis*, **32**, 563–67.

WHO classifies adults according to BMI:

- Underweight = < 18.50
- Normal range = 18.5–24.99
- Overweight = 25.00–29.99
- Obese = > 30.00
- Very severely obese = > 40.00

The value of these BMI levels probably has to be adjusted for ethnic groups because of differences in body composition. At a given BMI, South Asians and Indonesians have relatively more body fat, while Polynesians tend to have more muscle.

Assessing adult undernutrition, below a BMI of 18.5, Ferro Luzzi *et al.* (1992) suggest that severity of chronic energy deficiency is moderate down to 17.0, severe down to 16.0 and very severe below this.

In children, the BMI that corresponds to start of overweight in adults (i.e. 25) is lower. From surveys in different countries, Cole *et al.* (2000) estimate it should be 17.3 at age 5, 19.9 at 10 and 23.6 at 15 years.

29.3.4 Waist circumference

The metabolic complications of overweight and obesity (Chapter 16) have been found to be more likely if some of the adipose tissue is specially concentrated inside the abdomen (in the omentum, mesentery, etc.). This abdominal or visceral obesity can be estimated with a simple tape measure around the waist. Waist circumference correlates quite closely

Table 29.1 WHO recommendations for Caucasians

Risk of metabolic complications	Waist circumference (cm)	
	Men	Women
Increased	≥ 94	≥ 80
Severely increased	≥ 102	≥ 88

with BMI. Some authorities prefer measurement of the waist/hip ratio to allow for people with a heavy frame but it is more complicated to do and does not seem to have better predictive value.

Table 29.1 gives the WHO recommendations for Caucasians. The identification of risk using waist circumference is population-specific and depends on the levels of obesity and other risk factors for cardiovascular diseases and diabetes in the ethnic group.

29.3.5 Measuring children's growth

The primary index of growth, used universally, is *weight for age*. At any particular age, the infant's or the child's weight (unclothed) is compared against a reference, a sort of standard to see if its weight is at, below or above the average. If it is far off the average, percentile lines on the reference graph will show how it compares with the reference population.

The most used weight-for-age set is probably the US CDC growth reference. Graphs for boys and girls aged 2–20 years are reproduced in Chapter 32. There are also separate graphs for boys and girls from birth to 36 months. One reason for the separate graphs is that infants are weighed more frequently, so a broader horizontal scale is needed. The other is that infants' stature is measured lying down and length is 1.0–2.0 cm longer than height. The subjects were healthy and included all ethnic groups excluding those who had very low birth weights. In Britain, the current weight-for-age reference (Freeman *et al.*, 1995) is based on measurements of 25 000 white children between 1978 and 1990. These references replace earlier standards because more infants are now breast-fed and children have fewer infections and grow taller.

In weight-for-age graphs, the average is the 50th percentile (i.e. median) of the reference sample. An individual's difference up or down from this median can be read firstly from the *percentile lines*. A second way used for distance from the median is the *standard deviation* or *Z-score* above or below the median. A

third indicator used for undernutrition is not percentile of the reference children but *percentage of the median*, i.e. of the 50th percentile, the international standard. Below 80% of the median, a child is 'underweight'; this weight is near the 3rd percentile line and near a Z-score of −2. A child under 60% of the median is seriously underweight and has marasmus.

In developing countries, a simplified version of the weight-for-age graph; a 'Road to Health' card, can be kept by the mother for her child and brought back to the clinic on each visit (Chapter 18).

There is little difference in weight for age of modern children of the privileged class between different countries and ethnic groups. The reference data can thus be used internationally. If a child is somewhat heavy for age (say 80th percentile) or light (say 20th percentile), this does not mean overnutrition or undernutrition. The child may be larger (taller) or smaller (shorter) than average. The weight has to be judged against the height (or length).

Length-for-age (for infants) and *stature-for-age* references will show if a child's longitudinal growth is taller or average, or shorter than the reference population. In developing countries, stunting is an important measure of poor nutrition and/or other adverse environment. It is usually defined as 2 standard deviations below the international median reference height for age, i.e. a Z-score of −2.

Excessive thinness or *wasting* is recognized anthropometrically from *weight-for-height* of 2 standard deviations below the median for age, i.e. a Z-score of −2.

Some examples of wasting, stunting and underweight (as defined by WHO) in preschool children in different countries are given in Table 29.2. This shows the value of simple anthropometry in monitoring the world nutrition situation.

In adolescence, the growth references have to be used cautiously because there is a growth spurt around the time of puberty followed by slowing of growth, and some girls mature early and some late, with about 5 years between their peaks (see Fig. 32.1). There is the same sort of range in peak height velocity in boys.

Table 29.2 Wasting, stunting and underweight in 0–5-year-old children, 1998–2000 (%)

	Wasting	Stunting	Underweight
Afghanistan	16.1	47.6	49.3
Australia	0	0	0
Brazil	2.3	10.5	5.7
China	2.2	14.2	10.0
Cuba	2.0	4.6	3.9
Ethiopia	10.5	51.5	47.2
Guatamala	2.5	46.4	24.2
India	15.7	44.9	46.7
Papua New Guinea	5.5	43.2	29.9
South Africa	2.5	22.8	9.2
USA	0.7	2.0	1.4

Wasting < 2 SD below international reference median (WHO/NCHS) weight for height.
Stunting < 2 SD below reference median height-for-age.
Underweight < 2 SD below reference median weight-for-age.
Source: UN Standing Committee on Nutrition (2004) *Fifth report on the World Nutrition Situation*. Geneva, World Health Organization.

29.4 Estimating body composition: simple methods

The methods available that anyone can do to measure body fat or muscle at one or more sites and from there total body fat and/or muscle can be estimated approximately by clinical nutritionists, in systematic nutrition surveys and in athletic training. The following methods are used by clinical nutritionists.

29.4.1 Skinfold thickness

With special precision callipers (Fig. 29.6), a pinch of subcutaneous fat is gently taken up and the width measured. Caught between the jaws of the callipers is a double layer of fat and skin. This fold is measured in mm. Skinfolds could be measured at many sites but the best established are:

- *Triceps skinfold*: over the triceps muscle midway down the back of the upper arm.

- *Biceps skinfold*: measured as a vertical fold midway down the front of the upper arm, over the biceps muscle.

- *Subscapular skinfold*: a vertical fold taken just below and lateral to the inferior angle of the scapular, with shoulder and arm relaxed.

- *Suprailiac skinfold*: in the mid-axillary line immediately above the iliac crest, grasped obliquely.

The skinfold is first picked up between finger and thumb, clean away from the underlying muscle before closing the callipers on the fold.

Reference tables are published for triceps and subscapular skinfolds (see Gibson, 2005).

The above four skinfold sites are most commonly used partly because they are easily accessible and reference tables are available—partly because of the work of Durnin and Womensley (1974) who

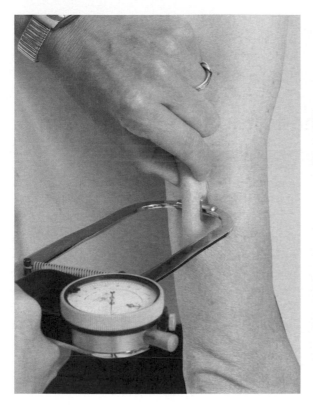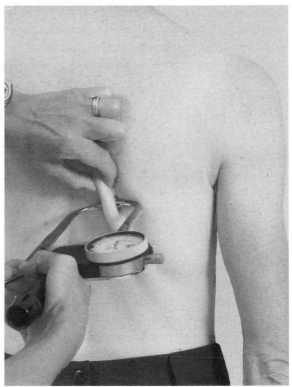

Fig. 29.6 Measuring skinfold thickness—triceps (left) and subscapular (right) sites with Holtain callipers.

Source: Truswell, A.S. (2003) *ABC of nutrition*. London, BMJ Books.

measured total body fat from body density by underwater weighing in 209 white men and 272 women ranging in age and fatness. They derived different equations to predict total body fat from the sum of four skinfolds in men and women at different ages. These were all arm or trunk skinfolds but the British Olympic Association recommends that addition of the anterior thigh skinfold improves the estimate of percentage body fat. In very fat people, skinfolds at some trunk sites are not practicable as it is impossible to take up and measure a fold or the fold is too large for the callipers.

29.4.2 Limb circumference

By simply measuring the circumference of an arm or leg and skinfolds at the same level, it is possible to calculate the circumference or the cross-sectional area of the limb's muscle. An assumption for the area of bone inside the muscle section improves the muscle area for estimating total muscle in the body.

Mid-upper arm is the usual site. The other two sites are mid-thigh and mid-calf. The arm is not always accessible. Heymsfield and Baumgartner (2006) found that the sum of limb muscle area for arm, thigh and calf predicted quite well the skeletal muscle measured by whole-body magnetic resonance imaging:

$$\text{Limb muscle circumference} = C - \pi \times SF$$

$$\text{Limb muscle area} = \frac{[C - \pi \times SF]^2}{4\pi}$$

where C is a limb circumference (upper arm, thigh or calf) and SF is the skinfold taken at the same level.

The uncorrected mid-upper arm circumference reflects muscle and fat in the limb and is used for screening preschool children in the field where no weighing scales are available. A tape is used, marked at 12.5 and 13.5 cm. From 12 to 60 months of age, the arm circumference of healthy children, boys and girls, stays the same. A circumference over 13.5 cm is normal, between 12.5 and 13.5 cm suggests mild undernutrition, and under 12.5 cm, and indicates definite malnutrition.

29.5　High technology methods for body composition

Total body water by isotope dilution　This method uses a tracer dose of water, labelled with deuterium ^{2}H, tritium ^{3}H or ^{18}O. After time for equilibration, the concentration of the label is measured in serum or urine.

Bone mineral density by DEXA　Dual energy X-ray absorptiometry (DEXA) scanning is usually of the lumbar spine and hip with X-rays at two energies. There is relatively more attenuation of the lower voltage rays by more dense tissue (i.e. bone mineral). Results are related to average bone mineral density for age. All major hospitals have this equipment. DEXA can also be used to quantify fat versus other tissue in regions of the body.

Underwater weighing using Archimedes principle The subject is weighed in air (i.e. in the usual way) and again when completely submerged in water in a large tank. Body volume is given by the apparent loss of body weight in water (i.e. the difference between weight in air and in water), which corresponds to the displaced water. Weight (in air)/volume gives body density. Knowing that the density of fat is 0.90, the percentage body fat can be calculated. Adjustments have to be made for residual air in the lungs.

Bioelectrical impedance　Relatively inexpensive equipment is used to measure the impedance of an electrical current (typically 800 microamps) passed between an electrode on the right foot and another on the right wrist where there is a voltage sensor. The fat-free mass is a good conductor of electricity, while fat is not. The voltage drop between foot and wrist is greater in subjects with more fat. A computer calculates fat-free mass and fat when data on weight, height, age, gender and level of physical activity are entered. A number of factors, including hydration state, meals and length of limbs affect the reliability of the results.

Total body potassium, by counting ^{40}K　This depends on the fact that 0.012% of potassium everywhere (and in our bodies) is the γ-emitting isotope ^{40}K. The amount of this can be counted in a whole-body counter from which background radiation has been screened with thick steel or lead. Potassium occurs in the body almost exclusively inside the cells so that from total body potassium the body's cell mass can be calculated.

Total body nitrogen by in vitro *neutron activation analysis*　This is an ingenious method for determining total body nitrogen and hence total protein in the body (N × 6.25). The patient is 'bombarded' while lying on a special table with a low neutron flux from a neutron source (such as californium-252). This converts a proportion of the nitrogen, ^{14}N, to a very short-lived state of ^{15}N, which emits a γ-ray at 10.83 MeV. This is counted with a gamma counter as the neutron source is moved over the subject's body on a motorized bed. The method is unfortunately very expensive; only a few institutions can use it, and it gives a significant radiation dose.

Ultrasound　This is harmless, not expensive and has some uses, e.g. in quantifying the size of the thyroid gland.

Magnetic resonance imaging and computed tomography　These have also been used for some research studies on body composition. Both use very expensive, bulky equipment.

29.6 Biochemical methods

A person may be ill from an inadequate diet and yet their body measurements can be within normal limits. The right biochemical test would show the deficiency. Anthropometry mostly reflects undernutrition or overnutrition, too little or too much food energy. Biochemical tests are needed to demonstrate micronutrient status. On the other hand, there is no biochemical test on a body fluid that gives a measure of carbohydrate or fat intake. Biochemical methods are an essential part of nutritional assessment. There are many more biochemical tests than anthropometric measurements. Each test costs money, for collecting the blood or urine, for the equipment and chemicals, and the skilled laboratory worker's time, and for reporting and interpreting the test. So tests have to be selected, based on the situation and the subject, that are likely to yield useful results.

29.6.1 Different situations for laboratory tests

Biochemical methods for nutritional assessment are used for several different purposes:

- To recognize acute malnutrition for which the clinical signs are non-specific, e.g. potassium deficiency.

- To confirm the clinical diagnosis of a deficiency disease, e.g. xerophthalmia, scurvy, beri-beri, rickets, Wernicke's encephalopathy, kwashiorkor.

- For monitoring nutritional management in intensive care, with parenteral nutrition and/or tube feeding.

- In haematological diagnosis, e.g. iron, folate and vitamin B_{12} estimations.

- In community nutrition surveys, to detect subclinical micronutrient deficiency, e.g. iodine deficiency, iron deficiency.

- For checking validity of food intake measurement: 24-hour urinary nitrogen indicates protein intake in people with stable dietary

pattern; carotenoids reflect fruit and vegetable intake.

- For reliability and convenience: biomarkers, for some nutrients, are more reliable and convenient than food intake estimations (e.g. 24-hour urinary sodium is better than trying to work out dietary salt).

- To demonstrate objectively the response to a nutrition education programme, e.g. reduction of plasma cholesterol or of urinary sodium.

- For biochemical confirmation of alcoholism.

- To diagnose nutritional supplement overdosing (e.g. with vitamin A, pyridoxine).

29.6.2 Stages of nutrient deficiency

When absorbed intake of a nutrient is less than the requirement, i.e. less than losses from metabolism and excretion, the depletion goes through four stages:

1. Reduced excretion of the nutrient, e.g. reduced urinary excretion but body pool maintained.

2. Body pool smaller but no disturbance of function.

3. Biochemical signs of impaired function: reduced activity of an enzyme or cell depletion.

4. Morphological changes and clinical signs of deficiency disease.

Obviously many more people are found at stage 1 than are found with obvious classic deficiency disease. In other words, biochemical tests usually show subclinical nutritional deficiency; the subject may or may not be ill and the illness may or may not be due to the nutritional depletion.

29.6.3 Which biochemical tests?

The principal biochemical tests for nutritional status are shown in Table 29.3. Most clinical biochemical

Table 29.3 Biochemical methods for diagnosing nutritional deficiencies

Nutrient	Indicating reduced intake	Indicating impaired function (IF) or cell depletion (CD)	Supplementary method
Protein	Urinary nitrogen	Plasma albumin (IF)	Fasting plasma amino acid pattern
Vitamin A	Plasma β-carotene	Plasma retinol	Relative dose–response
Thiamin	Urinary thiamin	Red cell transketolase and TTP effect (IF)	
Riboflavin	Urinary riboflavin	Red cell glutathione reductase and FAD effect (IF)	
Niacin	Urinary N' methyl nicotinamide or 2-pyridone, or both	Red cell NAD/NADP ratio	Fasting plasma tryptophan
Vitamin B_6	Urinary 4-pyridoxic acid	Plasma pyridoxal 5′ phosphate	Urinary xanthurenic acid after tryptophan load
Folate	Plasma folate	Red cell folate (CD)	
Vitamin B_{12}	Plasma holotranscobalamin II	Plasma vitamin B_{12} Plasma methylmalonate	Schilling test
Vitamin C	Plasma ascorbate	Leukocyte ascorbate (CD)	Urinary ascorbate
Vitamin D	Plasma 25-hydroxy-vitamin D	Raised plasma alkaline phosphatase (bone isoenzyme) (IF)	Plasma 1,25-dihydroxy-vitamin D
Vitamin E	Ratio of plasma tocopherol to cholesterol + triglyceride	Red cell haemolysis with H_2O_2 *in vitro* (IF)	
Vitamin K	Plasma phylloquinone	Plasma prothrombin (IF)	Plasma des-γ-carboxy-prothrombin
Sodium	Urinary sodium	Plasma sodium	
Potassium	Urinary potassium	Plasma potassium	Total body potassium by counting ^{40}K
Iron	Plasma iron and transferrin	Plasma ferritin (CD)	Free erythrocyte protoporphyrin
Magnesium	Plasma magnesium	Red cell magnesium (CD)	
Iodine	Urinary (stable) iodine	Plasma thryroxine (IF)	Plasma TSH
Zinc	Plasma zinc	Red cell zinc	
Selenium	Plasma selenium	Red cell glutathione peroxidase	Toenail selenium
Fluoride	Urinary fluoride	Plasma ionic fluoride	(Bone fluoride)

^{40}K = natural radioactive potassium; FAD = flavin adenine dinucleotide; NAD = nicotinamide adenine dinucleotide; NADP = NAD phosphate; TPP = thiamin pyrophosphate; TSH = thyroid stimulating hormone.

laboratories are set up for only some of the methods in the table as a routine, but others could be set up in special circumstances, or alternatively a laboratory specializing in nutrition research could be asked. It is usually easy to find methods for recent intake. Good methods for nutritional dysfunction or tissue depletion are not available for all nutrients. With reference to stores of a nutrient, the only method generally available is serum ferritin for iron stores.

29.6.4 Some problems with biochemical tests

Instability of the nutrient in vitro Vitamin C is the outstanding example. Plasma should be acidified with metaphosphoric or trichloracetic acid and analysed the same day or kept for a few days at −80°C.

Chemical specificity of the method Older methods were often not specific for the nutrient, e.g. DCIP or DNPH methods for vitamin C.

Other influences Non-nutritional influences can significantly raise or lower plasma concentrations of most, if not all, nutrients. Plasma albumin goes down

(without protein deficiency) with inflammatory disease or trauma. The liver switches to synthesis of 'acute-phase' plasma proteins and albumin may move to the extravascular space.

The relation between intake and plasma concentration This shows important differences among nutrients (Fig. 29.7). Plasma selenium increases in the expected linear fashion but serum calcium is homeostatically maintained the same over the range of usual calcium intakes. Plasma retinol also stays the same over most vitamin A intakes but it does go down at very low intakes, so this test is useful in low-income communities. Vitamin C concentration plateaus at intakes of about 150 mg/day so it is no higher in people who take megadoses than in those who eat a moderate amount of fruit.

Blood and urine tests cannot show calcium status (Calcium is not in Table 29.3.) This requires measurements of bone mineral. Biochemical tests for zinc are also unreliable. Serum zinc is affected by age, gender, acute inflammation, time of day, fasting status, oral contraceptives, storage, haemolysis, zinc contamination of collecting tube or anticoagulant. It therefore needs careful technique and interpretation.

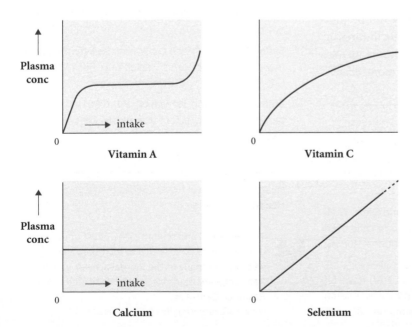

Fig. 29.7 Difference in relation of serum concentrations to intake of four nutrients: vitamin A, vitamin C, calcium and selenium.

29.6.5 Methods used

The previous edition of this book contained a table that gave the names of the methods then likely to be used for the different nutrients. However, such methods are constantly evolving, and the three main questions the nutritionist can ask the laboratory are: Is this specific for the nutrient? Is it a standard method? Is the laboratory experienced with using it?

Urine tests These should if possible be made on 24-hour urine collections. This may be rather inconvenient for the subjects; they have to carry a 2-litre bottle with them during the day. As second best, an early morning sample can be collected at home and the nutrient concentration related to the creatinine concentration, because creatinine excretion (in health) is assumed to be more or less constant from day to day. However, within subjects the coefficient of variation of 24-hour creatinine is 10% or more and it is larger between subjects because it depends on muscle mass and is increased after eating meat.

Hair is unreliable Researchers have sent hair samples from the same subjects for trace element analysis to several commercial laboratories and have received widely differing results. It is difficult to remove the many environmental contaminants that adhere to hair and the distribution of inorganics may not be uniform. Hair analysis may have some value in forensic work, for detecting toxic exposure to heavy metals, but for nutritional work urine analysis is more reliable.

FURTHER READING

1. **Cole, T.J.** (1991) Weight-stature indices to measure underweight, overweight and obesity. In: Himes, J.H. (ed.) *Anthropometric assessment of nutritional status*. New York, Wiley-Liss, pp. 83–111.

2. **Cole, T.J., Bellizzi, M.C., Flegal, K.M., and Dietz, W.H.** (2000) Establishing a standard definition for child overweight and obesity worldwide: international survey. *Br Med J*, **320**, 1240–43.

3. **Durnin, J.V.G.A., and Womersley, J.** (1974) Body fat assessed from total body density and its estimation from skinfold thickness: measurements on 481 men and women aged from 16 to 72 years. *Br J Nutr*, **32**, 77–97.

4. **Eston, R.G., Rowlands, A.V., Charlesworth, S., Davies, A., and Hoppitt, T.** (2005) Prediction of DXA-determined whole body fat from skinfolds: importance of including skinfolds from the thigh and calf in young, healthy men and women. *Eur J Clin Nutr*, **59**, 695–702.

5. **Ferro-Luzzi, A., Sette, S., Franklin, M., and James, W.P.T.** (1992) A simplified approach to assessing adult chronic energy deficiency. *Eur J Clin Nutr*, **46**, 17–86.

6. **Freeman, J.V., Cole, T.J., Chinn, S., Jones, P.R.M., White, E.M., and Preece, M.A.** (1995) Cross sectional stature and weight reference curve for the UK. *Arch Dis Child*, **73**, 17–24.

7. **Gibson, R.S.** (2005) *Principles of nutritional assessment*, 2nd edition. Oxford, Oxford University Press.

8. **Heymsfield, S.B., and Baumgartner, R.N.** (2006) Body composition and anthropometry. In: Shils, M.E. (ed.) *Modern nutrition in health and disease*. Philadelphia, Lippincott Williams, and Wilkins, pp. 751–70.

9. **Jelliffe, D.B.** (1966) *The assessment of the nutritional status of the community (with special reference to field surveys in developing regions of the world)*. WHO Monograph Series No. 53. Geneva, World Health Organization.

10. **Kukzmarski, R.J., Ogden, C.L., Grummer-Strawn, L.M.,** *et al*. (2000) CDC growth charts: United States. *Adv Data*, **314**, 1–27.

11. **Sauberlich, H.E.** (1999) *Laboratory tests for the assessment of nutritional status*, 2nd edition. Boca Raton, FL, CRC Press.

12. **Steindel, S.J., and Howanitz, P.J.** (2001) The uncertainty of hair analysis for trace metals. *J Am Med Assoc*, **285**, 83–5.

13. **World Health Organization** (2000) *Obesity: preventing and managing the global epidemic*. Report of a consultation. Technical Report Series 894. Geneva, World Health Organization.

 To see topical and scientifically robust updates on nutrition associated with this textbook, and active web links to many of the journal articles in the Reference areas, please see the dedicated Online Resource Centre at www.oxfordtextbooks.co.uk/orc/mann3e/.

PART 6

Life stages

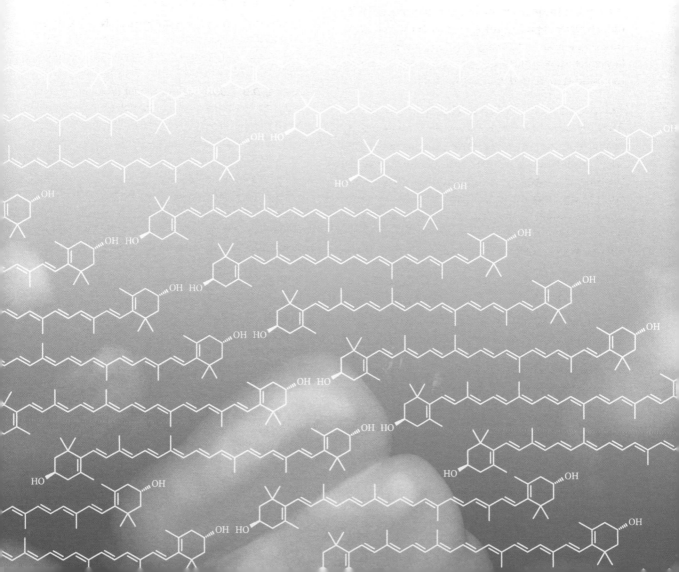

30 Pre-pregnancy, pregnancy and lactation

Annie S. Anderson

30.1 Pre-pregnancy

The lifelong nutritional status of a mother, from her own conception and throughout her life to the birth of her baby, will impact on the health and wellbeing of that baby. In addition, the particular importance of nutrition in the months before conception is now recognized. Here the emphasis is on the achievement of appropriate body weight and optimal nutritional status (and stores) for the months ahead. In addition, pre-pregnancy nutrition takes account of the needs of the very early stages of pregnancy (embryogenesis) when the woman may not be sure she is pregnant. Adequate intakes of folate are important during embryogenesis and avoidance of toxins such as alcohol and excess vitamin A need to be considered.

Maternal nutrition has a profound effect on all aspects of reproduction including fertility. When energy stores are low, menarche may be delayed, and if energy stores are diminished after menarche, menses are likely to become irregular, infrequent and possibly stop. Amenorrhea has been well described in excessive weight loss and in anorexia nervosa. It is estimated that where body fat is less than 22% of body weight, ovulation is unlikely. Healthy fertile young women have an average body fat proportion of 28%. Menarche can be delayed by athletic training or eating disorders and accelerated by excess nutrient consumption. It is thought this is due to a requirement for a certain energy store to be present to permit reproduction to occur. In natural settings where energy has been acutely restricted (e.g. due to famine), there has been a small reduction in birth weight if famine impacts on the last 3 months of pregnancy but, if it occurs prior to pregnancy, ovulation is likely to fail. Obese women are commonly infertile but simple weight reduction can bring about the return of ovulation, menstruation and fertility.

While there has been considerable speculation about the role of preconceptual nutrition and malformation, the only strong evidence relates to the benefit of folic acid supplements in minimizing neural tube defects (NTD). The neural tube, which will develop into the brain and spinal cord, starts as the neural fold in the ectoderm along the back of the embryo. Between days 21 and 28 after conception, it closes into a tube, the neural tube. If folate is inadequate, the tube may not close fully and spina bifida may result, or the brain may not develop at all. It is thought that NTDs arise from a combination of genetic and environmental components, both of which must be triggered for the defects to occur. An MRC trial demonstrated that a daily 4 mg folic acid supplement given around the time of conception to women at high risk (those who had already had one affected NTD pregnancy) was shown to prevent the disease (MRC Vitamin Study Research Group, 1991). The effect of multivitamins was also assessed but there was no indication that these conferred any preventive effect. From this work, it was concluded that folic acid should be given to all women with a previous affected pregnancy and that public health measures (e.g. supplements and/or food fortification) should be available to all women of childbearing age. In the UK, folic acid supplements are recommended to all women prior to conception so that folate status is adequate during the early embryonic stages. Surveys suggest that about 55% of women do take this action but figures are lower amongst the most socially deprived.

Additionally, around a half of all pregnancies are unplanned and therefore universal supplementation is unlikely to be achieved. Mean ($\pm$ SD) daily intake of folate in non-pregnant women from dietary sources in the UK is 290 $\pm$ 500 µg, which is lower than that provided by supplement use (400 µg) and likely to be insufficient to meet the requirements of women at risk of having an NTD-affected pregnancy. Some countries (USA and Canada) have now started fortifying key staple foods with folate, e.g. bread and cereals, and this is likely to become more widespread.

30.2 Pregnancy

Pregnancy is a period of rapid growth and development of the fetus, with high physiological, metabolic and emotional demands on the mother. Adequate nutrition during pregnancy is important to enable the fetus to grow and develop physically and mentally to full potential. It is widely believed that fetal nutrition plays a key role in the wellbeing of the newborn infant and further influences health during childhood and adulthood with possible effects into the next generation. In addition to fetal nutrient needs, food intake during pregnancy needs to be free from food safety hazards and contribute to the health and wellbeing of the mother, notably in the avoidance of inappropriate anaemia. Nutrition during pregnancy is especially important in adolescent mothers who have not yet completed their own growth.

Fetal growth is divided into three stages: the 2-week blastogenesis stage, where the fertilized ovum rapidly divides and implants itself in the endometrial lining of the uterus; the critical embryonic stage where the rudiments of all the principal organs and membranes develop (lasts for 6 weeks); and the fetal stage, which extends to term (40 weeks). During the embryonic stage, all the tissues and organs are defined. The fetus is particularly vulnerable to retarded development or abnormality at this stage if necessary nutrients are absent.

The gain in weight of the fetus is not uniform. By the end of the embryonic stage, the fetus weighs about 1 g and by the end of the first 3 months approximately 30 g, followed by a period of rapid growth in the last 6 months of pregnancy. During this time, growth accelerates to about 34 weeks, then slows. Normal birth weight averages around 3.3 kg.

30.2.1 Regulation of nutrient supply to the fetus

The relationship between fetal nutrition and maternal food intake is indirect. In addition to the quantity, quality and balance of maternal dietary intake, nutrient supply to the fetus will be influenced by a number of adaptive physiological processes that occur during pregnancy. These include increased maternal absorption of some nutrients (e.g. iron), increased bone turnover (facilitating calcium needs), an increase in circulating blood volume resulting in haemodilution of red cells (as plasma volume increases) and an accompanying fall in haemoglobin concentration. In general, maternal plasma levels of water-soluble vitamins fall with a relative rise in fat-soluble vitamins. The placenta is responsible for the exchange of nutrients between the mother and fetus, and nutrient supply will be influenced by an expanding uteroplacental blood flow (up to 800 mL/min at term), placental transfer mechanisms (by diffusion, facilitated diffusion and active transport) and fetal uptake. Thus, mothers have many protective mechanisms that will help to moderate the effect of poor diet and lifestyle (alcohol, activity, smoking) but these do not provide universal protection or guarantee life-long health.

30.2.2 The energy cost of pregnancy

Researchers who have investigated energy economics in pregnancy have found big differences between women in developing countries, who tend to be smaller and have to do more physical work, and well-nourished women in developed countries. In both settings, individual women vary considerably in their pre-pregnant size, in how much fat they put on during the pregnancy, in changes of basal metabolic rate and in reduction of their physical activity.

Recommendations for average energy intake are based on energy expenditure. In pregnancy, this is estimated from (i) the energy value of the fetus and placenta and the extra maternal tissues: uterus, breasts and adipose tissue, plus (ii) any extra energy expenditure (basal metabolic rate plus physical activity for the heavier body) at the different stages of pregnancy. The total energy cost of pregnancy is then distributed into the trimesters and it is agreed that there is little or no extra energy need in the first trimester. With the latest modern technology, including the use of doubly labelled water for total energy expenditure, the average energy cost of pregnancy for a women who gains 12 kg weight works out to 325 MJ. From this, the expert committees in North America and Australasia both recommend an extra 1.4 MJ/day in the second trimester and 1.9 MJ/day in the third trimester (Table 30.1).

However, many measurements of energy intake throughout pregnancy in women in ten different countries (nearly 1000 women in all) found that most of them ate less than one extra MJ/day and the average was + 0.3 MJ/day. This experience is the basis of the 1991 UK recommendation of (only) 0.8 MJ extra/day (only) in the third trimester (Table 30.1). However, the report states that 'women who are underweight at the beginning of pregnancy and women who do not reduce activity may need more'.

Weight gain during the first trimester is minimal, after which weight begins to accrue at a rate of

Table 30.1 Extra energy recommendations in pregnancy for the average woman (MJ/day)

	North American 2002 and Australasian 2006	WHO 2004	UK 1991
First trimester	0	+ 0.375	0
Second trimester	+ 1.4	+ 1.2	0
Third trimester	+ 1.9	+ 1.95	+ 0.8

350–400 g per week (about 1lb per week). Table 30.2 shows the distribution of maternal weight gain at birth. Increase in maternal tissue (i.e. uterine and breast tissue), blood and other body fluids, and adipose tissue occurs mainly in the second trimester, while growth of the fetus, placenta and amniotic fluid occurs mainly in the third.

Adequate maternal weight gain during pregnancy is the principal means of ensuring adequate fetal growth and, hence, infant birth weight. Excessive gain is associated with large infants (> 4200 g), increased likelihood of caesarean delivery and postpartum obesity. Because of the wide variation in weight gain among women who give birth to optimally grown infants, a range of weight gains is regarded as acceptable for

Table 30.2 The distribution of maternal weight gain at 40 weeks' gestation

Weight gain distribution (grams)	
Fetus	3300–3500
Placenta	650
Increase in blood volume	1300
Increase in uterus and breasts	1300
Amniotic fluid	800
Fat stores and additional fluid retention	4200–6000
Total	11 550–13 550

Table 30.3 Recommended weight gains for pregnant women[a]

Weight for height category	Recommended gain (kg)
Low (BMI < 19.8)	12.5–18.0
Normal (BMI 19.8 to 26.0)	11.5–16.0
High (BMI > 26.0 to 29.0)	7.0–11.5

[a]Young adolescents and black women should strive for gains at the upper end of the appropriate range. Short women (< 157 cm) should strive for gains at the lower end of the range. The target gain for women with BMI > 29.0 is ≤ 6.0 kg.
Source: Adapted from Institute of Medicine, Food and Nutrition Board (1990) *Committee on nutritional status during pregnancy and lactation*. Washington, DC, National Academy Press.

each body mass index (BMI). A normal weight gain for most healthy women is 11–15 kg, averaging about 12.5 kg. The US Institute of Medicine recommendations suggest that women who are underweight at the beginning of pregnancy or who do not reduce activity levels during pregnancy should gain more weight, and women who are overweight should gain less (Table 30.3). These tables were developed for women in the USA and have been shown to be applicable to all groups of women of European descent. However, maternal anthropometry differs among ethnic groups and separate tables should be used for other ethnic groups, such as Chinese and Polynesians.

30.2.3 Birth weight: the effect of maternal age, maternal weight and energy intake

Birth weight is regarded as one of the best indicators of overall nutritional status of the infant and its wellbeing. The normal birth weight range is considered to be between 2500 and 4200 g. Low birth weight (LBW) is a major cause of infant mortality and has been linked with long-term morbidity, including deficits in growth and cognitive development in childhood, and diabetes and heart disease in adult life. The

World Health Organization estimates that around 20 million LBW babies (< 2500 g) are born each year, 94% in developing countries. LBW is caused by preterm birth or intrauterine growth retardation, or both.

Adolescents who are still growing are one population subgroup at greater risk of having LBW babies. Even when their own weight gain is sufficient to ensure adequate fat stores, they do not appear to mobilize these stores to enhance fetal growth late in pregnancy. Fat stores are reserved for their own continued development. As a result, adolescents generally need larger weight gains to bear infants comparable in size with those of mature women. Consequently, their nutritional requirements are greater, and this is reflected in higher recommended energy intakes for younger pregnant women in the UK. Low maternal body weight is also associated with LBW. However, in the developed world, current evidence suggests that chronic low maternal energy intakes do not significantly contribute to LBW, and attempts to increase birth weight through energy supplements have had negligible effects. One (positive) potential nutritional influence on birth weight is a diet rich in long-chain ω-3 polyunsaturated (LCP) fatty acids, and randomized control trials have shown an increase in gestation (6 days) with LCP supplements, although overall the effects are rather modest. A wide range of nutrients has been examined in an attempt to influence birth outcomes (including iron, folate, zinc and vitamin D) but these have had little effect. Supplementation with magnesium from the 25th week of gestation has been shown to result in fewer preterm and LBW deliveries, but these results did not differ significantly from placebo groups. It should be noted that protein supplements have a negative effect on birth weight.

While it seems challenging to increase birth weight by increasing energy intake, it seems possible to decrease birth weight by decreasing energy intake, and therefore increase the risk of LBW. There has been considerable debate on the merit of reducing obesity risks by weight restriction during pregnancy versus increasing the risk of LBW. Maternal obesity increases the need for caesarean section and the risk

Table 30.4 Birth centile distribution (%) in obese primigravidae

	< 25	25–50	50–75	> 75
Diet-restricted (n = 51)	25.3	30.8	26.3	17.6
Controls (n = 51)	17.6	29.7	31.9	20.9

Source: Campbell, D., and MacGillivray, I. (1975) The effect of a low calorie diet or a thiazide diuretic on the incidence of pre-eclampsia and birthweight. *Br J Obstet Gynaecol*, **82**, 572–77.

of developing gestational diabetes, toxaemia and hypertension during pregnancy. The increased risk of gestational diabetes and hypertension in women who are overweight rather than obese emphasizes the importance of avoiding excess adiposity in women of childbearing age. Maternal obesity is also associated with a higher risk of neural tube defects, spina bifida and congenital malformations. However, the general consensus appears to be that dieting for weight loss during gestation should be discouraged and may result in a LBW infant if there is serious caloric restriction in the third trimester (as initially demonstrated from famine conditions). Table 30.4 shows a downward trend to lower birth weight with diet restriction, in research by Campbell (1975).

However, maternal concerns over pregnancy weight gain and slimming cannot be ignored. Many women want to know about dietary change during pregnancy and perceived loss of control of body shape and size, which may have a far greater influence on overall food intake than dietary advice on a healthy balanced diet. Clear, effective, practical advice and counselling on weight loss given in the postpartum period (and after lactation) would be appropriate for obese women.

30.2.4 Fetal nutrition, birth outcome and health in later life

An increasing body of evidence suggests that early nutritional status (as indicated by birth weight and other parameters) modifies the risk of disease (notably cardiovascular) in later life. Birth weight has been used as a proxy measure of fetal nutrient exposure, although it may not be a sensitive enough measure to describe inadequate or unbalanced maternal nutrition. The hypothesis for the relationship between nutrition and early origins of disease is based on the concept that, in fetal life, the tissues and organs of the body go through periods of rapid development, termed critical periods. Critical periods may coincide with periods of rapid cell division. Thus, if the fetus is deprived of nutrients or oxygen at such times, it may adapt by slowing the rate of cell division, especially in tissues undergoing critical periods. Even brief periods of undernutrition may permanently reduce the numbers of cells in particular organs. It is postulated that fetal undernutrition may change or programme the body with respect to distribution of cell types, hormonal feedback, metabolic activity and organ structure.

Extensive research by David Barker and colleagues (Barker, 1994) has related causes of adult mortality and morbidity to fetal and infant life. These observational studies have related LBW to adverse health outcomes in adulthood, including hypertension, type 2 diabetes and coronary heart disease. Variations in newborn ponderal index (kg/m^3) and placenta weight-to-birthweight ratios have also been related to sub-sequent hypertension. These observations have led to the fetal origins hypothesis, which states that fetal undernutrition in middle to late gestation leads to disproportionate fetal growth and programmes the later development of several diseases that are common in affluent societies and other groups undergoing rapid acculturation.

This hypothesis has been challenged by a number of researchers. Other studies only show a direct association between small size in early life and later adult health outcomes if body size at some intermediate period has been adjusted for. Researchers have suggested that this finding implies that it is probably the change in size across the whole time interval (postnatal centile crossing), rather than fetal biology, that is implicated. Thus, it remains to be resolved whether people who are small in early life and then grow rapidly are more at risk than those who remain small.

In an attempt to identify specific aspects of maternal nutrition that impact on adult disease, the balance of maternal macronutrient intake has been explored. In one British cohort study by Barker's group (Godfrey *et al.*, 1996), higher carbohydrate in early pregnancy and lower meat intakes in late pregnancy were followed by lower birth weights. But in another similar study by Mathews *et al.* (2000), after adjustment for maternal height and smoking, birth weight was only associated with vitamin C intake. It would seem therefore that macronutrient balance, at least in industrialized countries, has little influence on birth weight.

30.2.5 Nutrient requirements during pregnancy

Energy As we have seen (section 30.2.2) women do not eat or need to eat for two, but they do need to eat a high-quality nutritious diet to ensure they obtain their extra requirements for several essential nutrients.

Protein A summary of recommended intakes for protein and other nutrients for a number of countries is presented in Table 30.5. Additional protein is required during pregnancy to provide for the synthesis of fetal, placental and maternal tissue. Maternal and fetal growth accelerates in the second month of

Table 30.5 Recommended daily nutrient intakes during pregnancy

	USA[a]			Australia/ NZ[b]	UK
	Women NOT pregnant 2005	Change for pregnant	Pregnant 2005	Pregnant 2004	Pregnant 1991
Protein (g)	46	+ 54%	71	60	51
Vitamin A (μg)	700	+ 10%	770	800	700
Vitamin D (μg)	5	0	5	5	10
Vitamin E (mg)	15	0	15	7	—
Vitamin C (mg)	75	+ 13%	85	60	50
Thiamin (mg)	1.1	+ 27%	1.4	1.4	0.9
Riboflavin (mg)	1.1	+ 27%	1.4	1.4	1.4
Niacin (NE) (mg)	14	+ 29%	18	18	13
Folate (μg)	400	+ 50%	600	600	300[c]
Vitamin B_{12} (μg)	2.4	+ 8%	2.6	2.6	1.5
Calcium (mg)	1000	0	1000	1000	700
Magnesium (mg)	310	+ 13%	350	350	300
Iron (mg)	18	+ 50%	27	27	15
Zinc (mg)	8	+ 38%	11	11	7
Iodine (μg)	150	+ 47%	220	220	140

[a]Numbers for USA are recommended daily allowances (RDAs) from dietary reference intake (DRI) recommendations for females 19–50 years.
[b]These recommendations are RDIs 2004, except for vitamin D and vitamin E, which are adequate intakes.
[c]A supplement of 400 μg/day folic acid is now advised.
NE, niacin equivalents.

pregnancy and continues to increase until just before term. The need for protein follows this growth. However, the extra amount required is relatively small (6–10 g/day) and is usually readily provided in a normal pre-pregnant Western diet.

Folate Pregnancy is a period characterized by extra cell division and growth. This increases folate requirements more than for any other nutrient. Folate requirement is increased (as discussed in section 30.1) and supplements are recommended preconceptually and in the first 12 weeks of pregnancy. Increases in dietary intakes of folates are also recommended throughout pregnancy to avoid megaloblastic anaemia in late pregnancy or the puerperium. Rich sources are presented in Table 30.6. Differences in recommended dietary intakes by country (Table 30.5) have arisen due to differences in primary indicators of status.

Calcium Around two-thirds of the calcium in the fetus is deposited during the last 10 weeks of gestation, mostly in the fetal skeleton. Alterations in maternal calcium metabolism, including a substantial increase in the absorption of dietary calcium, occur early in pregnancy to facilitate this increase in fetal demand. There has been concern that inadequate dietary intake of calcium during pregnancy was compensated by mobilization of skeletal calcium, leading to an increased risk of osteoporosis in later life.

However, recent evidence suggests that the adaptation in calcium metabolism that occurs in pregnancy is sufficient to maintain fetal growth, even if dietary calcium is not increased. Current guidance promotes an adequate calcium intake throughout life rather than increasing dietary intake during the gestation period. A Cochrane review on calcium supplementation during pregnancy for preventing hypertensive disorders and related problems (Hofmeyr *et al.*, 2006) has reported that calcium supplementation appears to be beneficial for women at high risk of gestational hypertension and in communities with low dietary calcium intake, although optimum dosage requires further investigation.

Iron The demand for iron is not evenly distributed throughout gestation. During the first trimester, requirements are minimal, as iron is no longer lost during menstruation. Iron needs increase throughout the second trimester and reach a peak in the third trimester, when fetal demands are at their highest. Absorption increases as pregnancy progresses, from an absorption rate of around 7% at 12 weeks' gestation to 66% at 36 weeks. Many women enter pregnancy with low iron stores or even frank iron-deficiency anaemia (IDA). Maternal IDA may increase the risk of preterm delivery, resultant LBW and perinatal mortality. As well, evidence is accumulating that maternal IDA reduces infant iron stores postpartum leading to the

Table 30.6 Some food sources of folate

Food	Folic acid (μg)/100 g	Folic acid (μg)/portion
Bean salad	44	88 (200 g portion)
Spring greens (boiled)	66	63 (95 g portion)
Broccoli	64	54 (85 g portion)
Fortified breakfast cereals	167–350	50–100 (30 g portion)
Orange	31	50 (medium orange)
Granary bread	88	32 (medium slice)
Beef mince (cooked)	30	42 (140 g portion)
Orange juice	18	29 (glass)

possibility of impaired development in the infant. There remains considerable debate on the use of iron supplements during pregnancy with respect to whether this is an attempt to alter a natural physiological process that in some way enhances nutrient supply. Dietary guidance in the UK suggests that no dietary changes to iron intake are required due to physiological changes, although women with poor iron status at the time of obstetric booking may need iron supplements.

Zinc Zinc is necessary for DNA and RNA synthesis. Maternal zinc deficiency may be responsible for growth retardation, preterm delivery and abnormality in the fetus, and birth complications in the mother. Factors that limit the absorption of zinc such as high intakes of dietary phytate, calcium and iron supplements may cause secondary zinc deficiency. Recently published dietary recommendations include an increase of zinc intake in pregnancy. The extra zinc should come from foods (section 10.1.5). It is possible that iron supplements could reduce zinc intake.

Iodine Iodine deficiency during pregnancy remains a major public health problem in many areas of the world. Cretinism, caused by severe lack of iodine during fetal development, is characterized by both mental and physical retardation. Millions of babies are born each year at risk of mental impairment due to iodine deficient diets. Iodization of salt is commonly used to prevent deficiency. In areas where there is cretinism and extensive goitres, expectant mothers should be given an injection of iodized oil, preferably before conception (see section 10.3.5). However, overt iodine deficiency is not seen in developed countries among pregnant women.

Vitamin A Adequate vitamin A levels are essential because of the role of this vitamin in cell differentiation. Vitamin A deficiency, seen mostly in some developing countries, may be associated with blindness, depressed immune function, and increased morbidity and death from measles and other infectious diseases, as well as increased mother-to-child transmission of AIDS. Encouraging foods rich in this vitamin (see Chapter 11) is the most appropriate approach to ensuring adequacy. On the other hand, excessive intakes (> 3000 μg retinol daily) resulting from the use of supplements, excessive intakes of fortified foods and, occasionally, high intakes of liver can be teratogenic, causing central nervous and heart defects. High levels of vitamin A have been detected in the liver of farmed animals in the UK (due to the composition of animal feedstuffs); thus, all pregnant women are advised to avoid liver, liver products, vitamin supplements and fish oil supplements that are high in retinol. In developing countries where appropriate foods are not readily available, supplementation may be considered.

Vitamin D Populations at risk for vitamin D deficiency are those whose skin exposure to sunlight is low, particularly dark-skinned women living in northern climates such as ethnic minority groups in the UK. The infants born in such populations have low vitamin D stores. Vitamin D insufficiency during pregnancy is associated with lower maternal weight gain, neonatal tetany and biochemical evidence of disturbed skeletal homeostasis in the infant. In extreme situations, reduced bone mineralization, radiologically evident rickets and fractures may occur. In the UK, it is recommended that all pregnant women take a vitamin D supplement, although this rarely seems to be implemented.

Vitamin C It appears that the fetus concentrates vitamin C at the expense of maternal stores and circulating vitamin levels. Accordingly, it is recommended that dietary intake of foods rich in vitamin C are increased during pregnancy.

In summary, while mineral requirements increase during pregnancy, most of the extra nutrients can be attained through physiological adaptation rather than dietary change (in the well-nourished). With respect to vitamins, extra dietary intakes of vitamin C and vitamin A are required, which may mean increasing intakes by rich dietary sources (but not by supplements). Increasing intakes of folate and vitamin D should be met by increasing dietary sources (and sunlight for vitamin D), as well as by supplements.

30.2.6 Lifestyle factors that impact on pregnancy outcome

Alcohol Heavy drinkers have a greatly increased risk of inducing the fetal alcohol syndrome, with characteristic underdevelopment of the mid-face, small body size and mental retardation. Any effect of alcohol is likely to be greatest in the first few weeks after conception, the embryogenesis stage. Women who intend to become pregnant should not have multiple alcoholic drinks whatever the occasion; they could already be 2 or 3 weeks pregnant. Once pregnancy is established, the rule should be no more than one standard drink a day to be sure of avoiding minor effects, chiefly growth retardation.

Smoking Smoking causes retardation of fetal growth, thereby increasing the risk of producing a LBW baby. The older the mother and the more cigarettes smoked, the greater the effect. A decrease in birth weight of approximately 200–250 g is usually found in infants of mothers who smoke more than 20 cigarettes a day. Smoking also increases the risk of spontaneous abortion, preterm delivery and sudden infant death.

Exercise Most recent studies show that moderate exercise during pregnancy does not harm the fetus and benefits the mother. Benefits can include reduced fat gain, lower risk of gestational diabetes, maintenance of aerobic fitness, shorter labour, quicker delivery and fewer surgical interventions. However, high-impact exercise or hard physical work can affect fetal development and often results in LBW babies and a higher frequency of obstetric complications.

30.2.7 Other diet and health concerns

Coffee The rate of elimination of caffeine from the body decreases during pregnancy. Caffeine freely crosses the placenta. The risk of spontaneous abortion and LBW appears to increase with high maternal caffeine intake during pregnancy. It is sensible to limit caffeine consumption in pregnancy. However aversion to coffee is common so this advice is then not needed.

Oil-rich fish Due to contaminants such as mercury, which may be stored in high concentrations in fatty fish, pregnant women are recommended to restrict intake of oily fish. These recommendations will vary by region. In the UK, pregnant women are advised not to eat marlin, shark or swordfish, to limit tuna to four cans per week, and not to exceed oily fish consumption above two portions per week.

Food safety Pregnant women are unusually susceptible to infection with *Listeria monocytogenes*, which can contaminate uncooked foods. After an incubation period of 2–6 weeks, infection can result in a mild chill or more severe illness, premature birth or stillbirth. There can also be effects in the newborn, including meningitis. Listeriosis responds to antibiotics when it is diagnosed. In the UK, the incidence is estimated at 1 in 30 000 live and stillbirths. The government recommends that pregnant women avoid certain ripened soft cheeses, such as Brie, Camembert and blue-veined cheese and any type of paté.

Salmonella, Toxoplasma and food poisoning more generally also needs to be avoided with greater care during pregnancy than at other times.

30.2.8 Physiological effects of pregnancy that impact on dietary intake

Nausea and vomiting This is frequently experienced in the first trimester of pregnancy and, for an unfortunate few, lasts throughout pregnancy. It is hypothesized that nausea and vomiting are part of the maternal system to protect against toxins. In support of this hypothesis, a recent review reported that (i) symptoms peak when embryonic organogenesis is most susceptible to chemical disruption (weeks 6–18), (ii) women who experience morning sickness are less likely to miscarry than women who do not,

(iii) women who vomit suffer fewer miscarriages than those who experience nausea alone, and (iv) many pregnant women have aversions to alcoholic and non-alcoholic (mostly caffeinated) beverages and strong-tasting vegetables, especially during the first trimester. There is no generally effective remedy for morning sickness; however, small frequent meals and the avoidance of strong food odours appears to help. A recent Cochrane review using data from six double-blind randomized controlled trials with a total of 675 participants and a prospective observational cohort study (Jewell and Young, 2003) indicated that ginger was effective in relieving the severity of nausea and vomiting episodes with no significant side effects or adverse effects on pregnancy outcomes. The authors concluded that more observational studies are needed to confirm this encouraging preliminary data on ginger.

Hyperemesis gravidarum (HG) is a condition that causes severe nausea and vomiting in early pregnancy, often resulting in hospital admission. The incidence of HG varies from 0.1 to 1% and appears higher in multiple pregnancies, hydatidiform mole and other conditions associated with increased pregnancy hormone levels. Both the aetiology and pathogenesis of HG remain unknown, although a range of pregnancy hormones (progesterone, oestrogen and human chorionic gonadotrophin) and other hormones have been implicated. Infants from HG pregnancies have significantly lower birth weight and younger gestational age, and a greater length of hospital stay. The persistent vomiting can lead to Wernicke's encephalopathy so it is important that thiamin is given with replacement intravenous fluids.

Cravings and aversions Some change in liked and disliked foods is common in pregnancy. There can be cravings or aversions. Food cravings are popularly believed to be related to the nutritional needs of the mother, to have symbolic value, or to be related to sensory or physiological causes. Food aversions have been defined as 'a definite revulsion against food and drink not previously disliked'. Typical examples are tea, coffee and alcohol. The explanation for these cravings and aversions is incomplete. They may relate to changes in olfactory and taste sensitivity during pregnancy.

Constipation Around 40% of women reported having been constipated some time during pregnancy. Its aetiology is complex and includes depressed gut mobility in pregnancy, increased fluid absorption from the large intestine, decreased physical activity and dietary changes. However, an increase in fibre, from an average intake of about 18 g/day to 27 g/day, has shown to be effective in treating constipation.

30.3 Lactation

Lactation is the physiological completion of the reproductive cycle. The decision to breastfeed is influenced by psychobiological and psychosocial factors, which vary between and within cultures. Within Europe, rates vary by country and by baby age. For example, in Denmark 98% of babies receive some breast milk (initiation) with 75% still feeding at 4 months. In the UK, 69% of babies receive some breast milk with 21% still receiving breast milk at 6 months of age. In Australia in 2001, 89% of mothers started breastfeeding with 46% still providing some breast milk at 6 months. In most countries, initiation and duration of breastfeeding are positively associated with maternal education status, maternal income and marital status.

The physiology of lactation is complex, but may be briefly summarized as follows: the suckling infant stimulates the mother's pituitary gland to release prolactin, a hormone required for the synthesis of breast milk. Milk-producing cells synthesize most of the protein and some of the fats and sugars, which combine with other nutrients derived from the mother's circulation. A second pituitary hormone, oxytocin, is responsible for releasing the milk from the cells into the ducts that carry the milk to the nipples.

30.3.1 Composition of breast milk and implications for maternal nutrition

Human milk feeding is adequate as the sole source of nutrition for up to age 6 months providing that the maternal diet and stores are adequate and the milk is successfully transferred to the infant. The composition and volume of human milk progressively changes with the onset and duration of lactation and can be influenced by maternal nutritional factors. Current evidence indicates that infant demand is the major determinant of the quantity of milk produced. The nutritional demands of lactation on the mother are directly proportional to volume and duration of milk production.

The daily milk volume varies over the duration of lactation but is fairly consistent except in extreme maternal malnutrition or severe dehydration. Breast milk intake among healthy infants averages 750–800 g/day and ranges from 450 to 1200 g/day. The composition of milk will be influenced by time of day, gestational age (prematurity versus term) stage of lactation, parity, month (i.e. seasonal food intake), nutritional status of mother and maternal dietary intake. Lipids are the most variable constituent in human milk. In the first week after birth, colostrum is produced, which has a fat content of 2.6 g/100 mL. This is followed by transitional milk between days 7 and 14 and then finally mature milk, which has a fat content of 4.2 g/100 mL.

30.3.2 Maternal nutrient requirements to support lactation

During pregnancy, the mother's body prepares for lactation by storing some nutrients and energy. It is difficult to determine precisely nutrient requirements for lactation since there is variation in nutritional status before and during pregnancy, and limited knowledge about utilization of maternal nutrient stores and adaptations of maternal metabolism during lactation.

The total energy cost of lactation is derived from the energy content of the milk plus the energy required to produce it. The energy value of breast milk is between 2.7 MJ/L and 3.1 MJ per litre. The ratio between the energy content of milk and the total energy cost of lactation is the efficiency of milk production. Current estimates for exclusive breastfeeding suggest the energy cost of lactation is around 2.625 MJ/day based on a mean milk production of 750 g/day with an energy density of milk of 2.8 kJ/g and energetic efficiency of 0.80. In well-nourished women, this will be partially met by energy mobilization from fat tissues of about 0.65 MJ/day (for weight reduction of 0.5 kg fat/month), resulting in a net increment of around 2.0 MJ/day (= 480 kcal)) over non-pregnant, non-lactating energy requirements. This assumes the ideal situation where the new mother gradually uses up the extra 2–5 kg fat put on during pregnancy over 6 months of breastfeeding. The value will vary when complementary feeding is introduced or the baby becomes only partially breast-fed. Women who exclusively breastfeed for 6 months may require as much as 2.4 MJ extra/day.

Other nutrients

Table 30.7 shows recommended nutrient intakes for five countries. The north American recommended nutrient intakes were published between 1998 and 2002 and the Australasian in 2005–2006. The British recommendations date from 1991. In developed countries, there is sufficient protein and most other nutrients in usual diets so that the average extra 2.0 MJ of food per day will cover the extra nutrient needs with two exceptions. In the northern winter, a vitamin D supplement is advisable, and vegans must take a vitamin B_{12} supplement (these are available from microbiological, i.e. non-animal sources). Although some 260 mg of calcium are secreted per day in mother's milk, epidemiological studies have found no increase in osteoporosis or fracture in women who have breast-fed compared with those who did not.

The US Institute of Medicine sums it up:

' The loss of calcium from the maternal skeleton that occurs during lactation is not prevented by increased dietary calcium, and the calcium lost appears to be regained following weaning. There is no evidence that calcium intake in lactating women should be increased above that of non-lactating women. '

Table 30.7 Recommended daily nutrient intakes during lactation

Nutrient	USA Not pregnant Not lactating	USA and Canada, Australia/NZ[a] Lactating	USA and Canada % increase	UK 1991 Lactating
Protein (g)	46	67	+ 46	56
Vitamin A (µg)	700	1300 (1100)	+ 86	950
Vitamin D (µg)	5	5	0	10
Vitamin E (mg)	15	19 (11)	+ 27	—
Vitamin C (mg)	75	120 (80)	+ 60	70
Thiamin (mg)	1.1	1.4	+ 27	1.0
Riboflavin (mg)	1.1	1.6	+ 45	1.6
Niacin (NE) (mg)	14	17	+ 21	15
Folate (µg)	400	500	+ 25	260
Vitamin B_{12} (µg)	2.4	2.8	+ 17	2.0
Calcium (mg)	1000	1000	0	1250
Iron (mg)	18	9[b]	− 50	15
Zinc (mg)	8	12	+ 50	13
Iodine (µg)	150	290 (270)	+ 93	140

[a]Where the Australasian recommended dietary intake is different, it is shown in brackets.
[b]For first 6 months of lactation; figures assume menstruation has not re-started.
NE = niacin equivalents.

Some nutrients in the breast milk are increased if there is more of them in the mother's diet: water-soluble vitamins, vitamin A and polyunsaturated fatty acids. Most other constituents in the milk—protein, lactose, total fat and calcium do not appear to be influenced by maternal intake.

Certain foods and drinks may be undesirable. Foods with a strong flavour like garlic can carry into the milk and spoil the taste for baby. If there is a strong family history of allergy, it might be advisable for the mother to avoid peanuts or peanut butter in case the protein passes through to the milk. After a cup of coffee or, glass of wine the concentration of caffeine or alcohol in the milk is about the same as in the mother's plasma; the infant gets a lower dose per kg than the mother but has less metabolizing capacity.

30.3.3 Lactation and maternal obesity

Pregnancy is a risk factor for obesity. Some women put on more than the standard 2–5 kg of fat. The question arises whether milk production and the baby will suffer if the lactating mother restricts her food intake. Lovelady *et al.* (2000) tested this out in a randomized controlled trial in overweight (not obese) women. They lost approximately 0.5 kg per week between 4 and 14 weeks postpartum from moderate food restriction and exercise: their infants gained the same weight and length as the controls, but some of the control mothers put on weight.

FURTHER READING

1. **Allan, L.H.** (2005) Multiple micronutrients in pregnancy and lactation: an overview. *Am J Clin Nutr*, **81** (Suppl.), 1206S–1212S.

2. **Anderson, A.S.** (2001) Pregnancy as a time for dietary change. *Proc Nutr Soc*, **60**, 497–504.

3. **Barker, D.J.P.** (1992) *Mothers, babies and disease in later life*. London, BMJ Publishing Group.

4. **Bartley, K.A., Underwood, B.A., and Deckelbaum, R.J.** (2005) A life cycle micronutrient perspective for women's health. *Am J Clin Nutr*, **81** (Suppl.), 1188S–93S.

5. **Butte, N.F., and King, J.C.** (2005) Energy requirements during pregnancy and lactation. *Publ Hlth Nutr*, **8** (7A), 1010–27.

6. **Durnin, J.V.G.A.** (1987) Energy requirements of pregnancy: an integration of the longitudinal data from the five-country study. *Lancet*, **330**, 1131–33.

7. **Godfrey, K., Robinson, S., Barker, D.J. Osmond, C., and Cox, V.** (1996) Maternal nutrition in early and late pregnancy in relation to placental and fetal growth. *Br Med J*, **312**, 410–4.

8. **Hofmeyr, G.J., Atallah, A.N., and Duley, L.** (2006) Calcium supplmentation during pregnancy for preventing hypertensive disorders and related problems *Cochrane Database Syst Rev*, CD000145.

9. **Lovelady, C.A., Garner, K.E., Moreno, K.L., and Williams, J.P.** (2000) The effect of weight loss in overweight lactating women on the growth of their infants. *New Engl J Med*, **343**, 449–53.

10. **Mathews, F., Yudkin, P. Smith R.F., and Neil, A.** (2000) Nutrient intakes during pregnancy: the influence of smoking and age. *J Epidemiol Community Health*, **54**, 17–23.

11. **MRC Vitamin Study Research Group** (1991) Prevention of neural tube defects: results of the medical Research Council Vitamin Study. Lancet, **338**, 131–137.

12. **Prentice, A.M., Spaaij, C.J.K., Goldberg, G.R., et al.** (1996) Energy requirements of pregnant and lactating women. *Eur J Clin Nutr*, **50** (Suppl.), 82S–111S.

13. **Scholl, T.O.** (2005) Iron status during pregnancy: setting the stage for mother and infant. *Am J Clin Nutr*, **81** (Suppl.), 1218S–1222S.

14. **Scientific Advisory Committee on Nutrition** (2005) *Folate and disease prevention*—draft report. London, Food Standards Agency.

15. **Scientific Advisory Committee on Nutrition** (2006) Early nutrition and development of disease in later life—draft report. London, Food Standards Agency.

16 **Sulaimen, N.D., Florey, C., du, V., Taylor, D.J., and Ogston, S.A.** (1988) Alcohol consumption in Dundee primigravidas and its effects on outcome of pregnancy. *Br Med J*, **296**, 1500–03.

USEFUL WEBSITES

Scientific Advisory Committee on Nutrition (2005) Folate and disease prevention—draft report of the Food Standards Agency, London. http://www.sacn.gov.uk/reports/

Scientific Advisory Committee on Nutrition (2006) Early Nutrition and Development of Disease in Later Life—draft report. Food Standards Agency, London http://www.sacn.gov.uk/reports/

 To see topical and scientifically robust updates on nutrition associated with this textbook, and active web links to many of the journal articles in the Reference areas, please see the dedicated Online Resource Centre at www.oxfordtextbooks.co.uk/orc/mann3e/.

31 Infant feeding

Donna Secker and Stanley Zlotkin

Interest in infant feeding centres around two principal objectives: the promotion of normal growth and brain development, and the prevention of illness during the first years of life. Infants grow and develop rapidly in the first 2 years, making them particularly vulnerable to nutritional inadequacies. Breastfeeding, followed by the introduction of a wide variety of solid foods, provides the best opportunity for optimal growth and health during infancy. By 2 years of age, the infant should be consuming a variety of foods from the adult diet to ensure a nutritionally balanced intake.

Decades of animal experiments followed by recent studies evaluating the growth of human infants under varying environmental conditions suggest that early infant nutrition and postnatal growth are important factors for long-term health. Researchers have hypothesized that nutritional deficits that occur during fetal life predispose or program an individual towards a tendency to develop chronic diseases in later life. The original fetal origins hypothesis by Barker, proposing an association between low birth weight, accelerated postnatal growth and adult heart disease, has since been expanded to include chronic diseases such as hypertension, insulin resistance and obesity. More recently, researchers have proposed a postnatal programming hypothesis (the Lucas hypothesis), implying that it is early postnatal nutrition and growth that influences later health, rather than prenatal life. It has been suggested that altering dietary patterns in infancy could reduce the risk of developing these chronic conditions; however, there are no prospective studies that have evaluated the effectiveness of this strategy in infancy on outcomes during later adulthood. These types of study are nearly impossible to complete because of the length of time children would have to be followed (as much as 50 years or longer) and their extremely high cost. Hence, on the basis of current evidence, restriction of nutrition during infancy is not recommended, especially as undernutrition adversely affects brain growth.

31.1 Value of breastfeeding

Human milk is specifically composed to meet the nutritional requirements of the human infant and is considered the optimal nutrition source for healthy newborns, as well as many newborns with medical conditions. Breastfeeding provides immunological protection, which is greatest during the early months, but increases with the duration of breastfeeding. Although more difficult to quantify, the psychological benefit of early and prolonged physical contact contributes to the development of a strong mother–

infant bond. Other benefits include convenience, safety and cost. With the exception of vitamins D and K, breast milk produced by adequately nourished mothers provides all the nutrients needed by a normal healthy full-term infant for approximately the first 6 months of life. Water supplementation is unnecessary in the otherwise-healthy infant. The water requirements of infants in a hot, humid climate can be provided entirely by the water content in human milk. When it is hot, infants may just nurse more often.

Recent studies have provided good evidence that even in developed countries breastfeeding protects against gastrointestinal and respiratory infections, reduces the risk of otitis media (inflammation of the middle ear) and reduces the incidence of food allergy in infants with a genetic predisposition. Breastfeeding does not appear to decrease the incidence of atopy (clinical forms of inherited hypersensitivity) in infants not at increased risk. The evidence that breastfeeding may play a role in preventing type 1 diabetes (insulin-dependent diabetes mellitus), particularly for those with genetic markers of increased risk, is inconsistent. In addition, there is documentation that the mean values for cognitive development in populations of children who were breastfed are slightly higher compared with bottle-fed infants from similar environments. Breastfeeding is rarely contraindicated. Exceptions include infants with galactosaemia, or infants of mothers who are HIV-antibody-positive or have untreated, active tuberculosis. Neither smoking nor environmental contaminants are necessarily contraindications to breastfeeding. Moderate, infrequent alcohol ingestion, the use of most prescription and over-the-counter drugs and many maternal infections do not preclude breastfeeding.

31.2 Formula-feeding

When an informed mother chooses not to breast-feed, the only acceptable alternative is a commercial infant formula. Manufacturers continue to modify their products in an effort to emulate human milk, and although they provide less than the optimal benefits of human milk, they are nutritionally adequate for the first year of life. The standard formula choice is a formula based on cow's milk, containing skimmed milk powder, lactose and a variable blend of oils. These formulas are available in two versions: low iron (similar amounts to human milk, but with much lower bioavailability) or iron-fortified (10–12 mg/L elemental iron). Use of low-iron formulas is one of several risk factors implicated in the incidence of iron-deficiency anaemia, the most common nutritional deficiency among infants and toddlers. To provide the best guarantee of normal iron status, the use of iron-fortified formulas, not low-iron formulas, is recommended.

Soy-based formulas made from soy protein, vegetable oils and glucose polymers (with or without sucrose) are available for infants of vegetarian families, infants with galactosaemia or lactose intolerance, or infants with IgE-mediated allergy to cow's milk protein. Soy formulas are not indicated for low-birth-weight infants, prevention or management of colic, routine treatment of gastroenteritis, or treatment of infants with non-IgE-mediated allergy to cow's milk protein (i.e. enteropathy or enterocolitis). Recent concerns with respect to the safety of soy formulas are related to their content of phyto-oestrogens, which have been shown to slightly modify the menstrual cycles of premenopausal women and to alter reproductive behaviour in animals. Because phyto-oestrogens have oestrogen-like activity, it has been suggested that adverse effects on the developing endocrine system may occur in infants fed soy-protein-based formulas. The phyto-oestrogens present in soy-based infant formula are called isoflavones. Infants consuming soy-based infant formulas absorb and excrete isoflavones; however, the presence of isoflavones in human infants does not necessarily mean that they are biologically or clinically active. Although effects have been reported in animals, there are no reports that these chemicals cause any adverse effects in babies and young children in the early years of development. Current soy-based formulas have been used for almost 40 years without evidence of hormone-related adverse effects and infants fed soy-based formula have grown and developed normally.

Studies provide conflicting evidence about the importance of supplementing preterm and full-term infant formula with long-chain polyunsaturated fatty acids. Long-chain polyunsaturated fatty acids (docosahexanoic acid (DHA) in particular) accumulate in the brain and eye of the fetus, especially during the last trimester of pregnancy, and some studies suggest that infants, in particular preterm infants, may benefit from direct consumption. Infants receiving breast milk or infant formula supplemented with DHA and arachidonic acid (ARA) have higher levels of these fatty acids in the blood, brain and retina than infants fed regular formula. These higher levels are thought to have benefits related to visual acuity, growth, and psychomotor and mental development. Infant formulas supplemented with these long-chain polyunsaturated fatty acids are now available for preterm and full-term infants in many countries around the world. Current studies show no harmful effects of supplementing infant formula with DHA and ARA.

However, there are no published reports from clinical studies that address whether long-term beneficial effects exist.

Lactose-free cow's milk-based formulas are also available for infants with lactose intolerance. 'Follow-on' or transition formulas are designed for the second 6 months of life and although nutritionally superior to cow's milk during this time, they provide no nutritional advantages over regular iron-fortified infant formulas. Home-made formulas from evaporated milk are nutritionally incomplete and are not recommended. Specialized infant formulas are available for the small number of infants who cannot tolerate formulas based on intact cow's milk protein or soy protein. Most often, these infants have confirmed food allergies, malabsorption syndromes or carbohydrate intolerance.

Protein hydrolysate formulas, which have been heat-treated and enzymatically hydrolysed to produce free amino acids and peptides of various lengths, are designed for infants allergic to, or unable to digest, intact protein. Some protein hydrolysate formulas also contain medium-chain triglycerides; these formulas are designed for infants with protein and fat malabsorption due to gastrointestinal or liver failure.

31.3 Vitamin and mineral supplementation

With the exception of vitamins D and K, human milk from well-nourished mothers provides all the nutrients required for approximately the first 6 months of life. Routine administration of intramuscular vitamin K at birth has eliminated vitamin K deficiency. Commercial infant formulas are fortified with vitamins and minerals; therefore, supplements are unnecessary.

31.3.1 Vitamin D

The amount of vitamin D in human milk is insufficient to prevent rickets. Although vitamin D can be produced from exposure of the skin to sunlight (ultraviolet B rays), with increasing use of sunscreen and avoidance of sun exposure due to the risks of sunburn and skin cancer, the incidence of vitamin D-deficiency rickets is rising. Hence, a daily vitamin D supplement is now recommended for breastfed infants, beginning at birth and continuing until vitamin D intake from other dietary sources meets their recommended intake. Few foods contain significant amounts of naturally occurring vitamin D (e.g. liver and oily fish), whereas only milk and margarine are fortified with vitamin D in some countries. Infants at the highest risk for vitamin D deficiency and the development of nutritional rickets are those who are dark-skinned, exclusively breastfed, living at high northern or southern latitudes, or weaned to vegan diets. Due to the increasing incidence of rickets, some nations are recommending vitamin D supplements for all infants, continuing into childhood and adolescence. The typically recommended doses are between 200 and 400 IU/day.

31.3.2 Iron deficiency

Iron deficiency is most common among infants between the ages of 6 and 24 months. The major risk factors for iron-deficiency anaemia in infants relate to socioeconomic status and include the early consumption of cow's milk, use of non-iron-fortified infant formula, inadequate funds for appropriate foods and poor knowledge of nutrition. Other high-risk groups include low-birth-weight and premature infants and older infants who drink large amounts of milk (1 L/day) or juice and eat little solid food. The importance of preventing rather than treating anaemia has been accentuated by findings that iron-deficiency anaemia is a risk factor for developmental delays in cognitive function and that this delay is irreversible with iron therapy and persists into early childhood (see Box 31.1).

31.3.3 Fluoride

Fluoridation of the water supply has proven to be the most effective, cost-efficient means of preventing dental caries (see Chapter 10). In areas with low fluoride levels in the water source, fluoride supple-

> **BOX 31.1** Strategies for the prevention of iron-deficiency anaemia
>
> - Exclusive breast-feeding during the first 4–6 months
> - Introduction of iron-fortified infant cereal and/or other iron-rich foods (e.g. pureed meats) and enhancers of iron absorption (vitamin C, e.g. fruit) from approximately 6 months
> - Use of iron-fortified formula for infants weaned early from the breast or formula-fed from birth
> - Delaying introduction of unmodified cow's milk until at least 9–12 months of age

ments are recommended. The increased availability of fluoride (fluoridated water, foods or drinks made with fluoridated water, toothpaste, mouthwashes, vitamin and fluoride supplements) has resulted in an increasing incidence of very mild and mild forms of dental fluorosis in both fluoridated and non-fluoridated communities. This sign of excess fluoride intake has led to modifications in fluoride recommendations including later introduction and lower doses of fluoride supplements, and caution to parents of children to use small amounts and to discourage the swallowing of toothpaste. Dental fluorosis has not been shown to pose any health risks and while there may be mild cosmetic effects, the teeth remain resistant to caries.

31.4 Cow's milk

The use of unmodified cow's milk before 9–12 months of age is not recommended. In comparison with human milk and iron-fortified formula, cow's milk is higher in nutrients such as protein, calcium, phosphorus, sodium and potassium and significantly lower in iron, zinc, ascorbic acid and linoleic acid (Table 31.1). Nutrients in solid foods emphasize these excesses and deficiencies, so that infants fed on cow's milk receive a higher renal solute load and are at greater risk of eating an unbalanced diet. In particular, the

risk for iron depletion and iron-deficiency anaemia is higher because the iron content of cow's milk is low and not readily bioavailable, and its absorption may be impaired by the high concentrations of calcium and phosphorus and low concentration of ascorbic acid in cow's milk. In addition, intestinal loss of (blood) iron in the stool is associated with cow's milk-feeding in the first 6 months of life. Reduced-fat milks should not be given before 1 year of age because of insufficient essential fatty acid content and the high renal

Table 31.1 Nutrient content of human milk, formula and cow's milk per litre

Nutrient	Human milk mature	Formula			Cow's milk 3.3% fat
		Cow's milk[a]-based	Soy-based[b]	Follow-on[b]	
Energy (kcal)	680	670	670	670	640
Protein (g)	10	15	19	17	32
Fat (g)	39	36	37	33	36
Carbohydrate (g)	72	72	69	79	48
Sodium (mmol)	8	8	11	10	22
Potassium (mmol)	14	18	19	23	40
Chloride (mmol)	12	13	13	15	27
Vitamin D (μg)	<0.5	10	10	10	9[d]
Iron (mg)[c]	0.4	2.3/12	12	12	0.4

[a] Average value of seven brands.
[b] Average value of four brands.
[c] Non-fortified/iron-fortified.
[d] If fortified.

solute load that the infant receives when he or she drinks larger volumes to satiate hunger. Whole cow's milk (3.3% butterfat) continues to be recommended for the second year of life. Two per cent milk may be an acceptable alternative provided that the child is eating a variety of foods and growing at an acceptable rate; there is, however, a theoretical risk of growth faltering and essential fatty deficiency when partially skimmed milk provides a significant component of the infant's daily intake.

31.4.1 Association between cow's milk and incidence of diabetes

The aetiology of type 1 diabetes appears to require both genetic predisposition to an autoimmune destructive process and exposure to environmental triggers. Several infant-feeding practices have been investigated as possible environmental factors for genetically predisposed individuals, including early exposure to cow's milk protein (or early termination of breast-feeding) and solid food, and the ingestion of soy protein. The evidence remains unconvincing, however, and modification of current infant-feeding practices to avoid the disease is premature.

31.5 Goat's milk

For the same reasons as cow's milk, pasteurized goat's milk is not an appropriate milk choice for infants before 9–12 months of age. When goat's milk is used after this age, a product with added vitamin A, vitamin D and folic acid should be chosen. Infants who are allergic to cow's milk protein are also likely to have an allergic reaction to goat's milk.

31.6 Vegetarian beverages and herbal teas

Soy, rice and other vegetarian beverages, whether or not they are 'fortified', are inappropriate alternatives to breast milk or infant formula or to pasteurized whole cow's milk in the first 2 years. There are no minimum requirements for total fat or protein content of these products, and if used as a whole or major source of nutrition, they may result in marasmus and failure to thrive. Herbal teas are of no known benefit to an infant and may be harmful; toxic effects of herbal teas have been reported in infants fed herbal tea, as well as breastfed infants whose mothers were drinking large amounts of herbal tea.

31.7 Fruit juice

Infants may drink excessive amounts of fruit juice for a variety of reasons including their preferences, parental health beliefs, behavioural feeding difficulties and financial limitations. If juice consumption decreases the infant's appetite for solid foods, energy and nutrient intakes (e.g. fat, protein, calcium, vitamin D, iron, zinc) can be inadequate, leading to poor weight gain, nutrient deficiencies, and failure to thrive. Chronic diarrhoea can also occur in association with malabsorption of the juice's fructose and sorbitol and/or the low fat content of the infants' diets.

31.7.1 Nursing caries (decay)

The cause of extensive tooth decay in infants is multifactorial and includes feeding practices such as putting an infant to bed with a bottle of carbohydrate-containing liquid (including milk or formula), the frequent use of pacifiers dipped in sugar, syrup or honey, and bottle-feeding past 12 months of age. Acids produced by bacteria that ferment dietary carbohydrate attack the teeth, particularly during sleep when saliva secretion is decreased. Infection or severe tooth decay may warrant tooth extraction. Early loss of primary teeth can lead to problems with speech articulation and chewing. Bedtime bottles are unnecessary but if used should contain only plain water.

31.8 Introduction of solids

At some point in time, exclusive breastfeeding no longer meets a growing infant's energy and nutrient needs and complementary foods must be added. These additional foods are not intended to replace or interfere with breastfeeding. The timing and type of complementary foods is variable, reflecting the numerous cultural foods and practices of society. Recommendations that breast milk should be given exclusively for about the first 6 months and that complementary food should be introduced after this time are based on issues related to nutritional need, physiological maturation, behavioural and developmental aspects of feeding, immunological safety and environmental influences. Most evidence suggests that introduction before 2–3 months or later than 6 months has more risks than benefits. Individual infants may have unique needs or feeding behaviours that may require introduction of complementary foods as early as 4 months of age.

Scientific evidence in support of traditional recommendations for the order and progression of introducing solids is limited. Infants should be introduced to nutrient-rich solid foods, and because they require a good source of iron around 6 months of age, the most commonly used first food has been iron-fortified infant cereal. Iron-rich meat is also a good choice.

Although the permeability of the infant's intestinal tract to foreign proteins has diminished by this age, it is considered practical to reduce the allergenic load as long as possible, in particular for infants with a family history of allergies. Gluten, one of the more common allergens, is found in wheat, rye, oats and barley but not rice or maize. Therefore, for theoretical reasons, rice cereal has been considered the most appropriate first food. Because each new food constitutes a potential allergic challenge, the introduction of one new food every 2–3 days has been advised, using single rather than mixed foods initially. This is primarily important for infants at high risk for allergies, who are generally introduced to new foods more cautiously. Pureed or finely mashed vegetables and fruits, meats, fish, poultry, tofu, legumes and lentils are generally introduced after infant cereals. Although it is common practice in developed countries to offer bland foods, there is no evidence to suggest that infants are unable to tolerate spices or strong flavors. When an infant begins to make lateral motions of the jaw, chewing should be encouraged by increasing the texture of foods to include mashed table foods. An infant who is not encouraged to chew at this time may have trouble later accepting anything but fluids and purees. Between 9 and 12 months of age, finger foods should be introduced to encourage self-feeding. The size, shape and texture of the food should be considered because they influence the infant's ability to chew and swallow safely without choking (Table 31.2).

Table 31.2 Development of feeding skills and introduction of appropriate foods

Age	Oral-motor skills	Self-feeding	Foods to introduce
Birth–4 months	Well-developed sucking and rooting reflexes facilitate intake of human milk or formula Extrusion reflex causes tongue to protrude when solid food or spoon is put in mouth	Sees breast or bottle and becomes excited	Human milk or iron-fortified infant formula is all the infant needs
4–6 months	Sits up alone or with support Holds head up on own Indicates desire for food by watching spoon, opening mouth and closing lips over spoon, and swallowing Indicates disinterest in food or satiety, by leaning back, keeping mouth closed and turning head away Extrusion reflex decreases Able to depress the tongue and transfer semi-solids from spoon to back of mouth for swallowing Smacks lips	Pats or puts hands on breast or bottle	Iron-fortified infant cereal or puréed meat to introduce a supplementary source of iron
6–9 months	Teething starts Lips begin to move while chewing	Plays with spoon May help spoon find mouth	Plain, cooked, pureed or mashed vegetables to add new flavours and textures

Table 31.2 (*cont'd*)

Age	Oral-motor skills	Self-feeding	Foods to introduce
	Begins chewing up and down	Holds bottle	Plain, soft, pureed or mashed fruits
	Jaw and tongue move up and down	Feeds self crackers, toast, cookies, etc.	Plain, pureed, minced or finely chopped meat, poultry, fish, cooked egg yolk, cooked mashed legumes, lentils, tofu to provide additional iron, protein and B vitamins
	Lip closure achieved	Feeds from cup with help	Grains, toast, crackers and dry unsweetened cereals to provide opportunity for self-feeding
			Limited amounts of unsweetened fruit juices offered in a child-sized cup
9–12 months	Rotary chewing movement develops	Can hold own bottle well	Yoghurt, cheese and cottage cheese
	Rhythmic biting movements begin	Can hold cup but may spill contents	Soft, bite-sized pieces of vegetables, mashed potatoes, fruits, meats and alternatives; soft breads, rolls, plain muffins, rice and noodles to enhance chewing skills
	Licks food from lower lip	Picks up foods in fingers or palms	Finger foods: soft-cooked vegetables, cut into bite-sized pieces; soft, ripe, peeled fresh fruit, or canned fruits; strips of tender meat; soft, whole legumes or lentils; diced tofu to enhance motor skills and encourage self-feeding
	Fine motor skills improve	Puts food in mouth	

31.8.1 Safety issues around feeding

Infants are less immune to bacteria in the digestive tract than older children and adults. The risk of choking on foods with the potential for aspiration and asphyxia is highest for infants and toddlers. Therefore, foods provided to infants must be free of pathogens, appropriate in size and texture, nutritionally wholesome and fed safely (Box 31.2).

The greatest risk of choking and aspiration on food occurs in children under the age of 4 years, with a significant peak in the 12–24-month age group. Small, round, smooth foods such as smoked sausages, grapes, nuts, candies, raisins, seeds, peas, kernel corn and popcorn are the most dangerous as they can slip prematurely into the pharynx and with a quick gasp for breath be drawn downward and become lodged in the airway. These foods are not recommended before 3–4 years of age unless they are cut into pieces. Highly viscous foods, such as peanut butter, can plug the airway and should not be served by themselves. In addition to the shape and texture of foods, environmental factors such as distractions or inadequate supervision during eating increase the risk of food asphyxiation.

BOX 31.2 Guidelines for feeding infants safely

- Unpasteurized milk or unpasteurized food should not be fed to infants as they can introduce pathogens such as *Escherichia coli* 0157:H7, *Salmonella*, or *Cryptosporidium*, which cause diarrhoea or other more serious infections

- To prevent botulism, infants under 1 year of age should not be fed honey

- To prevent *Salmonella* poisoning, raw eggs and foods containing raw eggs should not be fed to infants

- Infant cereal or other solids should not be added to human milk or formula in a bottle as it may put the infant at risk for choking and aspiration

- To avoid burns to an infant's palate or face, formula or food warmed in a microwave should be shaken or stirred thoroughly, and the temperature tested, before serving

- Avoid hard, small and round, smooth and sticky solid foods, which may cause choking and aspiration

- Avoid feeding an infant using a 'propped' bottle

- Ensure that infants are always supervised during feeding

31.9 Assessing nutritional adequacy

In general, it is assumed that an infant's nutritional status is normal, and nutritional needs are being met, if he or she has a normal rate of growth, drinks adequate amounts of breast milk (or suitable formula or milk for age) and eats a variety of age-appropriate foods from each of the food groups. When nutritional status or growth is questionable, the infant's intake should be evaluated in comparison with established national or Food and Agriculture Organization/World Health Organization (FAO/WHO)-recommended nutrient intakes or allowances.

31.9.1 Energy and nutrient requirements

Due to their rapid rate of growth and higher metabolic rate, energy requirements for infants are higher than at any other time of life. Recent studies using the doubly labelled water technique have facilitated measurements of total energy expenditure of infants. Evidence from these studies resulted in a lowering of American and Canadian recommendations from approximately 120–95 to 107–81 kcal/kg/day.

When an infant's energy requirements are met from a well-balanced diet the risk of other nutri-

ent deficiencies is minimized. Intakes of individual nutrients that fall between 70% and 100% of recommended levels do not necessarily indicate a deficiency, as recommendations (with the exception of energy) are set at the mean requirement, plus two standard deviations, to ensure that the needs of almost all infants are met.

31.9.2 Monitoring growth

Postnatal growth and development of the central nervous system are most rapid during the first year of life. The typical infant doubles his or her birth weight during the first 4–5 months and triples it in the first year. By 2 years of age, a child has grown to half of their adult height. Plotting serial measurements of length-by-age and weight-by-length can be used to compare growth with normative values for healthy infants. In most children, height and weight measurements follow consistently along a channel (i.e. on or between the same centile(s)). Normal growth is indicated by weight-for-length and length-for-age tracking along similar percentiles or growth channels; however, it is common for infants to shift percentiles for both length and weight in the first 2–3 years of life with the majority settling into a channel towards the 50th percentile (i.e. regression toward the mean) rather than away. When length-for-age and weight-for-length percentiles are disproportional or weight and/or height measurements cross more than two percentiles downwards, investigation of potential nutritional imbalances is indicated.

Recent studies have demonstrated that the growth rate of infants who have been breastfed for more than 3 months is slower than that of formula-fed infants (or infants breastfed for less than 3 months)

from similar socioeconomic and ethnic backgrounds. Behavioural development, activity level and morbidity are not different between the groups of infants, suggesting the slower growth rate is of no nutritional significance. When this slower growth pattern of otherwise healthy and thriving breastfed infants is misinterpreted as growth faltering, it can lead to unnecessary concern about the adequacy of breast-feeding and interfere with the promotion of exclusive breastfeeding for approximately the first 6 months of life.

31.10 Common feeding problems

31.10.1 Food allergies

Adverse food reactions are divided into two general categories: food intolerance and food allergy. A true allergic reaction to a food involves the body's immune system. In the paediatric population, estimates of prevalence range from 1–8%, with the highest frequency in the first year of life. The risk of developing food allergies is largely related to genetic predisposition and the age at which the food is introduced, with the chance of sensitization greatest in the first year of life. Young infants are especially prone because their immature intestinal system is more permeable to absorption of food allergens and lacks local immunity defences. Most allergens are proteins of large molecular size. Therefore, food allergy commonly presents in infancy with the first introduction of milk, egg or peanuts. Along with soy, fish, nuts and wheat, these foods are responsible for about 95% of food allergies in infants and toddlers. It is rare for an infant to have allergies to more than two or three foods.

The issue of preventing allergy is controversial. There is good evidence that when there is a family history of atopic disease, exclusive breastfeeding for at least 4–6 months decreases the risk of food allergy. There is no scientific evidence that anyone without a close family history of allergic disease should make changes to the normal introduction of solid foods. In at-risk infants, there is not agreement about

the benefits of delaying introduction of, or the age at which to introduce, commonly allergenic foods. Avoidance of allergenic foods can postpone the development of allergic disease in individuals at risk, but not prevent it. Traditionally, parents have been advised to delay the introduction of allergenic foods such as egg white until 1 year of age (see Box 31.3). Management of food allergies involves strict avoidance of the allergenic food and requires careful reading of food labels to detect hidden sources. Sensitivity to many foods disappears within a few years; therefore, retesting and rechallenging with the offending food should occur at regular intervals. Allergies to peanuts, nuts, fish and seafood are the most severe and tend to be lifelong.

BOX 31.3 Strategies for reducing the incidence and severity of allergy in high-risk infants

- Prolonged breastfeeding
- Prolonged breastfeeding plus maternal avoidance of commonly allergenic foods during pregnancy and lactation
- Use of protein hydrolysate formulas in non-breast-fed infants
- Delayed introduction of solids until at least 4 months, and preferably 6 months, especially for foods that are hyperallergenic

31.10.2 Allergy to cow's milk protein

Cow's milk protein is the most important trigger of food allergy in infancy, with estimations of prevalence ranging from 1 to 5%. The decision of which formula to use should include consideration of the type of allergic reaction to cow's milk protein. Studies have revealed that 8–60% of milk-sensitive infants also react to soy. Although soy formulas are not hypoallergenic, they may be tolerated by infants with IgE-associated symptoms of cow's milk protein allergy (e.g. urticaria, wheezing, rhinitis, vomiting, eczema, anaphylaxis; see Box 31.3). In infants at high risk for allergy, identified by a strong family history of allergies, who are unable to be breastfed completely, there is no evidence that feeding with a soy formula compared with a cow's milk formula reduces allergies, whereas there is evidence that prolonged feeding with a hydrolysed formula compared with cow's milk formula reduces infant and childhood allergy and infant cow's milk allergy. Goat's milk has some similar antigens to cow's milk and is not recommended. Newer formulas with partially hydrolysed protein are less expensive and more palatable than the hypoallergenic hydrolysed formulas; however, they contain a significant percentage (approximately 20%) of peptides in the allergenic range. Further trials are required to determine whether partially hydrolysed formula is as effective as extensively hydrolysed formula in reducing infant cow's milk allergy. Rare reactions to extensively hydrolysed formulas have been reported in highly allergic infants who are then fed formulas based on free amino acids.

31.10.3 Lactose intolerance

The majority of adverse reactions to foods do not involve the immune system and are known as food intolerance. The most common food intolerance in infants is lactose intolerance, from lack of the lactase enzyme that normally splits lactose in the intestine. Congenital lactase deficiency is extremely rare while primary hypolactasia is more common due to a normal developmental decrease in lactase activity.

Lactose intolerance can develop in infants secondary to intestinal mucosal damage caused by gastroenteritis, malnutrition, cow's milk protein enteropathy, coeliac disease, giardiasis, bacterial overgrowth, inflammatory bowel disease or drugs. Common symptoms include gas, cramps and explosive diarrhoea. Diagnosis is best obtained using the non-invasive breath-hydrogen test; however, for practical reasons the test can only be performed starting around the age of 1 year. Infants with lactose intolerance should be changed from a cow's milk formula to either a lactose-free cow's milk formula or a soy formula. Infants beyond 9–12 months of age can be given cow's milk treated with β-galactosidase (LactAid®) or a soy formula. Soy milks, even those fortified with calcium and vitamin D, are inadequate in the first 1–2 years of life due to their low fat and energy content. Infants with primary intolerance may be able to tolerate small amounts of lactose-containing foods. Following secondary intolerance, reintroduction of small amounts of lactose should be tried at regular intervals to return to a balanced diet as soon as possible.

31.10.4 Dietary management of acute diarrhoea

In developed countries, the typical infant with acute diarrhoea is well nourished, presents with mild to moderate dehydration, and has a viral-induced diarrhoea with low stool electrolyte losses. In developing countries, children with acute diarrhoea are more likely to be malnourished and severely dehydrated with a viral- or bacterial-induced diarrhoea with high stool electrolyte losses. Oral rehydration therapy, which combines the use of oral electrolyte solutions with early refeeding, has proven to be safe and efficacious for restoring and maintaining hydration and electrolyte balance in infants with mild and moderate dehydration, including those with vomiting. Infants with severe dehydration should receive intravenous rehydration. Oral electrolyte solutions containing specific concentrations of carbohydrate, sodium, potassium and chloride promote fluid and electrolyte absorption whereas fluids such as juices, soft drinks, tea, jelly or broth do not. Human milk is well tolerated during diarrhoea and may reduce its severity and duration; therefore, breastfeeding should continue throughout the diarrhoea with additional fluids given as oral electrolyte solutions.

Early and rapid refeeding should occur as soon as rehydration is achieved and vomiting stops (ideally within 6–12 h of beginning treatment) as infants treated with oral rehydration therapy and early refeeding have reduced stool output, shorter duration of diarrhoea and improved weight gain. Routine change to lactose-free or diluted feedings is unnecessary in well-nourished infants with mild to moderate gastroenteritis. Factors that appear to increase the risk of developing lactose intolerance include younger age, malnutrition, bacterial diarrhoea, prolonged diarrhoea before treatment and a greater degree of dehydration on assessment. Infants and toddlers who were fed solid food before the onset of the diarrhoea should continue to receive their usual diet once rehydration occurs. The use of age-appropriate, nutrient-dense mixtures of common foods is recommended. These foods should be nutritious, easily digested and absorbed, culturally acceptable and should not have a deleterious effect on the illness. Although not based on strong science, starchy foods are generally well tolerated as the initial foods for refeeding. Use of a low-residue diet (commonly called the BRAT diet: bananas, rice, apple sauce or apple juice, and tea or toast) can theoretically worsen the clinical state as it supplies less than one-half of an infant's daily energy and protein needs.

New interventions for the control of diarrhoea

Recently, administration of certain strains of probiotic bacterium (e.g. *Lactobacillus*) to modify intestinal flora in diarrhoea treatment has been shown to be safe and to shorten recovery of acute diarrhoea managed by oral rehydration therapy and early refeeding.

It has been demonstrated that zinc supplements given during an episode of acute diarrhoea reduce the severity and duration of the episode and reduce the incidence of diarrhoea during the following 2–3 months. The WHO currently recommends at the start of an episode of diarrhoea to give 10–20 mg zinc/day for 10–14 days (10 mg for infants under 6 months of age).

31.10.5 Constipation

There is wide variation in the stooling patterns of infants, ranging from a bowel movement after each feed to one every few days. Stool frequency and consistency are influenced by the infant's type of feeding (e.g. human milk or formula, introduction of solid foods, transition from pureed foods to table foods). Bowel frequency decreases with age as a result of the maturing gut's ability to conserve water. After 3–4 years of age, the frequency of bowel movements does not change. Breastfed and non-breastfed infants receiving an adequate diet are rarely constipated. Although an infant may appear to be straining, it is normal for an infant to grimace or have a red face when having a bowel movement. Educating parents about the wide variation in stooling patterns is important for avoiding overtreatment of normal stooling habits. Hard and painful bowel movements, abdominal distension or blood in the stool may be signs of true constipation.

Approximately 90–97% of infants and children with constipation have idiopathic non-organic constipation, most often due to a decision made by the child to delay defecation after experiencing a painful or frightening evacuation (e.g. due to an anal fissure). This is known as *functional* constipation, functional faecal retention or withholding constipation. Functional constipation is uncomfortable but not dangerous, and therefore is considered benign. An infant of less than 6 months who is believed to be truly constipated should be referred to a physician for investigation of organic causes. The earlier constipation occurs, the greater the chance of an underlying problem (e.g. Hirschsprung's disease). Common recommendations regarding therapy for constipation in infants are based on theory, not scientific evidence. Practices such as adding sugar or corn syrup to formula to cause osmotic diarrhoea, or increasing free fluid intake by giving additional water or juice are safe, but without scientific support in the literature.

Fruit juices such as prune, apple and pear are also commonly suggested because of their high sorbitol content. However, there is no evidence to support the use of dietary factors to alleviate chronic constipation once stool withholding and stool retention have become a problem. In a small, select population of infants, chronic constipation can be a manifestation of intolerance or allergy to cow's milk. For children with constipation who do not respond to laxatives and dietary modifications, a trial of cow's milk elimination may be considered.

31.10.6 Fat intake

Dietary fat modifications recommended for adults are not applicable to infants. In contrast, a high-fat diet (approximately 50% of energy from fat) helps to meet the infant's requirements for energy and fatty acids. Restricting dietary fat may lead to inadequate energy intake and jeopardize growth and development. There is no consistent evidence that use of a fat-reduced, cholesterol-lowering diet in infancy decreases the risk of atherosclerosis in adulthood.

31.10.7 Vegetarianism

Signs of increased interest in vegetarianism can be found in the rising number of vegetarian websites, magazines and cookbooks, the addition of vegetarian entrees, including veggie burgers, to fast-food and other restaurant menus, and the wider choice of vegetarian options at supermarkets. The number of scientific articles on vegetarianism have also increased, with the focus switching from questions about nutritional adequacy to studies demonstrating benefits for disease prevention and treatment. Whether the beneficial effects observed in adults take root in infants and toddlers raised on vegetarian diets has not been investigated.

Although the low saturated fat and high fibre content of vegetarian diets offers advantages to the health of adults, their bulky nature and low energy density can restrict the amount of food energy that infants (with their limited stomach capacity and higher needs for accelerated growth) can consume. With careful planning, vegetarian infants fed adequate amounts of breast milk or commercial infant formula and a balanced, varied diet grow similarly to non-vegetarian infants. However, the risk of nutritional deficiencies increases if the variety of foods making up the diet is very restrictive (e.g. macrobiotic, Rastafarian, fruitarian, raw diets, etc.), and/or if supplementation and medical supervision is avoided. Key nutrients include energy, protein, fibre, vitamin B_{12}, iron, vitamin D, calcium, zinc and $n-3$ fatty acids. Because dietary practices among vegetarians are variable, assessment of dietary intake is important to determine whether fortified foods or supplements are needed to meet recommendations for individual nutrients.

Most vegetarians will continue breastfeeding well into the second year of life. Problems of nutritional inadequacy in the infant (e.g. vitamin B_{12}) are likely to occur if the mother's diet is very restricted, if prolonged breastfeeding is not supplemented around 4–6 months of age, or if infants are weaned prematurely on to an unsuitable breast-milk substitute. Vegan infants who are weaned from the breast before 1 year of age should receive a commercial soy formula until 1–2 years of age.

In infants consuming a macrobiotic diet, a clear relationship has been demonstrated between diet, nutrient intake, and physical and biochemical evidence of deficiency for several nutrients including iron, vitamin B_{12}, vitamin D and riboflavin. Slower growth rates (peaking between 6 and 18 months) and higher incidence of nutritional diseases such as rickets, kwashiorkor and anaemia have been reported. Macrobiotic diets consist of unpolished rice, pulses and vegetables with small additions of fermented foods, nuts, seeds and fruits; animal products are not consumed. Even less restricted vegetarian diets typically have a high content of phytates and other modifiers of mineral (e.g. iron, zinc, calcium) absorption, which are associated with a higher prevalence of rickets and iron-deficiency anaemia.

FURTHER READING

1. **A Collaborative Statement of Dietitians of Canada, Canadian Paediatric Society, College of Family Physicians of Canada, and Community Health Nurses Association of Canada** (2004) The use of growth charts for assessing and monitoring growth in Canadian infants and children. *Can J Diet Prac Res*, **65**, 22–32.

2. **American Academy of Pediatrics** (1994) Infant feeding practices and their possible relationship to the etiology of diabetes mellitus. *Pediatrics*, **94**, 752–4.

3. **American Academy of Pediatrics Section on Breastfeeding** (2005) Breastfeeding and the use of human milk. Policy Statement. *Pediatrics*, **115**, 496–506.

4. **American Dietetic Association and Dietitians of Canada** (2003) Position of the American Dietetic Association and Dietitians of Canada: vegetarian diets. *Can J Diet Prac Res*, **64**, 62–81.

5. **Baker, S., Liptak, G., Colletti, R.G.,** *et al.* (1999) Constipation in infants and children: evaluation and treatment. A medical position statement of the North American Society for Pediatric Gastroenterology and Nutrition. *J Pediatr Gastroenterol Nutr*, **29**, 612–26.

6. **Bock, A., and Atkins, F.** (1990) Patterns of food hypersensitivity during sixteen years of double-blind placebo controlled food challenges. *J Pediatr*, **117**, 561–7.

7. **Centers for Disease Control and Prevention** (2003) Managing acute gastroenteritis among children: oral rehydration, maintenance, and nutritional therapy. *MMWR Recomm Rep*, **52** (RR16), 1–16.

8. **Dewey, K.G., Peerson, J.M., Brown K.H.,** *et al.* (1995) Growth of breast-fed infants deviates from current reference data: a pooled analysis of US, Canadian, and European data sets. *Pediatrics*, **96**, 495–503.

9. **Gartner, L.M., Greer, F.R., and American Academy of Pediatrics, Section on Breastfeeding, Committee on Nutrition** (2003) Prevention of rickets and vitamin D deficiency: new guidelines for vitamin D intake. *Pediatrics*, **111**, 908–10.

10. **Health Canada** (2004) *Vitamin D supplementation for breastfed infants: 2004 Health Canada Recommendation.* www.hc-sc.gc.ca/fn-an/nutrition/child-enfant/infantnourisson/vita_d_supp_e.html.

11. **Health Canada** (2004) *Exclusive breastfeeding duration —2004. Health Canada Recommendation.* www.hc-sc.gc.ca/fn-an/nutrition/child-enfant/infant-nourisson/excl_bf_dur-dur_am_excl_e.html.

12. **Hendricks, K.M., and Badruddin, S.H.** (1992) Weaning recommendations: the scientific basis. *Nutr Rev*, **50**, 125–33.

13. **Huang, J., Bousvaros, A., Lee, J.W., Diaz, A., and Davidson, E.J.** (2002) Efficacy of probiotic use in acute diarrhea in children: a meta-analysis. *Dig Dis Sci*, **47**, 2625–34.

14. **Institute of Medicine** (2002) *Dietary reference intakes for energy, carbohydrates, fiber, fat, protein and amino acids (macronutrients).* Washington DC, National Academy of Sciences.

15. **Loening-Baucke, V.** (2005) Prevalence, symptoms and outcome of constipation in infants and toddlers. *J Pediatr*, **146**, 359–63.

16. **O'Connor, D.L., Hall, R., Adamkin, D.,** *et al.* (2001) Growth and development in preterm infants fed long-chain polyunsaturated fatty acids: a prospective, randomized controlled trial. *Pediatrics*, **108**, 359–71.

17. **Osborn, D., and Sinn, J.** (2003) Formulas containing hydrolysed protein for prevention of allergy and food intolerance in infants. *Cochrane Database Syst Rev*, **3**, CD003664.

18. **Osborn, D., and Sinn, J.** (2004) Soy formula for prevention of allergy and food intolerance in infants. *Cochrane Database Syst Rev*, **3**, CD003741.

19. **Sandhu, B., for the European Society of Paediatric Gastroenterology, Hepatology and Nutrition Working Group on Acute Diarrhoea** (2001) Practical guidelines for the management of gastroenteritis in children. *J Pediatr Gastroenterol Nutr*, **33** (Suppl. 2), S36–9.

20. **Setchell, K., Zimmer-Nechemias, L., Cai, J., and Heab., J.E.** (1997) Exposure of infants to phyto-oestrogens from soy-based infant formula. *Lancet*, **350**, 23–7.

21. **Singhal, A., and Lucas, A.** (2004) Early origins of cardiovascular disease: is there a unifying hypothesis? *Lancet*, **363**, 1642–5.

22. **Singhal, A., Morley, R., Abbott, R., Fairweather-Tait, S., Stephenson, T., and Lucas, A.** (2000) Clinical safety of iron-fortified formulas. *Pediatrics*, **105**, E38.

23. **Stallings Harris, C., Baker, S.P., Smith, G.P., and Harris, R.M.** (1984) Childhood asphyxiation by food. A national analysis and overview. *JAMA*, **251**, 2231–5.

24. **US Department of Health and Human Services. Centers for Disease Control and Prevention** (1998) Recommendations to prevent and control iron deficiency in the United States. *MMWR Recomm Rep,* **47** (RR-3), 1–30.

25. **Van Niel, C., Feudtner, C., Garrison, M.M., and Christakis, D.A.** (2002) Lactobacillus therapy for acute infectious diarrhea in children: a meta-analysis. *Pediatrics*, **109**, 678–84.

26. **Wharton, B.** (1999) Iron deficiency in children: detection and prevention. *Br J Haematol*, **106**, 270–80.

 To see topical and scientifically robust updates on nutrition associated with this textbook, and active web links to many of the journal articles in the Reference areas, please see the dedicated Online Resource Centre at www.oxfordtextbooks.co.uk/orc/mann3e/.

32 Childhood and adolescence nutrition

Colin Binns

Protein-energy malnutrition is covered in Chapter 18, nutritional consequences of poverty in developed countries in Chapter 38, eating disorders in Chapter 23, and obesity in Chapter 16.

Definitions Childhood and adolescence are defined by age:

- Childhood: aged 2–12 years.
- Adolescence: aged 12–18 years.

32.1 Introduction

Children are not small adults. Children are vulnerable to nutrition problems as they are dependent on adults for the provision of food. They have specific nutritional needs to maximize their health and well-being during childhood and subsequently as adults. Physiologically, the specific nutrition requirements result in children having a longer small intestine than an adult. Children need energy for growth, but this is only a surprisingly small proportion of their total energy intake. Most of the energy intake of children simply provides the energy needed to be a child—running, jumping and learning to explore the world. The added energy intake also provides the vehicle to bring sufficient micronutrients for growth and development.

One in four of the world's children still suffers from malnutrition. For at least one half, and perhaps the majority, the focus remains on getting enough food to grow adequately. For them, high-volume, low-nutrient-density diets are a major problem. For the remainder of the world's children, the focus starts on growth but quickly shifts to preventing obesity in the immediate and long-term future. The energy density of higher fat foods is a contributing factor to the obesity problem. Sometimes messages from society about body shape are misinterpreted and anorexia nervosa is the result.

Despite improvements in the world's economy and some progress in the alleviation of poverty, children around the world are still subject to a wide range of nutritional deficiencies, e.g. iodine and iron. Anaemia remains the most common nutritional problem in this age group, followed by protein-energy malnutrition.

The objectives for good nutrition during childhood include providing sufficient nutrients and energy for appropriate growth, not too little (which leads to undernutrition or stunting) or too much (obesity). Good nutrition is essential to minimize illness as a child, promote optimal health and also to minimize illness, including chronic disease, throughout adulthood. Cognitive development is influenced by nutritional factors including iron, iodine and

Table 32.1 Dietary guidelines for children and adolescents in Australia

Breastfeeding should be encouraged and supported

Children and adolescents need sufficient nutritious foods to grow and develop normally

Growth should be checked regularly for young children

Physical activity is important for all children and adolescents

Enjoy a wide variety of nutritious foods

Children and adolescents should be encouraged to:
– eat plenty of vegetables, legumes and fruits
– eat plenty of cereals (including breads, rice, pasta and noodles), preferably wholegrain
– include lean meat, fish, poultry and/or alternatives
– include milks, yoghurts, cheese and/or alternatives

Reduced-fat milks are not suitable for young children under 2 years because of their high energy needs, but reduced-fat varieties should be encouraged for older children and adolescents

Choose water as a drink
– Alcohol is not recommended for children

Care should be taken to:
– limit saturated fat and moderate total fat intake
– low-fat diets are not suitable for infants
– choose foods low in salt
– consume only moderate amounts of sugars and foods containing added sugars

Care for your child's food: prepare and store it safely

protein. In addition, children need sufficient energy to enable them to explore their environment, to respond to stimulation and hence to learn. Childhood is a time of learning. Eating habits established during childhood will last a lifetime. Children who learn to explore and enjoy a range of tastes and textures are more likely as adults to have a varied diet that meets dietary guidelines. Children who learn to drink water to quench their thirst are less likely to become obese by consuming sugar-rich carbonated beverages.

32.1.1 Food and nutrients for children

It is important for children to learn to eat healthy and varied diets that provide all of the nutrients required for growth and health. Typically, scientific advice on foods to consume is provided through dietary guidelines that should be evidence-based and also involve widespread consultation to ensure that they are prac-

tical in the community for which they are intended. In the developed countries, emphasis is shifting towards the prevention of obesity and there is increased emphasis on the introduction of lower-fat products and moderating sugar intakes by school-aged children. An example of a typical set of Dietary Guidelines for Children are shown in Table 32.1. Promoting daily exercise is an important part of nutritional guidance. Children's nutrition education and learning to follow examples of proper eating can be used to develop eating habits for a lifetime. Nutrient requirements are often proportionally greater for children than for adults, making it important to consume diets of high nutritional quality. (See Table 32.2 for a typical set of nutrient reference values.)

32.1.2 Growth

Measurement of weight and other anthropometric parameters remains central to the nutritional assess-

Table 32.2 Nutrient reference values for children and adolescents

Nutrient	Age group (years) and gender					
	Children		Boys		Girls	
	1–3	4–8	9–13	14–18	9–13	14–18
Protein (g/day)						
EAR	12	16	31	49	24	35
RDI	14	20	40	65	35	45
Calcium[a] (mg/day)						
EAR	360	520	800–1050	1050	800–1050	1050
RDI	500	700	1000–1300	1300	1000–1300	1300
Iron (mg/day)						
EAR	4	4	6	8	6	8
RDI	9	10	8	11	8	15
Vitamin C (mg/day)						
EAR	25	25	28	28	28	28
RDI	35	35	40	40	40	40
Vitamin A (µg/day)						
EAR	210	275	445	630	420	485
RDI	300	400	600	900	600	700

[a]For calcium, because of growth needs, there are separate recommendations for children aged 9–11 years and 12–13 years; 9–11-year-olds who are growing and maturing at much greater rates than average may need the intakes recommended for 12–13-year-olds.
EAR = estimated average requirement; RDI = recommended daily intake.
Source: Nutrient Reference Values for Australia and New Zealand, NH and MRC, Canberra, 2006.

ment of children. Parents often do not recognize overweight in themselves or their children and health professionals often do not recognize underweight, on casual examination, often assuming that the child is younger than they actually are.

Weight gain and an increase in body size during childhood and adolescence are integral parts of the normal process of growth and development. Important factors in growth include:

- genetic constitution
- nutrition
- endocrine function
- disease (recurrent infectious disease or chronic disease)
- an overall nurturing environment, including a stable family life, a peaceful community and good education.

Birth weight has an influence on growth during infancy and if growth should slow there is potential for some 'catch-up'. As nutritional status improves around the world, the differences in birth weight between racial groups is lessening and mean birth weights in countries such as China and Vietnam are now the same as in more developed countries. Genetic differences appear to be less important than nutritional status in determining growth rates and ultimate body size. There is more difference between children from well-nourished higher socioeconomic groups and disadvantaged children within the same country than there is between the higher socioeconomic groups in different countries. While ethnic differences in the growth of children may be fairly small, there are, however, body composition differences (percentage body fat) in adults, and probably children, which may have significance in the diagnosis of obesity.

In recent years, there has been increasing awareness through the fetal origins of disease hypothesis (the Barker hypothesis) of the importance of appropriate growth and nutrition, *in utero* and during childhood, and the development of disease in adulthood. In addition, there is increasing evidence of the importance of growth and nutrition in cognitive development and its importance in maximizing future bone mass.

Between birth and 18 years of age, body weight increases about 20-fold. During early childhood, the rate of increase in weight for length is essentially linear, i.e. the rate of increase in weight generally keeps pace with the rate at which length increases. Before puberty, children add about 6 cm to their height every year, increasing from 86 cm in girls (87.5 cm boys) at 2 years to 137 cm in girls (140 cm boys) at 10 years. During adolescence, the rate of growth accelerates over a period of 1 to 3 years (age of onset variable) and then decelerates rapidly until growth in height ceases at around 16 years of age in girls and 18 years in boys (see Fig. 32.1).

32.1.3 Growth references

The term 'growth reference' refers to the set of data used to compile a growth chart. The growth chart is used as a reference to plot the individual child's growth and not as an absolute standard for each child to achieve. In general, trends in growth are more important than the absolute position on the chart. In 1978, the World Health Organization (WHO) recommended universal use of the growth reference

produced by the US National Centre for Health Statistics for international use. These charts have been included in personal health records in many other countries for use by parents and health workers as a continuing record of a child's growth and health. Recently, the US data have been revised to eliminate some minor anomalies around 2 years of age (See Figs 32.2 and 32.3) (http://www.cdc.gov/nchs/data/ad/ad314.pdf). In particular, the data used for infants has been updated and the calculation of some percentiles has been revised.

Commonly used growth reference charts are prepared with a number of percentiles marked, usually ranging from the 3rd percentile up to the 97th percentile. Growth charts using Z-scores (standard deviations, above or below the mean; also see 29.3.5) are also available and are more commonly used in research studies and surveys. The 95th and 5th percentiles are approximately plus and minus 1.65 standard deviations, respectively (Z-scores of +1.65 and −1.65, respectively). Data must be plotted as accurately as possible on the chart for the correct gender. A note should be made on the chart of any potential source of error such as the child struggling or having been weighed clothed.

The international growth reference is derived from a mix of infants who were breastfed and fed on infant formula. Exclusively breast-fed babies may grow at a slightly lower rate than the reference, although if the charts are used as a reference (and not as a standard) the difference is not important (approximating a Z-score of −0.5). Children who have been breastfed during infancy, particularly for at least 6 months, will be leaner at the age of 2 years than their formula-fed cousins. While low birth weight influences infant size, after 12 months of age it is no longer necessary to allow for prematurity.

32.1.4 Assessment of body size and growth rate (see Box 32.1)

An accurate record of growth remains one of the most useful assessment tools for both the well child and the child suffering from disease. Growth trends reveal more about the child's nutrition or health than

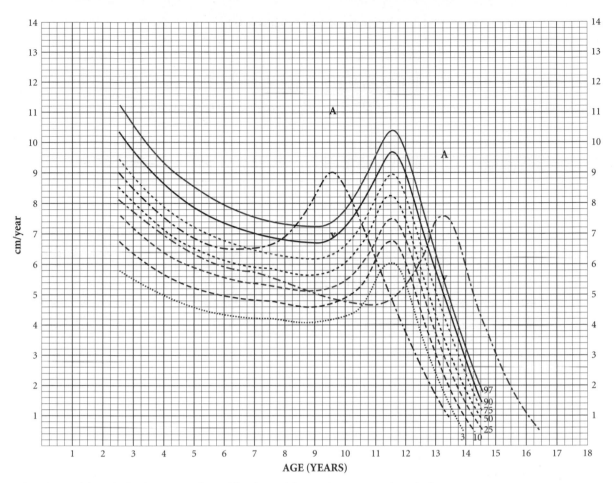

Fig. 32.1 Height velocity for N. American girls. The outlying peaks are an early and a late maturer.

Source: Used with permission from Tanner, J., and Davis, P.S.W. (1985), Clinical longitudinal standards for height and weight velocity for North American children. *J Pediat*, **107**, 317–29.

the position of one measurement on the chart. If weight and height are measured on several occasions, the measurements are most usefully interpreted by plotting them on reference growth charts. A child who is on approximately the same percentile for height and weight and who is growing at a rate parallel to the next percentile line is unlikely to have a serious nutrition or chronic health problem. Where a child's growth percentile is changing, or plotted values show a markedly irregular pattern, and particularly when near or crossing the upper or lower extremes, i.e. the 10th or the 90th percentiles, a reason should be sought. In all cases where a major discrepancy is found from the previous measurement, the accuracy of the measurement and recording should first be checked. The extent to which serial data for a child can deviate from a given percentile range before concern is warranted depends on the age of the child, the child's position in the percentile range, the length of time for which the rate of growth deviates from the norm and the coexistence of any medical condition. In general, the more pronounced the change in growth rate, the younger the child and the more extreme the percentile, the greater is the concern. In the current climate of our obesity epidemic, a rapid rate of growth may be of as much concern as growth faltering.

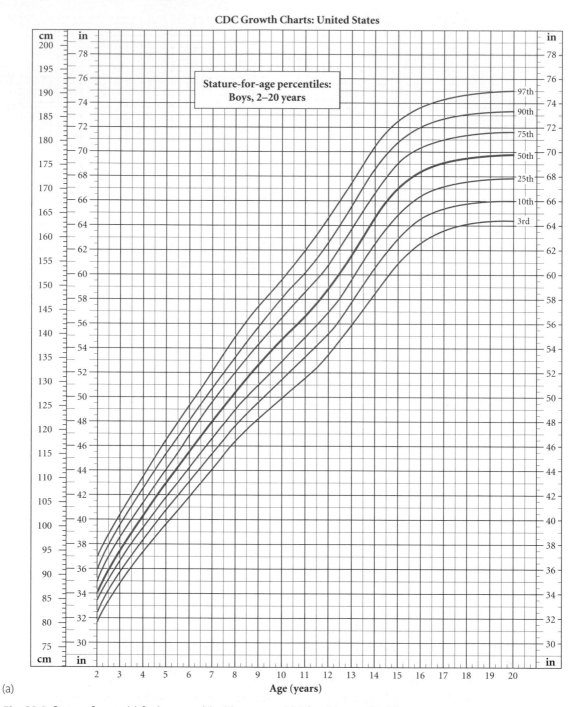

(a)

Fig. 32.2 Stature for age (a) for boys aged 2–20 years, and (b) for girls aged 2–20 years.

Source: National Centre for Health Statistics (NCHS)/National Center for Chronic Disease Prevention and Health Promotion (CDC), USA (2000).

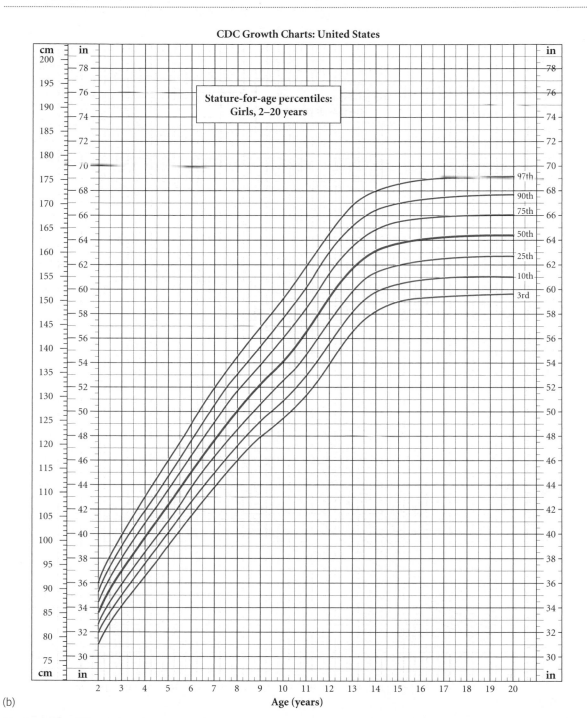

CDC Growth Charts: United States

Stature-for-age percentiles:
Girls, 2–20 years

(b)

Fig. 32.2 (cont'd).

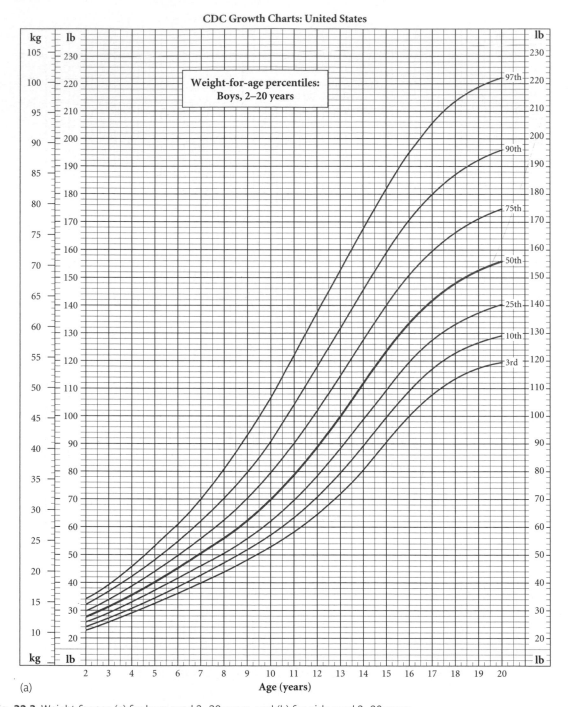

Fig. 32.3 Weight-for-age (a) for boys aged 2–20 years, and (b) for girls aged 2–20 years.

Source: National Centre for Health Statistics (NCHS)/National Center for Chronic Disease Prevention and Health Promotion (CDC), USA (2000).

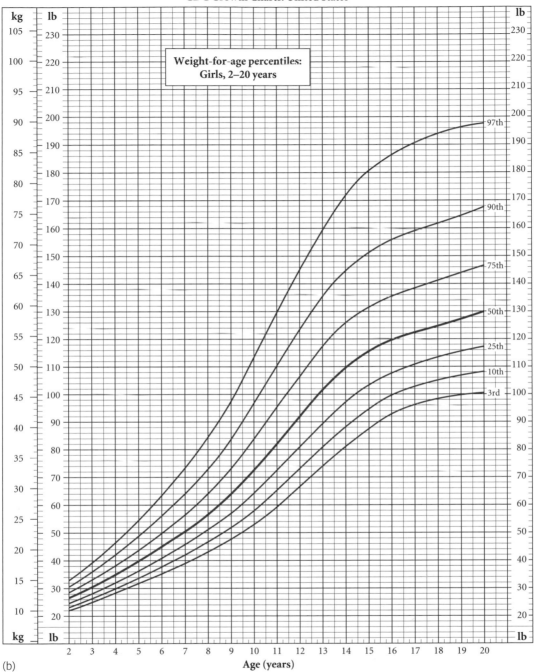

CDC Growth Charts: United States

Weight-for-age percentiles:
Girls, 2–20 years

(b)

Fig. 32.3 *(Cont'd)*

> **BOX 32.1 Measuring a child's growth**
>
> 1. Regular measurement of weight is the best way of assessing undernutrition or obesity
> 2. Growth trends give more information than one measurement
> 3. A child crossing the 90th or 10th percentiles should be assessed
> 4. Referral for treatment with growth hormone should only be made if the child is consistently below the 3rd percentile and there is no other cause to be found
> 5. Growth reference charts for use should be based on current CDC or WHO charts
> 6. Dietary guidelines provide advice on consuming a healthy, varied diet that will enable the nutrient reference values to be met

For example, a child who is moving toward or exceeding the 90th percentile of weight for age may require discussion with parents to implement an obesity prevention program. Similarly, a trend towards weight loss over 1 month or more should prompt efforts to establish a nutritional cause or the existence of an underlying disease. It is important to note any difference between the weight and height percentiles. In acute nutritional problems, weight is likely to be at a substantially lower percentile than height. For endocrine deficiencies or other long-term conditions or diseases, both weight and height will be substantially depressed.

Parental size also influences a child's measurements and where this is thought to be a significant factor, charts or tables adjusted for the average height of both parents are available. These charts are used only rarely.

What is the alternative to regular growth monitoring of children? There is no alternative—without accurate measurements health professionals are forced literally to guess the nutritional status of their clients. This has led to a reassessment of the value of growth monitoring and to the importance of regular measurement as a component of primary health care.

32.1.5 Undernutrition/failure to thrive

Failure to thrive occurs when a child of normal height and head circumference has a weight for age below the 3rd percentile. As well as this absolute definition, a child who was previously growing well who stops growing and plummets through several percentile lines might also be included in this group. In developing countries, the same children are usually called 'undernourished'. In these countries, the causes are usually insufficient food, shortage of specific nutrients important for growth and interaction with infectious disease. Often a high-volume, low-nutrient density limits the ability of a small child to consume sufficient energy and nutrients. The presence of pathogens in the gastrointestinal tract (bacteria, viruses and helminths) also interferes with absorption.

In the developed world about half of the cases are due to non-organic causes including psychosocial problems in carers (e.g. depression, child deprivation) or simply an inadequate diet due to ignorance, neglect or adherence to a strange dietary regime. Organic causes of failure to thrive are numerous and include chronic renal, cardiorespiratory and endocrine problems. Gastrointestinal abnormalities include coeliac disease, cystic fibrosis, Hirschsprung's disease and, during infancy, pyloric stenosis.

More than half of the children who are diagnosed as 'failure to thrive' in primary care or in a community clinic have a relatively simple nutrition problem —not enough food to meet their needs. For example, a child may be thought to have an 'allergy' and may have been placed on a very restrictive diet, or because the adults in the families are placed on a low-fat diet, the child may also be eating the same diet. Many chronic diseases cause growth retardation. In the absence of other symptoms or signs, it is usually appropriate to undertake a trial of improved nutrition rather than going immediately to further investigation. Referral to a specialist clinic for investigation of growth hormone deficiency is not necessary unless the child is consistently below the lowest percentile line and no other disease is present.

Children may develop food fads and be described by their parents as 'difficult eaters'. Prevention depends on the whole family eating a healthy diet and the children naturally falling into a pattern of good nutrition. The use of food, snacks and sweets in reward and punishment systems for inappropriate behaviour may lead to poor eating habits.

Diagnosis of failure to thrive includes careful review of accurate growth records and a full dietary and clinical history followed by medical examination. Management involves confirming the diagnosis and restoring proper nutritional habits.

32.1.6 Childhood overweight and obesity

The rapid increase in the prevalence of obesity in children and adolescents in all countries has serious public health consequences, including the development of diabetes and fatty infiltration of the liver (Table 32.3). Obesity during childhood is a significant risk factor for chronic disease (e.g. coronary heart disease, diabetes, hypertension) during adulthood. In many countries, the food supply and social environment could only be described as obesogenic. The prevention and treatment of overweight and obesity includes a review of the energy and macronutrient content of the diet, serving sizes of meals, meal pat-

terns, physical activity and the increasingly sedentary nature of modern society. Increased television viewing, computer-based activities, the lack of physical activity, and intake of fast food and the increasing substitution of water with higher-energy drinks all contribute to the obesity epidemic. The causation is multifactorial, and hence the prevention and treatment must also be multifactorial and should include an active debate of nutritional priorities within modern societies. Children should be encouraged to develop healthy nutrition and exercise habits early, since interventions are most effective when behaviours are still being formed. In countries such as Australia, one in four of all children are overweight or obese and the prevalence has been increasing every year. The irony is that obesity and undernutrition may exist side by side in many countries, regions, villages or even in the same family.

Overweight infants often become obese children who in turn can grow to obese adolescents; 80% of obese adolescents go on to become obese adults. In children, the growth chart remains the primary tool in the assessment of growth and the risk of obesity. Children heading above the 90 or 95th percentile are clearly at risk of obesity. Increasingly the body mass index (BMI) is also being used in the assessment and monitoring of obesity. Children above the 85th and 95th percentile of BMI for age and sex are recognized as being overweight and obese. Cole *et al.* (2000) used

Table 32.3 Age adjusted prevalence of overweight in children 6–11 years from national surveys in the USA

Dates	Boys		Girls	
	85th percentile	95th percentile	85th percentile	95th percentile
1963–1965 (NHES)	15.2	5.2	15.2	5.2
1971–1974 (NHANES I)	18.2	6.5	13.9	4.3
1976–1980 (NHANES II)	19.9	7.9	15.8	7.0
1988–1985 (NHANES III)	22.3	10.8	22.7	10.7

NHES = National Health Examination Survey; NHANES = National Health and Nutrition Examination Surveys.
Source: Adapted with permission from Troiano, R.P., Flegal, K.M., Kuczmarski, R.J., Campbell, S.M., and Johnston, C.L. (1995) Overweight prevalence and trends for children and adolescents. *Arch Pediatr Adolesc Med*, **149**, 1085–91.

Table 32.4 Body mass index levels to diagnose overweight and obesity in children

Age (years)	Overweight		Obesity	
	Boys	Girls	Boys	Girls
2	18.41	18.02	20.09	19.81
3	17.89	17.56	19.57	19.36
4	17.55	17.28	19.29	19.15
5	17.42	17.15	19.30	19.17
6	17.55	17.34	19.78	19.65
7	17.92	17.75	20.63	20.51
8	18.44	18.35	21.60	21.57
9	19.10	19.07	22.77	22.81
10	19.84	19.86	24.00	24.11
11	20.55	20.74	25.10	25.42
12	21.22	21.68	26.02	26.67
13	21.91	22.58	26.84	27.76
14	22.62	23.34	27.63	28.57
15	23.29	23.94	28.30	29.11
16	23.90	24.37	28.88	29.43
17	24.46	24.70	29.41	29.69
18	25	25	30	30

This table was developed by Professor Tim Cole using datasets from Brazil, Great Britain, Hong Kong, the Netherlands, Singapore and the USA. The columns show the levels of BMI equivalent to 25 and 30 in adults, which are the cut-off points for overweight and obesity.

growth data from a number of countries to develop BMI cut-off points for children of different ages for overweight and obesity. The Cole cut-off points are shown in Table 32.4 and are the equivalents of adult BMI levels of 25 (overweight) and 30 (obesity), respectively.

Recent research suggests there are differences in the percentages of body fat present in different ethnic groups at the same level of BMI. Thus, for Asian adults the BMI levels for diagnosis of obesity varied within the BMI range of 25–30. There is insufficient research available at present to set different levels of BMI for the diagnosis of childhood obesity in different ethnic groups, but evidence is accumulating.

32.1.7 At-risk families

The children most at risk of nutritional problems are those who live in poverty and whose parents, particularly mothers, have not benefited from modern education. The universal education of girls, the world's future mothers, should be promoted as one of the most important nutrition interventions. In modern Western families, the at-risk groups include children of single parents, of shift workers and those in long-day childcare while both parents work.

Childcare centres are increasingly important. Parents who work long hours may have insufficient time to prepare healthy meals for their children when they return home. Childcare centres must therefore take over the role of providing comprehensive nutritious meals and use these as the basis of nutrition education and cultivating appropriate food choices. Long-day childcare centres should aim to provide around 50% of the RDIs for those under their care.

32.1.8 Institutional meals

The demands of modern economies have changed the labour market in many countries, so many of the parents and carers of small children are involved in work that keeps them away from the family home. In previous generations, children were cared for by extended families, but in modern societies this function is given to childcare centres, often run by commercial organizations. As a child ages, food may be provided by school meal services or at boarding schools. Meals are also educational opportunities so it is important that these responsibilities are accepted, and there are specific guidelines to ensure that nutritious meals are provided. (Examples of nutrition resources can be found at: http://www.nutritionaustralia.org/ SNAC/snac_resource_reviews.asp.) School gardens are an excellent way of relating nutrition to practical aspects of the food supply. Advertising opportunities for fast-food suppliers should be limited. Reward programmes used in schools should not include vouchers issued by multinational chains peddling their products that do not meet standard nutritional guidelines.

32.1.9 Dental caries

Childhood is a high-risk period for the development of dental caries. Intact dentition is important throughout life. Historically, the prevalence of dental caries has increased in centuries where the diet changed to include more sugars and other refined foods. The relationship between sugar (sucrose) and dental caries was first documented in the scientific literature in the nineteenth century and confirmed in numerous studies since that time. Dental caries can be defined as a dietary carbohydrate and salivary-modified infectious disease. *Streptococcus mutans*, dietary sugars and a susceptible tooth surface are the important factors in dental caries. Dietary sugars, including sucrose, glucose and lactose, are involved in caries formation. Starch is less cariogenic than other dietary sugars because it does not readily diffuse into plaque and is less readily hydrolysed. If there is frequent exposure to sugars, the rate of demineralization of the tooth will exceed the rate of remineralization and dental caries will occur. The duration of exposure depends on the extent of retention of sugary foods in the mouth and the number of eating occasions and can be difficult to describe and quantify. Dental caries remains a significant public health problem in the Western world and is one of the more expensive diet-related health problems. Proper dental hygiene and the use of fluoridated toothpaste and water supplies have resulted in dramatic declines in average levels of dental decay. These improvements are obviously the starting point for future improvements in oral health in later life.

International comparative studies show that very few caries occur in children when the national per capita sugar (sucrose) consumption is below 10 kg per annum (approximately 30 g/day) but a steep increase may occur from 15 kg upwards. However, the frequency of eating sugar is related to dental caries rather than the amount. Sugars contained in the cellular structure of foods (such as the intrinsic sugars of fresh fruits and vegetables) have little cariogenic potential; it is foods high in extrinsic sugars that are most damaging to the teeth. Good oral hygiene is more likely to predict a low caries prevalence than a 'low cariogenic' diet. Prevention programmes to control and eliminate dental caries must focus on fluoridation and adequate oral hygiene, as well as moderating sucrose intake.

32.1.10 Food allergy

There are numerous reasons for reaction to foods. Food may contain toxic elements that cause rapid reactions, such as copper poisoning or the consumption of certain varieties of mushrooms that induce psychotropic reactions. In some children, gluten sensitivity or lactase deficiency (hereditary or transitory) may be confused with allergies. Children who drink large quantities of fruit juice may not be able to absorb the large quantities of fructose that it contains. The unabsorbed fructose is fermented in the gastrointestinal tract and causes osmotic diarrhoea. This is an important differential diagnosis in the assessment of allergy.

Food allergies that are common in childhood are caused by dairy products, egg, peanuts, other nuts, wheat, soy, fish and shellfish. While most food allergies decline after 5 years of age, those caused by peanuts, other nuts and shellfish tend to persist throughout life. Food allergies are usually classified into those that are IgE mediated and those that are non-IgE mediated. IgE-mediated food reactions generally occur soon after ingestion (1–2 hours). The types of reaction that occur include erythema if the food touches the skin or urticaria or angioneurotic oedema. Vomiting is the commonest gastrointestinal symptom. Severe reactions may occur; anaphylaxis can be life-threatening and needs immediate resuscitation. Peanut allergy can cause very severe reactions. Confirmation of the responsible food involves skin-prick testing and possibly food challenge under tightly controlled conditions. The suspected allergen should be totally withdrawn for 1 week prior to the challenge.

Non-IgE-mediated and mixed IgE/non-IgE reactions are less common and may cause delayed reactions after up to 24–48 hours. Gastrointestinal symptoms include vomiting, abdominal pains and diarrhoea. Eczema may be exacerbated.

Treatment of all forms of allergy involves careful elimination of that food from the diet. In severe cases of reaction to foods such as peanuts and shellfish, children may need to carry adrenaline (epinephrine) ready for injection. In families with a strong history of allergy, the introduction of cheese, yoghurt, ice cream, fish and wheat cereal should be delayed until 12 months of age. Cow's milk should not be introduced before 12 months, for the prevention of allergic gastrointestinal haemorrhage and because of its low iron content. If there is a strong history of peanut allergy, peanut products (including peanut butter) should be avoided until after 3 years of age. Peanut allergy is common and can be very severe. Peanut allergen can be found in breast milk, and if there is a family history of peanut allergy, breast-feeding mothers should avoid peanuts.

While food allergies are an important problem, they are now diagnosed more frequently than usually warranted. In some community studies, the prevalence of allergy is reported to be as high as 20%, but in reality it is probably only one-quarter of this figure. While trying to elucidate the cause of the allergy, children are regularly placed on restrictive exclusion diets. This should only be for a short period of time or it may place children at risk of nutritional deficiencies and undernutrition. Allergies to milk products are the most common group to be overdiagnosed but this food group is the major source of bioavailable calcium, needed for growth of bones. In some Western countries, food allergy and various degrees of anaphylactic reaction occur frequently enough for calls for teachers to be educated and provided with the means to deal with these reactions. The evidence linking food allergies and behavioural problems remains inconclusive.

32.1.11 Coeliac disease

Coeliac disease is an autoimmune enteropathy triggered by sensitivity to gluten in genetically sensitive individuals. Prevalence is estimated at 1% in the USA and western Europe. In first-degree relatives, the prevalence is as high as 10%. In its classic form, it causes poor growth, chronic diarrhoea, abdominal distension and anorexia. However, it can present just as growth retardation. The heterogeneous nature of the disease causes symptoms that range in severity and time of onset. Diagnosis rests on the presence of IgA and IgG antigliadin antibodies. Coeliac disease can be associated with other autoimmune diseases such as diabetes and Addison's disease. Small-bowel biopsy remains the gold standard for diagnosis. Treatment is with a gluten-free diet that completely excludes wheat, barley, rye and (usually) oats. Since these cereals are often included as ingredients in many varieties of food, this is a challenge to the family. Several dietetics websites maintain useful lists of foods that contain gluten:

- American Dietetic Association: http://www.eatright.org/
- British Dietetic Association: http://www.bda.uk.com/
- Dietitians Association of Australia: http://www.daa.asn.au/

32.2 Adolescence

There are more than 1 billion adolescents (aged 10–18) in the world, one in six of the total population. Adolescence is a time of rapid growth and transition from childhood to adulthood, from dependence to independent living in many societies. This period of life is often neglected by nutritionists, yet growth and development have a significant impact on health as adults. In particular, adolescent girls are often at nutritional risk.

Adolescence is a period of rapid physical, psychological and social growth when young people often gain 50% of their adult weight, more than 20%

of their adult height and 50% of their adult skeletal mass. Teenagers, particularly boys, are usually the biggest eaters in the family as energy and protein consumption reach a maximum. For many, this is a time of increased physical activity, yet it can be combined with poor diets due to the selection of inappropriate foods and increased consumption of high-energy, high-sugar drinks. For girls, menarche and the risk of pregnancy add to nutritional risk. Adolescents are subject to most of the nutrition problems that affect children but also face many adult problems in different parts of the world, including:

- undernutrition, underweight (thinness) and stunting
- anorexia nervosa
- unconventional and restrictive diets
- obesity and increasing rates of diabetes
- iron deficiency and anaemia (most common deficiencies, particularly in girls)
- other deficiencies (in some parts of the world) of calcium, vitamin D, iodine, vitamin A, folate and zinc
- pregnancy.

This is a period of considerable change in social attitudes towards food and drink.

- Adolescents assume major control over what they eat.
- Peer opinions are very important.
- There is pressure to begin to consume alcohol and perhaps smoke or use other substances.
- They may believe that the ideal body shape is very thin or, at the opposite extreme, may be training as elite athletes.
- They often adopt different diets or food habits due to fashion or ideological beliefs.

Food habits of adolescents are often contrary to those their parents consider appropriate for good nutrition. These include:

- Missing meals, especially breakfast.
- Increased drinking of soft drinks, flavoured waters and fruit juices instead of plain water.
- Eating snacks and confectionary.
- Increased consumption of fast foods and takeaway meals, often high in fat and salt.
- Eating unconventional meals (combinations of foods that other family members do not approve of).

The area of adolescent health is always difficult to manage as during this time of self-confidence, teenagers often consider themselves invincible. Late in adolescence, bone density should be approaching its maximum and calcium may be limited by restrictive diets. Adolescents need to be encouraged to drink more milk and consume more dairy products, such as yoghurt. At the same time, high-calorie soft drinks should be curtailed. As life expectancy increases, there is an increasing risk of osteoporosis in older women with resultant disability and increased healthcare costs. The control of osteoporosis must emphasize calcium intakes and exercise in childhood and adolescence. Vitamin D is also important and when skin synthesis is limited by lack of sunlight or complete coverage by clothing, provision in the diet or in supplements is essential. Dark-skinned races are more vulnerable to vitamin D deficiency.

Intake of bioavailable iron is often reduced by vegetarian or predominantly vegetarian diets. Menstruation leads to increased iron demands and may result in iron-deficiency anaemia. Consuming meat on several occasions per week or using foods fortified with iron is recommended.

Globally, WHO estimates that more than 1.9 billion individuals have inadequate iodine nutrition (defined as urinary iodine excretion $< 100\ \mu g/L$), and almost 300 million of these are school-aged children. In particular, children and adolescents in the developing world are at risk of iodine deficiency due to a less varied and lower iodine diet. Goitrogens present in vegetarian diets and contaminated water supplies can also block the uptake of iodine by the thyroid gland. The universal use of iodized salt is the best public health intervention available.

Adolescent girls need extra care to avoid nutritional deficiency, especially of iron and iodine because of menstruation and this time of rapid growth, respectively. Vitamin D deficiency is a risk if the adolescent female is clothed from head to toe. Where there is a risk of pregnancy folate supplementation or the fortification of the food supply with folate are important public health interventions to reduce the risk of neural tube defects.

32.2.1 Pregnancy

Adolescent pregnancy is a major nutritional challenge to the mother and her fetus, as the adolescent mother has not yet completed her own growth and in turn may lack the emotional and cultural maturity to provide adequate nutrition for her infant. Intrauterine growth retardation and low-birth-weight infants are more common in younger mothers. Nutritional problems in the mother may then lead to deficiencies, such as iron deficiency, in the infant and child. Breastfeeding initiation rates and duration are lower in younger and unmarried mothers. However, breast milk produced by teenage mothers is comparable in composition to milk produced by adults, and barriers to breastfeeding are more likely to be social and cultural. If teenage pregnancies is the beginning of frequent, closely spaced pregnancies, then both the mother and her infants are at nutritional risk. Family planning advice is an effective nutrition intervention.

32.2.2 Work

Adolescence is also often a time of entry to the workforce. The nutritional issues involved include the need for increased energy expenditure and the consumption of adequate nutritional meals during irregular working hours, often while the teenager is moving out of the home.

32.2.3 Alcohol

In many cultures, alcohol consumption commences during adolescence. Alcohol is a source of energy, but energy that is not accompanied by other nutrients and its regular consumption increases the risk of obesity. However, in adolescents, binge drinking is more common with all of the hazards that this brings. Driving and alcohol do not mix, even more so

in inexperienced drivers, and the combination is one of the major causes of death in young males.

32.2.4 Exercise

Exercise levels in children and adolescents vary widely in difference countries and cultures. In the Western world, the advent of easy transport, labour-saving devices, television, video games and computer-based games all serve to reduce levels of active energy expenditure. A minority of adolescents meanwhile are exercising hard, training to be elite athletes. In developing countries, children may walk many kilometres to school each day. Where children suffer from undernutrition, the amount of exercise may be severely limited by available energy, and this may decrease ability to explore the environment and reduce opportunities for cognitive development. In many societies, there is a need to increase exercise to build bone density and cardiorespiratory fitness and to control the risk of obesity.

32.2.5 Use of nutritional supplements

In Western cultures, adolescents often have irregular patterns of working, studying, sleeping and eating. Healthy regular meals are often replaced with 'fast foods' consumed outside the home. The more meals that are eaten outside the home, the higher the risk of obesity. In these situations, frustrated parents often resort to increased use of nutritional supplements. Indeed, teenagers themselves often become concerned about their body image and use a variety of nutritional supplements. However, the preferred option is to consume a varied and nutritionally adequate diet based on established dietary guidelines.

FURTHER READING

1. Cole, T.J., Bellizzi, M.C., Flegal, K.M., and Dietz, W.H. (2000) Establishing a standard definition for child overweight and obesity worldwide: international survey. *Br Med J*, **320**, 1240–43.

2. **Ebbeling, C., Pawlak, D., and Ludwig, D.S.** (2002) Childhood obesity: public health crisis, common sense cure. *Lancet*, **360**, 473–82.

3. **National Health and Medical Research Council** (2003) *Food for health: Dietary guidelines for children and adolescents in Australia—incorporating the infant feeding guidelines for health workers*. Canberra, National Health MRC.

USEFUL WEBSITES

Growth references of the Centre for Disease Control: http://www.cdc.gov/nchs/data/ad/ad314.pdf/

More detailed growth charts for clinical use: http://www.cdc.gov/nchs/about/major/nhanes/growthcharts/clinical_charts.htm/

Training module on the use of growth references: http://www.cdc.gov/nccdphp/dnpa/growthcharts/training/modules/module2/text/module2print.pdf/

To see topical and scientifically robust updates on nutrition associated with this textbook, and active web links to many of the journal articles in the Reference areas, please see the dedicated Online Resource Centre at www.oxfordtextbooks.co.uk/orc/mann3e/.

33 Sports nutrition

Louise M. Burke

There are few areas of nutrition in which the benefits of a well-chosen eating plan are as immediate and obvious as in the practice of sports nutrition. The principles of sports nutrition are underpinned by an increasingly sophisticated understanding of the physiology and biochemistry of exercise. Since they are related to basic principles of body function rather than the calibre of the person who is exercising, the goals of sports nutrition apply equally to the much larger number of highly motivated recreational athletes as they do to the elite performers.

Despite these benefits, sports nutritionists observe that many athletes do not achieve sound dietary practices for either optimal health or sports performance.

Factors include poor knowledge of nutrition and the practical skills needed to choose and prepare meals, dietary extremism, and reduced access to food due to the busy lifestyle and frequent travel that are typical of high-level athletes.

This chapter addresses the major issues in sports nutrition, incorporating updates to knowledge and practice that have occurred over the past decade. In particular, the reader will be directed to the outcomes of the 2003 International Olympic Committee (IOC) consensus on Nutrition for Athletes, published in the book *Food, nutrition and sports performance II* (Maughan *et al.*, 2004).

33.1 Goals for the everyday or training diet

Although exact nutritional needs vary among athletes, there are common goals for the everyday diet eaten in training (see Table 33.1). The achievement of most goals is underpinned by an adequate energy intake and a well-chosen variety of foods. Energy requirements are determined by a variety of factors including gender, age, size and the volume, intensity and frequency of the training programme. Athletes undertaking prolonged sessions of moderate–high intensity exercise can generally expect to have high energy requirements. Energy intake can be manip-

ulated to increase body size, for example during periods of growth and when attempting to achieve a gain in muscle mass, or to decrease body mass (BM) and body fat levels.

33.1.1 Achieving optimal physique

Physique plays a role in the performance of many sports, and elite competitors typically display the optimal physical characteristics for their event. This

Table 33.1 Sports nutrition goals for the athlete in training

The athlete should aim to:

Meet the energy and fuel requirements needed to support their training programme

Achieve and maintain an ideal physique for their event; manipulate training and nutrition to achieve a level of body mass, body fat and muscle mass that is consistent with good health and good performance

Refuel and rehydrate well during each training session so that they perform at their best at each session

Practise any intended competition nutrition strategies so that beneficial practices can be identified and fine tuned

Enhance adaptation and recovery between training sessions by providing all the nutrients associated with these processes

Maintain optimal health and function, especially by achieving the increased needs for some nutrients resulting from a heavy training programme

Reduce the risk of sickness during heavy training periods by maintaining healthy physique and energy balance and by supplying nutrients believed to assist immune function (e.g. consume carbohydrates during prolonged exercise sessions)

Make use of supplements and specialized sports foods that have been shown to enhance training performance or meet training nutrition needs

Eat for long-term health by paying attention to community nutrition guidelines

Continue to enjoy food and the pleasure of sharing meals

is the result of genetic factors that have helped to determine the athlete's pursuits combined with the conditioning effects of nutrition and training. Whereas some athletes achieve an ideal physique easily, others need to manipulate their training and dietary programs to achieve their desired size and shape.

In some sports, including combative events (such as boxing, wrestling and judo), weight-lifting and light-weight rowing, athletes compete in weight divisions, which attempt to match competitors based on size. Competition classification is decided at a 'weigh-in', undertaken in the hours prior to competition. 'Making weight' is a common activity whereby athletes, many of whom are already lean, shed kilograms in the hours or days prior to the weigh-in to qualify for a division that is lighter than their normal BM. Although this strategy is used to gain an advantage in strength or reach over a smaller opponent, it must be balanced against the problems of dehydration or suboptimal nutritional status that result from the rapid weight-loss techniques. The medical commit-

tees and governing organizations of many of these sports have issued guidelines to warn against extreme 'making weight' activities.

Low BM and body fat levels offer biomechanical and physical (power to weight) advantages in a range of other sports including distance running, uphill cycling, diving and gymnastics. Aesthetic considerations are important in sports such as gymnastics, figure skating and bodybuilding. However many athletes, often with pressure from coaches and parents, embark on extreme and rigid weight-loss schemes, often involving excessive training, chronic low energy and nutrient intake, and psychological distress. Problems arising from these activities include fatigue, inadequate intake of protein and micronutrients (especially iron and calcium), reduced immune status, altered hormonal balance, disordered eating and poor body image.

Targets for 'ideal' BM and body fat should be set in terms of ranges, and should consider measures of long-term health and performance, rather than short-term benefits alone. Athletes should be encouraged to set individual targets within these ranges, and where it is warranted, loss of body fat should be achieved by a gradual programme of sustained and moderate energy deficit. Each athlete should be able to achieve their targets while eating a diet that is adequate in energy and nutrients, and free of unreasonable food-related stress. Most importantly, the low body fat levels of elite athletes should not be considered natural or necessary for recreational and subelite performers. Expert advice from sports medicine professionals, including dietitians, psychologists and physicians, is important in the early detection and management of problems.

At the other end of the spectrum are athletes who are interested in gaining muscle mass and strength. The core components for success are genetic predisposition, a suitable resistance-training programme and adequate energy intake. However, these athletes often focus their dietary interests on protein intake and special supplements that claim to enhance the gain of lean body mass. Meanwhile, carbohydrate is the key nutrient needed to fuel training sessions and recovery, and an energy surplus is needed to support gain in BM or general growth. As discussed below, protein requirements are easily met within the high energy intakes that are typical of athletes undertaking heavy training.

33.1.2 Achieving fuel and fluid needs for training

Carbohydrate The energy for muscle contraction is provided by the breakdown of adenosine triphosphate (ATP). Since muscle ATP stores would be consumed in only a few seconds of high-intensity exercise, the body uses a range of energy pathways to regenerate ATP. In most situations of exercise or sport, the integration of the energy systems (non-oxidative pathways involving creatine phosphate and carbohydrate, and the oxidative pathways involving fat and carbohydrate) means that ATP replenishment matches ATP demand. A major advantage of the provision of ATP via anaerobic pathways is that the rate of ATP

synthesis is five or six times higher than that from aerobic pathways. However, oxidative metabolism of fat and carbohydrate provides an energy supply for longer-duration exercise. Several interrelated factors influence the selection of muscle fuel during exercise; these include availability of endogenous substrates (muscle glycogen and triglyceride stores), the training status of an individual, the intensity and duration of exercise, environmental conditions and nutrient intake during exercise.

Of these factors, the pre-exercise endogenous fuel stores (particularly carbohydrate) is an important determinant of the performance of many types of sport and exercise activities. The depletion of body carbohydrate stores is a cause of fatigue or impaired performance during prolonged sessions of submaximal or intermittent high-intensity activity. Unfortunately, total body carbohydrate stores are limited, and are often substantially less than the fuel requirements of the training and competition sessions undertaken by many athletes. Therefore, sports nutrition guidelines provide targets for adequate daily carbohydrate intake to support the needs of training and recovery. In the past, guidelines used the methodology of 'percentage of dietary energy intake' to describe the ideal carbohydrate intake of athletes. For example, athletes were commonly advised to consume more than 60% of dietary energy from carbohydrate with the target being raised for endurance athletes to greater than 70% of energy intake. However, the 2003 IOC consensus on sports nutrition included a recommendation that guidelines for carbohydrates (or other macronutrients) should not be provided in terms of contributions to total dietary energy intake. Such recommendations are not 'user-friendly'. Furthermore, when energy intakes are very high (growing athletes) or restricted (weight-loss diets), the same percentage of energy will translate into very different carbohydrate intakes and may not be related to the fuel needs of the muscle. Therefore, modern guidelines for carbohydrate intake are scaled to the size of the athlete and the volume of their training. General recommendations can be provided (see Table 33.3) but these figures should be fine-tuned with individual consideration of total energy needs, specific training needs and feedback from training performance.

In addition to meeting total carbohydrate needs over the day, athletes should practise a variety of strategies that ensure carbohydrate availability for exercise, particularly sessions that are longer than 1 hour in duration. Strategies to promote training performance and recovery include consuming carbohydrates before, during and in the period between prolonged exercise bouts. The immune system may also benefit from these practices, with some recent studies reporting that the post-exercise suppression of cellular immune parameters is attenuated when carbohydrate status is maintained during and after exercise. Whether this leads to an improvement in the immune status and health of athletes remains to be seen, but it could provide a useful tactic to support the athlete during periods of heavy training.

Fluid Fluid needs are also increased in response to training, with additional fluid losses from sweating being determined by factors such as the intensity and duration of exercise, the environmental conditions and the degree of acclimatization of the athlete. Athletes must make a conscious plan to increase their fluid intake to balance a sudden increase in sweat losses, such as that occurring when moving to a hot climate or undertaking a substantial increase in training load. Thirst does not provide an adequate guide to acute dehydration or sudden changes in fluid need. As well as looking after total fluid needs over the day, the athlete should take care to drink before, during and after each workout.

The strategies for fluid and carbohydrate replacement before, during and after exercise will be further examined in the context of the competition diet. However, it is important that they also be employed during the training programme to optimize the training response and to allow opportunities to fine tune the actual eating/drinking plan.

33.1.3 Achieving protein needs

Prolonged daily training may increase protein requirements, to meet the small contribution of protein oxidation to the fuel requirements of prolonged exercise as well as the protein needed to support muscle gain and repair of damaged body tissues. Athletes undertaking recreational or light training activities will meet their protein needs within population protein RDIs. However, the need for an increased protein intake for heavily training athletes, both endurance and strength training, is still debated. The finding from the 2003 IOC consensus is that evidence for increased protein needs in athletes habituated to heavy training is weak. However, the discussion may be unnecessary since calculations of any potential increases in protein need arrive at a figure of 1.2–1.6 g/kg BM/day for both strength and endurance athletes. Such intakes can generally be met within the increased energy allowances that accompany training; indeed dietary surveys show that most athletes report protein intakes within or above these goals. Athletes at risk of protein intakes below this range are those who restrict energy to lose weight—for example, male athletes in weight-division sports and weight-conscious females. Although strength-training athletes may eat large amounts of protein-rich foods or buy expensive protein supplements, this is considered unnecessary. In fact, a number of recent studies show that the *timing* of intake of protein in relation to training is more important than the total *amount* of protein in the diet. Early intake of protein after exercise (and perhaps in the case of resistance training *before* the session) has been shown to enhance protein synthesis and net protein balance. Such protein synthesis may help to enhance the adaptations to the training session, e.g. muscle mass, formation of new tissues and repair of muscle damage.

33.1.4 Micronutrient needs

The key factors ensuring the adequacy of vitamin and mineral intakes are a moderate to high energy intake and a varied diet based on nutrient-rich foods. Dietary surveys of athletes show that when these factors are in place, reported intakes of vitamins and minerals are well in excess of RDIs and are likely to meet any increases in micronutrient demand caused by training. On this basis, routine supplementation with vitamins is not justified, and research has failed to show evidence of an increase in performance following vitamin supplementation except in the case where a pre-existing deficiency was corrected. However, not all athletes eat varied diets of adequate energy intake, with energy restriction, fad diets and disordered eating being typical causes of reduced micronutrient intake. Food range may also be restricted by poor practical nutrition skills, inadequate finances and an overcommitted lifestyle that limits access to food and causes erratic meal schedules. The best management is to educate the athlete about the quality and quantity of their food intake. However, a low-dose, broad-range multivitamin/mineral supplement may be useful when the athlete is unwilling or unable to make dietary changes, or when the athlete is travelling to places with an uncertain food supply and eating schedule.

Minerals are the micronutrients at most risk of inadequate intake in the diets of athletes. Inadequate *iron status* can reduce exercise performance via suboptimal levels of haemoglobin, and perhaps iron-related muscle enzymes. However, it is often difficult to distinguish true iron deficiency from alterations in iron status measures that are caused by exercise itself (e.g. changes in plasma volume, acute-phase responses to training). Reduction of blood haemoglobin concentrations due to plasma expansion, often termed 'sports anaemia', does not impair exercise performance.

Nevertheless, some athletes are at true risk of becoming iron deficient. Iron requirements may be increased in some athletes due to growth needs, or to increased gastrointestinal or haemolytic iron losses. However, the most common risk factor among athletes, as it is in the younger general community, is a low-energy diet or low intake of available iron. Females, athletes who restrict dietary energy intake or variety, vegetarians and athletes eating high-carbohydrate/low-meat diets are most at risk. Evaluation and management of iron status should be undertaken on an individual basis by a sports medicine expert. Low iron status, indicated by serum ferritin levels lower than 20 ng/mL, should be considered for further assessment and treatment. Prevention and treatment of iron deficiency may include iron supplementation. However, the long-term management plan should be based on dietary counselling to increase the intake of bioavailable iron (increasing intake of heme iron sources and the complementary intake of vitamin C or meat foods with non-heme iron foods). These strategies can be integrated with the athlete's other dietary goals; this is where the expertise of a sports dietitian is most useful. Appropriate strategies to reduce any unwarranted iron loss should also be undertaken.

Previously, it was considered that low iron status without anaemia did not reduce exercise performance. However, recent studies have shown that it may interfere with desired training adaptations. In real life, many athletes with such low iron stores, or a sudden drop in iron status, frequently complain of fatigue and inability to recover after heavy training. Many of these respond to strategies that improve iron status or prevent a further decrease in iron stores.

Some athletes are at risk of problems with *calcium status* and bone health. Low body density in athletes seems contradictory, since exercise is considered to be one of the best protectors of bone health. However, a serious outcome of menstrual disturbances frequently reported in female athletes is the high risk of either direct loss of bone density, or failure to optimize the gaining of peak bone mass that should occur during the 10–15 years after the onset of puberty. Optimal nutrition is important to correct factors that underpin the menstrual dysfunction, as well as those that contribute to suboptimal bone density. Adequate energy intake and the reversal of disordered eating or inadequate nutrient intake are important. Adequate calcium intake is important for bone health, and requirements may be increased to 1200 mg/day in athletes with impaired menstrual function. Where adequate calcium intake cannot be met through dietary means, usually through use of low-fat dairy foods or calcium-enriched soy alternatives, a calcium supplement may be considered.

33.2 The competition diet

The nutritional challenges of competition vary according to the length and intensity of the event, the environment, and factors that influence the recovery between events or the opportunity to eat during the event itself. To achieve optimal performance, the athlete should identify factors that are likely to cause fatigue during the event, and undertake nutritional strategies before, during and after the event that minimize or delay the onset of this fatigue. In most cases, dehydration and/or depletion of body carbohydrate stores present the major nutritional challenges. Various goals of competition nutrition are summarized in Table 33.2.

Dehydration is a likely outcome in most sports events, with the effects being related to the degree of fluid deficit. Dehydration of as little as 2% of BM (1.5–2 L for most athletes) is sufficient to cause detectable changes to work output, and perception of effort, especially when exercise is carried out in a hot environment. Other penalties of fluid deficits include impairment of thermoregulation, reductions in skill and decision-making abilities, and an increased risk of gastrointestinal problems. Carbohydrate depletion can manifest as central fatigue (low blood glucose concentrations) and/or peripheral fatigue (glycogen depletion in the working muscle). When carbohydrate-intake strategies enhance or maintain carbohydrate status during exercise, they can be demonstrated to enhance endurance. Studies that measure the effect on exercise *performance* especially those involving field situations, unpredictable team games or sports involving complex decision-making and motor skills are much more difficult to conduct. Nevertheless, many of these studies have shown

---

Table 33.2 Sports nutrition goals for the athlete in competition

The athlete should aim to:
In weight-division sports, achieve the competition weight division with minimal harm to health or performance
'Fuel up' adequately prior to an event; consume carbohydrate and achieve exercise taper during the day(s) prior to the event according to the importance and duration of the event; and utilize carbohydrate-loading strategies when appropriate before events of greater than 90 minutes duration
Use opportunities to drink before and during the event to minimize dehydration by replacing most of the sweat losses, but without drinking in excess of sweat losses
Consume carbohydrates during events > 1 hour in duration or other events where body carbohydrate stores become depleted
Achieve pre-event and during-event eating/drinking strategies without causing gastrointestinal discomfort or upsets
Promote recovery after the event, particularly during multi-day competitions such as tournaments and stage races
During a prolonged competition programme, do not allow event nutrition to compromise overall energy and nutrient intake goals
Make use of supplements and specialized sports foods that have been shown to enhance race performance or meet race nutrition goals

benefits following various strategies to enhance carbohydrate availability.

33.2.1 Fuelling up before an event

Optimizing carbohydrate stores in the muscle and liver is a primary goal of pre-exercise preparation. The key factors in glycogen storage are dietary carbohydrate intake, and in the case of muscle stores, tapered exercise or rest. In the absence of muscle damage, muscle glycogen stores can be normalized by 24–36 hours of rest and an adequate carbohydrate intake (7–12 g/kg BM/day). Such stores appear adequate for the fuel needs of events of less than 60–90 minutes in duration.

Carbohydrate loading refers to practices that aim to supercompensate muscle glycogen stores; such protocols may elevate muscle glycogen stores by 125–200%. Pioneering studies undertaken in the late 1960s by Scandinavian sports scientists produced the 'classical' 7-day model of carbohydrate loading, involving a 3–4-day 'depletion' phase of hard training and low carbohydrate intake, and finishing with a 3–4-day 'loading' phase of high carbohydrate eating and exercise taper. Early field studies of prolonged running events showed that carbohydrate loading can enhance sports performance, not by allowing the athlete to run faster, but by prolonging the time that race pace can be maintained.

Studies extended to trained subjects have produced a 'modified' carbohydrate loading in which the depletion or 'glycogen stripping' phase is omitted. For well-trained athletes at least, carbohydrate loading may be seen as an extension of 'fuelling up' (rest and high carbohydrate intake) over 3–4 days. In fact, a recent study has shown that in well-trained subjects, glycogen supercompensation may be achieved in as little as 26–48 hours of such preparation. The modified carbohydrate-loading protocol offers a more practical strategy for competition preparation, by avoiding the fatigue and complexity of the extreme diet and training protocols associated with the previous depletion phase. Carbohydrate loading is useful for events of greater than 90 minutes duration

and will typically postpone fatigue and extend the duration of steady-state exercise by about 20%, or improve performance over a set distance or workload by 2–3%.

33.2.2 Pre-event meal

Food and fluids consumed in the 4 hours prior to an event may continue to fuel muscle glycogen stores if they have not been fully restored since the last exercise session, restore liver glycogen content after an overnight fast, and ensure that the athlete is well-hydrated. Gastric comfort issues must be balanced to prevent hunger, yet must avoid the gastrointestinal discomfort and upset often experienced during exercise. From the psychological viewpoint, the pre-event meal should include foods and practices that are important to the athlete's superstitions or feelings of wellbeing.

A carbohydrate-rich, low-fat meal is generally recommended as the ideal pre-event meal. Some experts have speculated, however, that the elevation of plasma insulin concentrations following pre-exercise carbohydrate feedings could be of potential disadvantage to exercise metabolism and performance. A rise in insulin suppresses lipolysis and fat utilization, accelerating carbohydrate oxidation and perhaps causing premature fatigue. This might be at most risk of occurring when small amounts of carbohydrate (e.g. < 1 g/kg BM) are consumed in the hour prior to exercise. One safeguard is to ensure that the amount of carbohydrate in the pre-event meal is substantial rather than minor; thus, any increase in carbohydrate utilization during exercise will be more than offset by the large increase in carbohydrate availability. Others have argued that low-GI (glycaemic index) carbohydrate foods provide a superior pre-event meal choice, since they provide a reduced insulinaemic response. In general, however, studies have failed to show that a low-GI pre-event meal produces a superior performance outcome. In fact, when carbohydrate is consumed during the event to maintain carbohydrate availability, the type of carbohydrate consumed before exercise may be largely irrelevant.

The type, timing and amount of food chosen for the pre-event meal will be determined by individual situations and experience. In general, meals that are low in fat and moderate in fibre and protein are recommended, especially for athletes who are at risk of gastrointestinal problems during their event. Fluid should be consumed in the hours prior to exercise to ensure that the athlete is well hydrated at the onset of the event. Above all, the athlete should experiment with their intended pre-event meal strategies to fine tune the plan that suits their individual needs.

33.2.3 Fluid and carbohydrate during the event

In events of greater than 30 minutes, there is likely to be both a need and opportunity for fluid replacement. Ideally, an athlete should drink at a rate that replaces most of their sweat loss; however, this is impractical and uncomfortable when sweat rates exceed 1 L/hour. There have been some recent changes in the education messages provided to athletes about fluid replacement during sports and exercise activities. Instead of receiving prescriptive advice (e.g. drink 150–250 mL of fluid every 15–20 minutes), athletes are advised to be aware of their own sweat losses, and use opportunities that exist within their activities to drink as often and as much as is practical to replace *most* of these losses. Since studies find that athletes typically replace only 30–60% of fluid losses across a range of sporting activities, most athletes can aim for an improvement in their fluid intake. However, recent observations from sporting events attracting large numbers of recreational participants have shown that there is a need specifically to warn against drinking excessively before and during exercise. Slower participants in running, cycling and triathlon races have been observed to consume fluids at rates that greatly exceed their sweat losses— combining low sweat rates with aggressive use of aid stations during the event. Such drinking patterns, which can lead to a weight gain over the race, are a major risk factor for the development of hyponatraemia (low plasma sodium concentrations). Several athletes have died in marathons as a result of severe hyponatraemia.

The literature clearly shows that the intake of carbohydrate during prolonged sessions of moderate-intensity or intermittent high-intensity exercise can improve work capacity and performance. Even when there is no significant positive effect of carbohydrate ingestion on exercise capacity, neither is performance adversely affected by increasing the availability of carbohydrates. The major mechanisms to explain the benefits of carbohydrate feedings during prolonged exercise are the maintenance of plasma glucose concentration and high rates of carbohydrate oxidation when muscle carbohydrate stores become depleted. Recently, a number of studies have shown that carbohydrate intake may benefit shorter-duration, high-intensity sports (of about 1-hour duration), even when carbohydrate stores are not thought to be limiting. This is thought to be a result of effects on the brain and central nervous system that promote enhanced pacing strategies.

In practice, athletes consume carbohydrates during exercise using a variety of foods and drinks, and a variety of feeding schedules. In general, a carbohydrate intake of 30–60 g/hour is recommended, with carbohydrate feedings starting well in advance of fatigue or depletion of body carbohydrate stores and being achieved according to the practical opportunities provided in each sport or exercise (see Table 33.3). The value of sports drinks (commercial solutions providing 4–8% carbohydrates, electrolytes and palatable flavours) is recognized since these allow carbohydrates to be delivered while attending to needs for fluid replacement. Such drinks have been shown to increase voluntary fluid intake during exercise, thus enhancing fluid balance as well as providing an additional source of fuel.

Table 33.3 General guidelines for carbohydrate intake for special situations during sport

Situation	Recommended carbohydrate intake
Athletes should aim to achieve carbohydrate intakes to meet the fuel requirements of their training programme and to optimize restoration of muscle glycogen stores between workouts. General recommendations can be provided, but should be fine tuned with individual consideration of total energy needs, specific training needs and feedback from training performance.	
Acute situation	
Pre-event meal to increase carbohydrate availability prior to prolonged exercise session	1–4 g/kg BM eaten 1–4 hours pre-exercise
Carbohydrate intake during moderate-intensity or intermittent exercise of > 1 hour	0.5–1.0 g/kg BM/hour (30–60 g/hour)
Rapid post-exercise recovery of muscle glycogen during the first 4 hours of exercise, where recovery between sessions is < 8 hours	1–1.2 g/kg BM immediately after exercise, repeated each hour until meal schedule is resumed

There may be some advantages to consuming carbohydrates as a series of small snacks every 15–60 minutes in the early recovery phase |
Chronic or everyday situation	
Daily recovery/fuel needs for athlete with moderate exercise programme (i.e. < 1 hour, or exercise of low intensity)	5–7 g/kg BM/day
Daily recovery/fuel needs for endurance athlete (i.e. 1–3 hours of moderate- to high-intensity exercise)	7–12 g/kg BM/day
Daily recovery/fuel needs for athlete undertaking extreme exercise programme (i.e. > 4–5 hours of moderate- to high-intensity exercise such as the Tour de France)	10–12+ g/kg BM/day

33.3 Post-exercise recovery

The main dietary factor in post-event refuelling is the amount of carbohydrate consumed, with a threshold for muscle glycogen storage being within the range of 7–12 g/kg BM/day. There is some evidence that moderate-GI and high-GI carbohydrate-rich foods and drinks may be more favourable for glycogen storage than some low-GI food choices. Since glycogen storage may occur at a slightly faster rate during the first couple of hours after exercise, athletes are often advised to begin refuelling immediately after exercise. However, the main reason for promoting carbohydrate-rich meals or snacks soon after exercise is that effective refuelling does not start until a substantial amount of carbohydrate (about 1 g/kg BM) is consumed. Rapid refuelling strategies are important when there is less than 8 hours between exercise sessions but when recovery time is longer, immediate intake of carbohydrate after exercise is unnecessary and the athletes should choose their preferred meal/snack schedule for achieving total carbohydrate intake goals. Whereas earlier research indicated that co-ingestion of protein with carbohydrate feedings may enhance glycogen synthesis, these findings have been refuted in recent studies in which the energy content of test meals was better matched. Nevertheless, the intake of protein in post-exercise eating is likely to benefit protein synthesis goals of recovery. Therefore, meals and snacks should be chosen from carbohydrate-rich food combinations that also provide a source of high-quality protein.

Rehydration is another issue in post-event recovery since athletes can expect to be at least mildly dehydrated at the end of their session. In essence, the success of post-exercise rehydration is dependent on how much the athlete drinks, and then how much of this is retained and re-equilibrated within body fluid compartments. It may take 6–24 hours for complete rehydration following fluid losses of 2–5% of BM. When it is important to encourage voluntary fluid intake, flavoured drinks have been shown to encourage greater intake than plain water. Urine losses appear to be minimized by the simultaneous replacement of lost electrolytes, particularly sodium. The inclusion of sodium in a rehydration drink is an important strategy in the rapid recovery of moderate to high fluid deficits. However, the optimal sodium level is about 50–80 mmol/L, as found in oral rehydration solutions used in the treatment of diarrhoea. This is considerably higher than the concentrations

found in commercial sports drinks and may be unpalatable to many athletes. Creatively planned meals and snacks may be consumed with fluids to fulfil all post-event recovery needs simultaneously; for example, salty carbohydrate-rich foods such as bread and breakfast cereals, or rice and pasta meals with added salt. These choices lend themselves to toppings and fillings of protein-rich foods.

Since alcohol promotes diuresis, consumption of large amounts of alcoholic drinks may interfere with speedy restoration of fluid balance. However, the most important problem with excessive intake of alcohol is indirect: it is likely to interfere with the athlete's commitment or interest in undertaking sound recovery practices. Caffeine has also been identified as a compound that causes diuresis. However, this effect has recently been reviewed, with the finding that it is overstated when consumed in small–moderate doses by habitual caffeine users. The value of the voluntary intake of well-liked beverages should not be forgotten. It is likely that athletes who are prevented from consuming their normal pattern of tea, coffee and cola drinks may not replace these fluids with an equivalent amount of another beverage.

33.4 Supplements and sports foods

The sports world is filled with supplements and sports foods that claim to make the athlete faster, stronger, leaner, better recovered, healthier, with greater endurance, or whatever other factors are important to performance. The ever-growing range of products can be divided into two separate categories: sports supplements and nutritional ergogenic aids. Sports supplements may be considered as products that address the special nutritional needs of athletes. This category includes sports drinks, sports bars, liquid meal supplements and micronutrient supplements that are part of a prescribed dietary plan. Many of these products are specially designed to help an athlete meet specific needs for energy and nutrients, including fluid and carbohydrates, in situations where everyday foods are not practical to eat. This is particularly relevant

for intake immediately before, during or after exercise. These supplements can be shown to improve performance when they allow the athlete to achieve their sports nutrition goals. However, they are more expensive than normal food, a consideration that must be balanced against the convenience they provide.

Nutritional ergogenic aids—products that promise a direct and 'supraphysiological' benefit to sports performance—are the supplements that seem most appealing to athletes. These products, which continually change in popularity, include megadoses of vitamins and some minerals, free-form amino acids, ginseng and other herbal compounds, bee pollen, coenzyme Q10, inosine and carnitine. In general, these supplements have been poorly tested, or have failed to live up to their claims when rigorous testing

---

BOX 33.1 Evidence for use of creatine by some athletes

Dose and mode of action	Supported uses

• Loading: 20–30 g taken in multiple doses (e.g. 4 × 5 g) for 5 days

• Maintenance dose 2–5 g/day

Creatine loading can significantly increase muscle creatine and creatine phosphate levels to reach the muscle storage threshold for these compounds. There is some variability in response to creatine loading, perhaps due to initial creatine stores (i.e. people with pre-existing high levels fail to respond, while those with low levels show the greatest response). Weight gain of about 1 kg occurs with loading due to fluid retention. New studies also show that prior creatine loading may assist the muscle to store glycogen or carbohydrate load more effectively.

   Creatine phosphate serves a number of important roles in exercise metabolism: the most well-known role is the rapid regeneration of ATP by the phosphagen power system. The long-term effects of creatine supplementation are not known; however, studies to date have not shown an increased prevalence of problems that are anecdotally linked to creatine use (e.g. muscle strains and tears, thermoregulatory problems). Even so, creatine supplementation is not recommended to young athletes, and athletes are reminded to adhere to the well-proven supplementation protocols. In real life, there have been anecdotal reports that some athletes take creatine in doses that far exceed the amounts that are shown to saturate muscle creatine stores.

Studies show that creatine loading enhances the performance of exercise involving repeated high-intensity bouts with short recovery intervals (< 2 minutes recovery). Performance benefits are seen only in subjects who experience significant increases in creatine stores following loading. Most studies have been undertaken in the laboratory and more research is needed to confirm the benefits of creatine loading by well-trained and elite athletes in sports-specific situations. No benefits to aerobic endurance have been reported, although protocols that involve the effectiveness of carbohydrate loading have not been undertaken. Creatine loading may enhance competition performance involving repeated short sprints (e.g. team games and racquet sports). It is also likely to assist interval and resistance training programmes, thus enhancing training adaptations and the gain of muscle mass and strength.

---

has been undertaken. Exceptions to this are creatine (Box 33.1), caffeine (Box 33.2) and bicarbonate and citrate (Box 33.3), each of which may enhance the performance of certain athletes under specific conditions. Athletes should seek expert advice about such supplements to see if their sport/exercise warrants experimentation with these products, and to ensure that a correct protocol is tried. The Sports Supplement Program of the Australian Institute of Sport provides information about many products, and rates supplements and sports foods into four categories based on the amount of scientific support for the claims made about the use of the product, and whether it is considered a banned substance (see http://www.ais.org.au/nutrition).

The decision to use a supplement or sports food should include consideration of the likely benefits and disadvantages (see Fig. 33.1). At best, most purported nutritional ergogenic aids offer a placebo to athletes, and at worst, they represent a waste of considerable amounts of money. Athletes will be better rewarded by investing their resources and interest in a more credible area of sports performance, such as better equipment, improved training techniques, or advice about nutrition or psychological preparation, before directing them to the majority of supplements on the market. Another disadvantage of the use of supplements is the possibility of contamination of products with substances that are illegal in sport, leading to a 'positive' doping offence for the athlete.

BOX 33.2 Evidence for use of caffeine by some athletes

Dose and mode of action

- Traditional protocol: 5–6 mg/kg BM taken about 1 hour prior to exercise
- New protocols: 2–3 mg/kg BM taken before exercise, or during prolonged exercise prior to the onset of fatigue

Caffeine affects numerous body tissues in a variety of ways, causing difficulty in isolating a specific mechanism for any observed changes in exercise performance and endurance. Possible effects include stimulation of the central nervous system and reduction in perception of effort or fatigue, an increase in adrenaline release and activity, and direct effects on muscle recruitment and contractility. New research shows that these effects occur at much lower levels of caffeine intake than previously suggested, and the benefits to performance of endurance exercise do not increase with increasing caffeine doses. Therefore, athletes may gain maximum benefit with a reduced risk of side effects such as sleep disturbances from using the low to moderate doses of caffeine found in a range of everyday foods, drinks and special sports foods. Previous beliefs that the intake of caffeine impairs hydration status, or that it achieves its effects by stimulating lipolysis leading to enhanced fat oxidation and glycogen sparing during prolonged exercise, are now discredited.

Supported uses

Studies show that caffeine intake is associated with performance enhancements in prolonged moderate-intensity exercise (> 90 minutes), prolonged intermittent events (e.g. team games), high-intensity events of around 20 minutes' duration and short very-high-intensity exercise of about 5 minutes' duration. Additional studies using sports-specific protocols and well-trained athletes are required, particularly using strategically timed intake of small to moderate doses of caffeine. Individual variability in beneficial response and side effects also warrants further research.

Caffeine was removed from the banned list of the World Anti-Doping Agency in January 2004.

BOX 33.3 Evidence for use of bicarbonate and citrate by some athletes

Dose and mode of action

- Acute protocol: 300 mg/kg BM taken 1–2 hours prior to exercise
- New research also suggests a chronic protocol may be effective: 500 mg/kg BM daily, split into four doses. Effects of buffering may be maintained for at least 24 hours after the last dose with this protocol

Increases blood bicarbonate levels and pH. May increase tolerance to production of H^+ ions from anaerobic glycolysis by enhancing extracellular buffering capacity. Gastrointestinal upsets are often reported and may be reduced by the intake of large volumes of fluid (1–2 L) with the bicarbonate/citrate dose, or the use of chronic protocols, which might allow the athlete to cease taking the buffer 24 hours prior to their most important event.

Supported uses

Meta-analysis of bicarbonate studies confirms that bicarbonate supplementation enhances the capacity for high-intensity exercise, which results in the production of high blood levels of lactate (and H^+ ions). Although some studies also show that citrate loading achieves a buffering effect, this outcome may be less effective for performance enhancement. Sports-specific studies are required to confirm use in competition situations. Events likely to benefit from bicarbonate/citrate loading are high-intensity events lasting 1–7 minutes, and perhaps prolonged events involving intermittent high-intensity bursts. Further study is needed to investigate buffering protocols for events in which a series of heats and finals are undertaken over a day or days to decide the final outcome. The protocol involving chronic bicarbonate supplementation may be useful for such sports.

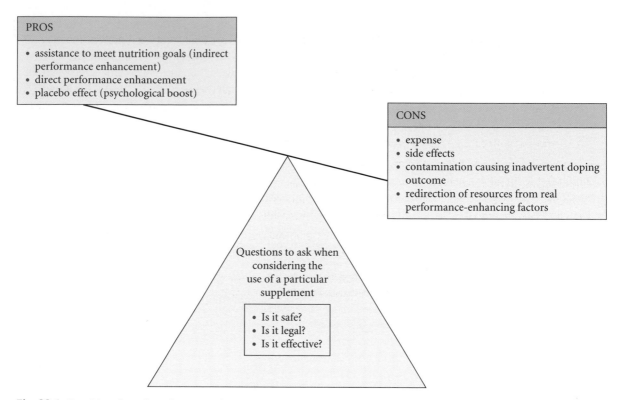

PROS

- assistance to meet nutrition goals (indirect performance enhancement)
- direct performance enhancement
- placebo effect (psychological boost)

CONS

- expense
- side effects
- contamination causing inadvertent doping outcome
- redirection of resources from real performance-enhancing factors

Questions to ask when considering the use of a particular supplement

- Is it safe?
- Is it legal?
- Is it effective?

Fig. 33.1 Considerations for using a supplement or sports food.
Source: Burke and Deakin (2006) p. 488.

BOX 33.4 Case study

Jack is a 16-year-old swimmer who recently moved to an elite training programme, effectively doubling the weekly training volume undertaken in his old squad. After 5 weeks, he was finding it hard to cope with this workload, finding that the excessive fatigue that he initially put down to the early morning starts had not abated. In fact, his times in the pool had gone backwards rather than improving with this new level of training. A loss of 2 kg in weight, despite taking up a programme of weight training, led him to consult a sports dietician.

The sports dietician's assessment of Jack's eating patterns and training programme was that he had failed to increase his energy and carbohydrate intake to cope with the new exercise demands. This was not due to poor commitment, or even poor nutrition knowledge. With Jack's busy schedule of school and training, it was difficult to find opportunities to consume his fuel and energy needs. Jack had been trying to increase the volume of his meals as his main strategy; this often meant that he left the table feeling uncomfortably full. Jack's mum is health conscious so that all their meals are based on high-fibre, low-fat cooking and food choices. Some creative strategies were needed to match this to Jack's new needs.

The sports dietician suggested a number of strategies to provide Jack with fuel for training, adequate energy for growth, and enhanced recovery between his 11 weekly workouts.

- Move to a pattern of six or seven meals and snacks each day rather than relying on three large meals; this will mean having foods available at school and while travelling in Jack's busy day

- Promote recovery after training sessions by consuming a snack providing carbohydrate and protein immediately after the session; in Jack's case, a liquid meal supplement or fruit smoothie could be consumed in the locker room, or in the car on the way home from training sessions before the next meal
- Provide extra fuel for each training session by having a quick snack on waking in the morning, and in the afternoon on the way to training; sports bars, or cereal bars and a yoghurt, accompanied by juice are convenient and portable snacks
- Add extra fuel during the session by drinking sports drink instead of water
- Add an extra snack before bed, maybe a late dessert or a fruit smoothie
- Be moderate in the use of high-fibre foods; while wholegrain cereals and fresh fruit and vegetables offer many nutritional advantages, it is not necessary for Jack to add additional fibre to his meals (e.g. adding bran to his breakfast cereal). Furthermore, there are advantages to reducing gastric 'fullness' by having some fruits in the form of juice
- In many of these strategies, the use of high-energy fluids provides an important tool in being able to increase total intake of carbohydrate or energy, or to consume nutrients straight after a heavy workout.

After 2 weeks of practicing these strategies, Jack regained his lost body weight and found new 'energy' for his training. His coach was impressed with his new-found enthusiasm in the pool, and the results of his recent time trial showed promise for the upcoming swimming titles.

Summary

The goals of sports nutrition vary according to the athlete and their event. However, these can be divided into issues of training and issues for optimal competition outcomes. Acute nutrition strategies can directly enhance performance by reducing or delaying the onset of factors that would otherwise cause fatigue. Competition performance also benefits when everyday eating strategies assist the athlete to stay healthy and in shape, and to optimize the adaptations from their training programme. The various strategies that make up these training and nutrition goals are summarized in Tables 33.1 and 33.2. The athlete can be assisted by the advice of a sports dietitian to adopt eating practices that achieve these goals, often integrating a number of goals into the same meal or snack.

FURTHER READING

1. **Burke, L., and Deakin, V. (eds)** (2006) *Clinical sports nutrition*, 3rd edition. Sydney, McGraw-Hill.

2. **Maughan, R.J., Burke, L.M., and Coyle, E.F. (eds)** (2004) *Foods, nutrition and sports performance II.* London, Routledge.

3. **Maughan, R. (ed.)** (2000) *The encyclopaedia of sports medicine. Vol VII: Nutrition in sport.* London, Blackwell Science.

USEFUL WEBSITES

Department of Sports Nutrition of the Australian Institute of Sport http://www.ais.org.au/nutrition/

 To see topical and scientifically robust updates on nutrition associated with this textbook, and active web links to many of the journal articles in the Reference areas, please see the dedicated Online Resource Centre at www.oxfordtextbooks.co.uk/orc/mann3e/.

34 Nutrition and ageing

Caroline Horwath and Wija van Staveren

Nutrition interacts with the ageing process in numerous ways and the risk of nutrition-related health problems increases in later life. This chapter provides an overview of why nutrition is important in old age, what happens to our bodies as we age (including how body composition and digestive function changes with advancing years), the nutritional needs and status of older adults, and some special issues arising in nutrition–disease relationships.

34.1 Why is nutrition important in old age?

As we entered the new millennium, the total number of people over 60 years reached 396 million, representing more than 13% of the total population in developed countries (167 million) and nearly 5% of that in developing countries (229 million). In some countries such as Sweden and Japan, almost 18% of the population is already aged 65 years and older, while in North America, Australia and New Zealand, the proportion is around 12–14%. The worldwide increase in the proportion of people in the older age groups is predicted to continue (see Fig. 34.1), and what is less known is the speed and significance of population ageing in less-developed countries. Fig. 34.2 shows regional differences in the world population over 60 years of age. It is estimated that around 70% of this age group lives in developing countries.

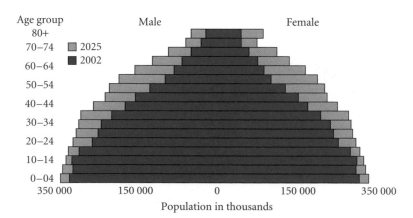

Fig. 34.1 Global population pyramids for 2002 and 2025. Note that as the proportion of children and young people declines and the proportion of people age 60 and over increases, the triangular population pyramid of 2002 will be replaced with a more rounded structure in 2025.

Source: WHO (2002).

An increasing number of people are also approaching the upper limit of the human lifespan (believed to be around 120 years), with currently over 100 000 centenarians worldwide. The dramatic increase in the proportion of older adults in the population results from a combination of lengthening life expectancy (in Western countries life expectancy has almost doubled last century) and declining birth rates. Gains in life expectancy are largely the result of better hygiene and nutrition, and advances in medical science (e.g. antibiotics).

Rapidly growing older populations have led to concern about whether or not a shrinking labour force will be able to support that part of the population who are commonly believed to be dependent on others, like disabled and older adults. In order to delay or even prevent disabilities and chronic diseases, active ageing policies and programmes focusing on lifestyle are required. But how?—and more specifically, can nutrition play a role in such an 'active ageing' programme?

Of the 20 leading risk factors for disability, chronic disease and death, a number are nutrition-related and may lead to cardiovascular diseases, type 2 diabetes and certain types of cancer (WHO, 2003). These global epidemiological data have motivated WHO/FAO to update dietary guidelines. The guidelines are evidence-based for younger adults, but may not have the same impact for elderly people. To get a better understanding of changing nutrient requirements in old age, we first have to answer the question: 'What happens to our body when we age?'

34.2 What happens to our bodies as we age?

Changes in body composition, physical performance and organ system function occur in all of us as we grow older. However, wide variation exists among people in the degree to which functions decline. As people become older, they become more dissimilar from their contemporaries of the same chronological age. There can also be considerable variability in the rate at which different changes occur within the same person. Some of this variability in functional decline may reflect heterogeneity in true rates of ageing; however, lifestyle and other factors that can accompany ageing seem to be of importance. These factors can contribute to deterioration in function (e.g. of cardiovascular, lung or endocrine functions), thereby accelerating one's apparent 'rate of ageing'. For example, decreased renal filtration rate and declining cardiovascular function have been observed in longitudinal studies such as the Baltimore Longitudinal Study of Ageing. However, after careful exclusion of people with kidney disease or heart disease, respectively, no consistent declines in function with age remained. Thus, the apparent declines in average

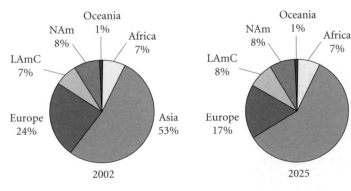

NAm: North America
LAmC: Latin America and the Caribbean

Fig. 34.2 Distribution of the world population over 60 years of age by region in 2002 and 2025.

Source: WHO (2002).

functional indices of the study group members as they aged were due to inclusion of people with defined disease, rather than to the ageing process *per se*. Never-theless, changes in body composition and changes in the gastrointestinal tract are at least partly due to ageing *per se*. Since they have an impact on nutritional requirements, these changes will be further discussed here.

34.3 Changes in body composition and energy balance

Changes in body composition during ageing include loss of lean body mass (LBM), bone mass, body water and a relative increase of fat mass. The latter also is redistributed from mainly subcutaneous to abdominal fat. The decrease in LBM is mainly caused by a loss in size and strength of skeletal muscle. On average, the marked decline in LBM begins around 60–70 years of age, approaching as much as a 40% loss compared with young adulthood (see Fig. 34.3).

A stable body weight during this process can be explained by a concomitant increase in body fat. This loss in muscle and in LBM is called *sarcopenia*. Together with age-related metabolic diseases, as well as the presence of individual handicaps, sarcopenia often coincides with a decline of physical activity. Moreover, due to diminished maximum oxygen intake and muscle fibre atrophy, a greater physical effort is required for the same task in older people. As a consequence, older people will reduce physical activity further and have lower energy expenditure. Fig. 34.4 shows how the physical activity level (PAL) (calculated as daily total energy expenditure divided by the resting metabolic rate) decreases with ageing.

(a)

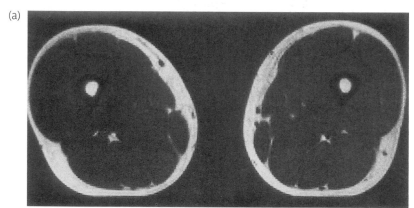

(b)

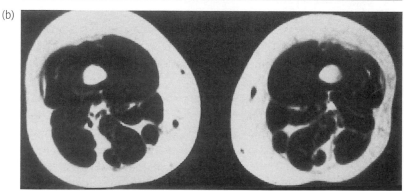

Fig. 34.3 Magnetic resonance images of the thigh showing differences in total muscles, intramuscular fat, subcutaneous fat and bone between (a) a young woman athlete (age 20 years, BMI 22.6) and (b) an elderly sedentary woman (age 64 years, BMI 30.7).

Source: Evans, W.J. and Meredith, C.N. (1989) Exercise and nutrition in the elderly. In: Monro, H.N. and Danford, D.E. (eds) *Nutrition, ageing and the elderly*. New York, Plenum Press.

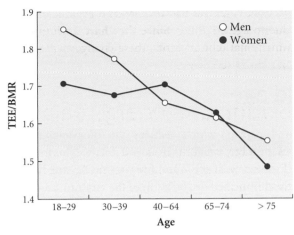

Fig. 34.4 Decrease of physical activity level (PAL) for men and women during ageing. PAL is derived as total energy expenditure (TEE; assessed by the doubly labelled water method) divided by basal metabolic rate (derived from proxy measures).

Source: Based on Black, A.E. (1996) Physical activity levels from a meta-analysis of doubly labeled water studies for validating energy intake as measured by dietary assessment. *Nutr Reviews*, **54**, 170–74.

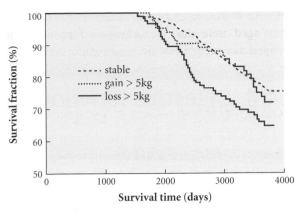

Fig. 34.5 Probability of survival for participants in the SENECA study with and without weight change.

Source: De Groot, C.P.G.M., and Van Staveren, W.A. (2002) Undernutrition in the European SENECA studies. *Clin Geriatr Med*, **18**, 699–708.

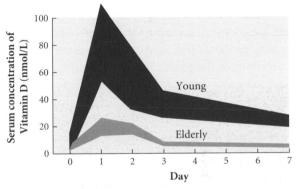

Fig. 34.6 Serum concentrations of vitamin D in healthy young and elderly adults in response to whole-body exposure to a dose of simulated sunlight on day 0.

Source: Holick, M. (1994) Vitamin D: new horizons for the 21st century. *Am J Clin Nutr*, **60**, 619–30.

Many nationwide food consumption studies have shown that older people respond to these changes with a lower energy intake and may even over-respond, which results in a negative energy balance. This phenomenon is called anorexia of ageing and is common in people over 70 years of age. In contrast to average younger adults, body weight tends to decrease in old age, even in healthy individuals. Weight loss in later life should be prevented, because it increases the risk of progressive malnutrition, micronutrient deficiency and nutrition-related diseases and is associated with frailty and increased mortality (Fig. 34.5).

Bone mass and bone density may start to decrease as early as age of 35–40 onwards (see Chapter 8). In women, bone loss accelerates during the menopause. They may lose half of their trabecular and about one-third of their cortical bone mass; in men, this loss is lower, only 50–70% that of females. The decrease in bone mass density is associated with risk of osteoporotic fractures. Osteoporosis is a multifactorial disease and inadequacy of the nutrients calcium and vitamin D are related to a decline in bone density and to fractures. Vitamin D deficiency is often observed in old age due to diminished synthesis in the skin (Fig. 34.6) as well as lack of sunlight exposure. Recommended intakes for the housebound elderly for vitamin D vary between 10 and 15 μg/day.

Dehydration is another problem that can occur in older adults. Due to less LBM, but also less interstitial fluid, the older adult contains less body water (< 50% versus 70% of total body mass in younger adults). Further decreased renal function, loss of thirst sensors, fear of incontinence and increased arthritic pain resulting from numerous trips to the toilet may interfere with an adequate intake of fluid. Dehydration may result in constipation, faecal impaction, cognitive impairment and even death. The recommended fluid intake is about 1500 mL/day, which should be taken during and between meals.

34.4 Digestive function in old age

Although for many years it was thought that the efficiency of the digestive and absorptive functions of the gastrointestinal tract declines with age, this is now known to reflect the effects of medications or disease states, rather than age itself. Where malabsorption occurs in an older adult, investigation of possible pancreatic or small intestinal disease is required.

Altered or reduced taste perception that occurs with ageing may influence enjoyment in eating. Although reduced salivary flow and a dry mouth can be a problem for some older people, these are usually the result of the side effects of drugs or the presence of disease, rather than being an inevitable part of the ageing process. Decreased thirst sensation can also contribute to the problem of a dry mouth. Difficulty in swallowing occurs in some older adults if neurological function is disturbed, e.g. after a stroke.

Perhaps the most important change in gastrointestinal function with ageing is the reduction in gastric acid output in a subgroup of older people who have atrophic gastritis. Atrophy of the stomach mucosa becomes more common with ageing and appears to affect about one-third of those over 60 years. The result is lowered secretion of acid, intrinsic factor and pepsin, which reduces the bioavailability of vitamin B_{12}, calcium, iron and folate. The implications are most profound for vitamin B_{12} due both to the diminished dissociation of the vitamin from food proteins, and binding of the small amount of freed vitamin B_{12} by the increased numbers of swallowed bacteria, which are able to survive in the low-acid environment of the proximal small intestine. In recognition of this and the prevalence of atrophic gastritis in the older population, the 1998 US dietary reference intakes (DRIs) recommend that older adults meet part of their vitamin B_{12} needs from supplements or foods fortified with crystalline, free vitamin B_{12}. Australia and New Zealand have adopted a similar recommendation; however, research is needed to determine whether functionality is improved by normalizing low vitamin B_{12} status, and the optimal dose required.

Another change is reduced intestinal motility, which may lead to constipation or diarrhoea—both disorders occur in later life. Constipation particularly contributes to morbidity and affects the individual's feeling of wellbeing. Sufficient fluid and dietary fibre may at least partly prevent this disorder.

34.5 Do nutritional needs change as we age?

Since the late 1990s, many countries have published nutrient recommendations with separate data for adults aged 51–70 years and ≥ 70 years. Until more specific information becomes available on the nutritional requirements of older adults, these broad age groupings will have to suffice for the entire heterogeneous older population (see Chapter 36 for more on recommended intakes). How are the nutritional needs of older adults currently thought to differ from those of younger adults?

Older adults have reduced needs for energy but presumably not for the B vitamins, which are involved in energy metabolism, and postmenopausal women have lower needs for iron, as a result of cessation of menstrual blood losses. These differences are reflected in lower recommended nutrient intakes for older adults. The lower energy needs of older adults are the result of declines in metabolic rate (secondary to reduced lean muscle mass) and in activity levels. Neither of these changes is inevitable; indeed, it can be argued that morbidity and mortality could be lowered if LBM and physical activity were maintained at more youthful levels rather than diminished in older persons. The greater food intake needed to balance higher energy expenditure is more likely to ensure adequate intakes of essential nutrients. If older adults consume low energy intakes, then it is important that most of the foods they eat are nutrient-dense, rather than of low nutrient density (high in sugars, fats or alcohol).

The body's requirements for iron are lowest in old age; however, other factors in the lives of many older people can increase the risk of iron deficiency. Such factors include chronic blood loss from ulcers or other disease conditions, poor iron absorption due to reduced stomach acid secretion, or medications like aspirin, which can cause blood loss.

Calcium needs are also higher in postmenopausal women (with low oestrogen) and this is reflected in increased recommendations for calcium intakes. An abundant calcium intake throughout life helps protect against osteoporosis, particularly in women (see Chapter 8).

There is also evidence accumulating that older adults have greater needs for vitamin D (discussed in section 34.3), riboflavin and vitamin B_6, and need higher doses of vitamin B_{12} to correct poor status.

The increase in vitamin B_6 requirement with age does not appear to be an absorptive problem, and subclinical deficiency of this vitamin may result in immune dysfunction. Also vitamin B_6, folate and vitamin B_{12} favourably affect serum homocysteine levels. Higher homocysteine levels are an independent risk factor for cardiovascular disease, impaired cognitive functions, osteoporotic fractures and other chronic diseases. The high levels generally observed in older adults may be reduced by an increased intake of folate, then vitamin B_{12} and vitamin B_6 (in that order of effectiveness). Riboflavin requirements, which had previously been thought to be lower in older than in younger persons, are now recognized to be higher in those over 70 years. Since vitamin E is the only lipid-soluble, chain-breaking antioxidant found in biological membranes, this vitamin might play an important role in maintaining neuronal integrity and preventing cell loss. Thus, it is logical to consider whether higher intakes may prove useful in neurological disorders where oxidative stress has been implicated. Current finding are inconclusive.

Overall, compared with younger adults, most older adults need to obtain the same or even higher intakes of several micronutrients, but usually in substantially lower overall food intakes. Thus, a nutrient-dense diet is a high priority in old age.

34.6 Secrets of long life?

For thousands of years the search for eternal life and youth has captured people's imagination. In about 1750, George Cheyne (physician to Samuel Johnson, David Hume and Alexander Pope) wrote *An essay of health and long life* in which he is emphatic that:

❛ Nothing conduces more to Health and Long Life, than Abstinence and plain Food, with due Labour. Most chronic diseases proceed from Repletion. Without due Labour and Exercise, the Juices will thicken, the Joints will stiffen, the Nerves will relax, and on these disorders, Chronical Distempers and a crazy old Age must ensue. This [lessening the diet gradually with age] is a powerful means to make their old age Green and Indolent, and to preserve the remains of their Senses to the very last. ❜

The similarities to recommendations derived from the latest research on ageing are remarkable! Currently Japan can still claim the greatest life expectancy in the world. It is theorized on the one hand that diet, particularly the low-fat intake amongst even Westernized Japanese people, may play a role. On the other hand, there are also theories that longevity-enabling genes protect against chronic disease and slow down the ageing process. At least one gene allele has been linked to increased longevity among centenarians. Conversely, lifespan does not appear to vary among populations. The extraordinary ages (150 years and older) claimed by inhabitants in several remote areas of Russian Georgia, southern Ecuador and in the

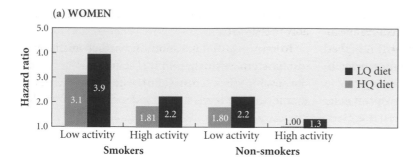

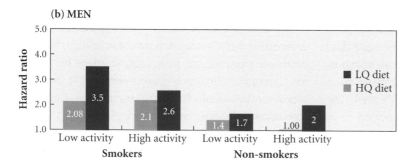

Fig. 34.7 Hazard ratios for single and combined effects of the lifestyle factors diet, smoking and physical activity in European women (a) and men (b) born between 1913 and 1918. The SENECA Study 1988–1999. LQ = low quality; HQ = high quality.

Source: Haveman-Nies, A., De Groot, C.P.G.M., Burema, J., Amorim Cruz, J.A., Osler, M., and Van Staveren, W.A. (2002) Dietary quality in relationships to 10-years mortality in older Europeans. *Am J Epidemiol*, **156**, 962–68.

Hunza River region of the Himalayan mountains in Pakistan have been found to be gross exaggerations.

Currently the only nutritional manipulation shown to increase lifespan has only been demonstrated in laboratory rats with a severe restriction of food intake. Beneficial effects of a moderate restriction of energy intake have also been observed in primates, but until now this has not been confirmed in (non-obese) humans. However, rather than focusing on the extension of longevity or 'adding years to life', WHO publications emphasize 'to add life to years', in other words to improve quality of life. The longitudinal survey SENECA (Survey in Europe on Nutrition and the Elderly, a Concerted Action) was designed to answer this question and to identify factors that contribute to healthy ageing. Adults aged 70–75 years living in centres in nine different countries participated in the study. Diet, physical activity, smoking, self-perceived health and wellbeing were examined at baseline in 1988–1989 and repeated in 1993 and 1999. Meal-time patterns as well as dietary intake varied across Europe, and geographical patterns were apparent. A healthy lifestyle was related to self-perceived health, a delay in functional dependence and mortality (see Fig. 34.7). Inactivity, smoking and

Table 34.1 Items in the Mediterranean Diet Score (MDS). Adapted for the SENECA study

Consumption
Vegetables and potatoes (g/day)
Legumes, nuts, seeds (g/day)
Fruit and fruit products (g/day)
Grains and bread (g/day)
Fish (g/day)
Monounsaturated/saturated fatty acid ratio
Milk and milk products (g/day)
Poultry and meat (g/day)

Note that for the first six items, consumption above median intake is beneficial, but for the last two items below median is beneficial.
Source: Trichoupoulou, A., Kouris-Blazos, A., Wahlqvist, M.L. *et al.* (1995) Diet and overall survival in elderly people. *Br Med J*, **11**, 1457–60.
Note: In the traditional Mediterranean diet only small amounts of dairy products and red meat are consumed, and consumption often goes together with a high amount of saturated fat. However, as stated in section 34.6 and Table 34.2, lean meat and (low-fat) dairy products are important sources of micronutrients and are recommended components of the daily food pattern of older adults.

a low-quality diet increased mortality risk. Dietary quality was based on an adapted Mediterranean Diet Score (MDS) as defined in Table 34.1. A higher consumption than average of high monosaturated/saturated fat ratio items, legumes, cereals, vegetables and fruits added positively to the score. In contrast, a lower consumption than average of the items meat and meat products and dairy products added favourably to the score.

To return to the question of whether nutritional changes can extend the human lifespan further, so far the answer is 'No'. However, if the question is 'Can we extend the number of healthy years lived?' then the answer is 'Yes'.

34.7 A look at the eating habits of older adults

A number of general conclusions can be drawn from studies of dietary intake conducted amongst older populations around the world. Contrary to the popular 'tea 'n' toast' myth, it appears that most older adults outside institutions eat reasonably well. The dietary patterns of older adults have generally been found to be similar to those of younger adults, but vary within and among different cultures and regions. Energy intake decreases with ageing, and when the intake level falls below 1500 kcal or 6.3 MJ it becomes difficult to fulfil the recommended daily requirements (see also Table 34.2).

Table 34.2 Daily consumption of type of foods and number of portions suggested in this table supply about 6.3 MJ and recommended daily intakes of micronutrients for populations over 70 years of age as suggested in several countries

Sandwiches with filling (margarine, cheese, meat, marmalade)	4 slices
Milk products (low fat)	3 cups
Fruit	1–2 pieces
Potatoes	1–2 pieces
Vegetables	4 serving spoons
Meat (lean) or fish	75–100 g
Oil for preparation of cooked meal	15 g
Fluid	8 servings
Vitamin D	10 μg

However, even with an apparently adequate food intake there are some nutrients for which there is a greater risk of inadequate supply. These nutrients are calcium, zinc, magnesium, vitamin B_6, folate, vitamin B_{12}, vitamin C and vitamins D and E. The low calcium intakes and vitamin D supply of many older people, particularly women, have important implications for bone health. Poor zinc status appears to contribute to delayed wound healing and impaired immune response in older adults. Both the SENECA study and the Boston Nutritional Status Survey have added considerably to our knowledge of the vitamin status of older adults. In the SENECA study, more than 20% had biochemical levels suggesting subclinical vitamin B_6 and—depending on the cut-off levels —also B_{12} deficiency. More than half of the people over 60 years in the Boston survey had vitamin B_6 intakes below two-thirds of the recommended allowance. Low folate intakes and inadequate absorption of vitamin B_{12} are common and might be linked via elevated plasma homocysteine with vascular and other chronic diseases. Vitamin C intake often seems to be adequate in older adults, but unfortunately vitamin C is readily lost from foods during storage and preparation. For the diet of Dutch and Danish participants, losses amounted to approximately 45% of the vitamin C content and consequently 30% of the subjects had low intakes. Low vitamin C intake, in addition to low intakes of other antioxidants (e.g. vitamin E and carotenoids), has been associated with increased risk for cataract and coronary artery disease. Also, a positive association between the plasma levels of these vitamins and memory has been observed.

Daily intake of fruits, vegetables, wholegrains and dairy products as well as the inclusion in the diet of lean meat, fish, poultry and legumes will ensure provision of those nutrients found to be most 'at risk' in the diets of older people. If older people eat these foods in amounts as suggested in Table 34.2, then about 6.3 MJ covers the daily recommended intake of most countries. However, with such a diet, there is no place for so-called social foods or snacks.

In the SENECA study, about 4% of men and 32% of women had an energy intake of less than 6.3 MJ. These people are vulnerable to malnutrition. Table 34.3 shows other factors contributing to nutritional problems in old age.

The two factors most consistently linked with poor dietary intake in old age are low socioeconomic status and social isolation. Compared with men living with a spouse, older men living alone tend to have a poorer fruit and vegetable intake, and more frequently choose less nutrient-dense, easy-to-prepare foods, which also tend to be higher in fat and lower in fibre. Limited cooking skills and reduced motivation when cooking just for one are probably important contributors. Institutionalized older people and those living independently in the community but restricted in their mobility also tend to be at higher risk of poor dietary habits. Lack of social contact, loneliness, being less active both socially and physically, and recent bereavement are also associated with poor dietary intake. It is probable that a rich and varied lifestyle and maintenance of positive interests lead to better dietary quality through an improvement in life satisfaction, a better social support network, and a lessening of the impact of some of the negative life events associated with growing older. In fact, participation in fewer activities outside the home is linked with higher mortality in old age. Other negative influences on dietary intake in old age are physical disability, shopping difficulties, depression and problems with chewing. Loss of teeth and poorly fitting dentures clearly reduce chewing efficiency.

Signs of poor nutrition in an older individual include recent weight loss, missing meals, infrequent grocery shopping, depression, loss of appetite or declining food intake due to digestive problems, taste changes, and chewing or swallowing difficulties.

Table 34.3 Potential contributors to nutritional problems in older people

Physical factors
Reduced total energy needs
Declining absorptive and metabolic capacities
Chronic diseases
Poor appetite
Changes in taste or odour perception
Poor dental health
Reduced salivary flow
Difficulty in swallowing
Lack of exercise
Physical disability (restricting the capacity to purchase, cook or eat a varied diet)
Side effects of drugs (anorexia, nausea, altered taste, drug–nutrient interactions)
Restrictive diets
Alcoholism
Social and psychological factors
Depression
Loneliness
Social isolation
Bereavement
Loss of interest in food or cooking
Memory loss
Food avoidances
Socioeconomic factors
Low income
Inadequate cooking or storage facilities
Limited nutrition knowledge
Lack of transport
Shopping difficulties
Cooking practices that result in nutrient losses (e.g. soaking vegetables)
Inadequate cooking skills (particularly in men)

34.8 Nutrition–disease relationships in old age

The role of diet in some chronic diseases is discussed elsewhere (in Chapters 20, 21 and 22, for example). Outlined here are some special issues in older adults and differences in nutrition–disease relationships from those in younger adults.

It is often assumed that lifestyle changes to improve health are no longer worthwhile in old age, that the remaining years are not sufficient to reap the benefits of modifications that are often thought to lead to a reduction in enjoyment of food. Certainly very restrictive diets may impair the adequacy of dietary intake. However, benefits can be gained from nutrition education and lifestyle change in older people. In several studies, a high proportion of older men and women have been found to make dietary changes, often for health reasons, thus challenging the stereotyped view of older adults being 'set in their ways'.

The incidence and prevalence of coronary heart disease are highest in the older population. Although long recognized as the leading cause of death in men, by age 65 years heart disease is also the primary cause of death in women. Smoking, hypertension and diabetes continue to be risk factors for heart disease during old age, and the prevalence of diabetes and impaired glucose tolerance rises steeply with age. Intervention trials clearly demonstrate that the health advantages of quitting smoking and managing hypertension remain in older people. Dietary approaches to the management of hypertension (i.e. weight reduction if overweight, salt restriction, limitation of alcohol) are particularly relevant for older adults who are more susceptible to severe adverse drug reactions and may be more responsive to salt restriction. There also appear to be even stronger grounds for salt restriction in older women on the basis of studies demonstrating a markedly increased obligatory urinary calcium loss on high sodium intakes. Halving salt intakes (currently around 140 mmol sodium/day) can lower dietary calcium needs by about a third.

Type 2 diabetes in older adults should be managed by weight reduction, mainly by increased physical activity, and hypoglycaemic agents. Even moderate weight reduction has been shown to have benefits for diabetic control in older people, when it occurred under professional guidance. The latter is important, because weight-loss programmes may result in mainly loss of LBM mass instead of fat mass, which is detrimental for health.

The relative risk associated with high versus low cholesterol levels diminishes with age because cardiovascular disease is highly prevalent, even in older adults with low cholesterol levels, and because those with the highest levels are more likely to have suffered early death. However, the absolute risk attributable to high cholesterol levels actually increases with age (i.e. the difference in absolute rates of disease between those with highest risk factor levels and those with lowest risk factor levels). Attributable risk infers the number of events or deaths that are avoided for people in the group with low exposure to the risk factor. All major risk factors, including elevated low-density lipoprotein cholesterol, show an increased attributable risk with advancing age. Evidence from statin trials suggests that older adults are as responsive to drug and dietary treatment of high cholesterol levels as younger adults. It seems appropriate to consider functional rather than chronological age when deciding whether an individual should be given dietary advice to lower cholesterol levels. Someone who is generally healthy and appears likely to have a reasonable life expectancy should not be denied dietary advice. However, more research is needed on the effects of cholesterol-lowering, particularly in those 70 years and older, and cholesterol-lowering in people over 80 years would not seem worthwhile.

In Western societies, the common pattern of weight gain up to the age of around 50–60 years means that overweight and obesity are common problems in old age. However, rather than being an inevitable part of growing older, this pattern is linked with sedentary lifestyles. The increase in abdominal or central obesity with advancing age is linked with greater risk of insulin resistance, hypertension and dyslipidaemia. Overweight and obesity also aggravate arthritis and impair physical mobility. Furthermore, among healthy adults who have never smoked, mortality is greater in those with higher body mass indices at least up until 75 years of age. Reflecting recent research, but in contrast with previous recommendations, the 1995 US Dietary Guidelines conclude 'health risks due to excess weight appear to be the same for older as for younger adults' and the 2000 guidelines write that 'like younger adults, overweight and obese older adults may improve their health by losing weight'. However, evidence regarding the consequences of weight *change* in old age is inconsistent. Although moderate intentional weight loss in overweight older adults appears to improve cardiovascular risk factors, the outcomes in terms of mortality are less clear. Weight loss in old age may be detrimental to health, particularly in the absence of other cardiovascular risk factors and in those who are not overweight. Heavier women also have a lower risk of hip fracture. This is partly due to 'padding' and better muscles, but may also be due to maintenance of higher oestrogen levels from the conversion of precursor steroids to oestrogen in adipose tissue. So perhaps the best advice is to avoid unwanted weight gain in mid-life, then maintain a lean body weight in old age.

Another link between nutrition and disease in older people is that between the antioxidant nutrients and risk of cataracts (a clouding of the lens of the eye resulting in diminished vision). Cataracts afflict nearly half of the American population aged 75–85 years and are a major cause of blindness worldwide. The main contributors to cataract formation appear to be photo-oxidative damage and osmotic stress in the lens of the eye. It has been found that the highest risk of cataract is among individuals with low intakes of vitamin C, vitamin E and carotenoids. Osmotic stress due to high glucose levels is believed to be why people with diabetes are particularly prone to cataracts.

The carotenoids lutein (xanthophyll) and zeaxanthin appear to be protective against degeneration of the macular lutea in the centre of the retina, a common cause of visual loss in old age. These two carotenoids are present in the normal macula and presumably function by protecting the photoreceptors from light damage. The best sources of lutein are dark green leafy vegetables and of zeaxanthin are orange capsicums and yellow maize.

Constipation and diverticular disease are common problems, and awareness of the need to increase fibre intake is high, as reflected in widespread use of unprocessed bran supplements in older populations. However, it is preferable for fibre intakes to be increased through the consumption of a variety of cereals and vegetables, rather than relying on extensive use of bran supplements. These may have adverse effects on the bioavailability of zinc and calcium, which may be marginally supplied in the diets of many older adults.

Severe nutrient deficiencies clearly impair both brain and immune function, and researchers are exploring the possibility that long-term moderate (subclinical) nutrient deficiencies also produce memory impairments or declining immunity in older adults. On the other hand, dementia can also have nutritional consequences. Early dementia may lead to difficulty in shopping or cooking, or a person with dementia may forget to eat or experience changes in taste, and may even not recognize food, or may eat non-food items.

For older adults, probably the single most important health message is to achieve or maintain at least moderate levels of physical activity combined with healthy eating. There are numerous health benefits from exercise in old age: cardiovascular, musculoskeletal and psychological benefits, improvements in fat and carbohydrate metabolism, and promotion of good bowel function. There are similarities between the deterioration that accompanies ageing and that which occurs with physical inactivity. Randomized controlled trials demonstrate that high-intensity strength training exercises are an effective and feasible means of preserving bone density while improving muscle mass, strength and balance in old age.

34.9 Supplements for older adults

The use of supplements in the USA, Canada, Australia and New Zealand is widespread amongst older men (35–60%) and women (45–79%). Advertisers often target older people, claiming their products prevent disease or promote longevity. Unfortunately, the nutrient supplements most commonly used are rarely those in shortest supply in the diet, and furthermore supplement users generally tend to have better dietary intakes than non-users. Particular concerns are the risk of supplement interference with drug absorption in an age group that heavily consumes both prescription and over-the-counter drugs.

There are, nevertheless, some indications for supplement use by older adults: vitamin D (10–15 μg/day) (countries differ according to whether supplements are recommended for *all* those over 60 years or *only*

for those with limited exposure to sunlight) or general multivitamins including folate and vitamin B_{12} and mineral supplements (at recommended intake levels) for those with very low food intakes (i.e. less than 6.3 MJ/day); B_{12} supplements or fortified foods may be indicated for those aged 70+; and calcium supplements for those women unable to meet the high recommended levels from foods alone. However, a well-balanced diet will provide most healthy older people with the nutrients they need (except vitamin D), and for those whose food intakes are very low, the more important priority is to identify and try to correct any underlying physical or psychosocial reasons for eating problems or poor nutritional state (see Table 34.3).

34.10 Drug–nutrient interactions

In developed countries where older adults comprise more than 12% of the population, they typically consume more than a third of all the country's prescription drugs, and are often taking several drugs at once. There are a number of means by which drugs can affect nutrition, usually increasing nutrient need. Many drugs can reduce appetite, produce nausea or gastro-

intestinal disturbances, or alter the senses of taste or smell and hence affect food intake; long-term laxative use can impair intestinal function; and laxatives and diuretics can lead to severe loss of potassium. As many as 30% of older adults complain that drugs change their sense of taste.

34.11 Conclusions

Logically, preventive measures to reduce diet-related disease should begin early in life; however, that is not to say that lifestyle modifications are worthless in old age. Improvements in diet and maintenance of exercise have been shown to benefit health, regardless of age. Behavioural risk factors (e.g. not regularly eating breakfast, lack of regular physical activity, unhealthy weight changes, smoking) remain predictors of 10-year mortality even at older ages (i.e. 70+). As the older population is more heterogeneous than any other age group, individual judgement is critical in

deciding on the advisability of dietary and lifestyle changes. Physiological, psychological and sociological factors need to be considered. At one extreme are independent, vigorous, healthy people in their 70s, 80s and even 90s; at the other extreme are patients who are dependent and have multiple diseases and limited reserves. For the latter, diet and lifestyle advice should focus on function and quality of life. However, it is often overlooked that, although life expectancy at birth may only be to the mid-to-late 70s, at age 65, men and women in developed countries still have a life expectancy of some 15 and 19 years, respectively. Furthermore, at age 75, these life expectancies are around 9 and 11 years, respectively, and recent studies have shown that a healthy diet and lifestyle may make these years healthier, more active and more independent.

FURTHER READING

1. **Binns, C. (ed.)** (1999) *Dietary guidelines for older Australians*. Canberra: National Health and Medical Research Council.

2. **Chopdar, A., Chakravarthy, U., and Verma, D.** (2003) Age-related macular degeneration. *Br Med J*, **326**, 485–88.

3. **De Groot, C.P.G.M., Verherheijden, M.W., De Henauw, S., Schroll, M., and Van Staveren, W.A.** (2004) Lifestyle, nutritional status, health and mortality in elderly people across Europe: a review of the longitudinal results of the SENECA study. *J Gerontol Med Sci*, **59A**, 1277–84.

4. **Finch, S., Doyle, W., Lowe, C., et al.** (1998) *National/diet and nutrition survey: people aged 65 years and over (Volume 1)*. London, HMSO.

5. **Hall, K.M., and Luepker, R.V.** (2000) Is hypercholesterolemia a risk factor and should it be treated in the elderly? *Am J Health Promot*, **14**, 347–56.

6. **Horwath, C.C.** (1989) Dietary intake studies in elderly people. *World Rev Nutr Dietet*, **59**, 1–70.

7. **Roubenoff, R.** (2000) Sarcopenia and its implications for the elderly. *Eur J Clin Nutr*, **54**, S40–S47.

8. **Solomons, N.** (2000) Demographic and nutritional trends among the elderly in developed and developing regions. *Eur J Clin Nutr*, **54**, S2–S14.

9. **Thomas, D.** (ed.) (2002) Undernutrition in older adults. *Clin Geriatr Med*, **18**, 661–91.

10. **WHO** (2002). *Ageing and life course program. Active ageing: A policy framework*. Geneva: World Health Organization.

11. **WHO** (2003) *Reducing risks, promoting healthy life*. Geneva, World Health Organization.

 To see topical and scientifically robust updates on nutrition associated with this textbook, and active web links to many of the journal articles in the Reference areas, please see the dedicated Online Resource Centre at www.oxfordtextbooks.co.uk/orc/mann3e/.

PART 7

Clinical and public health

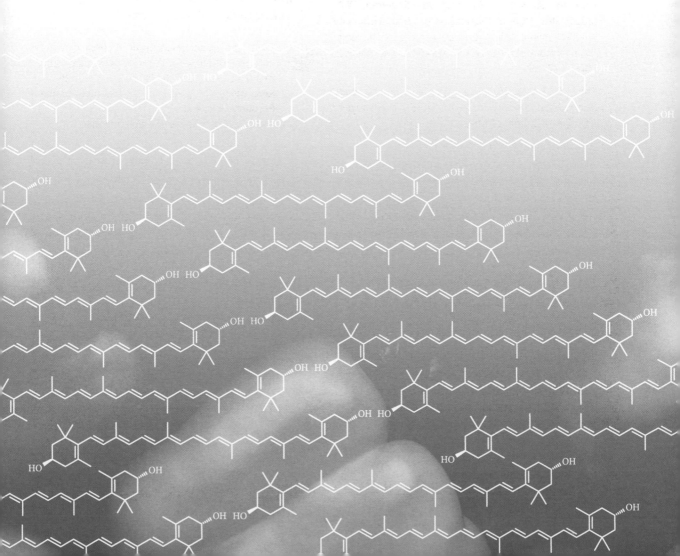

35 Food habits

Helen Leach

Many of the topics that form the chapters of this book represent specializations in the subject of human nutrition. Structurally speaking, they can be slotted into compartments within the overall framework of this scientific discipline. The study of food habits, however, might best be viewed as the exploration of a relatively unbounded field lying outside the construction of nutrition, but impinging on it at many points.

35.1 Studying food habits

A number of social scientists also locate their subject matter in this broad field of food habits: the American school of nutritional anthropology (e.g. Bryant, Fitzgerald, Jerome, Robson); a group of social anthropologists and sociologists interested in symbolism and structural order in food habits (e.g. Lévi-Strauss, Douglas, Nicod); anthropologists committed to more materialist explanations of food habits (e.g. Harris, Mintz); sociologists, economists and social historians concerned with explaining change in food habits (e.g. Mennell, Burnett, Charsley); and social psychologists who have an interest in the interface between cultural beliefs and individual behaviour, as they affect food preference (e.g. Rozin).

Historically, the science of human nutrition developed in tandem with other medical sciences. At a clinical level, therefore, it has concentrated on the individual, and at a policy level, on the population, using epidemiological studies as a starting point. It has made by far the greatest progress with the biological aspects of human nutrition, and with the development of effective treatment of nutritional disorders in individuals. But in those aspects of human nutrition where individuals cease to behave as biological organisms or as members of biological populations, nutrition as an explanatory and applied science has had much less success. Of course humans have to eat to survive, the environment constantly sets limits on food production, and populations will continue to show change in genetic factors affecting metabolism, but where humans exhibit any choice at all in what they eat, what they select is more likely to be socially influenced than the result of a biological craving, environmental determinism or idiosyncratic whim.

In discussing food habits, therefore, a definition must be used that stresses the socially influenced food-related behaviour of humans as members of groups. Murcott's usage of the phrase 'food habits' as 'a provisional, convenient and inclusive shorthand to cover the widest possible range of food choice, preferences, and meal patterns and cuisines' will be followed here.

35.2 Who chooses?

There can be no denying that in the course of a human lifetime, the decision whether to ingest a particular food item lies ultimately with the individual (except in cases of forced or tube feeding). Infants are particularly adept at exercising the right to reject food. But the power to decide what food items are made available for the selection process, and in what form, frequently lies beyond the individual. For the baby, the mother usually decides what should be offered, starting with the decision of either breast milk or formula. But her choice on behalf of the baby is usually influenced by advice from female relatives, or health professionals. In the case of the former, this permits a family tradition of infant feeding to be passed on, compatible with the beliefs of the family's ethnic group and with their religious affiliation. A nurse's or doctor's advice will normally reflect the society's prevailing scientific paradigm concerning infant nutrition, for example, that solids should not be introduced until a certain age or that certain foods should be avoided.

The growing child has little control over the household menu, though at certain times (such as illness or the celebration of milestones in development), the person responsible for food acquisition and preparation will deliberately produce an item known to be the child's favourite. In some cultures, gender and position in the family may affect what is offered to each child in both quantity and variety. Similarly, the menu selected for the household may be strongly influenced by the preferences of a senior adult member. In societies where it is traditional for women to cook for their families, the desire to please their husbands may dictate the dishes they prepare for the whole household. Finally, in old age, any former control over the menu may be lost through institutionalization or displacement from the kitchen by a younger household member. Thus, for many humans, selection of food is subject to significant constraints for much of their lifetime, despite the apparent freedom of the individual to eat as they choose.

35.3 Social and cultural influences on food choice

It is not surprising then that the cook, food purchaser, housewife or househusband, indeed any member of a group who makes food choices on behalf of that group, is sometimes referred to in research literature as the 'key kitchen person' (KKP), focal person, or gatekeeper, all terms that recognize a pivotal role in the diet and food habits of their group. What social factors influence their choice of food to prepare? The broad answer is that they select according to the unwritten rules or norms of the culture to which they belong. Even when they respond to the food preferences of a particular member of their group, they are choosing items, composing them into dishes, and combining the dishes into menus within particular culinary traditions.

Culinary traditions operate at many levels from small kin-based group traditions to the nearly global culinary styles of Western cultures. In some isolated Third World situations, only one culinary tradition may be relevant, but for most First World groups, food providers and KKPs choose to work within the tradition that they see as most appropriate for a particular eating situation. For many important social occasions, the family culinary tradition of the organizers and chief participants will be followed. The significance of the occasion (e.g. wedding breakfast, Christmas dinner, religious festival) and the desire for a successful outcome usually constrain the menu within the traditional family or community pattern.

Even at this lowest organizational level, the family pattern of eating may be distinctive from that of its neighbours, though both may belong to the same ethnic and religious group and occupy the same socioeconomic position. Family food habits may be comparatively resistant to change in places where culinary knowledge and skills are learned primarily within the household and passed down between generations. Marriage residency practices, such as the wife joining her husband's extended family in a single household, may work to suppress change and reinforce the distinctiveness of the family tradition. Non-Western societies incorporate many different forms of household structure, depending on family lifecycle and kinship system. Each type will have a distinctive pattern of decision-making relating to food.

Urbanized communities also feature a wide range of household arrangements, from two-parent, two-generational families to groups of unrelated young adults. Food habits here are influenced by the background and social network of the group member who becomes the KKP for each main meal. If that person learned culinary skills in his or her own family setting, many of these will be transferred to the new household and applied according to the type of meal. However, in urbanized Western societies, such knowledge is frequently acquired outside the home (e.g. from the formal education system). For most of this century, cooking training in schools has been motivated by the goals of 'good nutrition' and has been responsible for reinterpreting Western culinary traditions within a scientific paradigm. There is ample evidence, however, that after schooling is complete, recipe repertoire is influenced by interaction with peers, within social networks and by the media.

Magazines, newspapers and television reflect an amalgam of culinary traditions depending on the contributing sources. A locally based food writer for a monthly newspaper column may work within a regional food tradition, combining new variants with well-established and familiar dishes. A national or internationally distributed magazine may offer more cosmopolitan fare, strongly influenced by international food fashion trends. However, there is little research on whether these fashions have a lasting impact on household food habits. For example, will the currently fashionable grain couscous become an important cereal in cosmopolitan cuisine, or will it be as short-lived as the fondue party?

The twentieth-century trend to a cosmopolitan culinary repertoire has probably been influenced by the range of dishes cooked in the commercial kitchens of restaurants and fast-food outlets, and sampled as part of the phenomenon of 'eating out'. For the household member who is not actively involved in food preparation, eating out means more choice is possible from an extended menu. For the KKP, the responsibility for selecting food for others is removed, along with control over the dishes on the menu and their composition. However, the characterization of restaurants and other food outlets into well-defined categories, such as vegetarian, wholefood, seafood, Italian, Thai, Cantonese or other specified ethnic type suggests that consumers still prefer to choose their food from an identifiable culinary tradition, even if it is not that of their own birth culture.

Thus, for the purpose of food and menu selection, many Western households operate within multiple layers of culinary traditions, not simultaneously, but moving between them from meal to meal, through the weekly cycle and the annual calendar of festive occasions. Perhaps the unwritten rules for deciding which culinary tradition is appropriate are part of evolving culinary traditions in their own right.

35.4 Food habits in nutrition practice

From the viewpoint of the nutritionist offering clinical advice to an individual, it is clearly important to know how the patient relates to the KKP of the household where he or she normally resides. Without the informed support of the KKP, long-term dietary modification is unlikely to occur. And even with that support, pressure from other members of the household or a high-status member might frustrate any change.

It is also valuable for the nutritionist to have some knowledge of the culinary tradition from which most of the patient's meals are derived. Any modification of intake must be compatible with that tradition. We tend to categorize other traditions by their starch staple and typical flavouring substances. But culinary traditions are more than just the combinations of dishes/recipes that characterize and distinguish the eating patterns of particular human groups. They also include the rules for selecting and preparing food for consumption (such as butchering practices and preservation techniques), rules for composing the menu according to an acceptable structure of courses, and the rules or norms concerning eating behaviour (e.g. time, location, participants). As with all human social behaviour, these rules or norms are culturally transmitted. They are not immutable, but variation and innovation tend to take place more frequently within the structure than radical alteration of the overall framework. Culinary traditions also include the non-nutrient-related meanings of food, including those that concern ethnic identity, values and religious beliefs.

Within certain traditions, there is strong social pressure to prepare and serve more food on occasions than might be considered nutritionally desirable. In such instances, the food is satisfying more than biological needs, and the participants are well aware that it is carrying a coded message concerning social relationships and value systems. For example, the Oglala Sioux of Pine Ridge Reservation in South Dakota require participants at communal high feasts to eat beyond satiety, and to bring containers for the removal of leftovers. Since their culture values generosity as the most important of four cardinal virtues, overindulgence is a statement about the generosity of the host, and an affirmation that this virtue is more highly regarded by the Oglala than by Euro–Americans.

Similarly, on the Polynesian island, Tikopia, the anthropologist Raymond Firth observed that 'true hospitality consists in placing before a man more than he can possibly eat and then commanding him at intervals to continue when he shows signs of flagging'. In this Polynesian culture, which typically rates hospitality as an important virtue, the guest eats beyond satiety, regarding it as offensive to the host as well as shameful and embarrassing to confess to still being hungry. Food is used throughout Polynesia to confirm an agreement made between parties, and failure to partake could be interpreted as a sign that one party intends to break the contract.

Particular foods may encode metaphysical meanings that completely transcend any nutritional value. For the Christian taking communion, the wafer and the wine are clearly not food, but have been spiritually transformed. For modern Oglala Sioux Indians, ritual eating of dog involves equally complex rituals, reminding participants of the dog's role in Sioux cosmology and symbolizing all that is Indian in Oglala culture. The rejection of the dog as a food item by Euro–Americans adds to its symbolic importance for the Oglala, to the degree that the ceremonial stature of the dog feast has increased as Indian identity has been threatened. If dog consumption carried a health risk, a nutritionist who advised its avoidance would be threatening both group identity and religious belief.

Not all foods carry such complex spiritual meanings. However, under pressure, minority groups may encode particular items or dishes/recipes as markers of identity, when formerly they functioned simply as everyday food. Such is the case of 'soul food' in the USA. The pork and chicken products that provide the meat component of soul food, such as necks, backs, feet and giblets, were originally eaten because they were rejected by wealthier white consumers and were therefore cheaper. In one Southern case study, it was found that black households of middle socioeconomic class described them as 'black people's food' and ate them not for their cheapness but as a marker of ethnic identity. Black families from lower socioeconomic classes and middle-class white families classified them as 'poor people's food'. Lower-class white people avoided them. These food items have acquired a status ranking and racial connotation that is perceived differently according to the socioeconomic status and ethnicity of the various groups in the case study. It would be difficult for a nutritionist to change the usage or non-usage of these foods by any of the groups concerned because of their acquired load of non-nutritional meanings.

For many societies, food choice is constrained by religious proscription. Many of these food taboos are of such antiquity that they are written into the formal teachings of the religion (such as the Jewish and Hindu dietary laws that proscribe pork or beef). However, more recent dietary regimens based on particular philosophical or ethical principles have evolved food taboos of equal force for their adherents. As a secular movement, vegetarianism has been important for nearly two centuries, throughout this period drawing for justification on the accumulating data from the science of nutrition. Not surprisingly, nutritionists faced with evidence of health benefits from vegetarian diets for adults have treated the movement with respect. However, the twentieth century has seen the development of far more restrictive

dietary regimens allied to the 'health food' movement and the Western preoccupation with weight reduction. Food symbolism is highly developed in these regimens, with the polarization of 'natural' (= healthy) versus synthetic (= dangerous) constantly reworked and elaborated by those who benefit commercially from sales of diet books and the approved foods. For the clinical nutritionist, disentangling the pseudoscientific justifications and powerful symbolism of these restrictive and potentially damaging diets is a major challenge. Furthermore, the social networks into which adherents of 'fad' or extreme diets are drawn for mutual support are likely to counteract what is perceived as criticism by the health professionals.

35.5 Changing food habits in the modern world

So far, this introduction to food habits has stressed the inbuilt tendency to conservatism within a culinary tradition, the individual's lack of control over food choice at various periods in his or her life, and the symbolic loading on certain foods, which may exert powerful pressure against any change in usage or avoidance. Taken together, these factors explain why nutritional advice aimed at individual or group level may be listened to politely (because of the status of the health professional), but not subsequently acted upon.

At the same time, the success of multinational food companies provides ample evidence that throughout the world, even within highly conservative and symbol-rich culinary traditions, some substantial changes have occurred in diet during the twentieth century (see Box 35.1). These have included the introduction of many new food items, and even new menus borrowed from other traditions. Food manufacturers have invested heavily in research on food acceptance, and have realized that restrictive rules affecting food habits apply to meals rather than snacks. This observation, also made by Michael Nicod from his structuralist study of working class food habits in Britain (1974), led to his definition of the meal as a structured food event and the snack as an unstructured event. Although meals have courses that must be

served in a prescribed order and contain certain food categories, for snacks, consumers are free to eat the items in any order or combination, at any time and with or without company. It is not surprising then that snack-food manufacturers have had a global impact, because their promotional advertising does not have to confront long-established culinary norms. The lack of structure in snacking behaviour has allowed it to become a global arena where multinationals compete with new products, or old ones, newly packaged.

Nutritionists have had some success in promoting snacks with lower fat and sodium content, but realize that because snacking is usually supplementary feeding, their long-term objectives can only be met by dietary reform of meals, the area in which the multinationals have made much less headway. It has taken several decades to achieve public acceptance of pizza- or burger-based main meals, when these items were originally conceived of more as snacks. Fast-food outlets have had to supply additional items such as potatoes, salads and even desserts to meet the public's norms of what constitute 'proper' meals.

The key to effecting change in meal composition is to provide substitutions for existing elements without threatening the overall structure. Studies of dietary change in indigenous societies following contact with Europeans have shown that the way in

BOX 35.1 Food habits, modernization and globalization

The Samoan archipelago in the South Pacific provides a powerful example of the effects of modernization on food habits. Modernization is usually associated with the adoption of a cash economy, urbanization, formal education and increasing contact with the outside world. Globalization builds on those changes through the networks of multinational businesses and exposure to global media.

Although the recent arrival of fast-food outlets in the Samoan islands may be treated as a phenomenon of globalization, modernization began to affect Samoan people at least a century earlier. By the time that Paul Baker and his research team studied Samoan health in 1974–1983, modernization had already wrought significant changes.

Western Samoans and American Samoans share a Polynesian genetic heritage. Until the archipelago was partitioned in 1899, Samoans practised subsistence agriculture, obtaining most of their foodstuffs from fruit trees scattered through the landscape and from swidden gardens. Their staples (taro, breadfruit and bananas) were supplemented with sea foods and occasionally pigs and chickens. In the traditional division of labour, young untitled men were responsible for the harvesting of crops, their preparation and cooking. At times, this was strenuous activity and the gardens might be located some distance from the village. Women were responsible for childcare, mat weaving and village maintenance.

American Samoa was the first to begin the transition to a cash economy. Because Pago Pago Harbour on Tutuila Island was a strategic naval base, American Samoa was administered by the US Department of the Navy from 1900 to 1951. When the base closed, the territory was run by the US Department of the Interior. The naval base employed many Samoans and their wages allowed them to purchase imported foods, such as rice and canned meats. Improved health services and migration of relatives from Western Samoa fuelled a population boom. Fewer people engaged in gardening or fishing and Tutuila came to depend on food imports from Western Samoa, the USA and Tonga. After 1951, the establishment of two canneries and creation of more public service jobs completed the economic modernization of American Samoa; a cash economy prevailed and population density built up around Pago Pago. Despite the US investment in health services, American Samoans suffered rising rates of obesity, cardiovascular diseases and type 2 diabetes.

Were the same changes experienced in Western Samoa? After a short period as a German colony, it was administered by New Zealand, until it achieved independence in 1962. Until this time, most villagers practised subsistence agriculture, working unpaid with their extended families. There were only a few plantations employing wage labour, a small private sector and some public servants in the capital, Apia. From 1920, a rapid rise in population occurred. As in American Samoa, migration provided an outlet for large numbers of young adults. While American Samoans migrated to Hawaii or California, Western Samoans travelled to New Zealand. Such was the strength of the extended family and concept of *tautua* (service to elders) that cash remittances from overseas relatives became significant sources of income and purchasing power for village Samoans.

Paul Baker's team found that modernization was less advanced in Western Samoa than in American Samoa. They obtained health data from isolated villages and urban centres in both Western and American Samoa, and extended the survey to Samoans resident in Hawaii and California. In weight, they found that adult men from Western Samoa averaged 76 kg and displayed a good level of physical fitness, especially those engaged in food production. American Samoan men living on more 'modern' Tutuila averaged 86.3 kg, while those in Hawaii averaged 89.8 kg and the Californian Samoans 98.8 kg. As weight increased, physical fitness measures declined. Modernization of the diet and increasingly sedentary lifestyles were identified as the main factors in the obesity epidemic affecting American Samoans. Instead of the men growing, transporting and cooking their staple crops, waged workers (both women and men) increasingly purchased rice, mutton flaps, canned corn beef, chicken portions, bread and soft drinks. Samoan women have taken on the role of cooking non-traditional foods often with high fat and sugar content. Bottle-feeding has increased weight gains in infants as young women wean their babies in order to return to work.

Since the 1980s, globalization has accentuated the effects of modernization. With the arrival of fast-food outlets in American Samoa and recently Western Samoa, together with a dramatic increase in imported foods, traditional foods face greater competition than before, while imported four-wheel-drive vehicles now provide access to plantations formerly reached on foot.

which the new foods are slotted into existing native classification systems is a useful guide to their acceptability. The most rapidly accepted foodstuffs are those that are judged similar to existing foods, in attributes such as taste, appearance, style of preparation or growth habit. In many Pacific Island cultures, plants closely related to species already grown were the most rapidly incorporated, for example the West Indian root crop *Xanthosoma* spp., which was predictably classified as a form of taro (*Colocasia esculenta*). South American cassava (also known as manioc) and solanum potatoes were similarly acceptable because they could be grown like traditional yams, arrowroot and sweet potatoes. With no cereal precedent in Polynesia, maize took much longer to be slotted into local culinary and horticultural traditions. In most Pacific cultures, more than one starch staple was available, although they were seldom served at the same meal. This choice may have increased their readiness to accept the new staples introduced by Europeans. Monostaple cultures seem much more resistant to change. The depth of their attachment to their single staple may often be seen in the extension of the word used for the staple to mean food in general.

In some culture contact situations, foods that were initially disliked, but were essential to avoid starvation, eventually gained acceptance. This is reflected in the vernacular names, which give evidence of the crucial classification process. Faced by the loss of the symbolically and nutritionally important buffalo, the Oglala Sioux initially rejected government beef rations from cattle held in corrals as smelling offensive and no substitute for buffalo meat. Under pressure, they compromised by turning loose the cattle, and then hunting, butchering and ritually feasting on them as though they were buffalo. Cattle acquired buffalo terminology and became Indian.

The effects of globalization on developing countries constitute a special case of culture contact. The accompanying economic changes are of concern to nutritionists because they may lead to deleterious substitutions in traditional diets. These often involve replacement of higher-nutrient crops (such as millets in central Africa) with crops of lower nutritional value (such as cassava, which is more tolerant of drought and degraded soils). Studies have shown that given the local economic context, such diet shifts are based on rational choices designed to increase food security, even at the expense of optimal nutrition. Labour migration, pressure to produce cash crops and increasing poverty produce adaptations in traditional food systems, which can transform adequate nutrition into chronic undernutrition, or in the most vulnerable groups, even malnutrition. In these cases, nutritional reform is unlikely to succeed unless poverty can first be reduced.

The message for nutritionists from such studies of culture contact is that the structural elements of culinary traditions are highly resistant to change. It is precisely these elements that, in giving stability and continuity, define the tradition. Where dietary change has occurred, it has involved substitution of new foods for old within the indigenous food system, using the classification process as a guide to how the new food is to be used. Judging from historical studies, actual structural changes involving things like course order and essential elements may take a century or longer. If thought nutritionally desirable, reform at such a fundamental level might be expected to add a new dimension to the notion of long-term planning! Ultimately, nutritionists must translate their findings into recommendations that will work within the culinary tradition, not against it.

FURTHER READING

1. **Baker, P.T., Hanna, J.M., and Baker, T.S. (eds)** (1986) *The changing Samoans: behaviour and health in transition*. New York, Oxford University Press.

2. **Bryant, C.A., Courtney, A., Markesbery, B.A., and de Walt, K.M.** (1985) *The cultural feast: an introduction to food and society*. St Paul MN, West.

3. **Charsley, S.R.** (1992) *Wedding cakes and cultural history*. Routledge, London.

4. **Cox, D.N., and Anderson, A.S.** (2004) Food choice. In Gibney, M.J. *et al.* (eds) *Public Health Nutrition*, pp. 144–66. Oxford, Blackwell Science.

5. **Douglas, M. (ed.)** (1984) *Food in the social order: studies of food and festivities in three American communites*. New York, Russell Sage Foundation.

6. **Douglas, M., and Nicod, M.** (1974) Taking the biscuit: the structure of British Meals. *New Soc*, **30**, 744–7.

7. **Harris, M.** (1986) *Good to eat: riddles of food and culture*. London, Allen and Unwin.

8. **Leach, H.M.** (1993) Changing diets—a cultural perspective. *Proc Nutr Soc NZ*, **18**, 1–8.

9. **Lentz, C. (ed.)** (1999) *Changing food habits: case studies from Africa, South America and Europe*. Amsterdam, Harwood.

10. **Messer, E.** (1984) Anthropological perspectives on diet. *Annu Rev Anthropol*, **13**, 205–49.

11. **Murcott, A.** (1988) Sociological and social anthropological approaches to food and eating. *World Rev Nutr Diet*, **55**, 1–40.

12. **Robson, J.K.K. (ed.)** (1980) *Food, ecology and culture: readings in the anthropology of dietary practices*. New York, Gordon and Breach.

13. **Sharman, A., Theophano, J., Curtis, K., and Messer, E. (eds)** (1991) *Diet and domestic life in society*. Philadelphia: Temple University.

14. **Truswell, A.S., and Wahlqvist, M.L. (eds)** (1988) *Food habits in Australia*. Richmond, Victoria, Australia, Heinemann.

 To see topical and scientifically robust updates on nutrition associated with this textbook, and active web links to many of the journal articles in the Reference areas, please see the dedicated Online Resource Centre at www.oxfordtextbooks.co.uk/orc/mann3e/.

36 Nutritional recommendations for the general population

Katrine Baghurst

Nutrition research generates results that can often be translated by the media, or researchers themselves, into potentially confusing and conflicting messages. It is therefore critically important for governments, who develop food and nutrition policies, for those involved in health and nutrition education, and for consumers to have authoritative nutrition recommendations that represent consensus opinions of expert nutrition scientists. There are two major sets of recommendations: nutrient intake recommendations, and dietary guidelines and goals.

Nutrient intake recommendations were the earliest types of recommendations developed by governments and health authorities. They are based on authoritative quantitative estimates of human requirements for essential nutrients. The first set, which included only a few micronutrients, was issued by the nutrition committee of the old League of Nations in 1937. The best-known series of nutrient intake recommendations, the United States recommended dietary allowances (RDAs), were first published in 1943 and have been revised ten times since. Many other countries, groups of countries (e.g. Germany, Austria and Switzerland; the European Community) or health authorities (e.g. FAO, WHO) have their own sets of recommended nutrient intakes.

More recently, there has been the recognition that in most relatively affluent societies, and indeed even in more affluent groups within many developing countries, inappropriate intakes of macronutrients are adversely affecting health status through increasing the prevalence of chronic degenerative diseases. In response to this, some countries such as the USA and Canada have chosen to consider chronic disease prevention in setting their nutrient intake recommendations. Others, such as Australia and New Zealand, have chosen to retain a focus on nutrient essentiality for physiological requirement and/or prevention of deficiency states and to address chronic disease aspects of nutrition through supplementary nutrient recommendations as well as dietary guidelines and goals.

The distinction between chronic degenerative disease and deficiency disease is not always clear cut. Some conditions, such as osteoporosis, can be considered both a deficiency disease and a chronic degenerative disease, and it could be argued that certain aspects of coronary heart disease relate to nutrient deficiency (e.g. of fibre, antioxidants or long-chain ω-3 fats). One problem that arises in trying to set quantitative nutrient recommendations in relation to chronic disease prevention is the level of certainty surrounding the amount of a specific nutrient required for prevention of what is often a multicausal condition. Deficiency disease (e.g. scurvy, pellagra, beri-beri) is often, though not always (e.g. osteoporosis), related to a single nutrient and quantification is sometimes more clear cut.

In light of the increasing recognition of the role that diet plays in chronic disease aetiology, since the late 1960s many countries have developed *dietary goals*, which provide macronutrient targets aimed at achieving reductions of these diseases, and *dietary guidelines*, which help consumers to select, from the many available foods, a diet that will give them a better chance of long-term health. Dietary guidelines and goals should be predicated on knowledge about nutrient intake requirements. The guidelines generally address the balance of food groups required to attain a diet that will provide all the essential nutrients without the excesses that may increase chronic disease prevalence, or indeed overweight and obesity. The guidelines generally apply to total diet and not to the healthiness of particular foods. They are meant to be used as a framework for food choice at a time when the food supply in many affluent countries can be bewilderingly large and that in many developing countries can be changing rapidly.

36.1 Nutrient intake recommendations

Most developed and developing countries have a set of average daily nutrient intake recommendations for various groups within their population. Recommendations are generally given by age category, by gender, and for pregnancy and lactation. Until recently, these recommendations focused on a single value per nutrient per age/gender/lifestage group often called a recommended daily allowance (RDA) or intake (RDI) or a reference or recommended nutrient intake (RNI) that would be sufficient to cover the needs of most people in that population group.

The original 1943 US National Research Council's RDAs were defined as a 'tentative goals toward which to aim in planning dietaries'. They were later described in the 1964 edition as 'designed to afford a margin of sufficiency above average physiological requirements to cover variations among practically all individuals in the general population'. Essentially the same definition continued in the 1989 edition: 'RDAs are the levels of intake of essential nutrients that, on the basis of scientific knowledge, are judged by the Food and Nutrition Board to be adequate to meet the known nutrient needs of practically all healthy persons'.

The latest revision of the nutrient intake recommendations for the USA was undertaken jointly with Canada and published in a series of reports from 1997 to 2005, as dietary reference intakes (DRIs). In contrast to their earlier publications, the DRIs incorporated several reference figures for each nutrient along the same lines as the UK dietary reference values for food and energy (DRVs) published in 1991. This new approach involves defining a set of values for each nutrient for each age/gender group and for pregnancy and lactation, which may include (in the case of the UK) a lower reference figure covering the needs of the 2–3% of the population with the lowest requirement; a figure assessed as being the average requirement for a particular age/gender and pregnancy/lactation group; a figure (equivalent to the traditional RDA) that would cover the needs of the majority of the population (e.g. 97–98%); an optimal range of intake; and an upper level that may indicate a regular daily intake level above which harm might result (Table 36.1).

Many different names are used for these sets of nutrient intake recommendations such as dietary reference intakes (US/Canada); dietary reference values for food and energy (UK); nutrient reference values (Australia/New Zealand) or reference values for nutrient intake (Germany/Austria/Switzerland). In addition, different names may be used for the individual values within each set (Table 36.1). For example, in relation to estimates of the requirement to cover the needs of the majority of the population, the terms used include recommended dietary allowance (USA/Canada); recommended dietary intakes (Australia/New Zealand); recommended nutrient intake (FAO/WHO); recommended intake (Germany/Austria/Switzerland); or reference nutrient intake (UK). All these terms relate to the standard for a level of intake for each essential nutrient that will cover the needs of most people in that group in the population.

There has also been an increasing recognition that for some nutrients data is so limited or conflicting

Table 36.1 Different terms used for requirements of essential nutrients

R1	Lower diagnostic level of essential nutrient	EU: lowest threshold intake UK: lower reference nutrient intake (LRNI)
R2	Average nutrient requirement of a subgroup of an apparently healthy population	USA/Canada, Australia/New Zealand, UK and FAO/WHO: estimated average requirement (EAR)
R3	Amount to cover most members of the apparently healthy population	USA/Canada: recommended dietary allowance (RDA) Austria/Germany/Switzerland: recommended intake (RI) Australia/New Zealand: recommended dietary intake (RDI) FAO/WHO: recommended nutrient intake (RNI) UK: reference nutrient intake (RNI)
R4	Amount to cover most members of the apparently healthy population but where data is limited and certainty much less	USA/Canada, Australia/New Zealand: adequate intake (AI) UK: safe intake Germany/Austria/Switzerland: estimated values and guiding values (for certain nutrients)
R4	Suggested optimal range of intake	Intakes that give 'high-level' wellness or reduced risk of one, or more, degenerative diseases USA/Canada: acceptable macronutrient distribution ranges (AMDR) Australia/New Zealand: suggested dietary targets and acceptable macronutrient distribution ranges FAO/WHO: protective nutrient intake Germany/Austria/Switzerland: guiding values (for certain nutrients)
R5	Undesirably high intake or start of toxic level	USA/Canada, EU: tolerable upper intake level (UL) Australia/New Zealand: upper level (UL) UK: safe upper levels for vitamins and minerals

that the certainty with which recommendations can be made is much less than for other nutrients. In this case, some countries have used a different term such as adequate intake (US/Canada and Australia/New Zealand); estimated or guiding values for adequate intake (Germany/Austria/Switzerland) or safe intake (UK). Table 36.2 shows some international comparisons.

Why does each country have a different set of these numbers? When the figures are compared, it will be seen that many are similar, if not the same, as those from other countries. Some countries simply adopt the figures from another country or authority. For example, many developing countries will use figures published by FAO/WHO and indeed take part

in their initial development. Undertaking a major review of these figures is both time-consuming and expensive so many countries will use figures derived by another equivalent country (e.g. with a population with similar body size/culture/environment) but may vary their figures in the light of newer research data, a different philosophical approach, country-specific data, concerns about interpretation of the research data, or a perception that some key information was not considered. There may also be differences in the age groups used by different countries in relation to their own particular policy and assessment needs.

No matter what nomenclature is used, the purpose of the recommended figures is to set a standard

Table 36.2 Nutrient intake recommendations (per day) from four national sets and FAO/WHO, for selected nutrients for men: RDA/RDI/RNI, R3s in Table 36.1

Nutrient	USA/Canada 1997–2004 RDA or AI (31–50 years)	Australia/ New Zealand 2005 RDI or AI (19–51 years)	Germany/Austria/ Switzerland 2000 RI (25–51 years)	UK 1991 RNI (19–50 years)	FAO/WHO 2001 RNI (19–50 years)
Protein (g)	58	64	59	45	55[a]
Vitamin A (mg)	1.0	0.9	1.0	0.7	0.6
Vitamin D (μg)	10	5.0	5.0	—	5.0
Vitamin E (mg)	15	10.0	12	(7)	—
Thiamin (mg)	1.2	1.2	1.2	1.0	1.2
Riboflavin (mg)	1.3	1.3	1.4	1.3	1.3
Niacin (mg)	16	16	16	17	16
Vitamin B_6 (mg)	1.7	1.3	1.5	1.4	1.3
Folate (μg)	400	400	400	200	400
Vitamin B_{12} (μg)	2.4	2.4	3.0	1.5	2.4
Vitamin C (mg)	90	45	100	40	45
Calcium (mg)	1000	1000	1000	700	1000
Iron (mg)	10	8	10	8.7	9[b]
Zinc (mg)	15	14	10	9.5	7
Iodine (μg)	150	150	200	140	140[c]
Selenium (μg)	55	70	30–70	75	34

[a]1985 figures for protein.
[b]For diets with 15% bioavailability.
[c]2 μg/kg body weight (assuming body weight of 70 kg).

for an adequate intake (AI) of each essential nutrient for individuals or groups in the population. They advise people how much, on the average, they should aim to eat each day of these nutrients. They have a prescriptive or health promotion role. They also serve as the reference unit for each essential nutrient. We need them because adult human requirements for individual nutrients range 1 billion-fold from just over 1 μg for vitamin B_{12}, through 1 mg for thiamin, to 1 g for calcium and greater than 1 kg for water (Table 36.3).

The relationship among all the various measures is shown in Fig. 36.1.

Table 36.3 Range of requirements for selected essential nutrients

Adult daily requirements (rounded)	Essential nutrients
2–5 μg	Vitamin B$_{12}$, vitamin D
30–40 μg	Chromium, molybdenum, biotin
70–100 μg	Selenium, vitamin K
~150 μg	Iodine
~400 μg	Folate
1–3 mg	Vitamin A, thiamin, riboflavin, vitamin B$_6$, fluoride, copper
5–15 mg	Pantothenate, manganese, vitamin E, niacin (equivs), zinc, iron
50–100 mg	Vitamin C
400–500 mg	Magnesium, sodium
1–2 g	Calcium, phosphorus, essential fatty acids, potassium
~50 g	Protein
~2 kg (litres)	Water

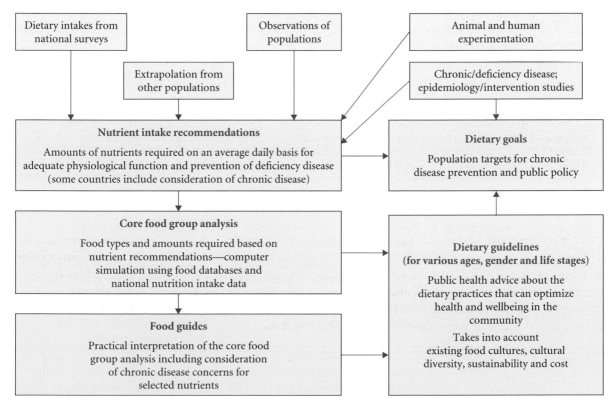

Fig. 36.1 Interrelationships between the evidence-based NIRs, Core Food Group Analysis food guides, dietary goals and dietary guidelines.

36.2 How should the various measures be used?

In the past, most countries published tables with only the single figure for population requirement (i.e. R3 in Table 36.1) variously known as the RDA, RDI or RNI, although an estimate of average requirement was generally necessary in order to derive the population figure. Since this 'population' figure is adequate to meet nutritional needs of practically all healthy people, it is more than most people need. It could not, therefore, be used directly to evaluate records of people's food intake for adequacy at the individual level, or if it was, there may be a misleading impression of inadequacy. Different approaches were used to define a diagnostic level for 'deficiency' with some people simply using two-thirds of the RDA, RDI or RNI.

In recent publications, an estimated average requirement figure has received the same prominence as the population recommendation. Although the average requirement was often to be found in the text of earlier publications, it rarely appeared in the tabular form that nutrition and health practitioners and consumers regularly used. For micronutrients, it is prudent to encourage people to eat more than the estimated average requirement for the group. Those with higher requirements should then get enough, while those with low requirements will come to no harm from eating a little more than needed. However, for energy, it is important for people to match their intake with their needs by adjusting their dietary intake and/or physical activity. Having a little more than needed each day can only increase body weight in the long term.

The availability of published and tabulated estimated average requirements helps to make assessment at the individual level more accurate than in the past. Table 36.4 shows how the various types of values now made available can be used to assess adequacy of either individual or group intakes. As part of the process of review for the US/Canadian DRIs, a statistical probability method was developed by Beaton in Canada, to assess more accurately the probability that a selected nutrient intake would be adequate for a particular person or group of people. A statistical estimate of degree of risk of inadequacy can be made

Table 36.4 Uses of the various values for assessing adequacy of intake in individuals and groups

Nutrient reference value	For individuals	For groups
Estimated average requirement (EAR)	Use to examine the probability that usual intake is inadequate	Use to estimate the prevalence of inadequate intakes within a group
Population recommendation (e.g. RDA, RDI, RNI)	Usual intake at or above this level has a low probability of inadequacy	Do not use to assess intakes of groups
Adequate intake (AI) or safe intake (population figure where data is limited or conflicting)	Usual intake at or above this level has a low probability of inadequacy. When the AI is based on median intakes of healthy populations, this assessment is made with less confidence	Mean usual intake at or above this level implies a low prevalence of inadequate intakes. When the AI is based on median intakes of healthy populations, this assessment is made with less confidence
Upper level of intake (UL)	Usual intake above this level may place an individual at risk of adverse effects from excessive nutrient intake	Use to estimate the percentage of the population at potential risk of adverse effects from excessive nutrient intake

Table 36.5 Proposed upper levels for essential nutrients for non-pregnant adults from three national sets of recommendations

	USA/Canada 1997–2000	Germany/Austria/ Switzerland 2000	Australia/New Zealand 2005
Vitamin A (mg)	3	3	3
Vitamin D (µg)	50	50	80
Vitamin E (mg)	1000	800	300
Niacin (mg)	35	35	35
Vitamin B$_6$ (mg)	100	100	50
Folate (µg)	1000	1000	1000
Vitamin B$_{12}$ (µg)	Not possible to set	5000	Not possible to set
Vitamin C (mg)	2000	1000	Not possible to set
Calcium (mg)	2500	2000	2500
Iron (mg)	45	—	45
Iodine (µg)	1100	500–1000	1100
Selenium (µg)	400	400	400

using Beaton's algorithms. The parameters used in Beaton's model are nutrient-specific, depending on the known variability in population needs for that particular nutrient (see Beaton, 1994).

Publication of an upper level of intake in some sets of recommendations has occurred partly in response to increasing interest in and use of nutrition supplements. It is difficult to overdose on vitamins and minerals from natural food sources; much easier if they are available as supplements. Consumers and pharmacists need guidance about a level that would be too much. It has long been known that vitamin A (retinol) and vitamin D can be toxic in some people at chronic intakes only ten times the RDA/RDI. It used to be acknowledged that fat-soluble vitamins could be toxic but that water-soluble vitamins would simply be excreted. The finding that vitamin B$_6$ in excess could cause peripheral neuropathy and that other water-soluble vitamins could be harmful in people with compromised kidney function changed this. Table 36.5 shows a comparison of upper intake recommendations from a number of countries. The US/Canadian DRI review defines this level as the highest level of a nutrient that is likely to pose no risk of adverse health effects for almost all individuals in the general population. As intake increases above the upper level, the risk of adverse effects increases. While there is general agreement for many nutrients, for some, estimates can vary quite widely because of the limited data.

36.3 Optimal intakes for chronic disease prevention

Although the RDAs or RDIs are traditionally determined on the basis of needs for sustenance and avoidance of deficiency disease, it is obviously most beneficial if nutrient intakes are also compatible with intakes that may reduce chronic disease risk. There is an extensive and growing database related to diet and

Table 36.6 Suggested dietary targets to reduce chronic disease risk—micronutrients, dietary fibre and long-chain n-3 fats from the Australian and New Zealand NRVs

Nutrient	Suggested dietary target[a] (intake per day on average)	Comments
Vitamin A	Vitamin A: —Men 1500 µg —Women 1220 µg Carotenes: —Men 5800 µg —Women 5000 µg	The suggested dietary target is equivalent to the 90th centile of intake in the Australian and New Zealand populations
Vitamin C	Men 220 mg Women 190 mg	Equivalent to the 90th centile of intake in the Australian/New Zealand populations
Vitamin E	Men 19 mg Women 14 mg	Equivalent to the 90th centile of intake in the Australian/New Zealand populations
Selenium	No specific figure can be set. There is some evidence of potential benefit for certain cancers but adverse effects for others	There are no available population intake data for Australia. New Zealand is a known low-selenium area; thus recommendations based on centiles of population intakes are inappropriate
Folate	An additional 100–400 µg DFE over current intakes (i.e. a total of about 300–600 µg DFE) may be required to optimize homocysteine levels and reduce overall chronic disease risk and DNA damage	Current population intakes are well below the new recommended intakes
Sodium/potassium	Sodium: —Men 1600 mg, 70 mmol —Women 1600 mg, 70 mmol Potassium: —Men 4700 mg, 120 mmol —Women 4700 mg, 120 mmol	An upper level of 2300 mg (100 mmol)/day was set for the general population, but it is recognized that additional preventive health benefits (in terms of maintaining optimal blood pressure over the lifespan and thus reducing stroke and heart disease) may accrue if sodium intakes are further reduced to about 1600 mg (70 mmol)/day, in line with WHO recommendations. Reducing intakes to this level may also bring immediate benefit to older and overweight members of the community with pre-existing hypertension. As potassium can blunt the effect of sodium on blood pressure, intakes at the 90th centile of current population intake may help to mitigate the effects of sodium on blood pressure until intakes of sodium can be lowered. At the level of 4700 mg/day for potassium, there is also evidence of protection against renal stones
Dietary fibre	Men 38 g Women 28 g	Upper level at 90th centile of intake for reduction in CHD risk
Long-chain n-3 fats (DHA, EPA, DPA)	Men 610 mg Women 430 mg	The suggested dietary target is equivalent to the 90th centile of intake in the Australian/New Zealand population

[a]For most nutrients, unless otherwise noted, this is based on the 90th centile of current population intake.
DFE = dietary folate equivalents.

chronic disease risk in humans, but the population methodologies generally employed have a number of limitations in relation to identifying a specific level of intake that is optimal for reducing the risk of chronic disease. With that proviso in mind, there is some evidence that a range of nutrients could have benefits in chronic disease aetiology at levels above the RDI/RDA/RNIs.

The nutrients for which higher-than-recommended population intakes have been linked to benefits for chronic disease include the antioxidant vitamins such as vitamin C, vitamin E and vitamin A (primarily its precursor, β-carotene) as well as selenium and nutrients such as folate, ω-3 fats and dietary fibre. For these nutrients, there is a reasonably large body of evidence of potential protective effects of higher than RDA/RDI levels for one or more chronic disease such as coronary heart disease, certain cancers, degenerative eye diseases (such as cataract formation or macular degeneration) and conditions like Alzheimer's or cognitive decline. In the case of folate, higher than RDA/RDI levels may also further decrease the occurrence of neural tube defects. There is also a lesser volume of evidence for a number of other nutrients. The 'suggested dietary targets' for micronutrients for prevention of chronic disease from the Australian/New Zealand nutrient reference values (NRVs) are shown in Table 36.6. As it is difficult to identify accurately the levels of intake that confer optimal protection, these Australian/New Zealand targets were generally set at the 90th percentile of current population dietary intake, on the premise that many epidemiological findings are based on observational data comparing upper and lower quintiles of intake in the population under study and that this level of intake is unlikely to cause harm.

In addition to micronutrients, the role of the various types of carbohydrates (starches, sugars, high-glycaemic versus low-glycaemic carbohydrates, resistant starch, dietary fibres), fats (saturated, polyunsaturated, monounsaturated) and protein (animal, plant-based) have been variously assessed in relation to risk of conditions such as coronary heart disease, certain cancers, diabetes or insulin sensitivity and risk of obesity. Unlike the micronutrients, the macro-nutrients (proteins, fats and carbohydrates) all contribute to dietary energy intake.

For a given energy intake, increases in the proportion of one macronutrient necessarily involves a decrease in the proportion of one, or more, of the other macronutrients—a high-fat diet is usually relatively low in carbohydrate and vice versa. A major imbalance in the relative proportions of macronutrients can increase risk of chronic disease and may adversely affect micronutrient intake. However, the form of fat (e.g. saturated, polyunsaturated or monounsaturated or specific fatty acids) or carbohydrate (e.g. starches or sugars, high or low glycaemic index) is also a major consideration in determining the optimal balance in terms of chronic disease risk.

There appears to be quite a wide range of relative intakes of proteins, carbohydrates and fats that are acceptable in terms of chronic disease risk. The risk of chronic disease (as well as the risk of inadequate micronutrient intake) may increase outside these ranges, but often data in free-living populations are limited at these extremes of intake. Much of the evidence is based on epidemiological studies with clinical endpoints but these studies generally show associations rather than causality and are often confounded by other factors that can affect chronic disease outcomes. The macronutrient recommendations from the US/Canadian DRIs and the Australian/New Zealand NRVs with respect to the acceptable range are shown in Table 36.7.

These acceptable macronutrient distribution ranges and the recommendations for micronutrient intakes for chronic disease prevention seem, on the surface, to resemble what are sometimes called 'dietary goals'. However, dietary goals are designed to direct national policy by outlining what nutrients or foods the nation should consume and provide, and are primarily addressed to bureaucrats and professionals. They are population targets whereas the 'acceptable macronutrient distribution ranges' and 'suggested dietary targets' for chronic disease prevention are aimed at individuals in the population.

One recent example of population dietary goals was produced by the WHO in 2003, in a report called *Diet, nutrition and the prevention of chronic*

Table 36.7 Acceptable macronutrient distribution ranges for macronutrients to reduce chronic disease risk while still ensuring adequate micronutrient status

Nutrient	Australia/New Zealand 2005	US/Canada 2005
Protein	15–25% of energy	10–35% of energy
Carbohydrate	45–65% of energy (predominantly from low energy density and/or low-glycaemic-index foods)	45–65% of energy
Fat	20–35% of energy	20–35% of energy
Linoleic acid (n-6 fat)	From 4–5% to 10% of energy	5–10% of energy
α-Linolenic acid (n-3 fat)	From 0.4–0.5% to 1% energy	0.6–1.2% of energy

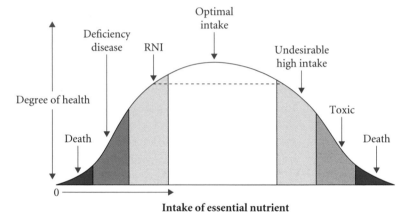

Fig. 36.2 The concept of optimal intake above the population recommended nutrient intake (i.e. RNI/RDA/RDI). Ingestion of the RNI/RDA/RDI should guarantee no deficiency disease, but beyond this there may still be additional health benefits (e.g. partial protection from a degenerative disease). The top of the dome beyond the RNI/RDA/RDI is then the optimal intake range.

disease. The WHO produced a suite of goals including some for percentage energy to be supplied by different macronutrients, for cholesterol (less than 300 mg/day) and sodium (less than 2 g/day) as well as for certain food groups (fruit and vegetable intake of 5400 g/day). When recommendations are made about nutrient intake for chronic disease prevention, it is thus important to be clear whether the cut-off numbers refer to populations or individuals. If the goal is set for the population, not every individual needs to conform for the population goal to be met.

Fig. 36.2 shows the general inter-relationships between the various levels of recommended intakes and health outcomes.

36.4 Recommendations for nutrient intakes, food labelling and standards

In many countries, labels on food packaging carry information relating the content of that food to a daily reference figure for intake derived from the nutrient recommendations. Because of the limitations of size in most instances, a single reference figure for a given nutrient is derived from the range available across gender and age bands. In the USA, this kind of figure is called a daily value (DV) and the nutrient content of a food may be expressed as % DV per serving or per unit weight, based on their 1968 RDAs.

With adoption of the new DRVs in the US and Canada, it has been recommended that the concept of expressing nutrient content as % DV be retained and that the DV be based on the population-weighted estimated average requirement. Where no estimated average requirement (EAR) could be set, the AI would be used as the reference. In addition, it was recommended that the acceptable macronutrient distribution ranges should be the basis for the DVs for the macronutrients protein, total carbohydrate and total fat; that 2000 calories should be used, when needed, as the basis for expressing energy intake when developing DVs; and finally that the DVs for saturated fatty acids, *trans* fatty acids and cholesterol should be set at a level as low as possible in keeping with an achievable health-promoting diet. For infancy, toddlers aged 1–3 years, pregnancy and lactation, dif-

ferent sets of DVs were recommended based on the EAR or AIs for those specific groups as their needs vary markedly from the general population.

In Australia and New Zealand, before the recent revision of NRVs (2005), the food law RDIs were based on the highest 1991 Australian/New Zealand RDIs for non-pregnant, non-lactating, younger adults. Thus, the RDI for younger adult men was generally used, with the exception of iron, for which the lower end of the range for younger women was used. This approach is likely to change with the advent of the new NRVs.

The wordings and the reference values used for food for labelling purposes are generally laid down by food law set by statutory bodies such as the Food and Drug Administration (FDA) in the USA or Food Standards Australia New Zealand (FSANZ) in Australia and New Zealand. The same reference value may be used in controlling permitted additions of micronutrients in food fortification (e.g. up to 50% DV may be added per reference quantity of food 'X').

36.5 Dietary guidelines

In contrast to dietary goals, 'dietary guidelines' are usually developed as advice to the general public about optimal food choices and consumption behaviours, written in reader-friendly language for ordinary people, although they are often backed up by a technical explanation, which may include quantitative expression of the guideline in the form of a food guide such as the US diet pyramid. Examples include statements such as 'enjoy a variety of nutritious food', 'eat plenty of vegetables, legumes and fruits', 'choose foods low in salt', 'care for your food, and prepare and store it safely' and 'encourage and support breastfeeding'. The dietary guidelines usually come as a set of recommendations that are meant to be adopted as a whole to produce an overall dietary pattern that will optimize health and wellbeing and prevent chronic disease, while providing all essential nutrients. Box 36.1 highlights some of the differences between dietary guidelines and goals, and nutrient intake recommendations.

In recent years, guidelines related to encouraging maintenance of desirable body weights and physical activity have been added to some countries suite of guidelines, in recognition of the intimate relationship between dietary intake of energy and appropriate physical activity in maintenance of appropriate body weight.

Dietary guidelines have been published in at least 35 countries, starting with the Nordic countries in 1968. As an example, Table 36.8 shows the headings of the *Dietary guidelines for Australian adults* published in 2003 and Table 36.9 shows a comparison of key messages related to cereal consumption from various countries. In many countries, there have been several new editions or publications since the first appearance.

Some countries produce a single set of recommendations for their population no matter what age or lifestyle; others (such as New Zealand and Australia) have developed different sets of recommendations

BOX 36.1 Comparison of nutrient intake recommendations (NIRs) and dietary goals and guidelines (DGGs)

- NIRs are primarily designed to ensure adequate intake of essential nutrients, while the focus of DGGs is promotion of general health as well as prevention of chronic disease. However, when developing dietary guidelines this is done in such a way as to also ensure adequate essential nutrient intake. Some countries (e.g. the USA and Canada) now include consideration of chronic disease prevention in setting their NIRs.

- NIRs deal only with essential nutrients. Dietary goals deal more with the balance of macronutrients (although some chronic disease-related micronutrients such as sodium may be included). Dietary guidelines have a whole-diet approach with a food group and dietary behaviour focus for optimal health and wellbeing, avoidance of deficiency disease and prevention of chronic disease.

- NIRs are expressed in terms of amounts of nutrients required per day (and right now) for optimal physiological function and prevention of deficiency in a specified age, gender or lifestyle group (e.g. an estimated average requirement of 5 mg/day for women aged 19–51 years). NIRs have both an individual (EAR) and a population (RDA/RDI/RNI) component. Dietary goals are traditionally population targets often expressed in relative terms (e.g. less than 10% energy as saturated fat). While being seen as appropriate for the here and now, they often have a time line attached for purposes of monitoring success of government initiatives to improve national dietary intake (e.g. a population mean intake of less than 10% saturated fat by the year 2010). Dietary guidelines are generally expressed qualitatively (e.g. 'eat plenty of fruits, vegetables and legumes'; 'choose foods low in salt') but may be quantified in an accompanying food guide giving recommendations as specified 'serves' per day of various food groups (e.g. the US Dietary Pyramid). As with NIRs, the dietary guidelines are for the here and now although it is recognized that it may take some time for people to fully adopt the recommendations.

- Although NRIs are relatively well established scientifically and usually depend on the results of short-term physiological experiments, DGGs are more provisional and are based on indirect evidence about the complex role of food components in multifactorial diseases with long incubation periods. They rely more on epidemiological evidence than NIRs.

Table 36.8 Dietary guidelines for Australian adults

Enjoy a wide variety of nutritious foods
Eat plenty of vegetables, legumes and fruits
Eat plenty of cereals (including breads, rice, pasta and noodles)—preferably wholegrain
Include lean meat, fish, poultry and/or alternatives
Include milks, yoghurts, cheeses and/or alternatives—reduced-fat varieties should be chosen where possible
Drink plenty of water
Take care to:
Limit saturated fat and moderate fat intake
Choose foods low in salt
Limit your alcohol intake if you choose to drink
Consume only moderate amounts of sugars and foods containing added sugars
Prevent weight gain—be physically active and eat according to your energy needs
Care for your food—prepare and store it safely
Encourage and support breastfeeding

Table 36.9 Comparison of guidelines mentioning cereals from various countries

Country, year	Guideline
Australia 2003	Eat plenty of cereals (including breads, rice, pasta and noodles)—preferably wholegrain
Denmark 1983	Eat more bread and corn products, potatoes, vegetables and fruit
France 1981	For sufficient fibre, take wholemeal breads, vegetables, cereals, (dry) legumes, dried fruits, etc.
Hungary 1988	Always have wholegrain bread on the table; choose potatoes over rice
Japan 1985	Eat 30 (different) foodstuffs a day; take staple food (i.e. rice) main dish and side dish together
Singapore 1989	Increase intake of fruit and vegetables and wholegrain cereal products, thereby increasing vitamins A and C and fibre
UK 1990	Eat plenty of food rich in starch and fibre (examples given)
USA 2005	Consume three or more ounce-equivalents of wholegrain products per day, with the rest of the recommended grains (depending on age, gender and activity category) coming from enriched or whole-grain products. In general, at least half the grains should come from whole grains

for various groups such as infants and toddlers, children, adults, the elderly and, in the case of New Zealand, pregnant and lactating women. This latter approach was encouraged by the WHO at a 1993 symposium, which concluded that guidelines would be most effective if targeted to defined groups.

The recently released revision of the *US Dietary guidelines* (2005) has also taken a slightly different approach to earlier versions, with two overarching general recommendations based on adoption of specific eating plans ('meet recommended intakes within energy needs by adopting a balanced eating pattern, such as the USDA Food Guide or the DASH Eating Plan') and a recommendation to 'consume a variety of nutrient-dense foods and beverages within and among the basic food groups while choosing foods that limit the intake of saturated and *trans* fats, cholesterol, added sugars, salt, and alcohol'. In addition, there are a series of key recommendations for specific population groups (e.g. people over age 50; women of childbearing age who may become pregnant and those in the first trimester of pregnancy; older adults; people with dark skin; and people exposed to insufficient ultraviolet band radiation).

There are also recommendations for specific amounts of foods and selected nutrients required in general or for specific groups in the population, and weight management and physical activity recommendations for the general population and for specific population groups. Alcohol consumption and food safety are also addressed. This set of guidelines seeks to be more comprehensive and tailored to the needs of various groups in the population than earlier versions of the US dietary guidelines, which were more generic.

In addition to the various national sets of dietary guidelines, organizations such as the WHO have been active in the development of food-based dietary guidelines, particularly aimed at assisting developing countries, and many health authorities such as heart, cancer, diabetes or vegetarian foundations or societies have also produced guidelines for their constituencies.

Among the various sets of recommendations, there are some common themes as shown in Box 36.2, although precise wording may vary.

Other guidelines that are more controversial and less widely recommended relate to issues such as polyunsaturated fats, dietary cholesterol and 'refined',

---

BOX 36.2 Dietary guidelines for which there is almost complete agreement across countries

- Eat a nutritionally adequate diet composed of a variety of foods
- Eat less fat (particularly saturated fat)
- Adjust energy balance for body weight control (match energy intake to physical activity)
- Eat more wholegrain cereals, vegetables and fruits
- Reduce salt intake
- Drink alcohol in moderation (if you drink at all)

'extrinsic', 'added' or 'concentrated' sugars (i.e. not the natural sugars found in fruits and milk). On sugar, there is the widest range of opinions. Some countries recommend that less than 10% of energy comes from refined sugars (e.g. Nordic countries and Singapore); others do not mention sugar at all (e.g. Japan and South Korea). There are many different guidelines related to sugar including:

- Do not increase sugar consumption.
- Decrease sugar (not quantified).

- Consume only moderate amounts of sugars and foods containing added sugars.
- Cut down on sugary snacks and sweets between meals.
- Eat sweets seldom.
- Reduce sugary snacks.

A third group of recommendations appear only in a few sets of guidelines:

- Quench thirst with water.
- Drink fluoridated water (or fluoride tablets).
- Make sure you get enough calcium or milk.
- Preserve (by good food preparation) the nutritive value of foods.
- Keep food safe to eat.
- Eat three good meals a day.
- Do not eat too much protein.
- Eat foods containing iron.
- Reduced intake of salt-cured, preserved and smoked foods.
- Limit caffeine intake.
- Eat happily for a happy family life.

36.6 How do the nutrient intake recommendations relate to the dietary goals and guidelines?

Recommendations about desirable intakes of essential nutrients and dietary goals and guidelines are often developed within countries or in international bodies at different times of the review cycle and by different committees. There is no need for this to occur, although the technical nature of the nutrient recommendations may require a rather different emphasis on nutrition science expertise, whereas the goals and guidelines have a broader social and public health aspect. While the assessment of essential nutrient needs is not reliant on the existence of dietary goals and guidelines, development of the latter are to some degree predicated on a knowledge of essential nutrient needs across the population.

It should go without saying that a diet that may lower the incidence of chronic disease (e.g. one lower in dietary fat or saturated) will not bring optimal health and wellbeing in the community if, in lowering the intake of fat or saturated fat, it compromises attainment of intake of essential fat-soluble vitamins, essential fatty acids or nutrients commonly found in foods also contributing to saturated fat intake (e.g. meats and milks). If goals aimed at reducing saturated fat result in people eating substantially less meat and milks, rather than choosing lower-fat versions, then intakes of certain nutrients that are borderline in the community, such as iron and zinc, which are primarily sourced from these food groups, may be compromised.

Thus, in order to develop goals and guidelines in such a way as to achieve the desired outcomes, consideration of essential nutrient needs is a necessary first step (see Fig. 36.1). It is a common misconception that dietary goals and guidelines are developed only from consideration of the evidence from chronic disease epidemiology. For example, in countries such as Australia and the USA, the more quantitative aspect of the certain guidelines are derived by a computerized modelling exercise linking nutrients to foods using national food databases to derive the amounts and types of various foods/food groups required to attain the nutrient needs of the various groups. Once basic requirements are met, this can then be refined and added to with reference to the evidence from chronic disease epidemiology.

36.7 Dietary goals and guidelines in developing countries

Dietary guidelines were originally introduced to address the nutrition problems of excess in affluent countries. In developing countries, the major nutritional problem is that large sections of the population cannot afford or cannot grow enough food to meet all their family's requirements for essential nutrients. There are, however, reasons why dietary goals and guidelines have a role in developing countries.

- Diet-related, non-communicable diseases in developing countries account for an increasing share of national mortality.

- Low-income countries cannot afford to add the burden of medical care of premature degenerative diseases to their already-overstretched health budgets.

- Preparation and production of dietary guidelines is a low-cost measure.

- The affluent middle-class in a country such as India or Indonesia may only be 5% of the population, but this means many millions of people (about 40 million in India—more than many whole nations). Many of these more affluent people in the community play a key role in the nation's development.

For India, Gopalan (1989) has proposed two sets of guidelines. For the 'relatively poor' majority, diets should be the least expensive and conform to tradition and cultural practice as far as possible. Some legumes (pulses) should be eaten along with the high-cereal diet, with some milk and leafy vegetable eaten each day. For affluent Indians, he recommends restriction of energy and of fat (especially ghee), sugar and salt, with emphasis on unrefined cereals and green leafy vegetables in the diet.

Consideration of the need for dietary guidance in developing countries has led to a move to coordinate development of food-based guidelines for specific sociocultural context that reflect the social, economic, agricultural and environmental factors affecting food availability and eating patterns in that particular community. It is envisaged that these will be primarily focused on food patterns and related to the key public health issues for that community.

36.8 The role of nutrient intake recommendations and dietary guidelines in nutrition promotion

In most countries, for the general community, the 'public face' of the national recommendations relating to nutrient intake and dietary guidelines takes the form of a food choice guide, which is generally summarized in a graphical form with some additional explanatory text.

Most countries base their guide on food groups but the number of food groups varies widely from as few as three, in countries such as Fiji and a number of African countries, to seven or eight in countries such as the Caribbean. In industrialized countries, food guides generally contain between four and six food groups. Three-group systems often group foods under the headings of 'energy' foods (grains, tubers, etc. and sometimes fats and oils), 'protein' or 'growth' foods (meats, milks, legumes, etc.) and 'sustenance' foods to provide additional vitamins and minerals (fruits and vegetables, etc.). Groupings commonly used in the more complex guides include meat/fish/poultry and alternatives (including legumes), milk and milk products, fruits, vegetables, cereals, fats and oils. Because of the degree of commonality in their nutrient profile, fruits and vegetables often form a single group. Sometimes, because of the importance of a particular staple, such as potato in Finland, that particular food alone constitutes one of the categories. Sometimes the 'starchy' foods such as potato, rice and other cereals are grouped together. Some countries also include an additional food group category of 'less healthy' extra or indulgence foods —generally these are energy-dense foods or drinks, high in fat, salt, sugar or alcohol. They are addressed in recognition that these foods and drinks do form part of the food supply in many countries and can form part of a healthy diet if consumed in small amounts.

The graphic display of food group recommendations also varies from country to country (see Fig. 36.3). In the USA, a pyramid form is used. The 1990s version showed breads and cereals at the base, with fruits and vegetables at the next level, followed by meat and alternatives and the milk group on the next level, and finally fats and sweets at the pinnacle. The most recent 2005 revision aligns all food groups

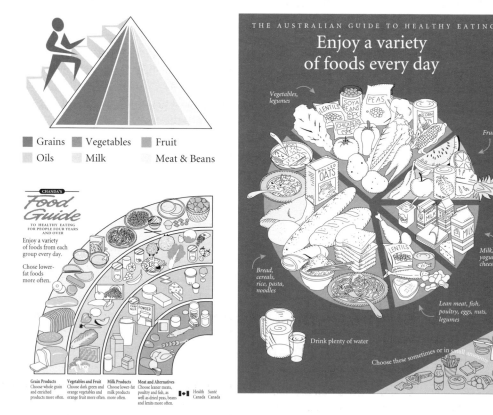

Fig. 36.3 Examples of three national food guides—the US Pyramid, the Canadian Rainbow and the Australian Guide to Healthy Eating.

vertically in a pyramid with the groups represented by different-coloured segments, displayed in proportion to the recommended amounts. There are no representations of foods *per se* in the new graphic. Some Nordic countries, together with health organizations in China, Australia and New Zealand, have also used pyramid or triangle designs. In the UK, Australia, many European countries and the Caribbean, the national food guide is depicted as a plate or in a

circular or semicircular design often divided up in proportion into the recommended amounts for the various food groups. Sometimes a food square is used in developing countries with each group equally represented (e.g. Iran). Other designs include a quarter-rainbow (Canada), steps (New Zealand), a wine glass (Israel) and a traffic light (UK Health Education Council), which is also often used in diabetic education materials.

36.9 Summary

In summary, there are a number of types of nutrition information and guidance that governments provide for their population to optimize health and address both deficiency and chronic disease prevalence. The information made available ranges from the more technical nutrient intake recommendations, which are now available both for individuals and for groups in the community, through to national food guides that attempt to summarize all these various recommendations in a user-friendly graphic mode. The various sets of recommendations are interrelated and dependent on one another to varying degrees, but each serves a specific purpose ranging from the setting and monitoring of national food and nutrition policy by bureaucrats to health promotion for the general public.

FURTHER READING

1. **Beaton, G.H.** (1994) Criteria of an adequate diet. In Shils, M.E., Olson, J.A. and Shike, M. (eds) *Modern nutrition in health and disease*, 8th edn, pp. 1491–505. Philadelphia, Lea & Febiger.

2. **Bengoa, J.M., Torun, B., Behar, M., and Scrimshaw, N.** (1988) *Guias de alimentacion bases para su desarrollo en America Latina*. Guatemala City, INCAP.

3. **Commonwealth Department of Health and Ageing, New Zealand Ministry of Health, NHMRC** (2005) *Nutrient reference values for Australia and New Zealand including recommended dietary intakes*. Canberra, National Health and Medical Research Council.

4. **Department of Health.** (1991) *Dietary reference values for food energy and nutrients for the United Kingdom*. Report of the panel on dietary reference values of the Committee on Medical Aspects of Food Policy. London, HMSO.

5. **Expert Group on Vitamins and Minerals** (2003) *Safe upper levels for vitamins and minerals*. London, Food Standards Agency.

6. **FAO/WHO/UN** (1985) *Energy and protein requirements*. Report of a joint FAO/WHO/UNU Expert Consultation. Technical Report Series No. 724. Geneva, World Health Organization.

7. **FAO/WHO** (1988) *Preparation and use of food-based dietary guidelines*. Report of a joint FAO/WHO Consultation. WHO Technical Report Series 880. Geneva, FAO/WHO.

8. **FAO/WHO** (2001) *Human vitamin and mineral requirements. Report of a joint FAO/WHO Expert Consultation in Bangkok, Thailand*. Rome, Food and Agricultural Organization.

9. **Food and Nutrition Board: Institute of Medicine** (1997) *Dietary reference intakes for calcium, phosphorus, magnesium, vitamin D and fluoride*. Washington, DC, National Academy Press.

10. **Food and Nutrition Board: Institute of Medicine** (1998) *Dietary reference intakes for thiamin, riboflavin, niacin, vitamin B$_6$, folate, vitamin B$_{12}$, pantothenic acid, biotin, and choline*. Washington, DC, National Academy Press.

11. **Food and Nutrition Board: Institute of Medicine** (1998) *Dietary reference intakes. A risk assessment model for establishing upper intake level for nutrients*. Washington, DC, National Academy Press.

12. **Food and Nutrition Board: Institute of Medicine** (2000) *Dietary reference intakes for vitamin C, vitamin E, selenium and carotenoids.* Washington, DC, National Academy Press.

13. **Food and Nutrition Board: Institute of Medicine** (2000) *Dietary reference intakes. Applications in dietary assessment.* Washington, DC, National Academy Press.

14. **Food and Nutrition Board: Institute of Medicine** (2001) *Dietary reference intakes for vitamin A, vitamin K, arsenic, boron, chromium, copper, iodine, iron, manganese, molybdenum, nickel, silicon, vanadium and zinc.* Washington, DC, National Academy Press.

15. **Food and Nutrition Board: Institute of Medicine** (2002) *Dietary reference intakes for energy, carbohydrate, fiber, fat, fatty acids, cholesterol, protein and amino acids (macronutrients).* Washington, DC, National Academy Press.

16. **Food and Nutrition Board: Institute of Medicine** (2003) *Dietary reference intakes: Guiding principles for nutrition labeling and fortification.* Washington, DC, National Academy Press.

17. **Food and Nutrition Board: Institute of Medicine** (2004) *Dietary reference intakes for water, potassium, sodium, chloride and sulfate.* Panel on the dietary reference intakes for electrolytes and water. Washington, DC, National Academy Press.

18. **German Nutrition Society/Austrian Nutrition Society/ Swiss Society for Nutrition Research/Swiss Nutrition Association** (2001) *Reference values for nutrient intake.* Frankfurt, Main, Umschau, Braus, German Nutrition Society. Translated by S. Sampe and A.S. Truswell.

19. **Gopalan, C.** (1989) Dietary guidelines from the perspective of developing countries. In: Latham, M.C., and van Veen, M.S. (eds) *Dietary guidelines: Proceedings of an International Conference. International Monograph 21.* Ithaca, NY, Cornell.

20. **Hunt, P., Gatenby, S., and Rayner, M.** (1995) The format for the National Food Guide: performance and preference studies. *J Hum Nutr Diet*, **8**, 335–51.

21. **Nordic Working Group on Diet and Nutrition** (1996) Nordic nutrition recommendations. *Scand J Nutr Naringsforskning*, **40**, 161–65.

22. **Truswell, A.S.** (1998) Dietary goals, and guidelines: national and international perspectives. In: Shils, M.E., Olson, J.A., Shike, M., and Ross, M.C. (eds) *Modern nutrition in health and disease*, 9th edition. Baltimore MD, Williams and Wilkins, pp. 1727–41.

23. **WHO** (2003) *Diet, nutrition and the prevention of chronic disease.* Report of a joint WHO/FAO Expert Consultation. WHO Technical Report Series 916. Geneva, World Health Organization.

 To see topical and scientifically robust updates on nutrition associated with this textbook, and active web links to many of the journal articles in the Reference areas, please see the dedicated Online Resource Centre at www.oxfordtextbooks.co.uk/orc/mann3e/.

37 Dietary counselling to change behaviour

Paula Hunt

In its broadest sense, the process of counselling enables clients to feel empowered to make decisions to help them live in a more satisfying and resourceful way. In *dietary* counselling, the specific aim is to change dietary behaviour to manage disease or improve risk factors for overall health.

37.1 Changing behaviour

It is clear from the literature and now generally accepted that information-giving alone is insufficient to achieve behavioural change. Eating is a behaviour influenced by a wide variety of factors and it is not surprising that simply telling someone what they must eat in order to improve their health will usually fail to achieve successful and sustained dietary change. Health professionals wanting to play a change-agent role will have to resist the 'medical model' of direct persuasion and coercion and adopt a client-centred approach. A professional-led persuasive approach assumes people will automatically be motivated enough to act on the information given, partly due to the credibility of the professional giving the advice and partly in response to health risk.

A considerable body of evidence suggests that the most effective types of dietary intervention are:

1. Client-centred.
2. Tailored according to the individual's:
   level of risk
   readiness to change
   present diet.
3. Intensive:
   longer rather than shorter sessions
   more than one session
   with repeated follow-up.
4. Actively involve the patient.

Standard advice given in a blanket form or a prescriptive manner to all patients and very short one-off and/or passive consultations are unlikely to have a successful outcome. Effective nutrition interventions need a behavioural approach.

37.2 Client-centredness

Communicating in a client-centred way is key to effective dietary change. Being client-centred shows acceptance and respect for people *as they are* and supports their self-esteem with the perhaps paradoxical consequence that they then seem 'freed up' to consider change. It begins with rapport-building and scene-setting and continues with the practitioner genuinely trying to understand the problem through the client's eyes and work on possible solutions together. It ends with the client feeling that they 'own' the plan for action because they have created it. Most importantly, they feel it is feasible and realistic.

Being client-centred in dietary counselling means more than smiling a lot and nodding kindly. It involves:

- demonstrating the three core practitioner qualities; unconditional acceptance, genuineness and empathy;

- using skills such as asking open questions, listening attentively, reflecting what you hear, summarizing accurately, offering rather than imposing information and presenting options for change rather than single solutions;

- adopting a medley of strategies borrowed from a variety of different therapies such as motivational interviewing and cognitive behavioural therapy.

Rollnick and colleagues (1999) have identified some common mistakes and dangerous assumptions made by health professionals who are not working in a client-centred way. Their list of things that can easily result in failed behaviour-change consultations includes: assuming that the person ought to or wants to change; that this is the right time for the person to change; that health is a prime motivating factor for the patient; and that because you are the expert the person must follow your advice. Ridding yourself of these assumptions will help greatly in your efforts to be truly client-centred. The key signals that you have got it right are summarized in Box 37.1.

> **BOX 37.1** Client-centredness: getting it right.
>
> Some of the key signals are:
>
> - You are speaking slowly
> - The patient is doing much more of the talking than you
> - The patient is actively talking about behaviour change
> - You are listening very carefully, and gently directing the interview at appropriate moments
> - The patient appears to be 'working hard', often realizing things for the first time
> - The patient is actively asking for information and advice
> - It feels as if you are holding up a canvas, and the patient is filling it with paint, in places sometimes selected by you, and sometimes by the patient
>
> Adapted from Rollnick *et al.* (1999) .

37.3 Understanding the change process

Part of understanding how best to help patients is to appreciate fully what happens from their own perspective, consciously or subconsciously, when they change a behaviour such as diet. To understand the change process better, a model described by Prochaska and DiClemente (1986), called the 'Stages of Change' is shown in Fig. 37.1. The model describes the different stages people typically go through, before successfully changing any behaviour. The model sees change as a process, which happens over time, rather than a single one-off event. Although not intended as a rigid tool to 'box' people in to stages, the general features of each stage are summarized in Table 37.1. By identifying what stage of change a person is in, a health professional will have a better indication of how best to steer the consultation.

The stages of change are usually shown as a circular model, like a revolving door. People can get stuck in different stages, move backwards or forwards or spiral onwards. Some people get stuck in 'contemplation' and are always thinking about changing but never quite get round to it. Others, for example, chronic dieters, constantly take 'action' but never progress to 'maintenance'. They are always making

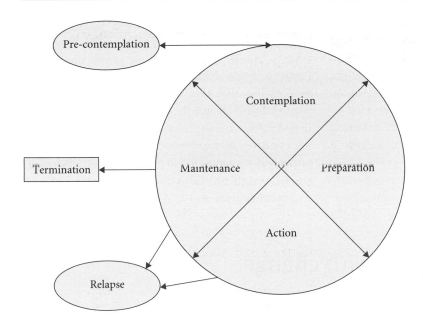

Fig. 37.1 The Stages of Change model.

Source: Prochaska and DiClemente (1986)

Table 37.1 Features of each stage of change

Stage	People in this stage are:
Pre-contemplation	Not seriously considering the possibility of change, either because they are unaware of it or because they resist confronting it
Contemplation	Aware of, or acknowledges, the existence of a problem Seriously considering the possibility of change but feel two ways about it (i.e. ambivalent) Able to see the benefits but distressed about what would have to be given up
Preparation	Decided in their commitment to change and will make a change in the very near future (within 3 months) Still ambivalent
Action	Actually starting to make changes in their behaviour May be very confident in their ability to sustain change at the start
Maintenance	Attempting to sustain the progress achieved during action Likely to be constantly struggling with thoughts about relapsing (lasts between 6 months and a lifetime)
Termination	Free from the temptation to return to old behaviours (the new behaviour is more habitual than the old)
Relapse	(not strictly a stage of change but a possible outcome of action or maintenance) Unsuccessful in their attempt at change Likely to go back into contemplation and seriously intend to make another attempt at change in the near future

a new attempt at losing weight without ever maintaining any losses achieved. Generally, people will go around the stages of change, making several unsuccessful attempts at change, before they finally go into maintenance and termination. Relapse (or recycling) is viewed positively; there are always reasons for relapse and these can be discussed with a view to having better success at the next change attempt. Relapse is always a learning experience.

Prochaska and DiClemente's model is transtheoretical. That is, it applies irrespective of the counselling/helping method being adopted. Whether you use a cognitive, behavioural, humanistic, psychoanalytic or experiential approach to helping, the Stages of Change model can apply to how people change. Its beauty is that it offers cues for the professional helper as to how to intervene, which will depend loosely on which stage of change the client is in. Two limitations in dietary counselling are (i) that because of the shifting nature of motivation and change it is not always possible to fix people into a particular stage of change, and (ii) people may be in different stages for different eating behaviours.

37.4 Skills for helping with change

It will now be clear that it is inappropriate to assume every patient is ready to change what they eat. Assessing whether the patient is ready to change first, then using the appropriate skills and strategies for helping, is a far safer approach. To establish a patient's readiness for change, the simplest approach is to ask, but this should be tentative and curious rather than a stark and direct question. Indeed, the question is most helpfully broken down into two parts, which assess important components of readiness; importance (in the value of changing) and confidence (in succeeding) and can be softened by preceding it with 'I'm wondering how you feel just now about changing your diet'. Rollnick and colleagues (1999) suggest offering patients a scale of 1 to 10, for where they see themselves in terms of, firstly, importance, then confidence.

'How important is it to you, personally, to eat differently? If "0" was "not important" and "10" was very important, what number would you give yourself?' Then 'And if you tried to change, how confident do you feel that you would succeed—again, on a scale of 0 to 10?'

Alternatively, a less-structured approach may feel more comfortable. For example, asking (with a hint of genuine curiosity) 'I'm not really sure *exactly* how you feel about changing your diet—what do you make of it all?' can reveal a lot. In some cases, it may even be appropriate to show the Stages of Change model to the patient and ask which stage they feel they are in. The main cut-off point is between those who are clearly not yet ready to change (precontemplators and contemplators) and those who are ready to change (in preparation or action).

In their work, Prochaska and DiClemente found that in order to prepare to change, clients need to believe that:

- Their current behaviour is 'bad for them' (change is for valid reasons).

- They will be better off if they change (change is worthwhile).

- They have a good chance of succeeding if they try to change (confidence).

Only a skilled practitioner can help patients identify with these beliefs or work towards them. Imposing them usually fails or backfires. Use of the following skills is central to creating a consultation within which clients truly feel they are being empowered to change:

- Listening.

- Asking open questions.

- Offering rather than imposing information.

Listen attentively, using reflective comments to show not only that you are listening but also that you have understood. 'So, it sounds as though you see the benefits in changing your diet, but on the other hand you're worried because of your long working hours and shift patterns and because you fear it might be more expensive to buy different foods. Have I got that right?'

Ask open questions along the theme of 'what', 'how' or 'where', which encourages patients to give more information about themselves. 'How do you see your diet and its links with your health?', 'What do you make of the things you've read about diet and diabetes?' These are much more helpful than closed questions (Do you . . . ? Have you . . . ? Are you saying that . . . ?) that need only a yes/no answer. 'Perhaps we can start by you telling me a bit about *how* food fits into your typical day. *How* has it changed over time?'

Offer information rather than imposing it. Patients will rarely refuse your invitation, but will respect the fact that you have asked. 'Your blood pressure is a little bit high. I wonder if you'd be interested in me talking a bit about blood pressure, your health and how diet might improve it?'

37.5 Strategies for helping people change

Although there is no clear-cut evidence to suggest that specific interventions only work for people in specific stages, some general themes apply. Some ideas to guide the practitioner in the type of help that may most match the various stages of change are summarized in Table 37.2.

37.6 Barriers to change

It seems reasonable (and much more client-centred) to assume that every patient has barriers to change. Few patients think it is going to be easy and those who do are perhaps being unrealistic. Barriers certainly need to be addressed as part of preparing to make a plan for change. For some patients, barriers instantly arise in the contemplation stage, as reasons against changing. For others, they will become cues for relapse if they are not thought through at the pre-paration stage. Common barriers to dietary change include:

- A perception that eating healthily will be prohibitively expensive.
- Having to give up favourite foods.
- Concern about having to eat differently from the rest of the family.
- A sense of poor 'willpower'.
- Busy lifestyle and irregular working hours.

- Having to use lengthy and different food preparation skills.
- Frequent eating outside the home.

Strategies to reduce the likelihood of barriers being an obstacle to change include:

- changing the external environment (e.g. driving home on a different route, which does not pass the fast-food store)
- learning to respond differently to cues (e.g. driving home as usual past the fast food store but noticing what a horrible smell it exudes)
- receiving positive reinforcement for the new behaviour (e.g. buying a new CD as a reward for not being tempted by fast food for a whole week)

Overcoming barriers is perhaps one of the import-ant reasons for offering individually tailored and personalized advice, rather than standard, blanket advice to every patient.

Table 37.2 Stage of change and the helper's role

Patient's stage of change	Helper's plan	Helper's aim(s)
Pre-contemplation	Neutral exchange of information offered (not imposed) in a way that avoids resistance (you know the client is resisting when they say 'Yes, but . . .')	Help the patient become more aware of the existence of the problem and its accompanying risks Encourage the patient to consider the possibility of change
Contemplation	Offer the space to discuss the pros and cons of change	Understand the client's ambivalence and tip the balance in favour of change Build confidence for change and achieve commitment to change
Preparation	Offer options for change (the client to choose the most realistic) and an opportunity to discuss (inevitable) barriers	Help the client explore options for change and choose the best course of action for them Strengthen commitment and confidence for change
Action	Offer positive reinforcement about change and raise the issue about coping with barriers and difficulties	Help clients to increase their confidence in changing and self-belief and to reward themselves for success Help develop coping strategies for inevitable triggers for relapse Support and reinforce convictions toward long-term change
Maintenance	Discuss progress and common cues for relapse	Help the client consolidate changes achieved in the action stage Identify high-risk situations and develop strategies for preventing relapse Increase self-belief in on-going change
Relapse	Offer an opportunity for a rational (and non-blaming) discussion about the circumstances that led to the slip or relapse and consider where this leaves them	Help the client re-enter the change cycle Take action more effectively on the next occasion

37.7 A structured approach

Unlike true Rogerian counselling in which the counsellors are non-directive and in which the agenda and direction are completely led by the patient, dietary counselling is active and directive, while also being client-centred. Thus, the practitioner has an agenda and needs a 'route map' to help steer the consultation. This structure is illustrated in Fig. 37.2.

1. *Assessment and information gathering*: an objective assessment of the patient's clinical state is needed to identify the case for a dietary intervention. Ensuring this information-gathering stage does not become an interrogation depends on skilled rapport-building and checking the patient's understanding or agenda at the outset.

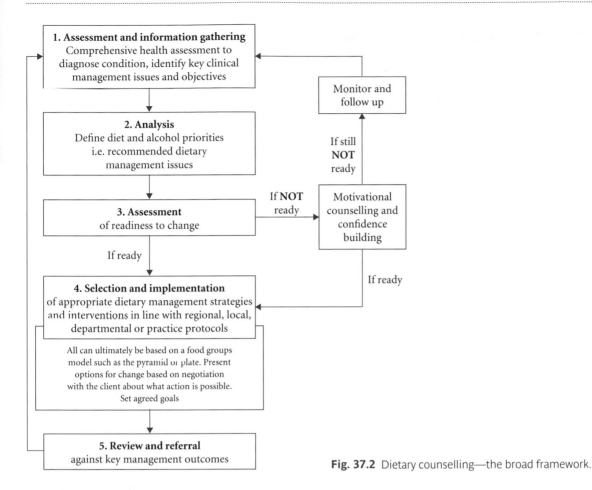

Fig. 37.2 Dietary counselling—the broad framework.

2. *Analysis of dietary priorities*: this stage identifies the dietary requirements based on the clinical and behavioural information gleaned above. Issues identified might be, for example, total energy, saturated fat, glycaemic index, sodium or alcohol.

3. *Assessment of readiness to change*: this is central to the progress of the consultation, irrespective of the condition. Patients who are not ready to change (for personal or external reasons) will not be successful in their attempt. Motivational counselling and confidence building is necessary. Discussion about barriers to change and possible ways of overcoming them will help free up the patient to feel ready and able to change their diet.

4. *Implementation of appropriate dietary management strategies*: traditionally the 'substance' of dietary counselling, offering practical, food-based options for achieving the desired diet. Goals must be agreed (or better still, suggested) by the patient.

5. *Review and referral*: good practice always builds in a review of progress against key management outcomes.

37.8 Summary

This chapter has introduced a general overview of dietary counselling as a process. The skills and strategies outlined are key for applying the nutrition science and clinical requirements to the real practicalities of dietary change. The constraints placed by patient's social, financial and environmental circumstances vary tremendously and mean that every patient scenario will be unpredictable.

The approach outlined requires the use of advanced skills and a medley of strategies that are not usually acquired during a health professional's training. Further professional development may well be necessary in order to effectively help patients change what they eat.

FURTHER READING

1. **Contento, J., Balch, G.I., Bronner, Y.L.,** *et al.* (1995) The effectiveness of nutrition education and implications for nutrition education, policy, programmes and research: a review of research. *J Nutr Educ*, **27**, Nov Dec Special Issue.

2. **Egan, G.** (1998) *The skilled helper. A problem-management approach to helping*, 6th edition. Pacific Grove, California, Brooks/Cole Publishing Company.

3. **Gable, J.** (1997) *Counselling skills for dietitians*. London, Blackwell Science.

4. **Glanz, K.** (1985) Nutrition education for risk factor reduction and patient education: a review. *Prevent Med*, **14**, 725–52.

5. **Greene, G., Rossi, S., Rossi, J.,** *et al.* (1999) Dietary applications of the Stages of Change Model. *J Am Diet Assoc*, **99**, 673–78.

6. **Hunt, P.** (1995) Dietary counselling: theory into practice. *J Inst Health Educ*, **33**, 4–8.

7. **Hunt, P., and Hillsdon, M.** (1996) *Changing eating and exercise behaviour: a handbook for professionals*. London, Blackwell Science.

8. **Kristal, A., Glanz, K., Curry, S., and Patterson, R.** (1999) How can stages of change be best used in dietary interventions? *J Am Diet Assoc*, **99**, 679–84.

9. **Miller, W.E., and Rollnick, S.** (2002) *Motivational interviewing: Preparing people to change addictive behaviour*. London and New York, The Guildford Press.

10. **Prochaska, J.O., and DiClemente, C.** (1986) Towards a comprehensive model of change. In: Miller, W.R., and Healther, N. (eds) *Treating addictive behaviours. Processes of change*. New York, Plenum.

11. **Rapoport, L., and Pearson, D.** (2006) Strategies for achieving dietary change. In: *Manual of dietetic practice*, 4th edition. London, Blackwell Science.

12. **Roe, L., Hunt, P., Bradshaw, H., and Rayner, M.** (1997) *A review of the effectiveness of health promotion interventions to promote healthy eating in the general population*. London, Health Education Authority (now Health Development Agency).

13. **Rollnick, S., Mason, P., and Butler, C.** (1999) *Health behaviour change: A guide for practitioners*. Edinburgh, Churchill Livingstone.

14. **Stewart, M., and Brown, W.** (2005) *Patient-centred medicine. Transforming the Clinical Method*. Thousand Oaks, California, Sage.

15. **Thorogood, M., Hillsdon, M., and Summerbell, C.** (2002) Changing behaviour. *Clin Evid*, **8**, 37–59.

16. **Truswell, A.S. (ed.)** (2005) International workshop. Empowering family doctors and patients in nutrition communication. Proceedings of a symposium held at Heelsum, The Netherlands, December 13–15, 2004. *Eur J Clin Nutr*, **59** (Suppl. 1), S1 – S196.

 To see topical and scientifically robust updates on nutrition associated with this textbook, and active web links to many of the journal articles in the Reference areas, please see the dedicated Online Resource Centre at www.oxfordtextbooks.co.uk/orc/mann3e/.

PART 8

Case studies

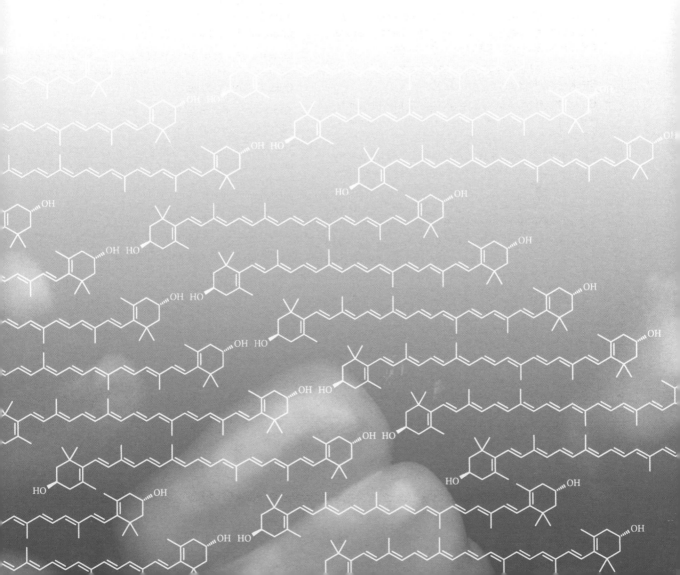

38 Nutritional consequences of poverty and food insecurity in developed countries

Winsome Parnell

❝ It upsets me that I'm not feeding the kids the food I want to and they want to eat. ❞

Traditionally, the many nutritional consequences of poverty have been identified and discussed in the context of developing countries. Recently, however, developed countries, particularly those with changes in their economic environments, have begun to identify an increasing prevalence of poverty-related health issues. Nutritionists recognize the overriding effects of the economic, social and educational factors, which together can influence nutritional status Research in this area has therefore had to encompass new definitions and methodologies to assess the magnitude of the problem and the multifaceted causes in order to develop strategies to alleviate them. Specific definitions of poverty and deprivation are always made in relative terms (between the haves and have-nots) and therefore only apply to the society or group under discussion. Poverty is defined in terms of money and equivalent income; deprivation refers to the lack of certain material items regarded as essential in that society. Different degrees of deprivation can occur over a range of income levels with low monetary income (below a defined poverty level) not necessarily being associated with severe deprivation.

Social and material circumstances are known to affect health outcomes. However, it is more difficult to ascertain whether food and nutrient intakes have actually been impaired by socioeconomic disadvantage and can therefore be viewed as a cause of poorer health. Research focus has mostly been to link socioeconomic factors with health outcome, and, to a limited extent, to link food and nutrient intake with poverty.

The major areas of nutritional concern, specifically found to be related to poverty in developed countries, include:

- energy intake – both undernutrition and overnutrition;
- insufficient intake of some micronutrients, such as iron;
- more babies with low birth weight and fewer babies being breastfed;
- lower intakes of vegetables and fruits.

38.1 Methodology

The selection of appropriate methodologies to study the nutritional consequences of poverty is not easy. Firstly, a definition of poverty needs to be developed that is appropriate to the specific population group under consideration. Many researchers have used purely economic definitions; for example, a percentage of mean equivalent disposable household income. Others recognize that deprivation criteria should be part of the definition of poverty, such as a lack of adequate housing, transport or clothing. The length of time a group or individual experiences deprivation will be a determining factor in the effects of poverty.

Secondly, in developed countries with adequate food supplies, it has been difficult to define the concept of hunger. It is not an isolated outcome, but one consequence of the larger problem of poverty. Hunger can be cyclical, short-term or long-term; it is not just physiological need. From the debate has emerged the term *food insecurity*. Food insecurity may be said to exist when the availability of nutritionally adequate and safe foods or the ability to acquire adequate supplies of culturally acceptable foods in socially acceptable ways is limited or uncertain.

Whereas most people living in poverty, defined in economic terms, are at risk of food insecurity, not all are food-insecure. Also, some households will experience food insecurity in the face of events such as sudden ill heath, job loss or unexpected expenses, even though income per se might place them well above a poverty line. National food and nutrition surveys often now include specific measures of food insecurity at household or individual level, which can potentially be correlated with food- and nutrient-intake data. Studies targeted at subgroups that are at risk require special consideration of their particular circumstances when developing the methodology and establishing sampling procedures. Participation may be affected by poor access to transport and telephones, language and literacy problems, along with a variety of other social stresses. Sensitivity to these issues, including those of confidentiality and privacy, must be taken into account.

A landmark study among an at-risk population was carried out in London, UK, by Dowler and Calvert. Their report *Nutrition and Diet in Lone-Parent Families in London* describes the socioeconomic circumstances, food-intake patterns and nutrient intakes of 200 lone-parent families, with the aim of identifying the most important factors that differentiate diets at higher or lower risk for long-term ill health. Data collected included 3-day weighed intake records for each lone parent and at least one child, a food-frequency questionnaire and a taped, semi-structured interview. The main conclusion from this work was 'that poor material circumstances combined with severe constraints on disposable income are the main factors characterising nutritional deprivation in lone parents, and sometimes their children'. The diets of parents (predominantly mothers) were affected more than children's diets, and patterns of food shopping and food-management skills had little effect on nutritional outcome. 'These mothers are not bad managers who do not know how to look after their children. They face impossible odds in making ends meet, and the aim of policy should be to help them, not to blame them.' This study encapsulates the root causes of food insecurity: inadequate financial resources and constraints on those resources that result in money not being available for food.

Further examples of studies of at-risk population groups have been carried out in Canada and New Zealand. In New Zealand, a convenience sample of 40 families receiving government benefits responded to a questionnaire developed to assess the aspects of food security relevant to them. Nutritional status was measured by means of weights and heights; nutrient intakes were measured by multiple 24-hour dietary recalls. Women in these families were the most nutritionally disadvantaged. In Canada, a study of women receiving emergency food assistance included assessment of dietary intake by three repeated 24-hour dietary recalls, and examination of dietary adequacy across levels of self-reported household-level hunger. The prevalences of inadequacy of nutrient intake of those reporting the most food insecurity were 'in a range that could put women at risk of nutrient deficiencies'.

Studies such as these have provided a step forward in the development of useful methods in this area. The surveillance of diets of people living on low incomes is important in developed countries.

38.2 Undernutrition and obesity

Studies of the growth rates and weight/height relationships of children in the 5–12-year age range, of varying socioeconomic circumstances, generally conclude that disadvantaged children have lower height-for-age and are more likely to have lower weight-for-height. This suggests that overt undernutrition (insufficient energy intake) over a period of time does have a negative effect on children's growth in developed countries.

However, it is clear that obesity also occurs in socioeconomically disadvantaged children, although to a lesser extent than among those of wealthier backgrounds. Evidence is emerging that food insecurity may contribute to overweight, particularly among girls. Further research is necessary and must include measures of dietary intake, along with measures of growth patterns and income, in order to determine the role of nutrition in growth in developed countries.

Few studies on adults in developed countries have linked poor socioeconomic status with frank undernutrition. Undoubtedly some extremely deprived men and women – for example, the homeless – exhibit clinical signs of undernutrition. Prevalence studies do not appear to have been conducted among these groups. In contrast, extensive work has documented

the inverse relationship between socioeconomic status and obesity among women; this relationship has not been shown in men. Whereas poverty has long been held to be a cause of obesity among women, recently the inverse has been suggested, that obesity will result in lower socioeconomic status, mediated through unequal work and partnership opportunities.

Although the relationship between obesity and lower socioeconomic status clearly exists, there is little evidence from food and nutrient data that excess energy intake is the main influencing factor.

Criticisms of the existing studies on the energy intakes of obese women focus on the fact that they are more likely than non-obese women to under-report food intake, and to eat less than their habitual intake during study periods. Until the problem of accurately determining energy intake among obese women is solved, no conclusions can be made about the primary cause of obesity in socioeconomically disadvantaged women. The applicability of standard cut-off values for the ratio of energy intake to estimated basal metabolic rate for estimating under-reporting has been questioned, as they were not developed for population subgroups so different from the populations on which the approach was developed. It seems also

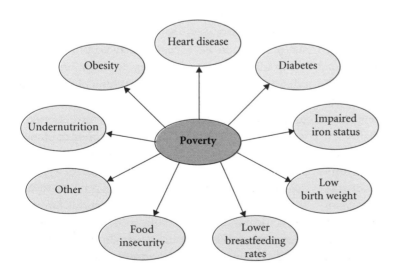

Fig. 38.1 Nutritional consequences of poverty.

that the notion of habitual intake is less applicable to socioeconomically disadvantaged women than wealthier women, because their economic resource base is not stable and they experience times of feast and famine. Food insecurity is associated with overweight, particularly among women. Given that food insecurity is characterized by an uncertain supply of food, this lends support to the point of view that fluctuations in energy intake and in body weight can contribute ultimately to accumulation of excess body fat. Whether obese women of low socioeconomic status are less physically active than obese women of wealthier backgrounds is not known. Economic deprivation is, however, known to affect motivation and self-esteem, and it limits opportunities for many forms of recreational exercise (Fig. 38.1 on p. 551).

38.3 Heart disease and diabetes

Research has shown that the prevalence of coronary heart disease and accompanying changes in risk and mortality rates appear to be influenced greatly by socioeconomic factors. Although coronary heart disease is more common in more affluent countries, it appears to have a higher incidence in less affluent subgroups of these countries. Overall, declining mortality rates have been largely at the higher end of the socioeconomic spectrum, and in some regions mortality has risen among lower socioeconomic groups of men and women. These differences have in part been attributed to differences in rates of blood pressure and obesity. Blood pressure, within average community levels, is influenced by sodium intake. Lower socioeconomic conditions in childhood have also been linked to increased risk of coronary heart disease in adulthood, in both women and men. This association has not been fully explained, but several studies provide some evidence to link nutritional status in childhood to subsequent coronary heart disease.

There is no obvious link between socioeconomic status and either quality or quantity of fat in the diets of men or women. However, there is clear evidence across all socioeconomic groups that fat intake, particularly intake of saturated fat, is a significant dietary factor associated with the incidence of coronary heart disease (see section 20.3). Many studies in developed countries document distinctive differences in eating habits and food choices between high and low socioeconomic groups, but this seldom has a profound effect on the contribution to energy intake from macronutrients, including fat. Indeed, some authors conclude that there is a general uniformity of nutrient-density consumption patterns across different socioeconomic groups. Evidence that the consumption of fresh vegetables and fruits is inversely related to socioeconomic indices is undisputed. Foods that are perishable and not nutrient-dense are less likely to be consumed in the context of food insecurity. If diets high in fruits and vegetables decrease degenerative diseases (e.g. by means of the antioxidative properties in these foods), then it may well be that their lack contributes to the burden of coronary heart disease and diabetes, as well as some cancers, among the poor.

Whereas obesity is one identified risk factor for coronary heart disease, it is also a major predictor in the onset of type 2 diabetes mellitus, with both the duration and magnitude of obesity increasing the risk of development of type 2 diabetes. Since obesity is associated with lower socioeconomic status, it would be expected that type 2 diabetes will occur more frequently in groups of lower socioeconomic status. The incidence of type 2 diabetes and impaired glucose tolerance was found to be inversely related to annual gross household income but not to an occupation-based index of socioeconomic status (the Elley–Irving Index) in a multi-racial workforce study in New Zealand. The prevalence of type 1 diabetes mellitus in children has been noted to be associated with material deprivation, but it has not been possible to link this with any particular nutrient. Recent research suggests that early exposure to cow's milk or diminished breastfeeding may be an important determinant of subsequent type 1 diabetes.

38.4 Iron deficiency

The aetiology of iron deficiency can be viewed as a negative balance between iron intake and iron loss. During the periods of rapid growth, iron balance is difficult to maintain; that is, during infancy, early childhood, adolescence and pregnancy.

In infancy, lower iron status is associated with lower socioeconomic status, although iron deficiency occurs in all strata of society. Low iron status among adolescent girls of all socioeconomic groups is largely attributable to their increased dietary requirement of iron to balance the needs of growth and menstrua-tion. Studies have not shown any difference in iron intakes among adolescent girls in low socioeconomic groups when compared with those from more affluent backgrounds.

Women of childbearing potential in the USA have lower intakes of some nutrients, including iron, if they are of lower socioeconomic status. This can con-tribute to low iron status during pregnancy. Iron-deficiency anaemia has been shown to be associated with poverty and to be linked with an increased risk of preterm delivery and low birth weight.

38.5 Low birth weight

Low socioeconomic status is predictive of low birth weight in most developed countries. A number of factors have been found to increase the incidence of low birth weight: cigarette smoking, low maternal weight gain during pregnancy, low pre-pregnancy weight, iron-deficiency anaemia, alcohol intake and possibly caffeine. Some of these factors are more pre-valent in lower socioeconomic groups and others are not. For example, cigarette smoking, which has a dir-ect effect on the flow of nutrients across the placenta, is higher among low socioeconomic groups. Smokers have also been shown to eat less than non-smokers. Alcohol intake, however, has in some studies been higher among the wealthy.

Women in whom birth outcome is most at risk from a nutritional cause enter pregnancy with a low body mass index and do not gain sufficient weight during their pregnancy. Poor socioeconomic circum-stances could contribute to this scenario, but no stud-ies show that it is confined to such groups. Future studies may be able to discern whether poverty has a significant influence on low birth weight because maternal nutrition has been impaired, rather than because, for example, smoking rates are higher, or other lifestyle factors, such as prenatal health care, are less than optimal.

38.6 Breastfeeding

Social class is an important marker of breastfeeding success, which is more common in mothers of high socioeconomic status. Solo mothers, who are over-represented in the lower socioeconomic groups, and obese mothers are less likely to initiate or continue breastfeeding. The reasons for this are complex, but it is generally acknowledged that women need adequate support and encouragement to breastfeed success-fully, and this help may be most limited among solo mothers. Infants who are not breastfed are at greater risk of respiratory illness and infections and are more likely to be subject to feeding practices that do not enhance iron status, and are at greater risk of child-hood obesity.

38.7 Behaviour

The issue of whether inadequate nutrient intake and particularly hunger affect behaviour has been most studied among school children. After World War II, policy-makers in the UK and USA felt that food programmes for lunches and/or breakfasts in schools would have a significant impact on school performance, including alertness, intelligence, educational attainment and general behaviour patterns. These programmes were made available regardless of socioeconomic circumstances, although those in higher socioeconomic groups were expected to pay. Fifty years on, when many such programmes have been reduced or dropped, hunger is again considered a problem among school children, and the reasons given are inadequate family income and lifestyle factors, such as time for food preparation and food habits. Thus, socioeconomic status is still believed to impact negatively on children's behaviour patterns. Whereas many believe that nutrition is a significant issue, it is very difficult to disentangle the effects of the many disadvantageous factors of low socioeconomic status and

how they impact on children's behaviour. Nutrition may well be one of these but few studies adequately address the issue in totality. For example, a study of 'perceived hunger' in schools in New Zealand found that the prevalence was higher in inner-city areas and where ethnic diversity was greatest. No measures of behaviour at school were made, or of nutritional status. Reviews of school feeding programmes in the USA conclude that they have positive nutritional impact, but have not adequately evaluated such programmes in terms of their effect on academic performance. Data from the USA have examined the ongoing effects of household food insecurity on children's academic performance and social skills and found that they are associated with developmental consequences. The fact that so many outcomes of poverty, in both the home and school environment, have the potential to influence behaviour of children means that adverse food patterns and nutrition will always be a part of the spectrum to a varying degree.

38.8 Food insecurity

From the above sections it can be concluded that it is difficult, in developed countries, to quantify the effect of poverty on nutritional status, both for methodological reasons and possibly because nutritional status is seldom profoundly affected, particularly in the short term. In addition, poor nutritional status is not confined to low socioeconomic groups.

Food security, however, is clearly difficult to achieve when economic status drops suddenly or when it is inadequate and remains so for long periods of time. To be food-secure, individuals need more than adequate disposable income. They may need to overcome obstacles such as lack of transport, inadequate cooking or storage facilities, and access to food that is culturally acceptable (Fig. 38.2).

❝I don't buy 5 kg of potatoes as I can't carry it. I hope my husband will agree to give us the car.❞

What is measurable is the growth of the many and varied programmes to alleviate shortage of food for groups of economically disadvantaged people. Food banks or pantries set up by charitable organizations continue to increase in number and size of operation in most developed countries. Their aim is to provide free food to the needy in an emergency or on a short-term basis. In some countries, government purchasing assistance such as food stamps serve as a permanent or semi-permanent source of food income. The efficacy of surplus-food redistribution is fiercely debated. Many consider that it perpetuates food poverty and provides no long-term solutions.

❝It's hard to ask people for help. I don't want to be a burden.❞

There is little dispute that the underlying causes of food insecurity are socioeconomic and political. These

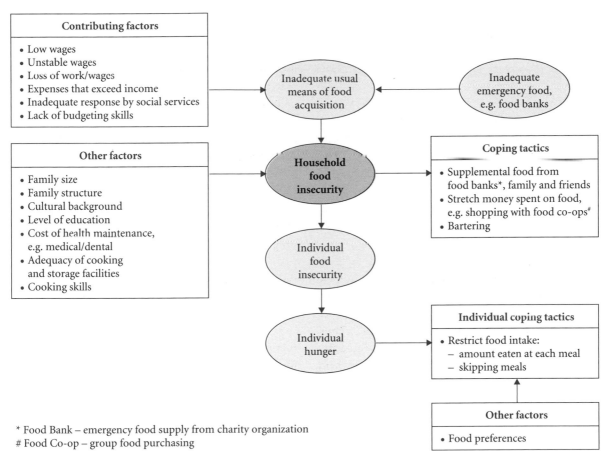

Contributing factors

- Low wages
- Unstable wages
- Loss of work/wages
- Expenses that exceed income
- Inadequate response by social services
- Lack of budgeting skills

Other factors

- Family size
- Family structure
- Cultural background
- Level of education
- Cost of health maintenance, e.g. medical/dental
- Adequacy of cooking and storage facilities
- Cooking skills

Inadequate usual means of food acquisition

Inadequate emergency food, e.g. food banks

Household food insecurity

Coping tactics

- Supplemental food from food banks*, family and friends
- Stretch money spent on food, e.g. shopping with food co-ops#
- Bartering

Individual food insecurity

Individual hunger

Individual coping tactics

- Restrict food intake:
  - amount eaten at each meal
  - skipping meals

Other factors

- Food preferences

* Food Bank – emergency food supply from charity organization
\# Food Co-op – group food purchasing

Fig. 38.2 Household food insecurity.

Source: Adapted from Williams, C., and Dowler, E.A. (1994) *A working paper for the Nutrition Task Force Low Income Project Team*. London, Department of Health.

must be addressed by economists and politicians. What can nutritionists do? Many have attempted an educational approach, on the premise that budgeting and food-preparation skills should be improved. In some instances, this is helpful. But many communities of people in constrained circumstances vocalize their need to find solutions and coping strategies using their own skills and resources, alongside appropriate professional input.

❝People are the experts on their own lives. ❞

Public health policy in many developed countries states that the effects of socioeconomic disadvantage on nutritional well-being is a public health priority. Australia's *Food and Nutrition Policy* document opens thus: 'The Government's food and nutrition policy is to facilitate and support action through the entire food and nutrition system, in order to achieve better nutrition for Australians, especially for those most disadvantaged'. New Zealand's National Plan of Action for Nutrition listed 'Improving household food security' as a first priority, noting the need to establish baseline information on the current situation with respect to accessibility, acceptability and affordability of food.

It is now apparent that developed countries cannot assume that all segments of their population are food-secure. Many are now developing tools to document the prevalence of food insecurity and monitor the nutritional outcomes. An example is in New Zealand, where eight indices of household food security were developed and ranked in order of severity.

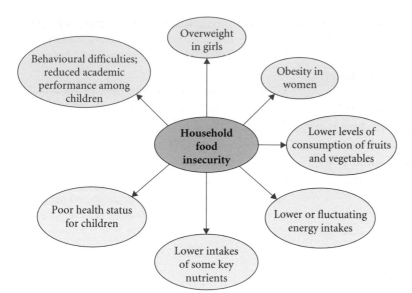

Fig. 38.3 Consequences of household food insecurity—emerging evidence.

Categories of food security (fully/almost fully secure, moderately secure and low security) have been shown to be associated with nutritional outcomes in the population. For adults, those with the lowest household food-security status have the highest intake of fats and the lowest intakes of glucose, fructose and vitamin C. For New Zealand children, those in households with lower food security have lower intakes of lactose, calcium, vitamin A and β-carotene. Such data confirm the hypothesis that without ready access to affordable and appropriate food, nutritional status will be compromised (Fig. 38.3). They also assist efforts to develop and coordinate economic policies, educational strategies and social action to alleviate the consequences of poverty, among which poor nutritional status is undoubtedly one.

38.9 Case study

Mary Smith is a 40-year-old solo mother (sole parent) with two sons aged 14 and 8 years. She has been co-owner/operator of a lunchtime cafe in a small town for a little over 1 year. She entered this venture after receiving money from a relative's estate, all of which was invested in the business. The cafe is making no profit. The local district Health Board schedule gall-bladder surgery without warning, which was necessitated by an acute attack of gall stones 6 months before. This obliges her to leave her partner to cope alone without arrangements for adequate cover. The surgery is followed by complications that delay her recovery and she is away from work for a month so that the partner demands the business

be sold. Debts have been incurred for intercity ambulance transport to enable urgent hospital re-admission in relation to the surgical complications and early discharge. Child-care costs for 2 months 'board' for her two sons have accrued.

Mary leaves the business with no assets and 2 months rent in her bank account. Her car requires repairs if it is to be roadworthy. She is not well enough to seek new paid employment for the forseeable future and anticipates eligibility for a government benefit in 2 months' time.

How should she provision her household until then? There are staple foods in the pantry: rice, pasta, some canned goods and condiments. Normally her garden would be a source of fresh vegetables but this has been neglected since she began to work in the cafe for 12 h each day.

Once the government benefit payments begin, they will need to stretch to service debts for her sons' school uniforms in addition to paying the debts for the ambulance and car repairs. Her immediate recourse is to the local food bank, which provides dried and canned foods. Neighbours supply some fresh vegetables. There is no money available to pay for fresh milk and fruit.

FURTHER READING

1. **Bailey, V.F., and Sherriff, J.** (1992) Reasons for the early cessation of breast-feeding in women from lower socio-economic groups in Perth, Western Australia. *Aust J Nutr Diet*, **49**, 40–3.

2. **Bartley, M.** (1994) Unemployment and ill health: understanding the relationship. *J Epid Comm Health*, **48**, 333–7.

3. **Dowler, E., and Calvert, C.** (1995) *Nutrition and diet in lone-parent families in London*. London, Family Policy Studies Centre.

4. **James, W.P.T., Nelson, M., Ralph, A., and Leather, S.** (1997) The contributions of nutrition to inequalities in health. *Br Med J*, **341**, 1545–9.

5. **Jyoti, D.F., Frongillo, E.A., and Jones, S.J.** (2005) Food insecurity affects school children's academic performance, weight gain and social skills. *J Nutr*, **135**, 2831–9.

6. **Miller, J.E., and Korenman, S.** (1994) Poverty and children's nutritional status in the United States. *Am J Epidemiol*, **140**, 233–43.

7. **Nelson, M.** (2000) Childhood nutrition and poverty. *Proc Nutr Soc*, **59**, 307–15.

8. **Nutrition Taskforce Low Income Project Team** (1996) *Health of the nation. Low income, food, nutrition and health: strategies for improvement.* Wetherby, Department of Health.

9. **Sobal, J., and Stunkard, A.J.** (1989) Socioeconomic status and obesity: a review of the literature. *Psychol Bull*, **105**, 260–75.

10.**Tarasuk, V.S., and Beaton, G.H.** (1999) Women's dietary intakes in the context of household food insecurity. *J Nutr*, **129**, 672–9.

 To see topical and scientifically robust updates on nutrition associated with this textbook, and active web links to many of the journal articles in the Reference areas, please see the dedicated Online Resource Centre at www.oxfordtextbooks.co.uk/orc/mann3e/.

39 Nutrition and HIV and AIDS

Hester Vorster

The raging global pandemic as a result of infection with the human immunodeficiency virus (HIV) and consequent development of acquired immunodeficiency syndrome (AIDS) first described in 1981 has been described as 'a human tragedy', 'one of the greatest calamities ever to befall humankind', one of the 'most devastating events in human history' and 'a threat to development, security and economic growth'.

The Joint United Nations Programme on HIV/AIDS (UNAIDS) reported that in 2004 globally between 35.9 million and 44.3 million adults and children were living with HIV and AIDS. Between 4.3 million and 6.4 million adults and children were newly infected with HIV during 2004, while between 2.8 million and 3.5 million died from AIDS in the same year. Sub-Saharan Africa has the highest prevalence (25.4 million people infected) while Eastern Europe and Central Asia (Russia, former Soviet republic, India and China) have the fastest growing epidemic of HIV and AIDS. The rate of increase in China is 25–30% per year with the doubling time of the epidemic only 30 months. It is estimated that since the beginning of the epidemic in the early 1980s until 2002, globally more than 65 million people have been infected with HIV and more than 25 million died of AIDS. The numbers in North America, Western and Central Europe and Oceania are lower (1.0 million, 610 000 and 35 000, respectively). The

consequences and impact of the pandemic are devastating. Life expectancy at birth in Southern Africa has already plummeted to levels last recorded in the 1950s (to 47 years) and infant mortality rates are severely affected in developing countries. It is predicted that the population in Africa in 2015 will be at least 60 million lower than it would have been in the absence of AIDS. In addition to the demographic impact of HIV and AIDS and its economic consequences, it is a disease with a profound social impact in the developing world. It turns grandparents into parents, and orphaned children into main breadwinners and heads of households, because it is usually young, sexually active adults in their reproductive years that are victims of the disease.

This chapter focuses on the role of nutrition in the prevention, progression, care and treatment of HIV and AIDS. Optimizing nutritional status is often the only option to assist infected people in poor, developing countries. To understand how nutrients, foods and diets influence the disease, and how to manage patients with HIV and AIDS, the virus, its transmission, the pathogenesis of the infection, clinical features and pharmacological therapy are briefly summarized in section 39.1 (see Boxes 39.1 and 39.2). The discussion of metabolic abnormalities associated with HIV and AIDS in section 39.2 leads into the discussion of the role of nutrition in HIV and AIDS in section 39.3.

BOX 39.1 Stages of HIV infection

Stage 1: *Acute infection (seroconversion)*

- rapid viral replication
- symptoms: fever, malaise, headache, myalgia, skin rashes, lymphadenopathy syndrome
- duration: 1 week to several months

Stage 2: *Asymptomatic HIV infection*

- none or only a few symptoms
- subclinical loss of lean body mass
- vitamin B_{12} deficiency
- changes in blood lipids and liver enzymes
- susceptible to pathogens in food and water
- duration: 10 years or longer (depending on nutritional status and drug treatment)

Stage 3: *Symptomatic HIV infection*

- CD4+ counts between 200 and 500 cells/μl
- symptoms: loss of appetite, white plaques in mouth, skin lesions, fever, night sweats, tuberculosis, shingles, other infections
- wasting: involuntary weight loss > 10% baseline body weight, caused by reduced food intake, malabsorption, nutrient losses and increased energy needs ('slim disease'); nutrition interventions may help to preserve lean body mass and strengthen the immune system

Stage 4: *AIDS*

- CD4+ cell counts below 200 cells/μL
- final, fatal stage if not treated by drugs
- immunosuppression leads to opportunistic (secondary) infections with fungi, protozoa, bacteria and other viruses
- malignant diseases and dementia may develop

BOX 39.2 Pharmacologic (drug) therapy of HIV and AIDS

Treatment of primary infection

- HAART: highly active antiretroviral therapy with at least three drugs (protease inhibitors such as amprenavir, indinavir, etc. and reverse transcriptase inhibitors such as abacavir, nevirapine, etc.)
- Slow progression of HIV to AIDS, restore immunofunction partially, decrease morbidity and mortality
- Start drug treatment with onset of symptoms or when CD4+ counts are below 200 cells/μL
- Individualize and monitor treatment to prevent drug resistance, interactions and side effects
- Daily, lifelong adherence required

- World Health Organization's '3 × 5' programme showed that drug treatment in developing countries is possible, affordable and sustainable

Treatment of wasting

- Megestrol acetate, testosterone, other metabolic steroids, growth hormone or thalidomide may be useful to use in adjunction to diet therapy and increased activity

Treatment of secondary (opportunistic) infections

- Individualized therapy of specific infections with fungi, protozoa, bacteria or other viruses, using appropriate drugs

39.1 HIV and AIDS

39.1.1 Human immunodeficiency virus characteristics

HIV is probably the most studied virus in human history. As yet, no vaccine against the virus is available, although many are now being tested. HIV is a member of the lentivirus family of retroviruses and was first isolated in 1983. Currently, six subtypes are known, with two major subtypes, HIV-1 the principal cause of the pandemic and HIV-2. Human beings are not the natural hosts of the virus. These viruses probably entered the human population as a result of cross-species transmission from chimpanzee species (HIV-1) and sooty mangabeys (HIV-2), possibly around 1930.

After HIV entry into the human body, it binds to the CD4+ receptor on the surface of CD4+ cells, part of the immune system. This allows the virus to penetrate the CD4+ cells and replicate, using reverse transcriptase to produce viral DNA. The new viral particles are secreted into the circulation and the CD4+ host cells are destroyed. The body produces new CD4+ cells to fight the HIV infection, but eventually the CD4+ cell counts drop, the immune system loses its ability to resist other infections, and signs of immune failure appear, namely mucocutaneous conditions, persistent generalized lymphadenopathy and high risk of infections and malignancies. At this stage, patients have

developed AIDS, and without effective antiretroviral therapy (see Boxes 39.1 and 39.2) will die within a few years.

39.1.2 HIV transmission

The virus is transmitted via certain body fluids: blood, semen, pre-seminal fluid, vaginal secretions and breast milk. Previously, and today in most developed countries, the principal modes of transmission were and are unprotected sexual contact between men and sharing of needles by intravenous drug abusers. The majority of infections globally, and especially in developing countries, are because of unprotected heterosexual contact and vertical transmission from an infected mother to her child antenatally, during labour or by breastfeeding. A small number have been infected by transfusion of contaminated blood or blood products. Extreme care when working with body fluids and the use of condoms reduces the risk of infection.

39.1.3 Stages of HIV infection and progression to AIDS

The destruction by the virus of the ability of the immune system to fight infections results in four stages of the disease (Box 39.1), which form the basis of clinical classifications.

39.2 Metabolic and endocrine abnormalities during HIV infection

The changes in metabolism and endocrine function during HIV infection, resulting from the primary and secondary infections, and the pharmacological therapy of the disease influence its nutritional management.

39.2.1 Changes in energy metabolism

Wasting associated with HIV and AIDS results from inadequate macronutrient and energy intake, malabsorption, increased losses and increased energy expenditure or needs. Most studies in adults show that resting metabolic rate (RMR) is about 10% higher in HIV-infected adults compared with healthy adults, especially when secondary infections occur. However, total energy expenditure is usually not raised, probably because of decreased activity. In asymptomatic HIV, energy intake is normal or slightly increased (15%), probably to compensate for malabsorption or increased RMR. Later, secondary infections lead to decreased intake. Antiretroviral drugs also cause anorexia, which disappears when clinical symptoms improve and drug therapy is established. HIV damages intestinal villi, causing malabsorption. Gut infections further exacerbate malabsorption through diarrhoea, all contributing to wasting. Energy needs during convalescence following severe infection may increase an additional 20–50%.

39.2.2 Changes in protein metabolism and turnover

Potential changes in protein metabolism and turnover are of importance to determine whether HIV and AIDS patients require higher-than-usual protein intakes. Some studies suggest that this may be the case. There is evidence of increased protein turnover (possibly explaining the increased RMR) and that on energy-deficient diets protein rather than fat stores may be preferentially metabolized. However, these are not consistent findings so that definitive recommendations regarding protein intake are not possible. It does seem that additional protein and amino acids are not utilized adequately until secondary infections have been treated.

39.2.3 Changes in lipid metabolism and development of the lipodystrophy syndrome

HIV increases lipid oxidation while carbohydrate oxidation in AIDS decreases. Fasting triglyceride and sometimes cholesterol levels increase, lipoprotein lipase activity and triglyceride clearance decrease and hepatic *de novo* lipogenesis increases. Severe hyperlipidaemia may occur in patients treated with antiretroviral drugs. The most striking abnormality of lipid metabolism is the development of the lipodystrophy syndrome seen in some patients treated with antiretroviral drugs. Body composition and shape changes include the development of a 'buffalo hump' (extra fat deposits in the dorsocervical fat pad), increased intra-abdominal fat deposition and loss of subcutaneous fat in the cheeks, arms and legs, leading to prominent veins and muscles. Some patients on HAART (see Box 39.2) develop insulin resistance and type 2 diabetes mellitus. It is not clear why and how antiretroviral therapy causes these abnormalities nor why they do not occur in all patients. Conventional dietary and drug treatments are recommended for the hyperlipidaemia and abnormalities of glucose metabolism.

39.2.4 Other metabolic and endocrine abnormalities

Raised levels of cytokines and disturbed levels of adiponectin, growth hormone, leptin, insulin-like growth factor and glycerol have all been observed in AIDS patients. Increased venous lactate levels (> 2.0 mmol/L) and low arterial pH (< 7.3) are potential consequences of antiretroviral therapy, especially in the presence of liver damage. Lactic acidosis is accompanied by nausea, abdominal pain, shortness of breath, fatigue and weight loss, and can be fatal. Hypogonadism occurs in 30–50% of men with AIDS, and the resultant male steroid hormone deficiency may play a role in HIV wasting.

39.3 Nutrition and HIV and AIDS

Appropriate nutrition cannot cure HIV and AIDS. However, based on the established relationship between nutrition and the immune system, it could enhance immune function and reduce the risk and severity of infections. Furthermore, there is evidence that improved nutritional status can reduce the risk of transmission, reduce HIV-associated wasting, slow progression of HIV to AIDS and optimize drug treatment of both the primary and secondary infections. Nutrition interventions can, therefore, help to improve the quality of life of infected people, promote a sense of wellbeing and keep them mobile and working. Unfortunately, HIV-infected persons are often exposed to inappropriate, untested and unproven advice regarding benefits of specific foods and supplements. This advice exploits ignorance and fear and raises false hope. In the following section, only nutrition interventions that have been proven and with a sound scientific basis are considered.

39.3.1 Specific nutrient requirements

Deficiencies of several nutrients including protein, essential fatty acids, vitamins A, B_6, folate, C and E, iron, zinc, copper and selenium, as well as an energy deficit, are associated with impaired immune function. This has led to speculation that some of these nutrients may have specific beneficial effects in HIV and AIDS. Attempts to definitively establish their roles have been hampered by a multitude of methodological problems and ethical considerations. Further studies are underway but in the light of existing knowledge, the following nutrients deserve attention.

Protein While there is no definitive evidence (see section 39.2.2) that the presence of HIV or AIDS *per se* warrants additional protein, there are some situations in which protein intake should be at the upper end of the recommended range (1.5–2.0 g/kg): presence of infection, catch-up growth in children, and wasting in adults. In such situations it is essential to optimize, as far as possible, conditions for the utilization of protein, e.g. by the treatment of infections. For most others, protein intake should be 1.0–1.4 g/kg body weight. Those with severe hepatic or renal disease should be recommended reduced protein intakes.

Fat Because of its high energy density, fat is a useful nutrient to include in small frequent meals of individuals with anorexia and others requiring increased energy intake. However, reduced fat diets are indicated for those with a decreased fat tolerance, fat malabsorption and diarrhoea. Medium-chain fatty acid oils may be better tolerated and absorbed than long-chain fatty acid oils by HIV-infected people. Supplementation with fish oils (ω-3 fatty acids) may be useful because they are less inflammation promoting than ω-6 fatty acids. Saturated fatty acids should be reduced in those with hyperlipidaemia as a consequence of antiretroviral treatment.

Fluids and electrolytes Fluid and electrolyte requirements of HIV-infected and uninfected individuals are similar: 30–35 mL/kg or 1.5 L/day for adults. However, additional fluids and electrolytes are often required because of losses during diarrhoea, vomiting and night sweats. These are replaced by oral dehydration solutions, which may be prepared at home (e.g. 1 L boiled, cooled water plus half a teaspoon of salt (sodium chloride) and 8 teaspoons of sugar or cooked cereal).

Vitamins Vitamin A supplementation is a key health intervention in developing countries. It reduces all-cause mortality and measles mortality in hospitalized children by 30% and 60–70%, respectively. There is also some evidence in children that larger doses will decrease HIV and AIDS morbidity and mortality. Vitamin A is necessary for maintaining epithelial integrity and is suspected to help prevent transmission of the virus. There is no convincing evidence that vitamin A supplementation decreases risk of transmission of HIV or slows the progression of the disease in adults. There is some evidence that several of the B vitamins may decrease transmission of the virus and that the antioxidant vitamins (C and E) may decrease progression of the infection, but the evidence is insufficient to recommend intakes greater than those usually recommended.

Minerals Iron stores decrease during the asymptomatic stages (1–3) of HIV infection, probably because of a decreased absorption. In the later stages of AIDS, iron accumulates in macrophages and other cells. Iron supplements are recommended in pregnancy and anaemia. However, iron may increase the risk of opportunistic infections. Moreover, the effects of iron on viral replication and load are not clear. Zinc deficiency is prevalent in many developing country populations, and supplementation with zinc is known to decrease the risk of diarrhoea and respiratory tract infections. It is also known that zinc is essential for the normal function of the immune system. However, in high doses, zinc has been shown to be immunosuppressive. There are conflicting results about the role of zinc in the progression and morbidity of HIV and AIDS. Selenium is another micronutrient (antioxidant) suspected to play a role in HIV. It seems that a selenium deficiency is associated with an increased virulence of the virus. There is, however, no evidence available on the effects of selenium supplementation on the course of HIV and AIDS.

Supplements From the above it is clear that there are gaps in our knowledge about the primary effect of HIV on micronutrient status and requirements and about the effects of supplementation with specific micronutrients on the course of the infection. Thus, at present the recommendations are that intakes of infected individuals should reach levels of intake that will prevent clinical and biochemical signs of any deficiency. A food-based approach with diversified diets is always the most appropriate. However, because of the effects of the infection on food intake, absorption and loss of micronutrients, and because of food insecurity in many infected individuals, the distribution and the use of fortified foods and

micronutrient supplements may be necessary. It has been shown that the daily intake of a broad-based or high-dose multivitamin supplement can reduce progression and mortality amongst infected adults and that vitamin A supplements can reduce morbidity and mortality in children. As in the case with antiretroviral treatment, the distribution of micronutrient supplements should be health-facility based and accompanied with detailed explanations on how to use them to prevent overdosage.

39.3.2 Public health versus therapeutic nutrition interventions

Fig. 39.1 gives a conceptual framework to help understand how targeted nutrition interventions leading to improved nutrition status can influence the outcomes of HIV and AIDS. The figure illustrates two important concepts: firstly, that poverty, underdevelopment and malnutrition, and the social dimensions of the disease, create ideal circumstances for the propagation of the HIV epidemic, which should be addressed by public health nutrition interventions. Secondly, the diagram illustrates that the biological dimensions of HIV infection call for individualized therapeutic nutrition interventions.

The top of the figure shows how the vicious circle of underdevelopment, food and nutrition insecurity, undernutrition, lack of education, poverty, inequity and lack of coping skills can lead to a lack of knowledge about HIV and AIDS, high-risk behaviours and increased exposure to the virus. At the same time, undernutrition will lead to a compromised immune system, damage to epithelial barriers, increased susceptibility and decreased resistance to infections. Collectively, these factors will all increase risk of transmission. The development of HIV will exacerbate the vicious circle by further worsening nutritional status and impact on all factors contributing to poverty in developing communities. The public health nutrition interventions needed should form part of other health, education and development programmes. The aims should be to educate people about AIDS; to

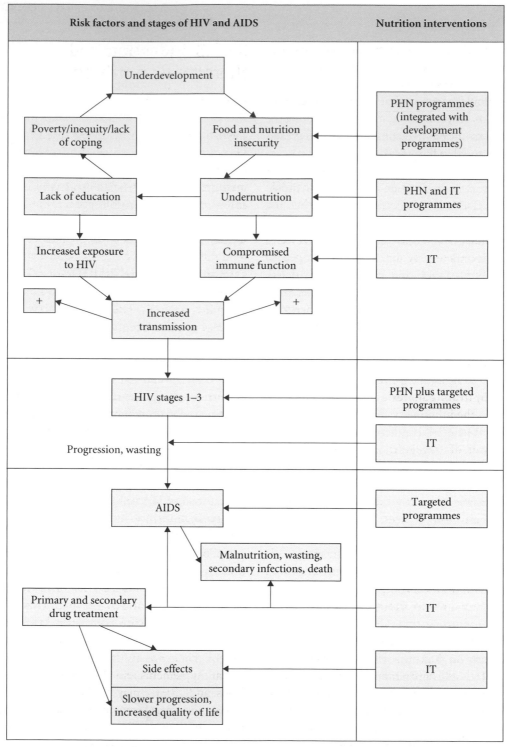

Fig. 39.1 A conceptual framework to show the role of public health nutrition (PHN) and individualized therapeutic (IT) nutrition interventions in HIV and AIDS. The top left section shows that increased transmission of HIV has a positive (+) feedback effect, exacerbating undernutrition and compromised immune function, as well as worsening the factors leading to increased exposure to HIV.

optimize nutritional status, immunity and resistance to infections; and to promote preventive behaviours, collectively to decrease transmission of the virus. Programmes should be targeted at specific risk groups. The approach, focus and programme content in the developed and developing worlds will differ and should be tailored to fit specific needs.

The middle of Fig. 39.1 shows the outcome of transmission, namely infection with HIV. The public health nutrition interventions needed during the progression of the infection should include specific nutrition guidelines to all people living with HIV and AIDS and food-aid programmes to assist people living with hunger and food insecurity. The deterioration of immune function, the effect of the virus on reduced food intake and absorption, and increased nutrient requirements and losses all lead to wasting, which requires individualized therapeutic nutrition interventions. The aims are to provide the needy with appropriate foods and supplements and to increase food intake by treating anorexia and wasting, in order to strengthen the immune system and slow the progression of HIV to AIDS.

The bottom of the figure shows that if stages 1–3 are not adequately managed, AIDS develops. If untreated, AIDS will lead to further malnutrition, wasting, secondary infections and death. If treated with a combination of antiretroviral drugs and appropriate individualized nutrition therapy, further progression of the disease, decreases in viral loads (and therefore less risk of transmission), improved immune function and an improved quality of life will result. The aims of nutrition therapy during AIDS are to address wasting, side effects of the treatment of primary (HIV) and secondary (opportunistic) infections, and to improve immune function. All AIDS patients should have written dietary and lifestyle guidelines and should be educated on how to avoid foodborne and waterborne pathogens, how to ensure nutrient adequacy by diet diversification, and how to use fortified foods and nutrient supplements.

39.3.3 Individualized, therapeutic nutrition interventions

The progression of HIV is associated with changes in nutritional status that require individualized, therapeutic nutrition interventions. The aims of these interventions should be to treat wasting (preserve and restore lean body mass), prevent nutritional deficiencies or excesses that may compromise immune function, minimize complications that interfere with food intake and nutrient absorption, and to support antiretroviral and other drug therapies. The standard components of nutrition therapy should be followed: screening, referral, assessment, intervention, outcomes evaluation and communication. Algorithms for the nutritional support, care and management of wasting and other symptoms are available in dietetic or clinical nutrition texts (see Box 39.3). Principles of nutrient–drug interactions should be applied. In addition to the general knowledge of food and nutrient effects on absorption and metabolism of drugs, some information is available on how antiretroviral treatment can be optimized. Table 39.1 summarizes practical dietary advice that can be followed to disguise the taste of these drugs, to avoid nausea and other symptoms, and to ensure optimal absorption. Patients should be counselled and issued with dietary guidelines and recommendations to help them cope with all the side effects and symptoms of both the primary and secondary infection drug therapies. The dietary advice should be based on the known effects of foods to alleviate these problems, but adapted and individualized to fit in with the patient's usual eating pattern. There are indications that some traditional herbal supplements and also garlic and caffeine-rich foods and drinks may inhibit antiretroviral drug absorption. These supplements and foods should be avoided until more scientific information on putative beneficial effects are available.

BOX 39.3

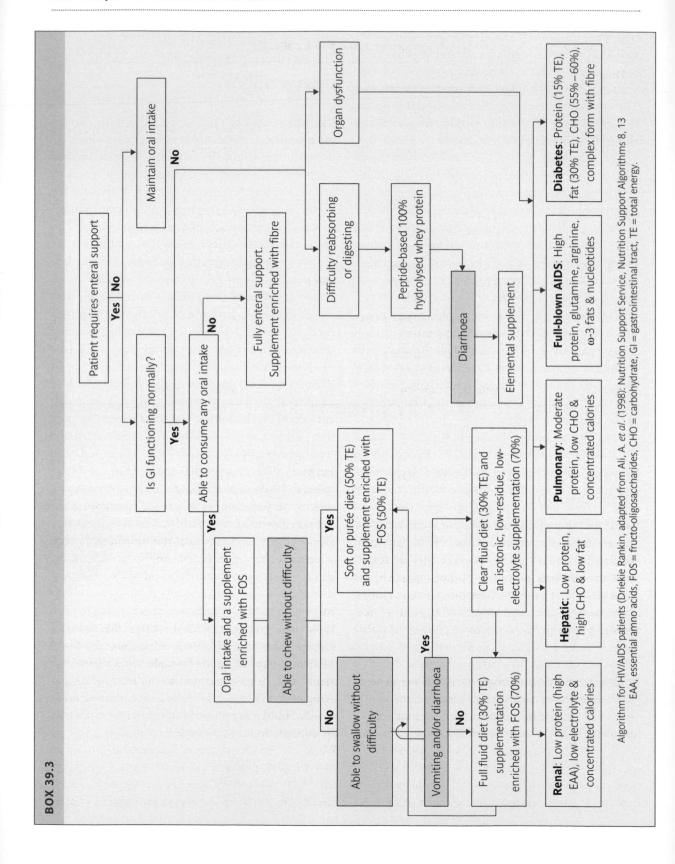

Algorithm for HIV/AIDS patients (Driekie Rankin, adapted from Ali, A. *et al.* (1998): Nutrition Support Service, Nutrition Support Algorithms 8, 13 EAA, essential amno acids, FOS = fructo-oligosaccharides, CHO = carbohydrate, GI = gastrointestinal tract, TE = total energy.

Table 39.1 Dietary advice to optimize drug treatment of HIV and AIDS

Drug	Objectives	Dietary advice
All drugs	Disguise taste Minimize side effects	Take drug with small quantities of honey, jelly, ice cream, yoghurt, milk shake, fruit juice, fruit ice or fruit purée
Neverapine	Avoid aggravating sore mouth	Can be taken with food or on empty stomach Use smooth and moist foods
Indinavir	Avoid nausea, vomiting, change in taste, diarrhoea Optimize absorption	Take on an empty stomach or with a low-fat snack, supplemented with fruit juice or other fluids taken in small regular amounts
Ritonavir	Avoid nausea, vomiting, diarrhoea, abdominal pain, burning and prickling sensations in mouth	Take with food
Nelfinavir	Avoid loose stools and diarrhoea Optimize absorption	Take with food
Saquinavir (contains lactose)	Avoid nausea, diarrhoea Optimize absorption	Take after a high-energy, high-fat meal
Etavirenze	Optimize absorption	Take with or after meals

39.3.4 Public health nutrition interventions

Two main types of public health nutrition intervention are needed to address the nutrition problems associated with HIV and AIDS. The first are integrated programmes aimed at optimizing nutrition status of whole populations, communities and groups of people. The second are targeted programmes that address specific needs of people living with HIV and AIDS.

Integrated nutrition programmes These general programmes form part of policies, strategies and services within countries aimed at improving the nutrition status of all, and are based on existing nutrition problems in these countries. In the developed world, examples would be programmes to address childhood and adult obesity, programmes to decrease risk factors of non-communicable diseases, efforts to increase fruit and vegetable consumption, and provision of food aid to the needy. In developing countries, these programmes will typically address food and nutrition insecurity and undernutrition. As indicated in Fig. 39.1, improvement of nutritional status of populations will indirectly and in the long-term influence the spread of the HIV and AIDS epidemic.

Targeted public health nutrition programmes These are programmes and efforts that address specific nutrition problems associated with HIV and AIDS in groups of infected people. An essential element of these programmes is education of people living with HIV and AIDS to understand the disease, its influence on nutritional status and how to choose appropriate foods to manage its complications. The World Health Organization has developed a set of user-friendly, practical guidelines for people living with HIV and AIDS. They can be adapted to local circumstances, basing advice on existing food-based dietary guidelines within countries. Such guidelines should also include advice on food safety, food preparation and healthy lifestyles. In countries where hunger and food insecurity are problems, the best advice can only be followed when recommended foods and supplements are available and affordable. Part of these programmes, therefore, should be food aid, providing energy-dense fortified products that are compatible with local culture and eating patterns.

39.4 HIV and AIDS during pregnancy, lactation and infancy

Without pharmaceutical intervention, the risk of vertical transmission of HIV from pregnant mothers to infants is between 15% and 20% and during breastfeeding between 20% and 45%. *In utero* and *post-partum* transmission can be reduced to less than 10% by treating pregnant women with oral antiretrovirals from 14 to 34 weeks of gestation, and with intravenous antiretrovirals during labour to reduce the viral load in blood and vaginal secretions. Ideally, infants born to infected mothers should also be treated for 6 weeks after birth. There are indications that poor nutritional status of pregnant women increases the risk of transmission.

Human milk can transmit the virus. The rate of HIV infection in breastfed infants increases with the duration of breastfeeding. The risk depends on the viral load and is increased during mastitis, nipple disease and when breast and bottle feedings are alternated. To reduce risk of transmission, HIV-infected mothers are advised to avoid breastfeeding. In the developing world, this may be difficult because replacement feeding is not always acceptable, feasible, affordable, sustainable or safe. A lack of clean water and unhygienic practices during replacement feeding are known causes of high rates of infant mortality. In these instances, exclusive breastfeeding is recommended for a few months to be replaced by altern-

ative feeding when it is available, affordable and safe. To assist mothers in this difficult choice between breast and replacement feeding, mothers from resource-poor developing countries should be supported with counselling and education regarding the risks to the infant.

Children born to HIV-infected mothers are mostly below the 50th percentile for weight and height. Uninfected, but not infected, children show catch-up growth. The poor growth in infected children not receiving antiretroviral therapy is reflected in their reduced survival rates. Energy and protein needs of infected children may be double that of uninfected infants. Increases in energy intake without antiretroviral treatment increase the weight but not the height of infected children. Antiretroviral treatment improves weight, height (growth), development and survival, provided that secondary infections are prevented or adequately managed. Infected babies, therefore, should be assessed at baseline, and nutritionally supported as necessary. All micronutrient intakes should reach dietary recommendations. There is some evidence that megadoses of vitamin A in children under 5 years decrease diarrhoea-related morbidity as well as all-cause and AIDS mortality. For further information and references, see Fawzi *et al.* (1999) as well as Coutsoudis *et al.* (1995).

39.5 Concluding comments

The experience with HIV and AIDS in the developed world has shown that it is a preventable and manageable disease. Unfortunately, in most developing countries, because of underdevelopment, poverty, malnutrition, a lack of education, lack of sufficient health infrastructures and services, a lack of informed, concerned and committed politicians, and the social stigma associated with the disease, the tide of the epidemic has not been stemmed. Hopefully, the future availability of an effective vaccine and the present efforts by international organizations and many governments to implement antiretroviral treatment in these resource-poor countries will help to prevent and manage the disease. There are huge gaps in our knowledge about the effects of HIV and AIDS on nutritional status (especially micronutrient status) and the benefits of specific nutrients in the management of disease. At present, the most responsible approach is to optimize nutritional status by diet diversification and the use of fortified foods and micronutrient supplements where indicated, to prevent signs and symptoms of nutrient deficiencies. Hopefully, these gaps in our knowledge will motivate more research in this area, providing results and nutrition tools to ensure better outcomes in the management as well as prevention of transmission of the disease.

FURTHER READING

1. **Anon.** (1999) The demographic impact of HIV/AIDS. New York, Population Division, Department of Economic and Social Affairs and the Joint UN Programme on HIV/AIDS (UNAIDS).

2. **Coutsoudis, A., Bobat, R.A., Coovadia, H.M.,** *et al.* (1995) The effects of vitamin A supplementation on the morbidity of children born to HIV-infected women. *Am J Public Health*, **85**, 1076–81.

3. **Fawzi, W.W., Mbise, R., Hertzmark, E.,** *et al.* (1999) A randomized trial of vitamin A supplements in relation to mortality among human immunodeficiency virus-infected and uninfected children in Tanzania. *Paed Infect Dis J*, **18**, 12–3.

4. **Fenton, M., and Silverman, E.** (2000) Medical nutrition therapy for human immunodeficiency virus (HIV) infection and acquired immunodeficiency syndrome (AIDS). In: Mahan, L.K., and Escott-Stump, S. (eds) *Krause's food, nutrition, and diet therapy*. Philadelphia: Saunders, pp. 88–11.

5. **Piwoz, E.G., and Preble, E.A.** (2000) HIV/AIDS and nutrition. Washington, US Agency for International Development.

6. **WHO** (2003) Scaling up antiretroviral therapy in resource-limited settings: treatment guidelines for a public health approach. Geneva, World Health Organization.

7. **WHO/FAO** (2002) Living well with HIV/AIDS. A manual on nutritional care and support for people living with HIV/AIDS. Rome, FAO.

8. **Zhu, T., Korber, B.T., Nahmias, A.J., Hooper, E., Sharp, P.M., and Ho, D.D.** (1998) An African HIV-1 sequence from 1959 and implications for the origin of the epidemic. *Nature*, **391**, 594.

 To see topical and scientifically robust updates on nutrition associated with this textbook, and active web links to many of the journal articles in the Reference areas, please see the dedicated Online Resource Centre at www.oxfordtextbooks.co.uk/orc/mann3e/.

40 Nutritional support for the hospitalized patient

Ross C. Smith

40.1 Enteral nutrition

Trainee surgeons in the 1960s and 1970s would provide puréed food directly through a large-bore gastrostomy tube into the stomach of patients who were unable to eat. The concept of 'enteral nutrition' is much more refined than this and has developed as a specialized form of nutrition therapy out of the space programme, where a balanced nutrition that resulted in minimal excretion was a distinct advantage. It is interesting that in the late 1960s the concept of parenteral nutrition was also at a phase of rapid development in the era of early space exploration, and this probably helped to evolve the use of 'space diets' as a type of complete nutrition in a liquid form that could be delivered by a tube directly into the gastrointestinal tract for the treatment of hospitalized patients. The first such product was an elemental formula, but there are benefits for polymeric products because of cost and more efficient metabolism. Following on from the success of enteral nutrition for complex hospitalized patients, the concept has been successfully evolved for nutritional treatment for nursing-home patients and outpatients who are otherwise unable to eat.

Currently, patients entering hospital are screened for nutritional status by admitting doctors, nurses and dietitians. The at-risk patient is referred to the ward dietitian who undertakes a more detailed nutritional assessment and considers the best method of treatment: specialized oral diet, enteral nutrition or parenteral nutrition. Nutritional support becomes indicated for all patients who are unable to nourish themselves with oral intake for more than 5 days or sooner if they are malnourished on admission. Because enteral nutrition is cheaper, more physiological and less complicated than parenteral nutrition, it should always be used in preference to parenteral nutrition when it can be safely administered. It is important to understand the safety issues when deciding on a patient's suitability for treatment.

40.1.1 Indications for enteral nutrition

Enteral nutrition is indicated as a means of nutritional support for patients who are unable to sustain themselves with an oral diet and there is a sufficient normal intestine available for absorption of enteral formula. The frequently quoted statement 'If the gut

---

BOX 40.1 Enteral nutrition

Feeding by tube directly into the stomach or upper small intestine by using a formula that is a mixture of nutrient sources that can be passed in water emulsion through a fine tube.

Table 40.1 Indications for enteral nutrition

	Examples
Anorexia due to illness	Eating disorders Weakness due to illness or surgery Cancer
Swallowing disorders	Cerebrovascular disease Motor neurone disease Oesophageal stricture
Gastric stasis (gastroparesis)	Post-operative, intensive-care patients
Inability to take sufficient oral nutrition	Burns Open infected wounds Trauma Inflammatory bowel disease Some patients with sepsis

works, use it!' should be remembered in all patients who are referred for nutritional therapy. There are many different clinical situations where enteral nutrition becomes the preferred method of feeding.

Patients with a stroke or other neurological deficit who are unable to swallow satisfactorily are a good example of a situation where enteral nutrition has been found to be invaluable. Critically ill patients who have a functioning gut are also suitable, but there may be an initial period when the gut is not functioning and parenteral nutrition should be considered.

40.1.2 Contraindications to enteral nutrition

The main contraindication to the use of enteral nutrition is poor functioning of the gastrointestinal tract. In general in this circumstance, the enteral nutrition causes vomiting, gastrointestinal distension or severe diarrhoea. Patients who are frail and have loss of sensation in the pharynx are at great risk of aspiration of enteral nutrition into the lung; an example of such a patient in this circumstance would be following a stroke involving the muscles of the pharynx. Aspiration should be particularly consid-

ered when patients are vomiting or have a respiratory disorder. This is a most important issue and needs to be emphasized.

Another important contraindication to the use of enteral nutrition is the presence of vascular compromise to the gut, which occurs during conditions such as septic shock and the use of high doses of vasopressor agents. Other extreme conditions, such as mesenteric artery thrombosis and abdominal compartment syndrome, cause gross impairment of absorption.

Ethical issues are also important when considering the need for enteral nutrition. Because enteral nutrition allows complete nutritional therapy, withholding such treatment can be seen as denying a patient their normal and natural requirements. Withholding nutritional support from a patient who is unable to eat is an emotionally charged ethical problem. It is inappropriate to withhold treatment from a patient who has reasonable potential for extended quality of life. Alternatively, it is unreasonable to extend a patient's life when there is no hope of relief from pain and suffering. Unfortunately these decisions are not always black and white and there are frequently discrepancies between the expectations of some relatives and of medical and nursing staff. Mostly these issues can be settled by discussion and by helping all parties understand the potential outcomes of the patient's condition. Funding issues are also an important consideration. In some communities, enteral nutrition is funded by government bodies, while in other communities the patients' families have to pay.

40.1.3 Access to the gastrointestinal tract

Enteral nutrition can be given by mouth as a bolus but, because it is unpalatable and uninteresting when repeated over a number of days, this is not frequently successful. It is therefore mostly given through a tube into the stomach or intestine (Fig. 40.1). The tube can be small and placed as a nasogastric tube. Because it is small and made of soft material, it is quite acceptable for many patients. Although these tubes are fine and

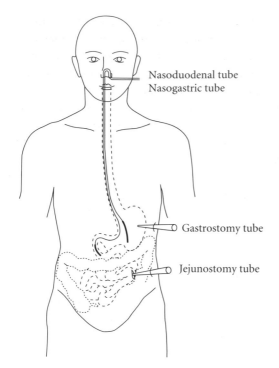

Nasoduodenal tube
Nasogastric tube

Gastrostomy tube

Jejunostomy tube

Fig. 40.1 Routes of enteral (tube) feeding.

can be used for bolus feeding to allow for disconnection and mobility of the patient free from the infusion, they are best tolerated as a continuous infusion over a 24-hour cycle. In some situations nutritional requirements are achieved as an overnight infusion to provide supplementation. Such a programme would require daily insertion of the tube, which would present difficulties.

A gastrostomy tube can be safely inserted through the skin into the stomach to allow for direct delivery of the nutrition. Gastrostomy tubes are most frequently placed with the aid of the endoscope. Under vision with an endoscope in the stomach, a needle is passed through the skin into the stomach and a guide is passed through the needle. This guide is pulled back into the mouth and attached to the tube. The tube is then pulled in through the mouth and pulled out of the stomach along the needle, leaving a bulbar portion of the tube in the stomach to anchor it in position. These tubes are designed to lie comfortably in the stomach and to be fixed to the skin. Such tubes are more easily used for intermittent feeding and can

be disconnected from the nutrition infusion to allow mobility.

Jejunostomy tubes can be placed to lie in the small bowel for conditions that result in poor gastric emptying. Again they can be inserted via the nose, via a gastrostomy or directly into the small intestine. When the tube is placed into the jejunum, it is best used for continuous infusion.

40.1.4 Enteral formulations

In each class of enteral nutrition formulation there are numerous commercial products. The reason for choosing one over the other often depends on the presentation or method of delivery. Some formulae are presented as dry powder while others are presented already prepared in a sterile container with easily connected delivery tubing. Therefore, the choice of solution is frequently not directly related to whether one formula has more or less than another of a particular nutrient. In early formulations, milk was a predominant protein source and with this, lactose was a significant carbohydrate; intolerance to lactose leads to diarrhoea in many patients. In general, lactose has been replaced by corn starch.

The majority of popular formulae use casein hydrolysates for protein and a mixture of different oils for the provision of lipid. They provide 1 kcal/mL of a solution containing about 110 kcal/g N (nitrogen) and have a balance of vitamins, trace elements and electrolytes with an osmolality of from 300 to 700 mOsm/kg.

Polymeric diets These are more commonly used because they are well utilized and are cheap to manufacture. They contain maltosedextrins, milk protein and vegetable oils. They provide recommended dietary intakes (RDIs) of vitamins and minerals and are presented in various manners for ease of clinical use.

Elemental diets Elemental diets were developed for space travel to have low residue. They mainly use amino acids and are enriched with glutamine. They have a low fat content but provide essential fatty acids along with the RDI of vitamins, trace elements and electrolytes. Although the amino acids are free, they are not necessarily absorbed more easily because the peptidases in the brush border improve the uptake of amino acids.

Added fibre Some enteral nutrition solutions contain a suitable form of added dietary fibre, which is important for some patients with diarrhoea. The fibre is also an important nutrient for the colonic mucosa and may be useful in patients with colitis.

Prebiotics, probiotics and synbiotics Some ill patients who are on long-term antibiotics have an alteration of the bowel flora that causes diarrhoea and may lead to endotoxaemia. Strains of lactobacilli, which are normal commensal organisms in the small bowel and may help with digestion of fibre, are able to compete with and reduce the effect of the pathogenic organisms. Different strains of lactobacilli have been recommended.

Special formulations

- *Immunonutrition*: these solutions contain added amounts of different nutrients considered to be useful in promoting the immune system. They include: ω-3 fatty acids and medium-chain triglycerides, L-arginine and L-glutamine and dietary nucleotides. These solutions have been shown to reduce postoperative wound infections.
- *Hepatic failure with encephalopathy*: these patients require solutions containing added branched-chain amino acids.
- *Renal failure*: it is important in these patients to reduce solute load to reduce the need for dialysis. The past concept of limiting protein is considered to lead to malnutrition, but there may be improvement in outcome by using a greater proportion of essential amino acids.
- *Acutely stressed patients*: these patients may need high-protein enteral nutrition.

40.1.5 Initiating enteral nutrition

Once the tube is in place, the enteral nutrition is commenced slowly to ensure that there is good tolerance.

It is recommended to reduce the rate rather than the concentration of the solution. This author's preference is for continuous feeding because bolus feeding can induce vomiting and dumping with diarrhoea. Monitoring of blood glucose, urea and electrolytes and liver function is important. After 12–24 hours, the rate can generally be increased to provide daily calorie and protein requirements. Frequent assessment of the patients for respiratory distress or abdominal distension should be part of routine care in these patients. Continuous enteral nutrition was not found to reduce the appetite in patients recovering from surgery.

40.1.6 Monitoring for efficacy

Monitoring of patients undergoing enteral nutrition therapy is not an exact science. It is important to monitor the amount that the patient receives and whether or not the patient has nausea, vomiting or diarrhoea. Patients should have urea, electrolyte, albumin and liver function monitored. By following weight each week, a judgement can be made as to whether more or less nutrition should be provided.

40.1.7 Complications and toxicity

Major complications include aspiration pneumonia, which is a particular threat in patients with weakness and reduced pharyngeal reflexes. It is particularly risky in patients with poor gastric emptying who may aspirate when vomiting. Other possible major complications are:

- acute intestinal distension and ischaemic damage to the intestine causing intestinal necrosis and disruption
- dislodgement of the catheter into the peritoneal cavity with spillage of nutrient solution into the peritoneal cavity
- severe diarrhoea causing electrolyte disturbances.

Moderate to minor complications include:

- diarrhoea
- metabolic complications

- glucose intolerance
- low serum sodium
- low serum potassium
- low serum phosphate
- low serum magnesium
- essential fatty acid deficiency
- low serum zinc.

Mechanical issues include:

- blocked feeding tubes
- dislodged feeding tubes
- bacterial contamination.

40.2 Parenteral feeding

Parenteral feeding is indicated when patients cannot be nourished with oral nutrition or enteral feeding for more than 5 days. Although the desire to feed directly into the vein had tempted doctors over the centuries, it was not until the development of pyrogen-free fluids in the 1920s and the development of protein hydrolysates and lipid emulsions by Arvid Wretland in the 1940s that this became possible. The technique of complete feeding was further advanced in 1968 by Stanley Dudrick and colleagues with central vein (line) placement and care, so that hypertonic glucose and amino acid solutions could be delivered. They neatly demonstrated that beagle puppies could grow with parenteral nutrition, and subsequently that human infants could develop at a similar rate to breastfed infants. The system of Dudrick was termed 'hyperalimentation' because it allowed the delivery of large amounts of nutrition that sometimes caused problems of overfeeding. There were fears about the use of lipid emulsions for many years but their safety with admixtures of amino acids and glucose in a three-in-one solution was demonstrated by French workers and this has gradually become a most common presentation. Three-in-one solutions allow the provision of the daily nutrient requirements in a 3 L bag with an osmolality of about 1000 mOsm/L. These solutions can be delivered into peripheral veins, particularly if a fine catheter is used in a larger vein such as the basilic vein. Parenteral nutrition also needs to provide all necessary electrolytes, trace elements and vitamins in a balanced manner.

40.2.2 Constituents of parenteral nutrition

The glucose concentration ranges from 10 % to 50 %, which is much higher then the usual 5 % of replacement intravenous fluids. One gram of glucose provides approximately 4 kcal (16.8 kJ) so 1 L of 25% glucose will provide about 1000 kcal (4200 kJ).

Lipid emulsions are presented as 10%, 20% and 30% solutions and provide about 8 kcal/g lipid so 500 mL of 20% solution provides about 1000 kcal (4200 kJ). It is generally considered that 'lipid burns in a carbohydrate fire' and therefore it is usual that no more than 50% of non-protein calories are given as lipid.

Amino acids are provided as crystalline *laevo* form in solutions providing from 5.5 to 11.4 g amino acid per 100 mL. This value needs to be divided by 6.25 to derive grams of nitrogen. The amino acid pattern corresponds to that of high-quality dietary protein.

The glucose, lipid and amino acid solutions are combined to provide between 110 and 150 non-protein calories to 1 g N in the final solution. Electrolytes, vitamins and trace elements are also necessary. It is particularly important to provide a balance of the intracellular electrolytes potassium, magnesium and phosphate because with the provision of nutrition there is an expansion of the intracellular compartment. If one nutrient is deficient, the response to nutrition is impaired.

An example of an adult formula is given in Table 40.2. This solution is run to provide about 0.25–0.3 g N/kg/day to the acute patient. Long-term patients may require less than this when they are not stressed. The maximum nutritional input that stressed hypermetabolic patients can metabolize is up to twice their basal metabolic rate, but there has been a tendency to be conservative to prevent the complications of overfeeding in these patients.

40.2.3 Methods of venous access

When solutions of glucose and amino acids are given, they have an osmolality of about 2000 mOsm and a pH approaching 5. This is therefore very irritating to the endothelium in veins and leads to *thrombophlebitis* in a short period of time if such solutions are delivered into small peripheral veins. However, when delivered into a large pool of blood it can be buffered and diluted. It therefore has to be delivered through a catheter placed in a large central vein like the superior

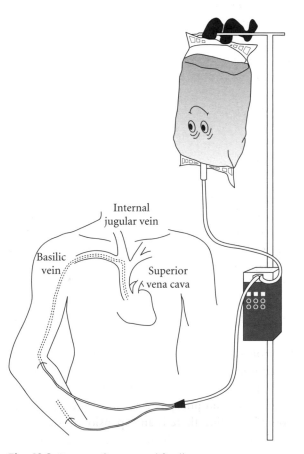
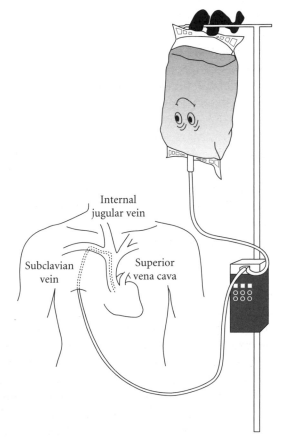

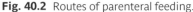

Fig. 40.2 Routes of parenteral feeding.

vena cava (Fig. 40.2). Central lines require special care to prevent sepsis and the catheter used for parenteral nutrition should be dedicated to this purpose. Antibiotics and other drugs should be delivered through a separate line. Apart from the risks of insertion of central lines, there is a constant risk of major sepsis either around or through a central line and it needs to be dressed and monitored carefully to prevent overwhelming sepsis. One always needs to be alert to the possibility of sepsis.

A three-in-one solution allows the buffering of the solution and a marked reduction of osmolarity. When this is at or below 1000 mOsm, it can be delivered into peripheral veins using normal cannulae, but these need to be rotated regularly to prevent thrombophlebitis. An improved thrombophlebitis rate can be achieved with a mid-line placed about 15 cm into the basilic vein (Fig. 40.2). There are a number of advantages to mid-lines because they can be placed without radiological guidance and can be monitored clinically for any tenderness over the vein. These lines need to be 2–3 Fr in size and can only be used for continuous infusion for rates up to 120 mL/hour. They cannot be used for resuscitation. Studies have demonstrated a reduced risk of sepsis with the use of mid-lines. Another advantage for these lines is that they can be safely managed by nursing staff without the need for referral to the radiology department.

A peripherally inserted central catheter (PICC) line is a further choice because it is safer to insert. It again has to be managed very carefully to ensure sepsis is not introduced around or through the catheter.

40.2.4 Monitoring when on parenteral nutrition

Monitoring of electrolytes in patients treated with parenteral nutrition is required more frequently in the acute setting because the introduction of nutrition can induce severe acute depression of blood values of many nutrients that are marginally deficient. The *refeeding syndrome* (Box 40.2) is prevented by the slow introduction of the parenteral nutrition and the provision of increased amounts of phosphate, potassium and magnesium. Patients at risk of refeeding syndrome may need to have their electrolytes checked twice daily until they are stable.

Blood glucose is also important to monitor to prevent hyperglycaemia. In intensive-care patients, this requires a 4-hourly finger-prick for blood glucose. In the more stable ward patient, a urinalysis is undertaken twice daily and followed by blood glucose measures if glucose is elevated.

Acid–base balance should be measured on arterial blood samples if the patient's condition suggests a metabolic disturbance. After the patient has reached goal amounts of parenteral nutrition infusion, the

---

Table 40.2 Parenteral nutrition, per day

Nitrogen 1 litre 18 g/L (114 g protein)
Glucose 1 litre 25% (1000 kcal)
Lipid emulsion 500 mL 20% (1000 kcal)
Sodium 70–100 mmol
Potassium 60–80 mmol
Magnesium 10–15 mmol
Phosphate 10–20 mmol
Balanced water-soluble and lipid-soluble vitamins
Balanced trace element solution (zinc, selenium, copper)

BOX 40.3 Daily requirements of micronutrients with total parenteral nutrition

Requirements of several *vitamins* given parenterally are approximately 2 × the RDI (i.e. food by mouth): thiamin, riboflavin, niacin, pantothenate, vitamin B_{12} and vitamin C. This is because of oxidation in the bag or faster urinary excretion when they go into a peripheral vein rather than the portal system. On the other hand, requirements are lower for several *inorganic* elements that are poorly absorbed when taken by mouth: about half or a third of the RDI for calcium, phosphorus, zinc and copper and about a tenth for iron.

frequency of blood electrolyte measures can be reduced to every other day if the patient is stable. Home parenteral nutrition patients are frequently sufficiently stable that electrolytes only need to be measured at monthly intervals.

Monitoring of vitamins and trace elements needs to be undertaken at weekly intervals in the acute setting and 3-monthly in the long-term patients. The vitamins and trace elements most frequently depressed during parenteral nutrition are folate, vitamin C and D, vitamin B_6, zinc, selenium and copper. Essential fatty acid deficiency occasionally occurred in patients who had glucose as the only non-protein calorie source and was prevented by twice-weekly lipid infusions. However, one needs to be aware that there may be depression of any nutrient that is not included in the parenteral nutrition formula.

Protein-calorie nutritional status is monitored with blood values that reflect protein metabolism, such as plasma proteins, albumin, transferrin and C-reactive protein. Serum creatinine and urea are depressed in patients with malnutrition and it is important to observe these return to the normal range. Measures of body composition can be simple by anthropometric measures of skin folds and arm muscle circumference. There are a number of techniques for estimating muscle and fat mass including electrical bioimpedence, DEXA, CT assessment and neutron activation analysis (see Chapter 29).

40.2.5 Complications

Complications include:

- Complications of venous catheter insertion. These are greatest when a central venous catheter is used; there is a risk of significant injury to the subclavian and related vessels or a pneumothorax can occur.

- Sepsis is a constant risk for patients with parenteral nutrition. Again this is greater with central venous access than with peripheral venous access, and any spike in fever or persistent fever has to alert the medical team to the possibility of line sepsis. Such events should be treated with removal of the line and blood culture.

- Metabolic complications are mostly related to hyperglycaemia. The many possible nutrient deficiencies are discussed in the monitoring section (section 40.2.4).

40.3 Nutritional support teams

Many studies have demonstrated the benefit of nutritional support teams. With complex medical treatment for patients in intensive care, gastroenterology, surgical, oncology and renal failure wards, many patients have poor nutritional status and the prevention of significant nutritional deficiency has been shown to improve outcome. Multidisciplinary teams help make this process happen in a complex tertiary hospital but all medical and paramedical staff need to be aware of the importance of good nutritional care.

40.3.1 Decision path for nutritional therapy

When a patient is at risk of developing malnutrition, Fig. 40.3 may help in considering nutritional therapy. Clearly it is unacceptable to allow patients to become malnourished in hospital when there are well-designed therapies that have proven efficacy for preventing this. There is a large body of evidence that malnutrition increases the risk of complication and death. Nutritional assessment of patients entering hospital is important, and there should be a greater stress on recording body weight and weight loss, plasma proteins, lymphocyte count and haemoglobin values on a nutritional assessment form.

Enteral nutrition should be used if the gut is available and functioning. Enteral nutrition is most commonly delivered through a fine-bore nasogastric tube. In complex patients in intensive care, it may be important to pass the tube into the jejunum. Long-term access may require the placement of a feeding

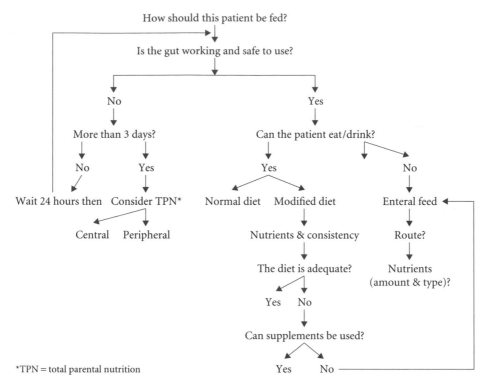

Fig. 40.3 Some factors in the decision process for providing nutritional support.

gastrostomy or jejunostomy tube. Enteral nutrition is frequently prescribed to provide 20–25 kcal/kg/day while the infusion rate for parenteral nutrition is frequently 30–40 kcal/kg/day. The decision to use either peripheral or central parenteral nutrition depends on the presence of suitable peripheral veins. Peripheral parenteral nutrition is preferred because the nutrient composition is satisfactory for repletion when given peripherally, and sepsis and complications of venous access are reduced. Infusion rates need to be individualized, depending on tolerance and complication and whether there is a positive response to treatment.

 To see topical and scientifically robust updates on nutrition associated with this textbook, and active web links to many of the journal articles in the Reference areas, please see the dedicated Online Resource Centre at www.oxfordtextbooks.co.uk/orc/mann3e/.

Index

W